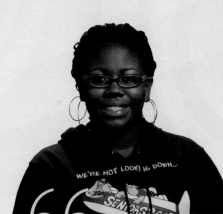

Hi, I'm Jasmine. I don't think I've gotten 8 hours of sleep since I was 13. I'm 19, so that's six years of not getting a full night's sleep. That takes a toll on your body and your mind."
(For more of Jasmine's story, turn to page 11.)

I'm Corey. I've had a total of three surgeries, which have left me with some scars. Growing up, I was always self-conscious, especially during the summer when everyone was out at the beach in swimsuits."
(For more of Corey's story, turn to page 4.)

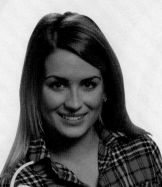

Hi, I'm Kristina. In my senior year of high school, one of my good girlfriends decided to take her own life. It was pretty devastating— emotionally, mentally, physically even."
(For more on Kristina's story, turn to page 35.)

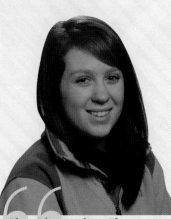

I'm Alexandra. I'm a vegetarian. I do it for my own personal reasons. I'm not trying to impose my beliefs on anyone else."
(For more on Alexandra's story, turn to page 82.)

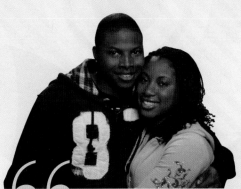

We're Jonathan and Yeani, and we've been a couple for six months. There are a lot of obstacles that we face in our relationship, especially when it comes to juggling our schoolwork in addition to all the other aspects of our lives."
(For more on Jonathan and Yeani's story, turn to page 196.)

My name is Holly. I am 45 years old. I was a single parent for about 12 years. I could not afford insurance for myself—it just wasn't in my budget. My kids always came first. If I got sick, I stayed at home and took care of myself."
(For more of Holly's story, turn to page 311.)

Student Stories Show the Relevance of Healthful Choices to Today's College Students

College students don't always believe that living a healthful lifestyle is something they need to start thinking about now. To drive home this point, we approached students around the country and asked them to share their health-related stories with us.

Student Stories throughout the book demonstrate that the lifestyle choices students make today can have lasting effects on the quality of their health tomorrow.

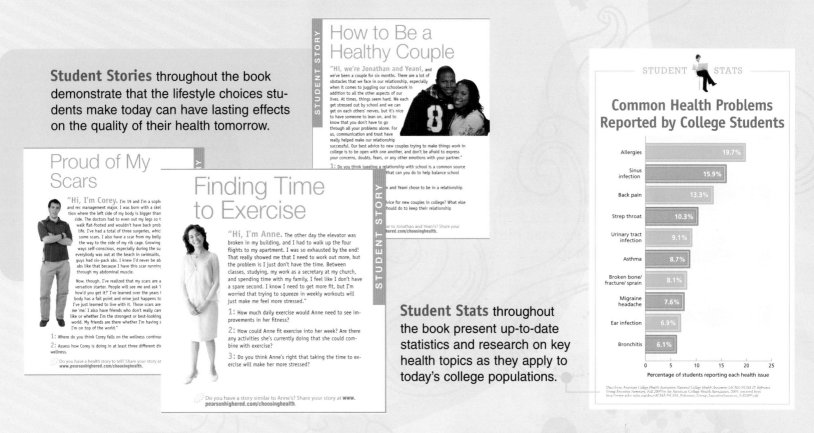

STUDENT STORY

How to Be a Healthy Couple

"Hi, we're Jonathan and Yeani, and we've been a couple for six months. There are a lot of obstacles that we face in our relationship, especially when it comes to juggling our schoolwork in addition to all the other aspects of our lives. At times, things seem hard. We each get stressed out by school and we can get on each others' nerves, but it's nice to have someone to lean on, and to know that you don't have to go through all your problems alone. For us, communication and trust have really helped make our relationship successful. Our best advice to new couples trying to make things work in college is to be open with one another, and don't be afraid to express your concerns, doubts, fears, or any other emotions with your partner."

1: Do you think juggling a relationship with school is a common source... What can you do to help balance school...

...n and Yeani chose to be in a relationship...

...vice for new couples in college? What else ...hould do to keep their relationship

...ar to Jonathan and Yeani's? Share your ...hered.com/choosinghealth.

Proud of My Scars

"Hi, I'm Corey. I'm 19 and I'm a soph... and rec management major. I was born with a skel... tion where the left side of my body is bigger than... side. The doctors had to even out my legs so t... walk flat-footed and wouldn't have back prob... life. I've had a total of three surgeries, whic... some scars. I also have a scar from my belly... the way to the side of my rib cage. Growing... ways self-conscious, especially during the su... everybody was out at the beach in swimsuits,... guys had six-pack abs. I knew I'd never be ab... abs like that because I have this scar running... through my abdominal muscle.

Now, though, I've realized that my scars are a... versation starter. People will see me and ask 'I... how'd you get it?' I've learned over the years t... body has a fail point and mine just happens to... I've just learned to live with it. Those scars are... me 'me.' I also have friends who don't really car... like or whether I'm the strongest or best-looking... world. My friends are there whether I'm having s... I'm on top of the world."

1: Where do you think Corey falls on the wellness continu...

2: Assess how Corey is doing in at least three different di... wellness.

Do you have a health story to tell? Share your story at www.pearsonhighered.com/choosinghealth.

STUDENT STORY

Finding Time to Exercise

"Hi, I'm Anne. The other day the elevator was broken in my building, and I had to walk up the four flights to my apartment. I was so exhausted by the end! That really showed me that I need to work out more, but the problem is I just don't have the time. Between classes, studying, my work as a secretary at my church, and spending time with my family, I feel like I don't have a spare second. I know I need to get more fit, but I'm worried that trying to squeeze in weekly workouts will just make me feel more stressed."

1: How much daily exercise would Anne need to see improvements in her fitness?

2: How could Anne fit exercise into her week? Are there any activities she's currently doing that she could combine with exercise?

3: Do you think Anne's right that taking the time to exercise will make her more stressed?

Do you have a story similar to Anne's? Share your story at www.pearsonhighered.com/choosinghealth.

STUDENT STATS

Common Health Problems Reported by College Students

Health issue	Percentage
Allergies	19.7%
Sinus infection	15.9%
Back pain	13.3%
Strep throat	10.3%
Urinary tract infection	9.1%
Asthma	8.7%
Broken bone/ fracture/ sprain	8.1%
Migraine headache	7.6%
Ear infection	6.9%
Bronchitis	6.1%

Percentage of students reporting each health issue
(0, 5, 10, 15, 20, 25)

Data from American College Health Association National College Health Assessment (ACHA-NCHA II) Reference Group Executive Summary, Fall 2009 by the American College Health Association, 2009, retrieved from http://www.acha-ncha.org/docs/ACHA-NCHA_Reference_Group_ExecutiveSummary_Fall2009.pdf.

Student Stats throughout the book present up-to-date statistics and research on key health topics as they apply to today's college populations.

In addition, **videos of real college students** talking about their health lets students see that they're not alone in facing health issues—and learn about strategies their peers are using to deal with problems. View these videos on the *Choosing Health* website at **www.pearsonhighered .com/choosinghealth**. We will also screen featured student videos on our **YouTube channel** at **www.youtube.com/ ch00singhealth**.

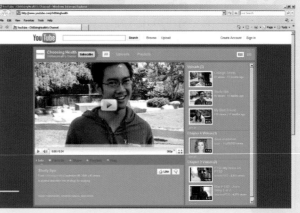

Cutting-Edge Technology Allows Students to Track Their Health in Real Time...and Stay Up to Date on the Latest Health News

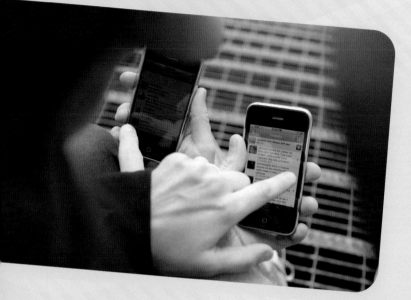

tweet your health

TweetYourHealth

Students using *Choosing Health* will have access to TweetYourHealth (**www.tweetyourhealth.com**), a Twitter-based application that allows them to:

- Keep an online log of their health-related activities, such as diet, exercise, weight management, smoking, and drinking
- Post real-time updates to their online journal through text messaging or by using the TweetYourHealth mobile website
- Upload photos of their activities and include comments to share with their friends
- Receive automated health tips that can be sent to their mobile phones via Twitter direct message or via email at user-specified times
- Take advantage of an online community forum to support them in their health and wellness goals

Visit Our Facebook and Twitter Pages and Stay Up to Date

Visit our Facebook page (**www.facebook.com/ChoosingHealth**) or our Twitter page (**www.twitter.com/choosing_health**) to stay up to date on health-related topics in the news. Additionally, learn about opportunities to contribute to future editions of *Choosing Health*!

twitter

Choosing_Health

Follow

have you checked out choosing health's facebook page yet?
http://bit.ly/arPSRX #fb
4:08 PM Apr 13th via Echofon

How will health care reform affect you? (NYTimes):
http://www.nytimes.com/interactive/2009/09/29/health/health-care-conversations.html#/26/
3:18 PM Mar 22nd via web

Coming up soon on most campuses - #midterms. Cue scary

Facebook (1) | Choosing Health - Windows Internet Explorer

http://www.facebook.com/pages/edit/picture.php?id=372825281390&success=1#!/ChoosingHealth

File   Edit   View   Favorites   Tools   Help

Facebook (1) | Choosing Health

facebook   Search   Home   Prof

Choosing Health

Wall   Info   Discussions   Video   Polls   Submit!   +

What's on your mind?

Attach: Share

Choosing Health + Others   Choosing Health   Just Others   Settings

Edit Page
Promote with an Ad
Suggest to Friends

Submit your stories, videos, photos, and questions at http://www.pearsonhighered

Choosing Health The New York Times Magazine recently published a cover story about 20-somethings, asking "Why are so many people in their 20s taking so long to grow up?" http://www.nytimes.com/2010/08/22/magazine/22Adulthood-t.html?_r=1&src=me&ref=homepage

What Is It About 20-Somethings? - NYTimes.com
www.nytimes.com
They move back in with their parents. They delay beginning careers. Why are so many young people taking so long to grow up?

Actions
block Choosing_Health
report for spam

Following

RSS feed of Choosing_Health's tweets

Behavior Change Tools Help Students Put Plans into Practice

In the textbook...

Behavior Change Workshops

Changing long-ingrained behaviors is tough. This worksheet-style feature steps students through behavior change for topics in every chapter of the book. Workshops ask students to articulate realistic goals, assess their current stage of readiness for behavior change, and complete activities that help them determine and follow through with appropriate next steps.

Behavior Change Workshop

To complete this workshop online, visit www.pearsonhighered.com/choosinghealth.

Changing long-ingrained behaviors is one of the toughest things to do. Consider the student case studies presented throughout this chapter, and then think about your own life. What stressors can you reduce or eliminate? How can you change the way you respond to the stressors that remain? What stage of behavior change are you in? Given your current stage of change, what is an appropriate goal you can set to reach the next stage?

Part I. Assessing the Stressors in Your Life

1. What are the main sources of stress in your own life? List the top five.

2. Mark one of the stressors above that you want to target. Ask yourself honestly: How ready are you to commit to a behavior change that will help you reduce or eliminate that stressor? What stage of behavior change are you in?

Target stressor:

Current stage of behavior change:

3. Keeping your current stage of behavior change in mind, describe what you might do or think about as a "next step" to reduce or eliminate that stressor in your life. Also list your timeline for making your next step.

Next step:

Deadline for next step:

4. Consider the stressors that you have some control over. Now consider the stress management techniques introduced in this chapter. Which techniques can you try to better respond to and manage the stress you feel over those stressors?

Chapter 3 • Stress Management 61

Behavior Change Workshop

To complete this workshop online, visit www.pearsonhighered.com/choosinghealth.

Changing long-ingrained behaviors is one of the toughest things to do. Consider the student stories presented throughout this chapter, and then think about your own life. What can you do to manage your weight? What stage of behavior change are you in? Given your current stage of change, what is an appropriate goal you can set to reach the next stage?

Part I. Creating a Weight-Management Plan

1. What does your BMI and waist-to-hip ratio tell you about the effect of your weight on your health? How do you feel about your weight when you look in the mirror? Do you want to maintain your current weight? Gain weight? Lose weight? By how many pounds? Write down exactly what you want to accomplish with your weight-management plan.

BMI and waist-to-hip ratio:

Weight-management goal:

2. Ask yourself honestly: How ready are you to commit to a behavior change that will help you manage your weight? What stage of behavior change are you in?

3. Keeping your current stage of behavior change in mind, describe what you might do or think about as a "next step" to manage your weight. Which side of the energy balance equation do you want to change: energy in or energy out? You can also modify both.

4. Consider that a healthful prescription for weight loss is cutting 500 to 1,000 calories a day, through reduced calorie intake or increased exercise. This typically leads to a weight loss of 1 or 2 pounds a week. To gain weight, you would add a similar amount of calories daily. Now, consider the weight-management techniques introduced in this chapter. Which techniques can you try to better manage your weight? Keep in mind that you should not cut calories below the recommended MyPyramid levels shown in Table 4.3 on page 000.

Chapter 6 • Weight Management 137

Behavior Change Workshop

To complete this workshop online, visit www.pearsonhighered.com/choosinghealth.

You may not realize how many drugs you already take on a daily basis. When you think of "drugs," you may only think of illegal drugs such as marijuana or cocaine or perhaps prescription medications. However, common substances such as alcohol, caffeine, and nicotine are also drugs. Try monitoring your drug use for one day.

	What Did It Do for You?
	Helped me wake up

	What Did It Do for You?

Choose To... Cards

Magazine-style tear-out cards let students post behavior change tips to their fridge or bulletin boards, or take them on the go. Featuring everything from recipes for cheap, nutritious meals to easy ways to get a cardiovascular workout, the Choose To. . . cards provide practical strategies for making change easier. Downloadable versions of the Choose To. . . cards are also available for use with mobile phones.

Choosing Health Stress Management

Reduce Stress Through Wellness Habits

www.pearsonhighered.com/choosinghealth

Choose To...
Reduce Stress Through Wellness Habits

You can reduce stress by following these basic guidelines. See pages 11–12 for more information.
- Manage your time effectively.
- Get enough sleep.
- Eat well.
- Exercise.
- Strengthen your support network.
- Communicate.
- Take time for hobbies and leisure.
- Keep a journal.

Online...

Interactive Tools for Behavior Change

Access interactive tools for behavior change on the Choosing Health Companion Website. The **Live It** section provides behavior change tools for each chapter of the book. Access the companion website at **www.pearsonhighered.com/choosinghealth**.

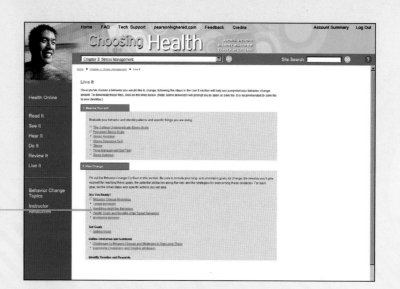

Name: _____
Date: _____
Click on the gray boxes to fill out the worksheet. Remember to save your answers.

✓ SELF-ASSESSMENT

Perceived Stress Scale
Instructions: The questions in this scale ask you about your feelings and thoughts during the last month. In each case, please indicate with a check how often you felt or thought a certain way.

1. In the last month, how often have you been upset because of something that happened unexpectedly?

☐ 0 = never
☐ 1 = almost never
☐ 2 = sometimes
☐ 3 = fairly often
☐ 4 = very often

2. In the last month, how often have you felt that you were unable to control the important things in your

Step 1: Assess Yourself
Access electronic versions of the Self-Assessments from the book, along with a host of additional assessments.

Step 2: Plan Change
Here are all the tools needed to successfully plan for change and fill out a behavior change contract.

Examining Attitudes and Creative Strategies

Place your

Setting Goals

Place your cursor in gray boxes to fill out worksheet. Remember to save your answers.

Name:

Underst
better u

Name: Date:

Now that you have examined your current behavior you can begin to plan a chang

---

Budget Worksheet

Wonder
break?
determi
money.

Journal Topic: Managing Stress

Place your cursor in gray boxes to fill out worksheet. Remember to save your answers.

Step 1:
Here, lo
loan che

Name: Date:

Think about the major stressors in your life: classes, work, relationships, and
What is a concrete step you can take now to cope with one aspect of the mo

Step 3: Implement Change
Track and log progress with the tools provided here.

Weekly Behavior Change Evaluation

Place your cursor in gray boxes to fill out worksheet. Remember to save your answers.

Name: Date:

DIRECTIONS: Answer the following questions for each week of your behavio

Step 4: Evaluate Change
Here are tools to reflect on the changes made.

Course Management That Makes It Easy for Your Students to Choose Health (and for You to Teach It)

MyHealthLab™

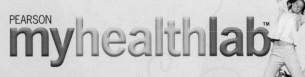

www.pearsonhighered.com/myhealthlab

MyHealthLab™ is an online course management system with a rich suite of assignable and gradeable content for teaching and learning about health. For each chapter, MyHealthLab offers the following resources:

Health Online

A chapter-specific guide to the text's Health Online features is available here, including:

- Weblinks from the book
- Links to podcasts related to chapter topics
- Videos related to chapter topics
- A link to TweetYourHealth
- Links to our Facebook and Twitter pages
- A link to our YouTube channel with featured student videos

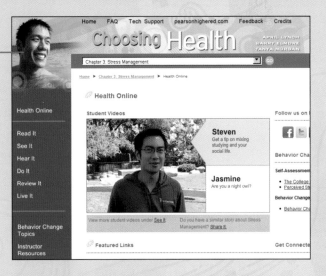

It's the one-stop shop where students can find everything online related to the chapter they're studying.

Read It

The Read It section contains:
- *Choosing Health* Twitter feed by author April Lynch
- Chapter-specific RSS feed of the most current health-related news articles
- Chapter objectives that direct student learning
- The Pearson eText, a full-featured electronic book
- Assignable and gradeable pre- and post-reading quizzes

See It

The See It section contains:
- Student-generated videos for every chapter
- A link to the *Choosing Health* YouTube channel with featured student videos
- 30 ABC News videos, each 5–10 minutes long, that cover a variety of important health topics

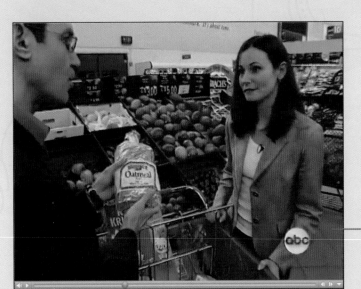

Note: Student videos and ABC News videos can be assigned with multiple-choice quiz questions that feed to the instructor gradebook.

Hear It

The Hear It section contains:
- MP3 Tutor Sessions that explain the big picture concepts with assignable and gradeable quizzes
- Audio case studies that encourage students to think about real-life health choices
- Links to podcasts discussed in the book that give students another avenue to learn about health.

Do It

The Do It section contains:
- Mobile phone resources, including Tweet Your Health and downloadable Choose To... cards
- Author Barry Elmore's video responses to student-generated Ask an Expert questions
- Forms that can be submitted to instructors with student responses to the Get Critical questions in each chapter

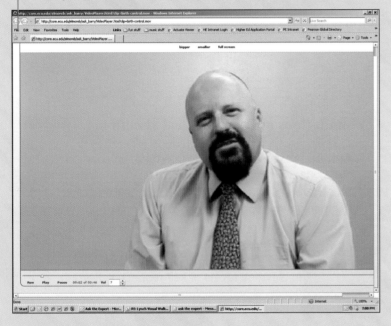

Review It

The Review It section contains:
- Online glossary
- Flashcards for use online or downloadable to mobile phones
- Crossword puzzles
- 25-question quiz for each chapter

Live It

This electronic toolkit helps jumpstart your students' behavior change project.

Behavior Change

This section helps students understand their current health status and which of their behaviors are risky before they decide on a behavior change project.

Additional Resources

● Companion Website
www.pearsonhighered.com/choosinghealth

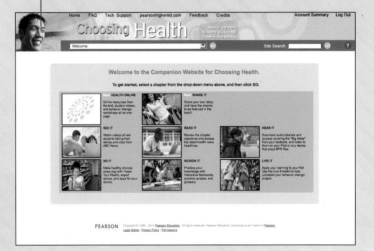

Health & Wellness Teaching Community Website
www.pearsonhighered.com/healthcommunity

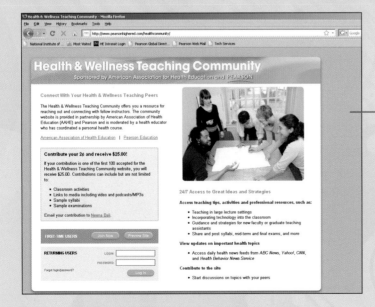

Connect with other health instructors!
The Health & Wellness Teaching Community website, sponsored by AAHE and Pearson, serves instructors like you by offering teaching tips and ideas, as well as a forum for peers to talk to one another about health-related issues. Submit a great idea and receive a $25 gift card!

The Teaching Toolbox:
Everything You Need in One Spot

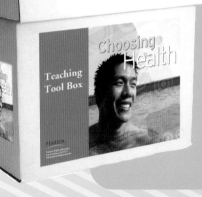

Teaching Toolbox 0-321-72083-0 / 978-0-321-72083-2
Save hours of valuable planning time with this comprehensive course planning kit. Adjunct, part-time, and full-time faculty will find a wealth of resources in one handy box. The Teaching Toolbox provides all the prepping and lecture tools an instructor needs.

Complete Contents of Toolbox:

- Teaching with Web 2.0
- Instructor Resource and Support Manual
- Printed Test Bank
- Instructor Resource DVD
- Great Ideas in Teaching Health
- MyHealthLab Instructor Access Kit

- Course-at-a-Glance Quick Reference Guide
- Take Charge! Self-assessment worksheets
- Behavior Change Log Book
- Eat Right!
- Live Right!

Instructor Resource DVD
The IRDVD includes 30 ABC News Lecture Launcher video clips; selected student videos; Web 2.0 teaching ideas; clicker questions; quiz shows; PowerPoint Lecture Outlines; Computerized Test Bank; TA masters; jpegs and PowerPoint files of art, tables, and some photos from the text; and Word files of instructor resources.

Foundations of Psychological Health

- **Autonomy**: capacity to make informed, un-coerced decisions.
- **Assertiveness:** making your needs and wants clear to others in an appropriate way.
- **___**: ability to perceive life as it really is so that ___ rationally respond to its demands.
- **___em:** a sense of positive self-regard, ___ in elevated levels of self-respect, self-worth, ___dence, & self-satisfaction.

Copyright © 2011 Pearson Education Inc.

Category 4: Diabetes
$300 Question

A risk factor for type 2 diabetes is _____.

a. sedentary lifestyle
b. frequent snacking
c. regular physical activity
d. weight control

ANSWER
BACK TO GAME

Copyright © 2009, Pearson Education, Inc., publishing as Pearson Benjamin Cummings.

Instructor Resource and Support Manual
Easier to use than a typical instructor's manual, this guide provides a step-by-step visual walkthrough of all the resources available to you for preparing your lectures. Also included are tips and strategies for new instructors, sample syllabi, and suggestions for integrating MyHealthLab into your classroom activities and homework assignments.

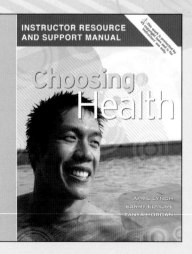

Teaching with Web 2.0
Twitter, Facebook, YouTube, Google—it's a new world out there. Learn strategies for incorporating web 2.0 technologies into your classroom in a meaningful manner with our Teaching with Web 2.0 booklet.

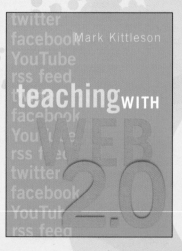

Choosing Health

APRIL LYNCH

BARRY ELMORE, M.A.
EAST CAROLINA UNIVERSITY

TANYA MORGAN, PH.D.
WEST CHESTER UNIVERSITY

WITH CONTRIBUTIONS BY
KAREN VAIL-SMITH, M.S., M.P.A.
EAST CAROLINA UNIVERSITY

SANDRA M. WALZ, PH.D., R.D.
WEST CHESTER UNIVERSITY

JULIE SEVRENS LYONS

Benjamin Cummings

Boston Columbus Indianapolis New York San Francisco Upper Saddle River
Amsterdam Cape Town Dubai London Madrid Milan Munich Paris Montréal Toronto
Delhi Mexico City São Paulo Sydney Hong Kong Seoul Singapore Taipei Tokyo

Executive Editor: *Sandra Lindelof*
Director of Development: *Barbara Yien*
Senior Project Development Editor: *Marie Beaugureau*
Development Editor: *Laura Bonazzoli*
Art Development Manager: *Laura Southworth*
Associate Editor: *Emily Portwood*
Media Producer: *Sarah Young-Dualan*
Assistant Media Producer: *Molly Crowther*
Assistant Editor: *Brianna Paulson*
Editorial Assistant: *Meghan Zolnay*
Senior Marketing Manager: *Neena Bali*
Market Development Manager: *Brooke Suchomel*

Senior Managing Editor: *Deborah Cogan*
Production Supervisor: *Beth Collins*
Production Management and Composition: *S4Carlisle Publishing Services*
Manufacturing Buyer: *Jeffrey Sargent*
Senior Photo Editor: *Donna Kalal*
Photo Research: *Regalle Jaramillo*
Text and Cover Designer: *Riezebos Holzbaur Design Group*
Art House: *Precision Graphics*
Cover Photo Credits: *Tim Kitchen/Getty Images; Brad Wilson/Getty Images*

Library of Congress Cataloging-in-Publication Data

Lynch, April.
    Choosing health / April Lynch, Barry Elmore, Tanya Morgan; contributions by Karen Vail-Smith, Sandra Walz, Julie Sevrens Lyons.
      p. cm.
    Includes bibliographical references and index.
    ISBN 978-0-321-51618-3 (alk. paper)
    1. Health—Popular works. I. Elmore, Barry. II. Morgan, Tanya. III. Title.
RA776.5L96   2012
613—dc22   2010042144

Benjamin Cummings
is an imprint of

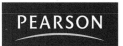

www.pearsonhighered.com

ISBN 10: 0-321-51618-4; ISBN 13: 978-0-321-51618-3 (Student edition)
ISBN 10: 0-321-72071-7; ISBN 13: 978-0-321-72071-9 (Exam copy)

1 2 3 4 5 6 7 8 9 10—CRK—14 13 12 11 10

This book is dedicated to my husband, Colin, daughter, Ava, and son, Van. In the ever-changing love and laughter project that is our family, I'm inspired to reach for better choices, every single day.

—April Lynch

To Billie, Sudie, Rick, my colleagues at ECU, and my students. Without you this book would not have been possible.

—Barry Elmore

This text is dedicated to my husband, Tom. Your strength and courage continue to amaze me. To my students, it's my hope that you, too, make the best decision of your life by *Choosing Health*.

–Tanya Morgan

About the Authors

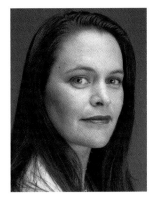

April Lynch

April Lynch is an award-winning author and journalist who specializes in health, science, and genetics. During her tenure with the *San Jose Mercury News,* the leading newspaper of Silicon Valley, she served as the Science and Health editor, focusing the paper's coverage on personal health and disease prevention. She has also worked as a writer and editor for the *San Francisco Chronicle*. April has written numerous articles on personal health, medical and scientific advances, consumer issues, and the ways that scientific breakthroughs are redefining our understanding of health. She has been a frequent contributor to leading university textbooks covering applied biology, nutrition, and environmental health and science. Together with a leading genetic counselor, April is the co-author of *The Genome Book,* a hands-on guide to using genetic information in personal health decisions. Her work has won numerous awards from organizations such as the Society of Professional Journalists, the California Newspaper Publishers Association, and the Associated Press. Her current interests include personal genomics, personalized medicine, and a focus on how people receive and interact with health information online. She lives in San Francisco with her husband and children.

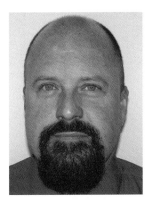

Barry Elmore, M.A.
East Carolina University

Barry Elmore is a faculty member at East Carolina University in the College of Health and Human Performance. He obtained a B.S. from Mount Olive College and an M.A. in Health Education at East Carolina University, where he was a merit scholar. Barry has extensive experience in the field of community health, with particular focus on sexually transmitted infections. He served as the Executive Director of the Pitt County AIDS Service Organization, the third largest AIDS service organization in North Carolina, before beginning his teaching career and worked as a health educator in the nonprofit sector for nearly 20 years. He is a member of the American Public Health Association (APHA), the Society for Public Health Education (SOPHE), and the North Carolina Association for Research in Education (NCARE). Barry has been recognized for outstanding teaching by his department, college, and university.

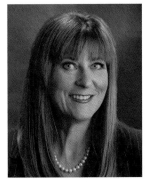

Tanya Morgan, Ph.D.
West Chester University

Tanya Morgan is an Associate Professor and Masters of Public Health Program Director for Health Care Management at West Chester University. She received her Ph.D. in Health Policy and Administration from the University of North Carolina at Chapel Hill. Tanya has traveled around the world to teach and consult in the development of health curricula, in locations as diverse as Oxford University, England; Guizhou University, China; and La Paz, Bolivia. In addition to her global interests, Tanya's research focuses on health assessment of college students, examining underserved populations, women's health issues, and health-care access. In honor of her research efforts, Tanya was awarded the Southern Academy of Women in Physical Activity, Sport, and Health (SAWPASH) Young Scholars Award. Most recently, she was recognized by the Rural Liberia Children's Educational Program for her support. She is actively involved in health advocacy and serves as chairperson for the Society for Public Health Education (SOPHE) Health Advocacy Committee and is a member of the Health Promotion Advocates Grassroots Committee. Tanya's interaction with her students in the classroom continually encourages her work. It is her desire that this textbook will help motivate the health behavior change that will increase the longevity of the millennial generation. She lives in Downingtown, Pennsylvania, with her husband, Tom, and her dog, Furio.

About the Contributors

Karen Vail-Smith, M.S., M.P.A.

East Carolina University

Karen Vail-Smith received a B.S. from The University of North Carolina at Chapel Hill and a M.S. and M.P.A. from East Carolina University. She has been a faculty member in East Carolina University's Department of Health Education and Promotion for 22 years. She specializes in personal health and human sexuality. She has received numerous teaching awards, including the prestigious UNC Board of Governor's Distinguished Professor for Teaching award. She has published more than 25 articles in health professional journals.

Sandra M. Walz, Ph.D., R.D.

West Chester University

Sandra M. Walz, a Registered Dietitian, is an Associate Professor in Nutrition and Dietetics at West Chester University. She teaches foods, nutrition, and dietetics management courses. Sandra earned a B.S. in both Nutrition and Corporate and Community Fitness from North Dakota State University, a M.S. in Food and Nutrition from North Dakota State University, and a Ph.D. in Hospitality Management from Kansas State University. She has worked in medical nutrition therapy, community nutrition, food service, and education settings. Sandra was the Founder and Director of a summer youth fitness and weight management program for 8- to 12-year-olds and has earned certificates of training in childhood and adolescent weight management, and Level 2 adult weight management from the Commission on Dietetic Registration. Her research interests include pedagogy (problem-based, experiential, and accelerated learning), adolescent obesity, and hospitality management. Sandra is devoted to engaging students in life-long learning.

Julie Sevrens Lyons

Julie Sevrens Lyons is a communications expert based in the San Francisco Bay Area. She has worked as a Personal Health and Science reporter at a number of publications, including the *San Jose Mercury News* and the *Contra Costa Times*. Her articles have been recognized by the Society of Professional Journalists and California Newspaper Publishers Association, as well as by many leading health organizations. Julie received her M.S. in Mass Communications from San Jose State University—graduating with honors—and lives with her husband and young son.

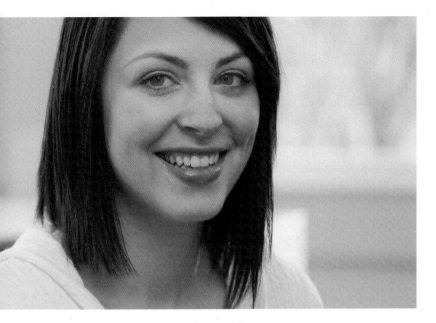

Chapter 5
Physical Activity for Fitness and Health 89

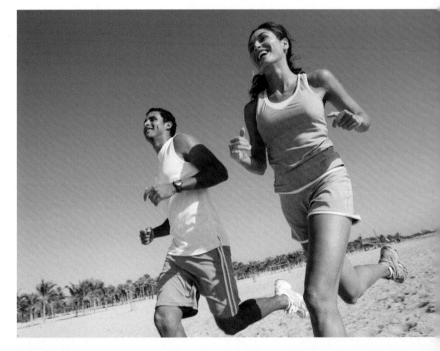

Chapter 6
Weight Management 116

Chapter 3
Stress Management 44

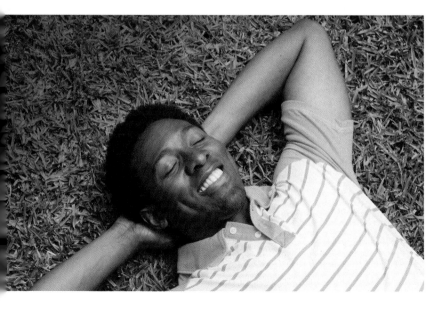

Chapter 4
Nutrition and You 65

Contents

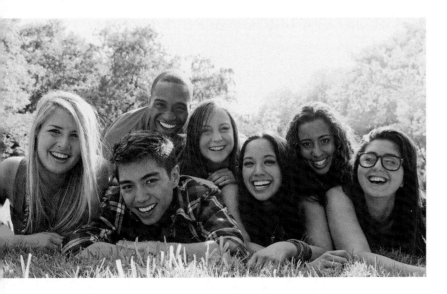

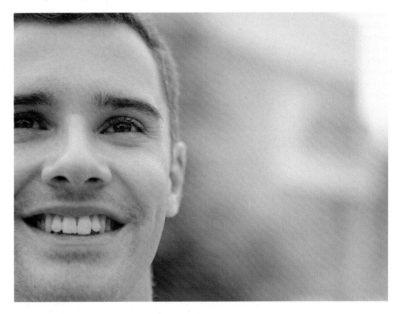

Brief Contents

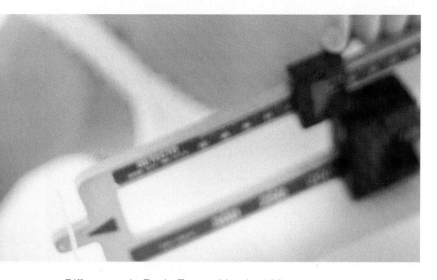

Chapter 7
Drug Use and Abuse 142

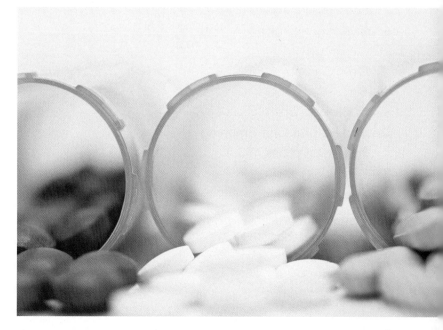

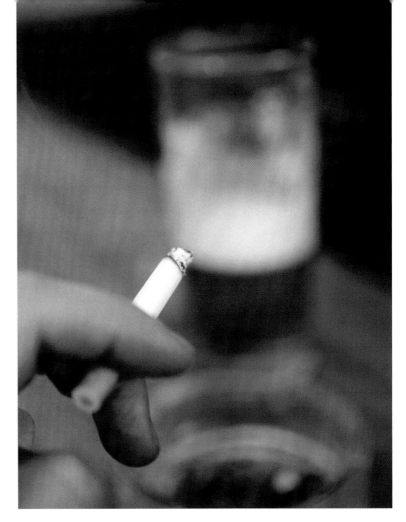

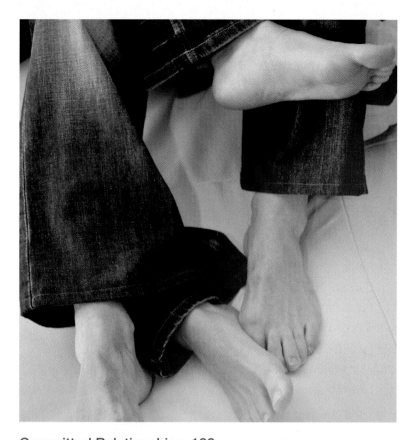

Chapter 10
Sexuality, Contraception, and Reproductive Choices 209

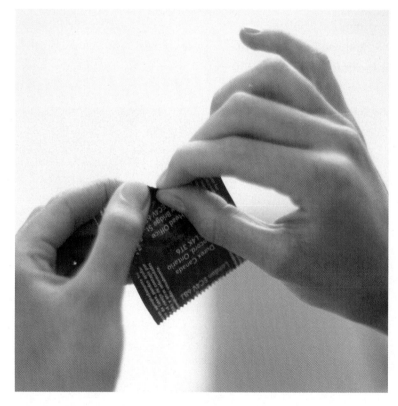

Chapter 11
Preventing Infectious Diseases and Sexually Transmitted Infections 244

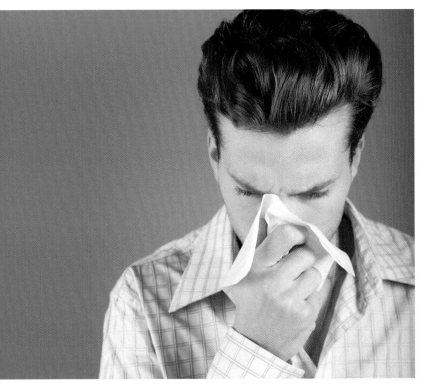

Chapter 12
Preventing Cardiovascular Disease, Diabetes, and Cancer 271

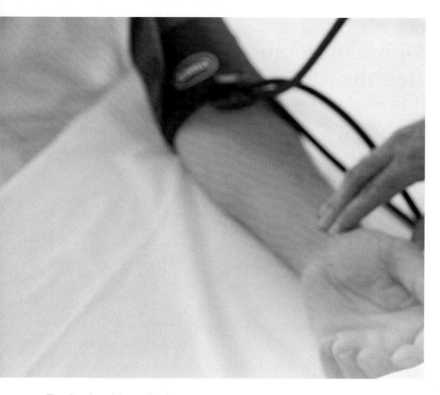

Chapter 13
Consumer Health 303

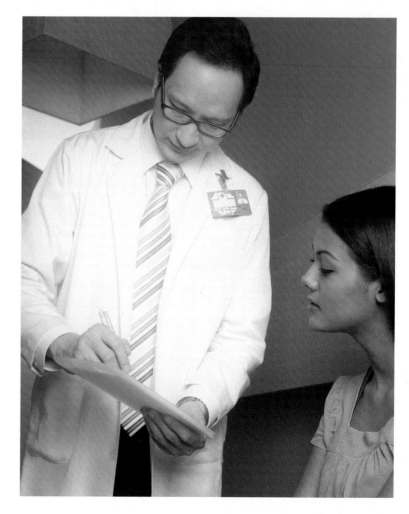

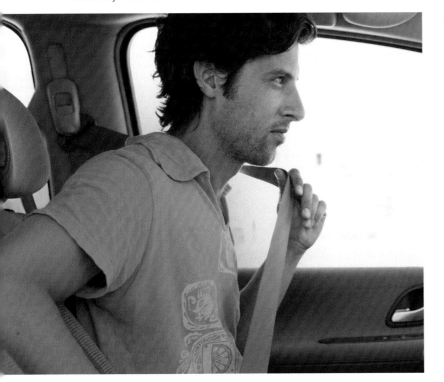

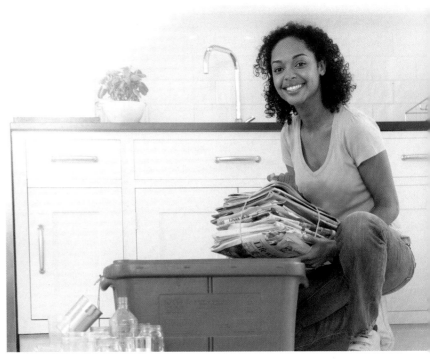

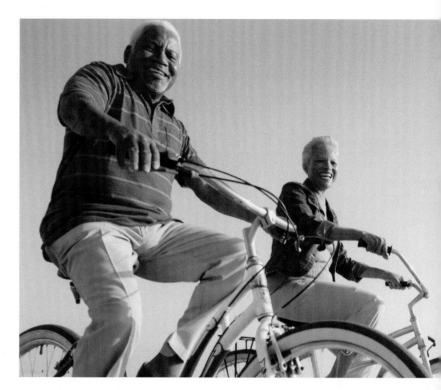

Feature Boxes

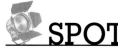

MYTH OR FACT?

DIVERSITY & HEALTH

CONSUMER CORNER

Preface

When it comes to your health, what will you choose?
You might think that question pertains to something in your future,
such as who your next doctor should be, or how you can avoid
illness down the road.

But the truth is you will also answer that question several times today, in ways both large and small. Did you get enough sleep last night? What will you have for lunch? Will you really hit the gym this afternoon, or just think about it? Are you waiting until the last minute to begin that paper due next week, or are you planning ahead so that you don't get overwhelmed?

In an era filled with medical innovations and high-tech health care, it's easy to overlook the fact that much of your health still rests in your hands. We all have to live with some factors we can't immediately control, such as our genetics or the physical environment that surrounds us. But beyond these more fixed elements, your decisions and lifestyle habits count for a lot. This book is called *Choosing Health* to underscore that your actions and behavior *matter*. You can consciously make decisions now that greatly reduce your chances of developing health problems later. The health you choose is an essential part of creating the life you want, both on campus now and in the years ahead.

Key Features of this Text

We wrote this book to help you make the best possible health choices, using the most recent and scientifically accurate information available. Other textbooks provide plenty of health information, but offer little guidance for actively making choices to improve your health. *Choosing Health* makes health information more relevant for students, with unique features such as:

- **Behavior Change Workshops** in every chapter that help you target a behavior you want to change, think through the steps necessary to make that change, and put yourself on a path to success.
- **Student Stories** throughout the text, along with videos of real college students telling health-related stories on our

companion website (www.pearsonhighered.com/choosinghealth). These stories reveal how students have dealt with health challenges, and may inspire you to make changes in your own life.

- **Health Online** links throughout the book that guide you to relevant health-related websites, videos, and podcasts. These links can also be found on the companion website, where they will be updated as needed.
- **Full-color, tear-out Choose To. . . cards,** which provide quick, handy health tips, such as recipes for cheap nutritious meals or ideas for easy ways to get a cardiovascular workout.
- **Self-Assessments** (also available online), which enable you to evaluate your current health behaviors and identify areas you may wish to work on.
- **A magazine-style design** that makes it fun to read!
- **Lively, engaging writing** that's still informative, scientifically reliable, and authoritative.

You will also find the following features:

- **Student Stats** throughout the book show you how health issues affect the college student population. Colorful graphs display statistics compiled by national surveys of college students.
- **Practical Strategies for Health** and **Practical Strategies for Change** provide you with specific, concrete tips you can use to develop and maintain healthful behaviors.
- **Consumer Corner** boxes examine consumer-related issues such as evaluating online health information, using over-the-counter medications safely, choosing athletic shoes, and deciding on whether to purchase organic produce.
- **Diversity & Health** boxes highlight how health issues can affect certain populations disproportionately, depending on

sex, racial/ethnic background, socioeconomic class, and other factors.

- **Myth or Fact?** boxes debunk common health myths by providing the scientific evidence against them.
- **Special Feature** boxes highlight hot topics in health, including getting enough sleep, the effect of Facebook on social relationships and communication, emerging infectious diseases, and what health-care reform means for you.

Student Supplements

The student supplements for this textbook include:

- **The *Choosing Health* Companion Website** (www.pearsonhighered.com/choosinghealth), where you can view a complete set of student videos; view health-related ABC News videos; access online behavior change tools; access practice tests and self-assessments; view videos of author Barry Elmore responding to questions about health-related issues; find links to updated websites, videos, and podcasts; and access a rich suite of additional study tools, including MP3 audio files, downloadable mobile versions of the Choose To. . . cards, audio case studies, an online glossary, and flashcards. You can also **send us your own videos, stories, or questions** via this website. If we decide to use your video or story for a future edition of *Choosing Health,* you will receive both payment and publication credit!
- ***Choosing Health* Facebook** (www.facebook.com/ChoosingHealth) **and Twitter** (http://twitter.com/choosing_health) **pages,** which provide up-to-the-minute health news as well as keep you informed of opportunities to submit your own videos and student stories.
- **A *Choosing Health* YouTube channel** (www.youtube .com/ch00singhealth), which features selected student videos. If you send us a student video of your own that we like, you just might find it on this channel!
- **Access to TweetYourHealth** (www.tweetyourhealth .com), a powerful, easy-to-use, Twitter-based application that allows you to track and keep an online journal of everyday health behaviors (such as what you eat, how often you exercise, and how much sleep you get) via any mobile device with text messaging or Internet capabilities.
- **Behavior Change Log Book and Wellness Journal,** a booklet you can use to track your daily exercise and nutritional intake and create a long-term nutrition and fitness prescription plan.
- **Digital 5-Step Pedometer,** which measures steps, distance (miles), activity time, and calories.

- **MyDietAnalysis** (www.mydietanalysis.com), an online tool powered by ESHA Research, Inc., that features a database of nearly 20,000 foods and multiple reports. It allows you to track your diet and physical activity, receive analyses of what nutrients you may be lacking, and generate and submit reports electronically.
- **Eat Right! Healthy Eating in College and Beyond**, a guidebook that provides practical tips, shopper's guides, and recipes so that you can start putting healthy principles into action. Topics include healthy eating in the cafeteria, dorm room, and fast food restaurants; eating on a budget; weight management tips; vegetarian alternatives; and guidelines on alcohol and health.
- **Live Right! Beating Stress in College and Beyond**, a guidebook that provides useful strategies for coping with a variety of life's challenges, during college and beyond. Topics include sleep, managing finances, time management, coping with academic pressure, relationships, and being a smart consumer.
- **Take Charge! Self-Assessment Worksheets**, a collection of 50 self-assessment exercises that students can fill out and assess their health and wellness. Worksheets are available as a gummed pad and can be packaged at no additional charge with the main text.

Instructor Supplements

This textbook comes with a comprehensive set of supplemental resources to assist instructors with classroom preparation and presentation.

- **The Teaching Toolbox** contains everything you need to teach your course, all in one place. It includes *Teaching with Web 2.0,* a booklet of ideas for incorporating Web 2.0 technologies into your classroom; an *Instructor Resource and Support Manual;* a printed *Test Bank;* an *Instructor Resource DVD* containing PowerPoint lecture outlines, PRS-enabled active lecture "clicker" questions, quiz show questions, computerized Test Bank, transparency acetate masters, jpeg and PowerPoint files of all the art, tables, and selected photos from the book, ABC News video clips, and student story videos; *Great Ideas! Active Ways to Teach Health and Wellness*; a *MyHealthLab* Instructor Access Kit (see below for details on *MyHealthLab*); *Take Charge! Self-Assessment Worksheets; Behavior Change Log Book and Wellness Journal; Eat Right! Healthy Eating in College and Beyond;* and *Live Right! Beating Stress in College and Beyond.*
- **MyHealthLab** (www.pearsonhighered.com/myhealthlab) provides a one-stop shop for accessing a wealth of

preloaded content and makes paper-free assigning and grading easier than ever. MyHealthLab contains all of the resources found on the *Choosing Health* companion website, along with the Pearson eText version of *Choosing Health* (which allows for instructor annotations to be shared with the class).

- **Health & Wellness Teaching Community Website** (www.pearsonhighered.com/healthcommunity) provides a convenient forum for connecting with other health instructors. Sponsored by the American Association for Health Education (AAHE) and Pearson, the website allows instructors to exchange teaching tips and ideas, as well as communicate with each other about issues related to health education.

Electronic Editions

Choosing Health is available in two electronic versions:

- **The Pearson eText** gives students access to the text whenever and wherever they can access the Internet. The eText pages look exactly like the printed text, and include powerful interactive and customization functions. Students can create notes, highlight text, create bookmarks, zoom in and out, click hyperlinked words and phrases to view defi-

nitions, and search quickly and easily for specific content. Instructors can add notes to guide students, upload documents, and customize presentations using Whiteboard mode. Contact your local Pearson sales representative for more information.

- **CourseSmart eTextbooks** are an exciting new choice for students looking to save money. As an alternative to purchasing the print textbook, students can subscribe to the same content online and save 40% off the suggested list price of the print text. Access the CourseSmart eText at www.coursesmart.com.

We are a team of health educators and communicators whose work reflects our deeply held belief that discussions of health are always a dialogue in progress. We hope this book will help you make changes toward better health. We also hope you'll let us know how those changes are going, and how we can make *Choosing Health* even more useful. Find us on Facebook, Twitter, or our Companion Website, and share your stories with us!

April Lynch
Barry Elmore
Tanya Morgan

Acknowledgments

Authoring a new textbook can feel like a solitary job during countless hours alone researching topics or drafting chapters. But in reality, we as authors were supported not only by each other, but by an amazing team of editors, publishing professionals, content contributors, supplement authors, and reviewers.

Collectively, the authors would like to thank everyone at Benjamin Cummings for their support and belief in our vision and our book, and call out a few of the key players for special thanks. First off, this book would not be possible without the support of Vice President and Editorial Director Frank Ruggirello, who was always there to provide backing and funds for the project and to be our advocate to the highest reaches of the organization. Another lifeline for the book was Executive Editor Sandra Lindelof, who believed in our team from the start, provided creative and enthusiastic guidance for the book as a whole, and really fostered our student-centric approach to teaching health. This book would not be what it is today without the razor-sharp, insightful, and deeply knowledgeable edits, feedback, and management of Director of Development Barbara Yien. Senior Project Development Editor Marie Beaugureau stepped in and supplied even more editorial guidance, feedback, coordination, and management—her continuous contact with the team and good cheer in the face of tight schedules kept us all happy and on-track. We'd also like to thank Project Editor Emily Portwood, who commissioned and managed the impressive print supplement package for the book, and Molly Crowther, Assistant Media Producer, and Sarah Young-Dualan, Media Producer, for their creativity and know-how in creating the robust and innovative interactive media and applications for the book. Assistant Editor Brianna Paulson and Editorial Assistant Meghan Zolnay commissioned hundreds of reviews and provided administrative assistance that none of us could have done without. Beth Collins, Production Supervisor, expertly coordinated the production aspects of the book, from coordinating the design to making sure manuscript was being sent to the correct places to double-checking all aspects of page proofs. We must also thank everyone at S4Carlisle Publishing Services, especially Senior Project Editor Norine Strang, for their wonderful work on the production and composition of the book—no matter how tight the schedule, they were always able to turn out the next round of page proofs. Manufacturing Buyer Jeffrey Sargent researched all types of paper and printing methods for us, to help us produce the most beautiful printing of the book possible. And speaking of beautiful, a million thanks to Yvo Riezebos, who designed the modern, engaging, and lively cover and interior for the book. Regalle Jaramillo and Donna Kalal provided invaluable expertise in the researching and coordinating of hundreds of photos for the book. A huge thanks goes out to Neena Bali, Senior Marketing Manager, who has worked tirelessly to get the message of *Choosing Health* out to instructors across the country. In addition, we as authors would not be nearly as informed about what health instructors from all over the nation want and need from a textbook were it not for the work of Market Development Manager Brooke Suchomel.

We would also like to thank our contributors, all of whom truly left their stamps on the book and whom we can't thank enough for their time and expertise. Karen Vail-Smith at East Carolina University provided help with every chapter of the book, and was invaluable at creating and editing Behavior Change Workshops and finding truly helpful Self-Assessments from valued sources for many of the chapters. Sandra Walz at West Chester University wrote the nutrition and weight management chapters—bringing her considerable expertise to these important topics. Julie Sevrens Lyons wrote the initial drafts for the chapters on drugs, alcohol, and tobacco, relationships, sexuality, and infectious diseases, and sexually transmitted infections; her skilled treatment of these topics really brings them to life. We'd also like to thank Mary Jane Niles at University of San Francisco for her careful check and editing of the immunity content for the infectious diseases chapter; with her help we feel that this potentially confusing information has been presented in the most accurate and crystal-clear manner possible. We'd also like to give special thanks to Laura Bonazzoli, who revised and polished several key chapters in the manuscript, and to Laura Southworth, who developed a beautiful and engaging art program.

The creation of the instructor and student supplements for *Choosing Health* could not have been completed without the excellent work of our supplement authors. The Test Bank was created by Natalie Stickney at Kennesaw State University, Teresa Snow at Georgia Institute of Technology, and John Kowalczyk at the University of Minnesota, Duluth. The PowerPoint Lecture Slides were written by Sloane Burke at East Carolina University. Cheryl Cechvala authored the Instructor Resource and Support Manual. Many thanks to all of them.

And finally, we'd like to thank all the reviewers who spent their time reading and commenting on our chapters—we listened to each and every one of your comments and are extremely grateful for your feedback. A full list of reviewers begins on the next page.

From April Lynch

I have countless people to thank, beginning with those who helped with the heavy lifting of putting words to page. I'll always be grateful to long-time colleague and fellow writer Julie Sevrens Lyons. Julie's prose has a deft, highly approachable touch, and this book is far the stronger for her contribution.

This project would have never gotten off the ground without the deep knowledge, health expertise, teaching wisdom, and killer sense of humor held by my co-author Barry Elmore. It wouldn't have stayed off the ground without the up-front advice of fellow textbook author Jay Withgott or the support of my former editorial director at my "day job," David Ansley. For particular guidance on the topic of human and clinical genetics, I'm indebted to Vickie Venne, M.S., C.G.C., an excellent genetic counselor, advisor, and friend. And for some occasional real-world perspective, student-style, there's no one I'd turn to before my niece Emma Marini, whose insights and help on this book have always been smart, funny, and spot-on. Maybe, Emma, you'll use this book when you reach college!

From Barry Elmore

I have so many people to thank for their hard work and contributions to this book. Thanks to Matt Cox, for his help with the initial research. Thank you to all of the people at Benjamin Cummings who worked so diligently on this book. I'd like to offer my sincere appreciation to Karen Vail-Smith, Dr. Sloane Burke, Sandra Walz, Julie Sevrens Lyons, Mary Jane Niles, and Laura Bonazzoli for their varied and invaluable contributions. It took a talented team of many players to bring this book to press, and I'd like to thank everyone who was a part of the effort.

From Tanya Morgan

There are so many people to thank for the efforts they put forth to produce this text. I want to begin by thanking the staff at Benjamin Cummings who had the unbelievable talent of taking words and magically transforming them into the beautiful pages that are depicted in this book. Very special thanks are extended to Dr. Sandra Walz. Not only is she an expert dietitian, but she is a dear friend. She never hesitated when asked to author the chapters on nutrition and weight management and willingly sacrificed many nights and weekends to complete the work. And, whenever I needed support, she was always there for me as a professional and a friend. Last, but not least, I would like to thank my students who have been my inspiration from the beginning. It has always been my dream to educate as many as possible about the benefits of a healthy lifestyle, and this text is a way of making my dream come true.

REVIEWERS

Katherine Lewis Allen
Northern Arizona University

Elizabeth Barrington
San Diego Mesa College

Linda Beatty
McLennen Community College

R. Cruz Begay
Northern Arizona University

Robin Benton
Salem State College

James Brenner
West Chester University

Liz Brown
Rose State College

Jocelyn Buck
Wake Technical Community College

Ni Bueno
Cerritos College

Sloane Burke
East Carolina University

Angela Burroughs
North Carolina Central University

Annette Carrington
North Carolina Central University

Dusty Childress
Ozarks Technical Community College

Fay Cook
Lock Haven University of Pennsylvania

Jane Curth
Georgia Perimeter College

Dan Czech
Georgia Southern University

Asad Dalia
University of Cincinnati

Brent Damron
Bakersfield College

Kathleen Dayton
Montgomery College, Rockville

Jennifer Dearden
Morehead State

Jacqueline Dove
Baylor University

Maureen Edwards
Montgomery College

Paul Finnicum
Arkansas State University

Ari Fisher
Louisiana State University

Kelly Fisher Shobe
Georgia Perimeter College

Autumn Hamilton
Minnesota State University

Chris Harman
California University of Pennsylvania

Valarie L. Hilson
Arkansas State University

Yvonne Hilton
Lincoln University

Kathy Hixon
Northeastern State University

Angela D. Holley
Georgia Perimeter College

Jane House
Wake Technical Community College

Guoyuan Huang
University of Southern Indiana

Hollie Huckabee
Arkansas State University

Emogene Johnson-Vaughn
Norfolk State University

Aaron Junta
Shasta College

Patricia Kearney
Bridgewater College

Bill Kernan
William Patterson University

Brian Kipp
Grand Valley State University

John Kowalczyk
University of Minnesota, Duluth

Gary Ladd
Southwestern Illinois College

Ellen Larson
Northern Arizona University

Ayanna Lyles
California University of Pennsylvania

Debbie Lynch
Rose State College

Bridget Melton
Georgia Southern University

Roseann Poole
Tallahassee Community College

Mary Jo Preti
MiraCosta College

Elizabeth Ridings
Montgomery College

Albert Simon
Jackson State University

Becky Slonaker
McLennen Community College

Carol Smith
Elon University

Deborah Stone
Louisiana State University

Nancy Storey
Georgia Perimeter College

Cody Trefethen
Palomar College

Sandra Walz
West Chester University

Lesley Wasilko
Montgomery College

Linda White
Metropolitan State College

Sharon Woodard
Wake Forest University

CLASS TESTERS

Fran Babich
Butte College

Elizabeth Bailey
Elon University

Stephanie Bennett
University of Southern Indiana

Tina Cummings
Bakersfield College

Dan Czech
Georgia Southern University

Kathy Deresinski
Triton College

Melody Durrenberger
Georgia Perimeter College

Max Faquir
Palm Beach State College

Renee Fenwick-Frimming
University of Southern Indiana

Kendra Guilford
University of Alabama, Tuscaloosa

Essam Hamido
Tennessee State University

Chris Harman
California University of Pennsylvania

Guoyuan Huang
University of Southern Indiana

Hollie Huckabee
Arkansas State University

Emogene Johnson-Vaughn
Norfolk State University

Tim Jones
Tennessee State University

Walt Justice
Southwestern College

September Kirby
South Dakota State University

Ayanna Lyles
California University of Pennsylvania

Bridget Melton
Georgia Southern University

Susan Milstein
Montgomery College

Kim Queri
Rose State College

Lesley Rennis
Borough of Manhattan Community College

Bernard Smolen
Prince George's Community College

Resa Walch
Elon University

Sharon Woodard
Wake Forest University

PERSONAL HEALTH FORUM AND FOCUS GROUP PARTICIPANTS

Kim Archer
Stephen F. Austin State

Brian Barthel
Utah Valley University

Laura Blitzer
Long Island University

Dan Czech
Georgia Southern University

Jennifer Dearden
Morehead State

Joel Dering
Cameron University

Joyce Fetro
Southern Illinois University

Paul Finnicum
Arkansas State University

Teresa Hardman
Moorehead University

Emogene Johnson-Vaughn
Norfolk State University

Andrew Kanu
Virginia State University

Patricia Marcum
University of Southern Indiana

Bridget Melton
Georgia Southern University

Maria Okeke
Florida A&M University

Dana Sherman
Ozarks Technical Community College

INTERVIEWEES

Duro Agbede
Southwestern College

Mike Basile
Borough of Manhattan Community College

Philip Belcastro
Borough of Manhattan Community College

Rebecca Brey
Ball State University

Elaine Bryan
Georgia Perimeter College

Ni Bueno
Cerritos College

Laura Burger-Simm
Grossmont College

Lynda Butler-Storsved
Elon University

Michael Calhoun
Elon University

Cheryl Campbell
Grossmont College

Doug Casey
Georgia Perimeter College

Steve Chandler
Florida A&M University

Kim Clark
California State University, San Bernardino

Mary Conway
Sierra College

Marianne Crocker
Ozarks Technical Community College

Paula Dahl
Bakersfield College

Brent Damron
Bakersfield College

James Deboy
Lincoln University

Eva Doyle
Baylor University

Melanie Durkin
Southwestern College

Maureen Edwards
Montgomery College

Kelly Falcone
Palomar College

Paul Finnicum
Arkansas State University

Barb Francis
Metropolitan State College

Valerie Goodwin
Southwestern College

Michelle Harcrow
University of Alabama, Tuscaloosa

Chris Harrison
Montgomery College

Bryan Hedrick
Elon University

Casie Higginbotham
Middle Tennessee State University

Valerie Hilson
Arkansas State University

Yvonne Hilton
Lincoln University

Kris Jankovitz
California Polytechnic State University, San Luis Obispo

Carol Jensen
Metropolitan State College

David Jolly
North Carolina Central University

Shannon Josey
Middle Tennessee State University

Beth Kelley
Grossmont College

Jerome Kotecki
Ball State University

Aaron Krac
Queensborough Community College

Randy Maday
Butte College

Rick Madson
Palm Beach State College

Vance Manakas
Moorpark College

Patricia Marcum
University of Southern Indiana

Mitch Mathias
Arkansas State University

Connie Mettille
Winona State University

Gavin O'Connor
Ozarks Technical Community College

Maria Okeke
Florida A&M University

Kevin Petti
San Diego Miramar College

Rod Porter
San Diego Miramar College

Regina Prodoehl
James Madison University

Elizabeth Ridings
Montgomery College

Karla Rues
Ozarks Technical Community College

Todd Sabato
James Madison University

Dana Sherman
Ozarks Technical Community College

Agneta Sibrava
Arkansas State University

Jeff Slepski
Mt. San Jacinto College

Nancy Storey
Georgia Perimeter College

Debra Sutton
James Madison University

Amanda Tapler
Elon University

Karen Thomas
Montgomery College

Silvea Thomas
Kingsborough Community College

Iva Toler
Prince George's Community College

Tim Wallstrom
Riverside Community College

Lesley Wasilko
Montgomery College

Patti Waterman
Palomar College

Linda White
Metropolitan State College

Susanne Wood
Tallahassee Community College

LaShawn Wordlaw-Stinson
North Carolina Central University

Bonnie Young
Georgia Perimeter College

Thank You to Our Student Advisory Board

The *Choosing Health* Student Advisory Board consists of students who submit stories, videos, questions, or feedback to us about *Choosing Health.* Many of them are thanked on the Student Advisory Board page at the beginning of the book. The *Choosing Health* team is constantly speaking to more health students and receiving more contributions from them. A continuously updated list of student advisors appears at **www.pearsonhighered.com/ choosinghealth.**

Choosing Health

Health in the 21st Century

1

- The current life expectancy at birth in the U.S. is 77.7 years. [i]

- Heart disease, cancer, and stroke are the top three causes of death in the U.S. [ii]

- Just four bad habits—eating poorly, being physically inactive, smoking, and drinking too much—can prematurely age you by up to 12 years. [iii]

- A growing number of consumers—at least 70 million in the U.S. alone—are seeking health information on the Internet. [iv]

What is health?

LEARNING OBJECTIVES

IDENTIFY and describe the multiple dimensions of health.

DISCUSS how lifestyle choices can affect health.

DESCRIBE how age, sex, racial and ethnic background, geography, income, and sexual orientation can affect health.

DISCUSS the *transtheoretical model* and the *health belief model* of behavior change.

LIST strategies for critically evaluating health information online and in the media.

Health Online icons are found throughout the chapter, directing you to web links, videos, podcasts, and other useful online resources.

In the past, the term **health** meant merely the absence of illness or injury. Today, however, the term has a much broader meaning, encompassing many different aspects of your life. The World Health Organization defines health as "a state of physical, mental, and social well-being, and not merely the absence of disease or infirmity."[1] This holistic view of health acknowledges that many different factors can affect your sense of well-being. In this textbook, we will discuss not only physical health, but also social, psychological, spiritual, intellectual, environmental, and even occupational dimensions of health.

Another running theme of this textbook is that *your lifestyle choices can have a profound influence on your health*. Whereas you can't control your age or genetics, you have the power to make behavioral decisions such as whether to eat nutritiously, be physically active, manage your stress level, prioritize sleep, and refrain from smoking or excessive drinking. On a day-to-day basis, these may seem like mundane decisions. Over the long term, however, the cumulative effects of these decisions can greatly increase or decrease your risk of developing serious diseases such as cancer, heart disease, and diabetes. The results of a recently published 20-year study has found that just four bad habits—eating poorly, being physically inactive, smoking, and drinking too much—can prematurely age you by up to 12 years.[2] This book is called *Choosing Health* to underscore that your actions and behavior <u>matter</u>, and that you can consciously make decisions today to greatly reduce your risk of developing health problems tomorrow.

Another goal of this text is to provide you with strategies to critically evaluate all the health information that you are exposed to—whether from books, magazines, newspapers, television, advertisements, or the Internet. Online search engines like Google are increasingly the first place many people turn when seeking health information, but search results don't distinguish between sites that provide unbiased, up-to-date, scientifically sound information and sites that contain inaccurate or misleading content. This chapter—along with the "Consumer Corner" and "Health Online" features you'll find throughout this book, and Chapter 13, Consumer Health—will help you sort through the maze of information in today's intensely media-saturated world.

Let's begin by returning to the concept of *health*—and an important related concept: *wellness*.

Dimensions of Health and Wellness

As we've noted, health encompasses multiple dimensions of well-being. Closely related to health is the concept of *wellness*. **Wellness** is the process of actively making choices to achieve optimal health.[3] People who have a high level of wellness have achieved their goals in multiple dimensions of health, by continually making behavior decisions that promote health. On the other hand, poor behavior decisions are likely to lead to low levels of wellness, and increase the risk of illness, injury, and premature death.

The Illness-Wellness Continuum

In 1975, wellness pioneer John W. Travis, M.D., published the *illness-wellness continuum*. He envisioned a continuum with two extremes: premature death at one end and high-level wellness on the other **(Figure 1.1).** Most of us fall somewhere in between, shifting between states of feeling sick, "neutral," and vibrantly healthy. Your general direction on the continuum (either toward optimal wellness or toward premature death) matters more than your place on it at any given time. You may have a cold, for instance, and not feel particularly well—but if you take care of

health More than merely the absence of illness or injury, a state of well-being that encompasses physical, social, psychological, spiritual, intellectual, environmental, and occupational dimensions.

wellness The process of actively making choices to achieve optimal health.

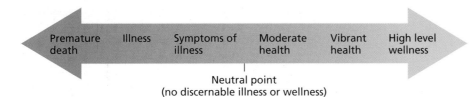

| Premature death | Illness | Symptoms of illness | Moderate health | Vibrant health | High level wellness |

Neutral point
(no discernable illness or wellness)

Figure 1.1 The illness-wellness continuum. Your general direction on the continuum matters more than your specific point on it at any given time.

Reprinted with permission, from Travis, J. W., & Ryan, R. S. (2004). *Wellness workbook* (3rd ed.). Berkeley: Celestial Arts. www.wellnessworkbook.com.

yourself, eat nutritiously, exercise, and have a positive attitude, your general direction will be toward greater wellness. Likewise, you may consider yourself physically fit—but if you are under a great deal of stress, eating poorly, not getting enough sleep, and drinking excessively, your general direction on the continuum will edge toward reduced wellness.

Dimensions of Health

We've mentioned that health is multidimensional. These dimensions include physical, intellectual, psychological, social, spiritual, environmental, and occupational health **(Figure 1.2).** (Note that because wellness is the process of achieving optimal health, wellness, too, is multidimensional.) Let's take a closer look at each of these dimensions.

Physical Health
Physical health focuses on the body: how well it functions, and how well you care for it. Optimal physical health includes being physically active, eating nutritiously, getting enough sleep, making responsible decisions about sex, drinking, and drugs, and taking steps to avoid injuries and infectious diseases.

Intellectual Health
Intellectual health is marked by a willingness to take on new intellectual challenges, an openness to new ideas and skills, a capacity to think critically, and a sense of humor and curiosity. People who have a high level of intellectual health not only recognize problems quickly, but also seek and create solutions.

Psychological Health
Psychological health is a broad category that includes *mental health, emotional health*, and aspects of *spiritual health*. Mental health describes a person's ability to perceive reality accurately and respond to

> *You can consciously make decisions today to greatly reduce your risk of developing health problems tomorrow.*

its challenges rationally and effectively. Emotional health refers to the subjective side of psychological health, and includes a person's feelings and moods. Spiritual health contributes to psychological health by providing a sense of connection to a larger purpose.

Social Health
Social health describes the quality of your interactions and relationships with others. How satisfying are your relationships with your family, your friends, your professors, and others in your life? How do you feel about your ability to fulfill social roles, whether that role be as a friend, roommate, or community volunteer? Good social health is also characterized by an ability to provide support to others and receive it in return.

Spiritual Health
As we've noted, aspects of *spiritual health* can affect psychological health—but spiritual health is a significant enough topic to be considered a dimension of health on its own. Spiritual health centers on

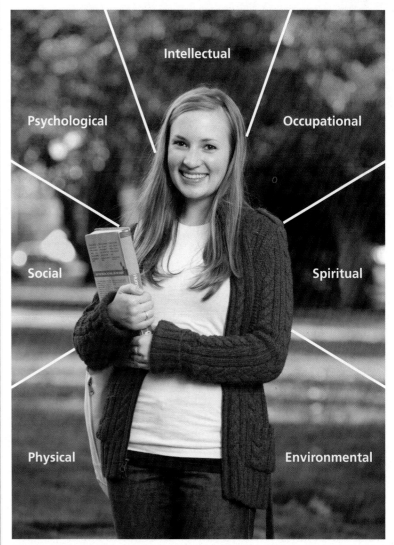

Figure 1.2 Dimensions of health. Health is more than just the absence of injury or illness; it encompasses multiple dimensions.

Proud of My Scars

"Hi, I'm Corey. I'm 19 and I'm a sophomore park and rec management major. I was born with a skeletal condition where the left side of my body is bigger than the right side. The doctors had to even out my legs so that I could walk flat-footed and wouldn't have back problems later in life. I've had a total of three surgeries, which left me with some scars. I also have a scar from my belly button all the way to the side of my rib cage. Growing up, I was always self-conscious, especially during the summer when everybody was out at the beach in swimsuits, and all these guys had six-pack abs. I knew I'd never be able to have abs like that because I have this scar running straight through my abdominal muscle.

Now, though, I've realized that my scars are a great conversation starter. People will see me and ask 'Oh, cool scar, how'd you get it?' I've learned over the years that everybody has a fail point and mine just happens to be physical. I've just learned to live with it. Those scars are what make me 'me.' I also have friends who don't really care what I look like or whether I'm the strongest or best-looking guy in the world. My friends are there whether I'm having surgeries or I'm on top of the world."

1: Where do you think Corey falls on the wellness continuum?

2: Assess how Corey is doing in at least three different dimensions of wellness.

Do you have a story similar to Corey's? Share your story at **www.pearsonhighered.com/choosinghealth.**

the beliefs and values we each hold that lend meaning to life. We may each define and express those beliefs and values in our own way—perhaps in the form of organized religion, or in respect for nature and the environment. Regardless of how it is expressed, spiritual health and the values that shape it contribute to a sense of place and purpose in life, and can be a source of support when we face challenges.

Environmental Health

Environmental health describes the quality of our home, work, school, and social environments—as well as the health of our planet. Air quality, availability of clean water and nutritious food, crime rates, weather, pollution, and exposure to chemicals are just a few of the variables that factor into environmental health.

Occupational Health

Occupational health describes the quality of your relationship to your work. How happy and fulfilled do you feel by your work? Do you feel respected by your coworkers? Do you have opportunities to advance and learn? Consider that "work" may consist of your studies, a job, an athletic endeavor, or an artistic pursuit—whatever it is that you consider to be your primary occupation. Challenges to occupational health include stress, poor relationships with coworkers, lack of fulfillment in the work, and sudden unemployment. *Financial wellness*—or lack thereof—can play an undeniable role in our overall sense of health and wellness.

How Healthy Are We?

By one very basic measure of health—how long the average person born in the United States can expect to live—we are in far better shape than our predecessors. The current **life expectancy** at birth in the United States is a record 77.7 years—nearly 15 years longer than it was in 1940.[4] The causes of death have also changed dramatically over the years. In 1900, the leading causes of death were infectious diseases such as pneumonia, influenza, and tuberculosis, frequently claiming victims at a relatively early age.[5] Today, the leading causes of death in the U.S. are chronic diseases such as heart disease and cancer that tend to strike older adults (see **Table 1.1**).[4] Note that among those aged 15–24, the leading causes of death are accidents, homicide, and suicide.

life expectancy The average number of years a person may expect to live.

To be sure, the monumental public health innovations and initiatives of the last 100 years—including a reduction in smoking rates, widespread vaccinations, advances in antibiotics, and safer food handling practices—have brought about vast improvements in health. However, important challenges remain. In a recent national health survey of more than 75,000 U.S. adults:[6]

- More than 60% said they never participated in vigorous leisure-time exercise.
- More than 35% were overweight, and 26% were obese.
- About 23% said they had been told by a healthcare professional that they had high blood pressure.
- About 20% were current smokers.
- About 10% reported feelings and symptoms linked to depression.
- About 13% reported feelings and symptoms linked to anxiety.
- About 15% said they had no regular place where they sought or received health care, a significant obstacle to preventing illness and maintaining good health.

Table 1.1: Top Five Causes of Death in the U.S.

	Cause of Death
All Ages	1. Heart disease
	2. Cancer
	3. Stroke
	4. Chronic lower respiratory disease
	5. Accidents/unintentional injuries
15–24 years old	1. Accidents/unintentional injuries
	2. Assault/homicide
	3. Suicide
	4. Cancer
	5. Heart disease

Data from "Deaths: Final Data for 2006" by Heron, M., Hoyert, D., Xu, J., Scott, C., & Tejada-Vera, B. 2009, *National Vital Statistics Reports,* 57(14), pp. 1–135.

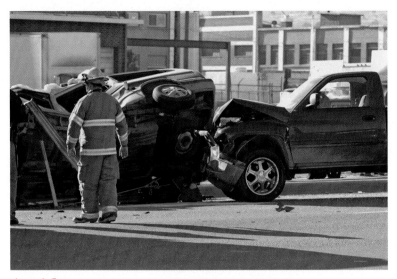

Accidents are the leading cause of death among people aged 15–24 in the U.S.

Table 1.2: **Healthy People 2010: A Progress Report on Selected Leading Indicators**

Objective	Estimated percentage of population meeting objective	2010 target for percentage of population meeting objective
Engage in regular moderate or vigorous physical activity	32	50
Be a healthy weight	32	60
Don't smoke	79	88
Don't use illicit drugs	92	97
Stay within low-risk guidelines for drinking	45 (female), 39 (male)	50 (female and male)
Possess health insurance	84	100

Data from *Data2010: The Healthy People 2010 Database* by the Centers for Disease Control, 2010, retrieved from CDC Wonder, http://wonder.cdc.gov/data2010, May 5, 2010.

Healthy People 2010 and Healthy People 2020

To address these challenges, the U.S. government launched the **Healthy People initiative.** Every decade since 1980, federal health officials have published reports outlining the nation's progress in meeting national health goals over a 10-year period. The most recent effort, Healthy People 2010, focused on two primary goals: (1) helping people in the U.S. improve the length and quality of their lives and (2) eliminating significant **health disparities,** or differences between various segments of the population. The initiative also identified ten *leading health indicators* that represent the nation's top health concerns:

- Physical activity
- Overweight and obesity
- Tobacco use
- Substance abuse
- Responsible sexual behavior
- Mental health
- Injury and violence
- Environmental quality
- Immunization
- Access to health care

Table 1.2 illustrates a progress report for how well the 2010 goals were met for selected leading indicators.

> **For the latest updates on Healthy People 2010 and Healthy People 2020, visit www.healthypeople.gov.**

In the meantime, Healthy People 2020 has already begun. This initiative seeks to build on the goals and objectives set for Healthy People 2010. The top goals for Healthy People 2020 include:

- Increase public awareness and understanding of the underlying causes of health, disease, and disability.
- Eliminate preventable disease, disability, injury, and premature death.

Healthy People initiative A federal initiative to facilitate broad, positive health changes in large segments of the U.S. population every 10 years.

health disparities Differences in quality of health among various segments of the population.

Healthy Campus An offshoot of the Healthy People initiative, specifically geared toward college students.

- Create social and physical environments that promote good health for all.
- Promote healthy development and healthy behaviors across every stage of life.

Healthy Campus

Promoting good health also extends to college campuses across the nation. In conjunction with Healthy People 2010, the American College Health Association adapted the initiative for use in student settings. As part of the **Healthy Campus** program, participating colleges and universities could choose to focus on improving health topics most relevant to them, such as:

- Reducing stress and depression
- Decreasing student abuse of alcohol and drugs
- Improving opportunities for daily physical activity on campus
- Improving sexual health among students

Healthy People 2020 may also receive a similar adaptation so that campuses can apply the goals in ways that best meet their needs.

> **For more information on the Healthy Campus initiative, visit www.acha.org/Topics/HC2010.cfm.**

How Healthy Are College Students?

The creation of the Healthy Campus initiative reflects the growing focus on health at colleges and universities across the country. Stress, depression, anxiety, alcohol and tobacco use, and sexual health are just a few of the issues that can affect your academic performance and achievement. Centers of higher learning, as microcosms of our larger society, have come to recognize that when assessed collectively, student health can shape how well a campus performs and meets its goal of providing the best education possible.

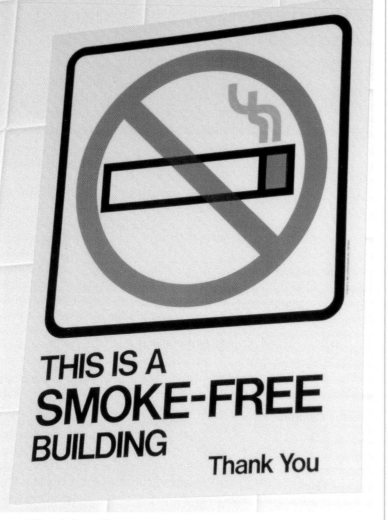

THIS IS A
SMOKE-FREE
BUILDING
Thank You

The **Healthy Campus** initiative aims to improve the health of college students nationwide.

The **Student Stats** box lists common health issues reported by students in a recent nationwide study, and includes allergies, sinus infection, back pain, and strep throat as among the most common health concerns.[7] Stress, sleep difficulties, and colds/flu/sore throats topped the list of factors that most affected students' academic performance (see the Student Stats box in Chapter 3). The same study reported that 61.8% of students described their health as either "very good" or "excellent."

Students tend to be younger than the general population, and so do not experience the same high rates of chronic illnesses (such as heart disease and cancer) seen in the adult population as a whole. However, the behaviors that increase the risk of developing these diseases—including unhealthy eating habits and a lack of physical activity—are common among college students. Although 61.8% of students reported being at a healthy weight, 21.2% were overweight, and more than 10% were obese.[7] Furthermore, although 43.6% of students met the American Heart Association's recommendations for physical activity (moderate exercise at least 5 days per week or vigorous exercise at least 3 days per week), 56.4% did not.[7]

STUDENT 🪑 STATS

Common Health Problems Reported by College Students

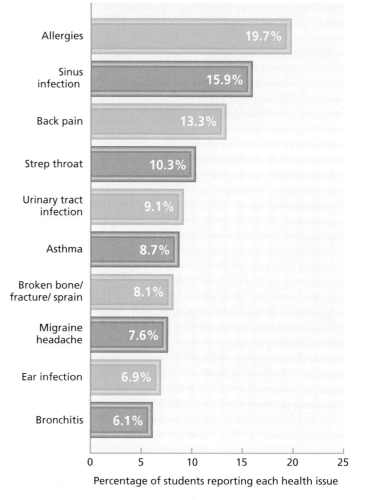

Data from *American College Health Association National College Health Assessment (ACHA-NCHA II) Reference Group Executive Summary. Fall 2009* by the American College Health Association, 2009, retrieved from http://www.acha-ncha.org/docs/ACHA-NCHA_Reference_Group_ExecutiveSummary_Fall2009.pdf.

Interestingly, research has shown that students tend to vastly overestimate how many of their peers are regularly using alcohol, tobacco, or other drugs.[7] For example:

- Students believed that 93% of their peers consumed alcohol during a given 30-day period. The actual percentage was 59.2%.
- Students believed that 81.2% of their peers had smoked cigarettes during a given 30-day period. The actual percentage was 13.8%.
- Students believed that 76.6% of their peers had smoked marijuana during a given 30-day period. The actual percentage was 12.5%.
- Students believed that 76.2% of their peers used illicit drugs (excluding marijuana) during a given 30-day period. The actual percentage was 13%.

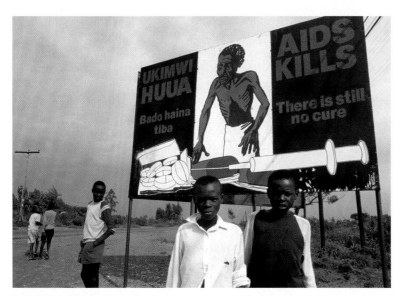

HIV/AIDS continues to be a serious concern worldwide, especially in sub-Saharan Africa.

The lesson here: When it comes to drugs and alcohol, it's simply not true that "everyone is doing it."

Health Around the World

In our increasingly mobile and connected world, where a country experiencing a dangerous infectious disease is just a plane ride away, global health has become a top concern.

Some countries with lower levels of economic development and less stable political systems continue to experience diseases that have largely been eradicated in other parts of the world. Parts of the African continent, for example, have continued to grapple with preventable infectious illnesses such as polio and cholera. Many parts of Africa, Asia, and South America continue to face malaria. Although infections from the human immunodeficiency virus (HIV) have dropped in number in more developed countries, HIV/AIDS continues to be a serious concern worldwide. More than 33 million people around the world are living with HIV infection, according to international health statistics; more than 67% of them live in sub-Saharan Africa. China, India, and Russia have seen a substantial increase in HIV infections in recent years.[8]

> For more information on infectious diseases around the world, visit the World Health Organization website at www.who.int/topics/infectious_diseases/en.

To address these global disparities, a number of privately funded international health organizations have joined with public efforts in recent years. Groups founded by prominent business leaders such as Microsoft founder Bill Gates and former U.S. president Bill Clinton now provide funds for public health initiatives such as improved vaccination campaigns or cleaner drinking water. In the next decade, it will become clear how well these initiatives improve global health, and how well they complement the public health efforts carried out by long-standing international agencies such as the United Nations and the World Health Organization.

Factors That Affect Personal Health

To some extent, we all have the same basic health needs. We need a nutritious diet, regular exercise, safety from physical injury, access to medical care, protection from infectious disease, and supportive emotional relationships. But each of us also has factors in our lives that make good health a more individual matter. Some of these factors are beyond our power to control. Others, however—such as lifestyle choices—are very much within our ability to control, and are the emphasis of most personal health courses.

Factors that influence health include:

- **Lifestyle choices.** Four key behaviors with a profound ability to influence your health are to (1) eat nutritiously, (2) be physically active, (3) not smoke, and (4) not drink excessively. Making these four behaviors a part of your regular lifestyle can greatly decrease your risk of developing serious illnesses later in life.

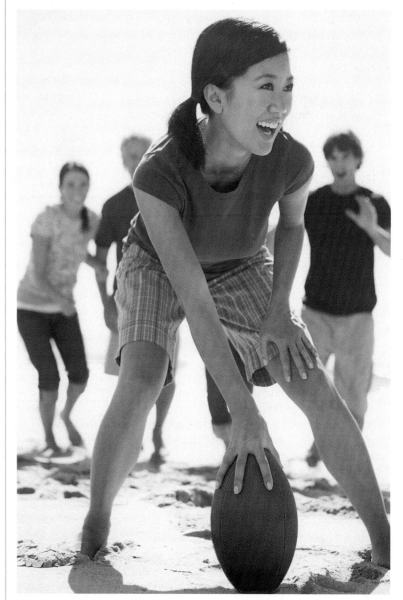

Regular **physical activity** is a key component of staying healthy.

Other lifestyle choices that play a key role in promoting health include managing your stress level and getting enough sleep (Chapter 3), maintaining a healthful weight (Chapter 6), refraining from illicit drug use (Chapter 7), developing supportive relationships with others (Chapter 9), making responsible sexual health decisions (Chapter 10), and taking basic steps to ensure your personal safety, such as wearing a seat belt and avoiding high-risk behaviors (Chapter 14).

- **Age.** Our health concerns change with age. Think back to childhood and your visits to the pediatrician. The kinds of health issues your doctor likely focused on then—frequent immunizations, treating ear infections, tracking your growth in height and weight—are probably not the same priorities that your doctor would have for you today. As we grow older, we become more susceptible to some diseases and less susceptible to others. Influenza, for example, tends to be more of a health concern for very young children and for the elderly (although the recent epidemic of the H1N1 influenza virus, which affects younger adults more so than it does the elderly, is a notable exception). Chronic illnesses like cancer and heart disease, meanwhile, are more common concerns for older adults than younger ones.

- **Sex. Sex,** or the biological and physiological features that differentiate a male from a female, is determined at conception. Sex has a powerful role on health, with biological differences between men and women resulting in many different health outcomes. Women tend to live about 4 years longer than men, for example, but have higher rates of some disabling health problems, such as arthritis and osteoporosis. Men are more likely to experience other serious chronic conditions, such as high blood pressure and cancer.[9]

- **Racial and ethnic background.** Health disparities exist among different racial and ethnic populations. Some of these disparities are tied to socioeconomic causes, while others may be cultural, biological, or still not well understood. This **Diversity & Health** box examines some of these differences.

- **Geography.** Where you live can increase your vulnerability to certain health risks. Americans living in rural areas (that is, places with fewer than 2,500 residents) have less access to specialized medical care or emergency services, and are more likely to die from serious injuries or other medical emergencies. People living in regions with high levels of air pollution, such as Detroit, Michigan, or California's Central Valley, are more likely to experience higher rates of asthma and other respiratory ailments.[10] The southeastern United States includes an area known as the "stroke belt" because of its higher incidences of stroke compared to the rest of the country, most likely due to regional differences in diet, smoking, and access to health care.[11]

- **Income and health insurance.** People with lower incomes and inadequate or no health insurance are less likely to have a regular doctor or place of care, and less likely to receive a wide range of health services. One recent study found that while higher-income Caucasians have enjoyed a wide range of health gains, these improvements have not been shared by lower-income Caucasians

and ethnic minorities.[12] Chapter 13, Consumer Health, covers health insurance in more detail, including the main points of the health reform legislation signed into law by President Obama on March 23, 2010, which aims to substantially reduce the number of Americans who do not have health insurance.[13]

- **Sexual orientation.** Some adults self-identify as gay, lesbian, bisexual, or transgender, while others may avoid formal labels but have same-sex relationships. While statistics on sexual orientation often vary, several studies have found that significant percentages of people pursue same-sex relationships. One international study, for example, found that 6.2%, 4.5%, and 10.7% of males and 3.6%, 2.1%, and 3.3% of females in the United States, the United Kingdom, and France, respectively, reported having had sexual contact with someone of the same sex in the previous five years.[14] This diverse group faces a wide range of health concerns. Gay and bisexual men are at higher risk for contracting HIV/AIDS and drug-resistant staphylococcus infections.[15] Gay, lesbian, bisexual, and transgender teens face emotional challenges and sometimes violence or physical abuse if they share their orientation with their peers or family. As adults, members of the gay, lesbian, bisexual, and transgender communities continue to face societal pressures and challenges to their emotional wellness as they form partnerships, establish households, and have families of their own.

- **Health literacy. Health literacy** is the ability to evaluate and understand health information and to make informed choices for your own health care. It includes the ability to read, understand, and follow instructions in medical brochures and prescription drug labels; the ability to listen to health care providers, ask good questions, and analyze the information you receive; and the ability to navigate an often-confusing and complex health care system.[16] Increasingly, health literacy also requires a degree of computer literacy and media awareness, which we will discuss shortly in more detail. Chapter 13, Consumer Health, also discusses several strategies for becoming a savvy health consumer.

Given that health disparities arise from a variety of causes—including differences in income, education, access to health care, lifestyle choices, genetics, and discrimination—there is no single solution to resolve them. But the decades of research behind the Healthy People initiative have clarified some of the improvements that are possible and how to achieve them. The goals include:

- **Improving everyone's access to health insurance.** Members of ethnic minorities are generally less likely to have health coverage than the general population.

- **Improving everyone's access to health services.** Health insurance is just one part of the answer. Greater geographic and cultural diversity of health services is also important. More isolated areas, such as rural regions, need quicker access to a broader range of health services. Once a person has arrived at a care center, he or she needs care provided by staff who understand any relevant cultural concerns and can address the language needs of patients who speak limited English. Medical translation

---

sex The biological and physiological features that differentiate a male from a female.

health literacy The ability to evaluate and understand health information and to make informed choices for your health care.

How does your state compare to others in terms of heart disease incidence and mortality? View side-by-side maps at the CDC website at **http://apps.nccd.cdc.gov/giscvh2/.**

Health Disparities Among
Different Racial and Ethnic Groups

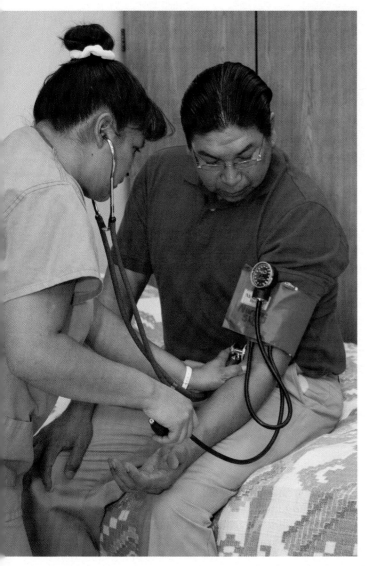

Native Americans have the highest rate of diabetes in the world.

Whether the causes are socioeconomic, biological, cultural, or still not well understood, health disparities exist among different racial and ethnic populations. For example:

- As a group, Hispanics are more likely to be overweight or obese than Caucasians, more likely to die from complications of stroke or diabetes, less likely to receive all recommended childhood vaccinations, and less likely to receive prenatal care early in pregnancy.[1]

- African-Americans experience the same leading causes of death as the general population, but tend to experience these illnesses and injuries more often and die of them at younger ages and higher rates than other groups. These differences start in infancy, when African-American babies experience a higher infant mortality rate. Later in life, issues such as injury, violence, being overweight and obese, and chronic illnesses become especially pressing concerns. When it comes to cancer care, for example, African-Americans are less likely to be diagnosed with many types of cancer early, when the disease is easier to treat, and less likely to survive 5 years after diagnosis.[2]

- Asians and Asian-Americans, overall, tend to have a life expectancy longer than that of the general population. But as a highly diverse group with ancestries encompassing dozens of countries and regions throughout Asia and the Indian subcontinent, there are also significant differences in health concerns among subgroups of Asians. For example, people from parts of northeast Asia with high levels of hepatitis B tend to experience higher rates of this infectious illness (and the liver damage and liver cancer that follows it) than other Asian subgroups.[3]

- Native Americans experience some of the more common health concerns in the United States at lower rates, such as heart disease or cancer.[4] But they also tend to have a shorter life expectancy than the general population, due to factors including accidental injuries, substance abuse, and suicide.[4] Diabetes and its complications are an especially important concern—Native Americans as a group have the highest rate of diabetes in the world.[4]

- Caucasians are more susceptible to cystic fibrosis (a genetic disease) than other populations.[5] In addition, Caucasian women have a higher incidence of breast cancer than other racial or ethnic populations.[6] One recent study found that middle-aged white men and women had the fastest-growing rates of suicide compared to other ethnic groups, whose rates were holding steady or declining.[7]

References: **1.** "Health Disparities Experienced by Hispanics – United States," by Centers for Disease Control and Prevention, 2005, *Morbidity and Mortality Weekly Report, 53*(4), pp. 935–937. **2.** "Health Disparities Experienced by Black or African Americans – United States," by Centers for Disease Control, 2005, *Morbidity and Mortality Weekly Report, 54*(1), pp. 1–3. **3.** "Hepatitis B" by S. Chavez, 2009, *Travelers' Health – Yellow Book,* retrieved from the Centers for Disease Control, http://wwwnc.cdc.gov/travel/yellowbook/2010/chapter-2/hepatitis-b.aspx. **4.** "Health Disparities Experienced by American Indians and Alaska Natives," by Centers for Disease Control and Prevention, 2003, *Morbidity and Mortality Weekly Report, 52*(30), p. 697. **5.** "Cystic Fibrosis," by the U.S. National Library of Medicine, 2008, retrieved from http://ghr.nlm.nih.gov/condition/cystic-fibrosis. **6.** "Breast Cancer Rates by Race and Ethnicity," by the Centers for Disease Control and Prevention, 2009, retrieved from http://www.cdc.gov/cancer/breast/statistics/race.htm. **7.** "Mid-life Suicide: An Increasing Problem in U.S. Whites, 1999–2005" by G. Hu, H. Wilcox, L. Wisslow, and S. Baker, 2008, *American Journal of Preventive Medicine, 35*(6), pp. 589–593.

services, available with a quick phone call, now help many medical centers care for patients who otherwise might not be able to communicate with doctors or staff effectively.

- **Increasing awareness.** New health programs aimed at specific communities help build knowledge of important health needs. In communities with sizeable Asian-American populations, for example, targeted public awareness campaigns are emphasizing the need for screening and treatment for hepatitis B, which is more prevalent in several Southeast Asian countries and is often acquired in infancy or early childhood.[17]

- **Boosting medical training.** When caregivers see patients from diverse backgrounds, better training can result in better care. Since African-American men tend to develop aggressive prostate cancer at a higher rate than the general population, informed doctors may start screening these men for the condition earlier than others. Since Caucasians are more likely to carry genetic mutations for cystic fibrosis, doctors may consider making genetic screening before or during pregnancy a priority. Groups such as the National Coalition for Health Professional Education in Genetics are working to make medical professionals more aware of these diverse needs.

Although eliminating health disparities remains a challenge, health professionals believe that steps such as these, combined with ongoing research into the problem, is putting the United States on a path toward a system where we all have an equal chance at better health.

Choosing Health: Achieving Successful Behavior Change

We can't change our age or genetics, but we can modify and change our behavior. Every day, we encounter opportunities to make choices that will benefit our health. Making the right choices, however, can be a challenge. We often have a good idea of what choices we *ought* to be making—for instance, eating more fruits and vegetables, setting aside time each day to exercise, or getting more sleep—but actually doing these things and achieving true **behavior change** is the hard part.

Factors That Influence Health Behavior

Let's begin our discussion of behavior change by taking a look at three factors that influence health behavior: *predisposing factors, enabling factors,* and *reinforcing factors.*

- **Predisposing factors** are the physical, mental, emotional, and environmental factors that shape behavior. They include your knowledge of health issues, your beliefs about how susceptible you are to illness or injury, and your attitude toward how behavior change can benefit your health. Your age, sex, race, income, and family background can also be predisposing factors in your health behavior. If you have a history of cancer in your family, for instance, and you believe in the wisdom of early screenings to detect and prevent cancer, you may be predisposed to schedule and obtain these screenings yourself. On the other hand, if you grew up in a family of smokers, you may be predisposed to view this behavior as "normal" and be more likely to take up smoking yourself.

- **Enabling factors** are the skills, assets, and capacities that shape behavior. They include the capabilities and available resources you have at your disposal to make lasting changes. If you want to eat more nutritiously and have access to a neighborhood grocery store stocked with fresh, affordable produce, that is an enabling factor that can help you change your behavior in a positive direction. Other examples of enabling factors include strong personal motivation and willpower, the physical health necessary to embark on a regular exercise program, or the ability to afford health care when you need it.

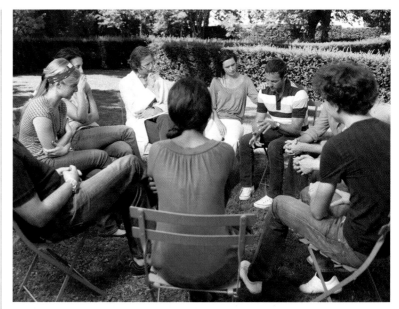

Support groups for quitting smoking or drinking can play a key role in lasting behavior change.

- **Reinforcing factors** are encouragements and rewards that promote positive behavior change. They include support and praise from others around you. A support group for quitting smoking or drinking, encouragement from family members if you are trying to lose weight, or the companionship (and positive peer pressure) of a workout partner are all examples of reinforcing factors.

Think about a health behavior you'd like to change in your own life, and then consider the predisposing, enabling, and reinforcing factors that may affect your attitude and/or ability to implement that change.

Models of Behavior Change

There are a number of models that focus on how effective behavior change occurs. Two of the more prominent are the *transtheoretical model of behavior change* and the *health belief model.*

The Transtheoretical Model

The **transtheoretical model of behavior change,** also called the *Stages of Change* model, was developed by psychologist James Prochaska and his colleagues. This theory proposes that a person progresses through six stages of change before achieving sustained behavior change (see **Figure 1.3**).[18]

- **Precontemplation,** during which a person may or may not recognize a health challenge, and in either case has no intention of making changes to address it in the near future (that is, within the next 6 months).

behavior change A change in an action or habit that affects health.

predisposing factor A physical, mental, emotional, or surrounding influence that shapes behavior.

enabling factor A skill, asset, or capacity that shapes behavior.

reinforcing factor An encouragement or a reward that promotes behavior change.

transtheoretical model of behavior change A model of behavior change that focuses on decision-making steps and abilities. Also called the *Stages of Change* model.

Precontemplation → Contemplation → Preparation → Action → Maintenance → Termination

Figure 1.3 **The transtheoretical model of behavior change.** Developed by James Prochaska, this model outlines six stages of behavior change.

- **Contemplation,** during which a person acknowledges the health challenge and thinks about making a change within the next 6 months. At this stage, the person is still not ready to take action but is thinking about it.
- **Preparation,** during which a person intends to change the behavior within the next month and has a plan of action in mind (such as enrolling in a class or joining a support group).
- **Action,** during which a person has modified the behavior in an observable way: for example, quit smoking, begun jogging each week, cut down on fatty foods, etc.
- **Maintenance,** in which a person has maintained the new behavior for six months or more, and continues to actively work to prevent relapse (reverting to old habits). Maintenance can last months or even years, and relapse is not unusual.
- **Termination,** during which a person has successfully achieved behavior change to the point where he or she is completely confident that relapse will not occur.

The transtheoretical model has its share of critics. The research is inconclusive, for instance, on whether application of the model truly results in lasting changes in behavior. However, the model is widely studied and referenced in academic papers in the field, and can be useful to consider when you think about embarking on a behavior change plan in your own life.

The Health Belief Model
Another model of behavior change is the **health belief model.** This model identifies six factors as being instrumental in explaining or predicting your health behavior:

- **Perceived threat.** The belief that you are at risk of a threat (such as illness or injury) and perceive that threat to be a real one.
- **Perceived benefit.** The belief that making a behavior change will help reduce the perceived threat.
- **Perceived barriers.** Your assessment of the potential negative consequences of changing the behavior.
- **Cues to action.** For example, events that would motivate you to make a change, such as witnessing a friend or family go through a health problem that you may face yourself.
- **Self-efficacy.** Your belief in your ability to make a lasting change in behavior.
- **Other variables.** Other social or personal factors that may affect your attitude toward making the behavior change.

Like the transtheoretical model, the health belief model has been widely studied. One survey looked at how useful this model is in weight management, and found that the greatest motivation came from the perceived threat of obesity, while the greatest resource for change came from a person's belief in his or her ability to lose weight or to maintain a healthy weight.[19] Critics, meanwhile, say the model does not adequately gauge the effect that a person's family or friends have on his or her ability to make successful changes. In any case, it may help to consider the health belief model when you are assessing your own readiness for changing a health behavior.

Behavior Change Techniques

Even when we have factors in our lives that make successful change more likely, and even when we believe we need to change, effec-

Sleep Deprived

"Hi, I'm Jasmine. I'm a freshman and I'm a child development major. Each night, I'm very lucky if I get four hours of sleep. I'm just a night owl. I like staying up at night. My father's the exact same way. It's like 3 o' clock in the morning and we'll still be up watching the food channel. Around exam time, I find myself awake at 7:30 in the morning, still up—knowing that I have a test at 9:30. Why, I don't know.

I don't think I'm doing my best right now because when I drag myself to class, I'm half asleep. I do need to change and get better rest so that I can do better in school. I don't think I've gotten 8 hours of sleep since I was 13. I'm 19, so that's six years of not getting a full night's sleep. That takes a toll on your body and your mind."

1: What stage of the *transtheoretical model of behavior change* would you guess that Jasmine is in?

2: Apply the health belief model to Jasmine's situation. What is the perceived threat? What is the perceived benefit to changing her behavior? What are the perceived barriers she may face?

Do you have a story similar to Jasmine's? Share your story at **www.pearsonhighered.com/choosinghealth.**

tively modifying our habits is still tough. Why? Changing behavior requires more than positive factors or an ideal set of beliefs. It also requires a determined attitude and a systematic approach that enables us to implement change one step at a time.

Self-Efficacy and Locus of Control
Perhaps the most important personal factor each of us brings to the process is self-efficacy. As described in the health belief model, self-efficacy is the conviction that you can make successful changes. But self-efficacy is also more than a belief—it is the ability to take action demonstrating a sense of personal control over a situation. If you believe in your own ability to get in better shape, you'll keep exercising, even if a few workouts leave you tired or frustrated. If you have low self-efficacy, you may give up, or never attempt an exercise program in the first place.

Your sense of self-efficacy, and the actions that stem from it, are closely tied to your **locus of control.** If you have a stronger *internal* locus of control, you are more likely to believe that you are the master of your own destiny and exert more control over your life. If you have a stronger *external* locus of control, you are

health belief model A model of behavior change emphasizing personal beliefs in the process of creating effective change.

locus of control A person's belief about where the center of power lies in his or her life; can be external or internal.

more likely to believe that events are out of your hands and that you can do little to shape some situations.

As with other aspects of your health, your sense of self-efficacy and your locus of control are not set in stone. By turning to clearly defined techniques that help change behavior in positive ways, you can increase your own sense of self-efficacy. That greater sense of empowerment, in turn, can help you make even more changes.

Basic Behavior Change Strategies

The following are some basic behavior change strategies:

- **Modeling,** or learning behaviors by watching others. This strategy enables you to learn from the experiences of others who have already made successful change. If you'd like to eat less junk food, for example, but don't know where to find healthier choices during your busy day, you can learn a great deal from watching the habits of a friend who has already made a similar change and found healthy options on campus.

- **Shaping,** or breaking a big task into a series of smaller steps. If you'd like to eventually run a 10k, for instance, you might begin by setting yourself a goal of a smaller distance at first, and then gradually increase your distance a little bit each week.

- **Reinforcement,** or establishing rewards that keep you motivated to sustain change. For example, you might buy yourself new clothing after you have reached a target weight goal. However, reinforcement doesn't have to be a material object. For instance, the natural "high" people often feel after physical exercise can be its own positive reinforcement.

- **Changing self-talk,** or rewriting your own internal dialogue in a more positive way. When you find yourself saying "I can't do this," stop and think about a different way to approach the problem. Talk to yourself in more constructive, supportive ways by changing "I can't" to "I can." Look for solutions, rather than dwelling on roadblocks. The result will help you feel better about yourself and solve problems more effectively.

- Drafting a *behavior change contract.* The act of identifying a particular behavior to change, listing obstacles to making that change, brainstorming strategies to overcome those obstacles, making an inventory of the resources you have available, setting achievable short-term goals for your long-term objective, and putting all of it in writing can be a powerful first step to lasting change. See the **Behavior Change Workshop** on page 15 for an example of a behavior change contract. You will find Behavior Change Workshops throughout this book to help you take the first steps toward modifying health habits in various dimensions of health and wellness.

Evaluating Health Information in the Media

Is the health information you just researched on the Internet accurate? Can you trust your favorite actor's television advertisement

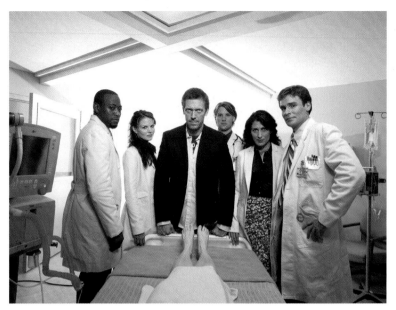

Can you trust **medical information** from doctors (real or fictional) on TV?

modeling A behavior change technique based on watching and learning from others.

shaping A behavior change technique based on breaking large tasks into more manageable parts.

reinforcement A motivational behavior change technique that rewards steps toward positive change.

changing self-talk Shifting one's internal dialogue in a more positive, empowering direction.

for a weight-loss product? Was last week's episode of *House, M.D.* based on any kind of medical reality? How can you make sense of the endless stream of news headlines trumpeting health studies that sometimes contradict one another?

As we discussed earlier, health literacy is the ability to evaluate and understand health information and to make informed choices for your health care. Increasingly, health literacy also requires some degree of computer literacy, as well as an awareness of how print, television, and online media present (and often distort) health information. We are surrounded by more health-related information than ever before, and must be able to distinguish useful, scientifically and medically sound information from poor or biased advice.

The term *media* can mean a variety of different things. We use it here to include books, newspapers, magazines, television, and Internet/web programming, as well as advertisements. To get a sense of how frequently you are inundated with health information from the media, consider the following:

- How often have you watched or seen an advertisement promoting prescription drugs—for everything from insomnia and social anxiety to weight loss and erectile dysfunction?

- How often do you encounter an advertisement for prepackaged snack foods or meals? In contrast, how often have you encountered an advertisement for fresh fruits and vegetables?

- How regularly are you exposed to images of seemingly physically perfect celebrities? How does this affect your feelings about your own body and your self-esteem?

- How frequently do you come across a health-related news headline, either on the radio, in a printed newspaper, on TV, or on the Internet?

Evaluating Health Information Online

When evaluating health information online, consider the following questions to help evaluate whether the information is credible:

- Is the sponsor of the site identified? Is it a commercial, nonprofit, academic, or government site? In general, sites with URLs ending in ".gov" (signifying a U.S. government site) or ".edu" (signifying an educational institution) are more likely to provide credible information than those that end in ".com." Note that the domain ".org" is used by many credible, nonprofit, noncommercial sites, but it is sometimes used by commercial entities as well.

- What is the purpose of the site? Is it to inform and educate, or is it to sell you something? If it is to sell you something, be aware that the information presented is more likely to be biased or one-sided to paint the product in a favorable light.

- Does the site tell you where the information it presents is coming from? If so, is the content based on scientific evidence, or was it written by someone hired by the site to produce marketing information? Sites that are able to provide citations and links to scientific studies and journals are more likely to be credible than sites lacking these references.

- Does the site specify when its content was last updated? Health information can sometimes change quickly, so you want to seek out information that is as current as possible.

- Does the site list a reputable professional accreditation? Many reputable health sites, for example, are accredited by the Health on the Net Foundation, and bear an insignia reading "HON."

See the **Get Connected** feature on page 17 for a list of general health-related websites that are good starting points for obtaining health information. Keep in mind that information on the Internet is <u>never</u> a substitute for consulting a health care professional. Do not rely solely on online information to make important decisions about your health! Make an appointment with your doctor and don't be afraid to ask questions to be certain that you are receiving the most accurate information about any health issue you may be facing.

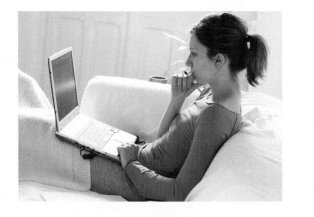

Visit the Health on the Net Foundation's search engine at **www.hon.ch/HONsearch/Patients/index.html** to search for health information from vetted, reputable sources.

Whenever you encounter information from the media, critically assess it by keeping the following in mind:

- Is someone trying to sell you something? Are there other ways to solve problems like insomnia or a desire for weight loss without resorting to drugs and pills?

- Do you realize that many of the images of celebrities you see in magazines have been digitally altered to make models look slimmer and more physically flawless than they really are?

- When you come across an article about the results of the latest health-related study, consider: Was the study conducted by an unbiased source, or was it carried out by an individual or organization with a vested interest in the outcome? Have the results been replicated by other researchers? Was the sample size of the study large or small? Was the study conducted over a short or long period of time? Is the study only showing what may be a coincidental *correlation* between two things, or is it truly showing that one variable is the direct result of another variable?

The Internet deserves special attention in discussions of health in the media, as it is increasingly where people turn for information. In one survey of more than 70,000 college students, students listed the Internet as their second most-often used source of health information.[20] The only source they turned to more often was their parents. The box **Consumer Corner: Evaluating Health Information Online** provides guidelines for assessing health content on the Internet. In addition, Chapter 13, Consumer Health, delves into a wide variety of consumer health topics in more detail.

> **"***In one survey, college students listed the Internet as their second-most-often used source of health information.***"**

Creating Your Personal Plan for Health

By enrolling in a personal health course and reading this textbook, you have already taken the initial step toward achieving better health and wellness. Throughout this book you will find **Self-Assessments** that will help you assess your current health status, as well as **Behavior Change Workshops** that guide you on how to set appropriate goals and implement plans for behavior change. You can also find online versions of all of these worksheets at www.pearsonhighered.com/choosinghealth.

Self Assessment: How Healthy Is Your Current Lifestyle? is a general self-survey evaluating your current health behaviors.

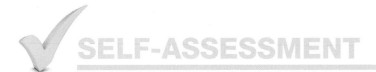

SELF-ASSESSMENT

To complete this self-assessment online, visit www.pearsonhighered.com/choosinghealth.

How Healthy Is Your Current Lifestyle?

Complete one section at a time by circling the number under the answer that best describes your behavior. Then add the numbers you circled to get your score for that section. Write the score on the line provided at the end of each section.

Cigarette Smoking	Almost Always	Sometimes	Almost Never

If you are currently a non-smoker, enter a score of 10 for this section and go to the next section on Alcohol and Drugs.

	Almost Always	Sometimes	Almost Never
1. I avoid smoking cigarettes.	2	1	0
2. I smoke only low tar and nicotine cigarettes or I smoke a pipe.	2	1	0

Smoking Score _____

Alcohol and Drugs

	Almost Always	Sometimes	Almost Never
1. I avoid drinking alcoholic beverages or I drink no more than 1 (for women) or 2 (for men) drinks a day.	4	1	0
2. I avoid using alcohol or other drugs (especially illegal drugs) as a way of handling situations or problems.	2	1	0
3. I am careful not to drink alcohol when taking certain medicines (for example, medicine for sleeping, pain, colds, and allergies) or when pregnant.	2	1	0
4. I read and follow the label directions when using prescribed and over-the-counter drugs.	2	1	0

Alcohol and Drugs Score _____

Eating Habits

	Almost Always	Sometimes	Almost Never
1. I eat a variety of foods each day, such as fruits and vegetables; whole grain breads and cereals; lean meats; low-fat dairy products; beans and legumes; nuts and seeds.	4	1	0
2. I limit the amount of fat, saturated fat, *trans* fat, and cholesterol I eat (including fat on meats, eggs, butter, cream, shortenings, and organ meats such as liver).	2	1	0
3. I limit the amount of salt I eat by cooking with only small amounts, not adding salt at the table, and avoiding salty snacks.	2	1	0
4. I avoid eating too much sugar (especially frequent snacks of sticky candy or soft drinks).	2	1	0

Eating Habits Score _____

Exercise/Fitness	Almost Always	Sometimes	Almost Never
1. I do vigorous exercises for 30 minutes a day at least 5 times a week (examples include jogging, swimming, brisk walking, or bicycling).	4	2	0
2. I do exercises that enhance my muscle tone for 15–30 minutes at least 3 times a week (examples include using weight machines or free weights, yoga, calisthenics).	3	1	0
3. I use part of my leisure time participating in individual, family, or team activities that increase my level of fitness (such as gardening, dancing, bowling, golf, baseball).	3	1	0

Exercise/Fitness Score _____

Stress Control

	Almost Always	Sometimes	Almost Never
1. I have a job, go to school, or do other work that I enjoy.	2	1	0
2. I find it easy to relax and express my feelings freely.	2	1	0
3. I recognize early, and prepare for, events or situations likely to be stressful for me.	2	1	0
4. I have close friends, relatives, or others whom I can talk to about personal matters and call on for help when needed.	2	1	0
5. I participate in group activities (such as religious worship and community organizations) and/or have hobbies that I enjoy.	2	1	0

Stress Control Score _____

Safety/Health

	Almost Always	Sometimes	Almost Never
1. I wear a seat belt while riding in a car.	2	1	0
2. I avoid driving while under the influence of alcohol and other drugs, or riding with someone else who is under the influence.	2	1	0
3. I obey traffic rules and avoid distractions like texting and talking on the phone when driving.	2	1	0
4. I am careful when using potentially harmful products or substances (such as household cleaners, poisons, and electrical devices).	2	1	0
5. I get at least 7 hours of sleep a night.	2	1	0

Safety Score _____

HOW TO INTERPRET YOUR SCORE

Examine your score for each section and refer to the key below for a general assessment of how you are doing in that particular area of health.

Scores of 9 and 10

Excellent. Your answers show that you are aware of the importance of this area to your health. More important, you are putting your knowledge to work for you by practicing good health habits. As long as you continue to do so, this area should not pose a serious health risk. It's likely that you are setting an example for the rest of your family and friends to follow. Since you got a very high test score on this part of the test, you may want to consider other areas where your scores indicate room for improvement.

Scores of 6 to 8

Good. Your health practices in this area are good, but there is room for improvement. Look again at the items you answered with a "Sometimes" or "Almost Never." What changes can you make to improve your score? Even a small change can help you achieve better health.

Scores of 3 to 5

At Risk. Your health risks are showing. Would you like more information about the risks you are facing? Do you want to know why it is important for you to change these behaviors? Perhaps you need help in deciding how to make the changes you desire. In either case, help is available. You can start by contacting your health care provider or a registered dietitian.

Scores of 0 to 2

Seriously at Risk. Obviously, you were concerned enough about your health to take this test. But your answers show that you may be taking serious risks with your health. Perhaps you were not aware of the risks and what to do about them. You can easily get the information and help you need to reduce your health risks and have a healthier lifestyle if you wish. Are you ready to take the next step?

Source: Linda Bobroff, Ph.D., *"Healthstyle: A Self-Test,"* Department of Family, Youth and Community Services, University of Florida, http://edis.ifas.ufl.edu/he778, adapted from U.S. Department of Health and Human Services, DHHS Publication Number (PHS) 81-50155. Used by permission of the University of Florida, Institute of Food and Agricultural Services.

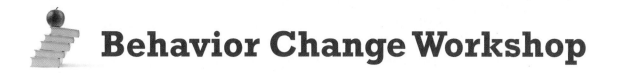

Behavior Change Workshop

To complete this workshop online, visit **www.pearsonhighered.com/choosinghealth.**

After you have completed the Self-Assessment in this chapter, select one behavior you would like to target for change over the next few months. Next, fill out the Behavior Change Contract below, sign it, and either tape it to your wall or discuss it with your health instructor as part of your work toward your long-term goal.

Behavior Change Contract

1. My behavior change will be:

_____

_____

_____

_____

2. My long-term goal for this behavior change is:

_____

_____

_____

_____

3. Barriers that I must overcome to make this behavior change are:

a) _____

b) _____

c) _____

4. The strategies I will use to overcome these barriers are:

a) _____

b) _____

c) _____

5. Resources I will use to help me change this behavior include:

- a friend, partner, or relative: _____

- a school-based resource: _____

- a community-based resource: _____

- a book or reputable website: _____

6. In order to make my goal more attainable, I have devised these short-term goals:

Short term goal: _____   _____   _____
                                                      Target date   Reward

Short term goal: _____   _____   _____
                                                      Target date   Reward

Short term goal: _____   _____   _____
                                                      Target date   Reward

When I make the long-term behavior change described above, my reward will be:

_____   _____
                                                      Target date

I intend to make the behavior change described above. I will use the strategies and rewards above to achieve the goals that will contribute to a healthy behavior change.

Signed: _____   Witness: _____

Chapter Summary

- *Health* is more than merely the absence of disease or injury. It also encompasses physical, social, psychological, spiritual, intellectual, environmental, and occupational dimensions of being.
- *Wellness* is the process of actively making choices to achieve optimal health.
- Although life expectancy in the United States is much greater than it was in the past, many health challenges remain. Initiatives such as Healthy People and Healthy Campus seek to raise public awareness of health, decrease the incidence of preventable disease and injury, and eliminate health disparities among different demographic groups.
- Stress, depression, anxiety, alcohol and tobacco use, and sexual health are all common health concerns faced by college students.
- Four key lifestyle behaviors that have a profound ability to affect your health are: (1) eating nutritiously, (2) being physically active, (3) not smoking, and (4) not drinking excessively.

- Other factors that can affect health include age, sex, racial or ethnic background, geography, income, access to health insurance, sexual and gender orientation, and health literacy.
- *Health literacy* is the ability to evaluate and understand health information and to make informed choices for your health care.
- *Predisposing, enabling,* and *reinforcing* factors can all affect health behavior.
- The *transtheoretical model of behavior change* proposes six stages of behavior change.
- The *health belief model* identifies six factors as being instrumental in explaining or predicting health behavior.
- Basic behavior change strategies include modeling, shaping, reinforcement, changing self-talk, and drafting a behavior change contract.
- It is important to critically assess the health information you encounter in the media.

Test Your Knowledge

1. Which dimension of health is characterized by the quality of your interactions and relationships with other people?
   a. physical health
   b. intellectual health
   c. social health
   d. environmental health

2. What is the process of actively making choices to achieve optimal health?
   a. psychological health
   b. wellness
   c. self-efficacy
   d. precontemplation

3. Which of the following behaviors can have profound consequences for health?
   a. eating nutritiously
   b. being physically active
   c. not smoking and not drinking excessively
   d. all of the above

4. The ability to read, understand, and follow instructions in medical brochures and prescription drug labels is an example of
   a. health literacy
   b. wellness

   c. behavior change
   d. occupational health

5. A support group for quitting smoking is an example of
   a. a predisposing factor for behavior change.
   b. an enabling factor for behavior change.
   c. a reinforcing factor for behavior change.
   d. none of the above.

6. In James Prochaska's transtheoretical model of behavior change, which stage indicates the period during which a person has modified the behavior in an observable way?
   a. precontemplation
   b. contemplation
   c. preparation
   d. action

7. According to the health belief model, self-efficacy is exemplified by which of the following?
   a. your belief that you are at risk of illness or injury
   b. your belief that making a change will reduce a threat to your health
   c. your belief in your own ability to make a lasting behavior change
   d. your assessment of the potential negative consequences of changing a behavior

8. The belief that events are out of your control is characteristic of
   a. a strong internal locus of control.
   b. a strong external locus of control.
   c. the maintenance stage of behavior change.
   d. the termination stage of behavior change.

9. Adopting a behavior by watching and learning from others is characteristic of
   a. modeling.
   b. shaping.
   c. reinforcement.
   d. changing self-talk.

10. Which of the following is most likely to be scientifically objective and reliable?
   a. a study about the effects of a new drug, funded and conducted by the drug's manufacturer
   b. a study about the effects of a new drug, conducted by independent researchers over a short period of time
   c. a study about the effects of a new drug, conducted by independent researchers over a short period of time on a small group of people
   d. a study about the effects of a new drug, conducted by independent researchers over a long period of time on a large group of people

Get Critical

What happened:

In the fall of 2009, British celebrity chef Jamie Oliver arrived in Huntington, West Virginia, and declared a "food revolution." With its soaring obesity rates, Huntington had recently been named the unhealthiest city in the United States by the Centers for Disease Control. Oliver's goal was to educate the residents of Huntington on the basics of good nutrition and to encourage behavior change at both the community level (for example, making school lunches more nutritious) as well as at the individual level, and to film his efforts for a nationally broadcast reality television show. While the project had many supporters, critics charged that Oliver was a celebrity opportunist with a condescending attitude toward the citizens of Huntington.

What do you think?

- What's your opinion of Jamie Oliver's "food revolution"? Are you in favor of his efforts or do you find them offensive?

- Does a celebrity-driven health campaign make you more motivated to change a health behavior? Why or why not?

Get Connected

Health Online Visit the following websites for further information about the topics in this chapter:

- Centers for Disease Control and Prevention
  www.cdc.gov
- Go Ask Alice (answers to health questions, sponsored by Columbia University)
  www.goaskalice.columbia.edu/index.html
- U.S. Department of Health and Human Service's healthfinder.gov
  http://healthfinder.gov
- Medline Plus
  www.nlm.nih.gov/medlineplus

- Mayo Clinic
  www.mayoclinic.com
- World Health Organization
  www.who.int/en
- New Mexico Media Literacy project
  www.nmmlp.org/media_literacy/index.html

Website links are subject to change. To access updated web links, please visit ***www.pearsonhighered.com/choosinghealth.***

References

i. Heron, M., Hoyert, D., Xu, J., Scott, C., & Tejada-Vera, B. (2009). Deaths: Final data for 2006. *National Vital Statistics Reports, 57*(16), 1–135.

ii. Ibid.

iii. Kvaavik, E., Batty, G., Ursin, G., Huxley, R., & Gale C. (2010). Influence of individual and combined health behaviors on total and cause-specific mortality in men and women. *Archives of Internal Medicine, 170*(8), 711–718.

iv. Tu, H., & Cohen, G. (2008). Striking jump in consumers seeking health care information. *Center for Studying Health System Change: Tracking Report No. 20.* Retrieved from http://www.hschange.com/CONTENT/1006

1. World Health Organization. (2010). What is the WHO definition of health?, in *Frequently asked questions.* Retrieved from http://www.who.int/suggestions/faq/en/index.html

2. Kvaavik, E., Batty, G., Ursin, G., Huxley, R., & Gale C. (2010). Influence of individual and combined health behaviors on total and cause-specific mortality in men and women. *Archives of Internal Medicine, 170*(8), 711–718.

3. National Wellness Institute. (2010). *Defining wellness.* Retrieved from http://www.nationalwellness.org/index.php?id_tier=2&id_c=26

4. Heron, M., Hoyert, D., Xu, J., Scott, C., & Tejada-Vera, B. (2009). Deaths: Final data for 2006. *National Vital Statistics Reports, 57*(14), 1–135.

5. Centers for Disease Control. (2000). *Leading causes of death, 1900–1998.* Retrieved from http://www.cdc.gov/nchs/data/dvs/lead1900_98.pdf

6. U.S. Department of Health and Human Services. (2008). *Vital and health statistics, Summary health statistics for U.S. adults: National health interview survey, 2007.* Series 10, No. 240.

7. American College Health Association. (2009). *ACHA-NCHA II: Reference group executive summary, Fall 2009.* Retrieved from http://www.acha-ncha.org/docs/ACHA-NCHA_Reference_Group_ExecutiveSummary_Fall2009.pdf

8. Joint United Nations Program on HIV/AIDS. (2009). *09 AIDS epidemic update.* Retrieved from http://data.unaids.org/pub/Report/2009/JC1700_Epi_Update_2009_en.pdf

9. Williams, D. R. (2008). The health of men: Structured inequalities and opportunities. *American Journal of Public Health, 93,* 150–157.

10. American Lung Association. (2010). *State of the air 2010.* Retrieved from http://www.stateoftheair.org/2010/assets/SOTA2010.pdf

11. Reasons for Geographic and Racial Differences in Stroke (REGARDS). (2010). *UAB study shows African-Americans have highest stroke rate, southerners more likely to die.* Retrieved from http://main.uab.edu/Sites/MediaRelations/articles/74036/

12. Krieger, N., Rehkopf, D., Chen, J., Waterman, P., Marcelli, E., & Kennedy, M. (2008). The fall and rise of U.S. inequities in premature mortality: 1960–2002. *Public Library of Science Medicine, 5*(2), e46.

13. The Henry J. Kaiser Family Foundation. (2010). *Focus on health reform: Summary of patient coverage provisions in the patient protection and affordable care act.* Retrieved from http://www.kff.org/healthreform/upload/8023-R.pdf

14. Sell, R., Wells, J., & Wypij, D. (1995). The prevalence of homosexual behavior and attraction in the United States, the United Kingdom and France: Results of national population-based samples. *Archives of Sexual Behavior,* 24(3):235–48.

15. Gay and Lesbian Medical Association. (2001). *Healthy People 2010 companion document for lesbian, gay, bisexual, and transgender (LGBT) health.* Retrieved from http://www.lgbthealth.net/downloads/hp2010doc.pdf

16. National Network of Libraries of Medicine. (2010). *Health literacy.* Retrieved from http://nnlm.gov/outreach/consumer/hlthlit.html

17. American Liver Foundation. (n.d.). *Hepatitis B and Asian Americans.* Retrieved from http://www.thinkb.org/professionals/asianamericans/

18. Prochaska, J., & Velicer, W. (1997). The transtheoretical model of health behavior change. *American Journal of Health Promotion, 12*(1), 38–48.

19. Daddario, D. (2007). A review of the use of the health belief model for weight management. *Medsurg Nursing, 16*(6), 363–366.

20. The American College Health Association. (2008). American College Health Association – National College Health Assessment spring 2007 reference group data report (abridged). *Journal of American College Health, 56*(5), 469–479.

2 Psychological Health

- Mental disorders affect **more than 25%** of Americans over the age of 18—almost **60 million** people—every year.[i]

- During the **college years** (late adolescence/young adulthood) the first symptoms of **panic disorder, bipolar disorder,** and **obsessive–compulsive disorder** may begin to appear.[ii]

- **One in 10** college students report being recently diagnosed or treated for **depression.**[iii]

The **third** leading cause of death among 15- to 24-year olds is **suicide.**[iv]

DEFINE *psychological health, mental health, emotional health,* and *spiritual health.*

IDENTIFY the characteristics of psychological health.

UNDERSTAND common psychological problems and describe ways to address them.

DESCRIBE the characteristics of depression, bipolar disorder, attention disorders, anxiety disorders, and schizophrenia.

LIST the warning signs of suicide and describe suicide prevention methods.

UNDERSTAND the different types of treatments for psychological problems and mental disorders.

Health Online icons are found throughout the chapter, directing you to web links, videos, podcasts, and other useful online resources.

Look at a brochure advertising any college campus in the country, and you'll find photos

of happy students enjoying their studies and having fun. But as you know, real life for college students is much more complicated than those images suggest. At some point in your college life, you are likely to feel pressure, anxiety, loneliness, or sadness. When these types of problems surface, good psychological health can help you maintain your balance. Being psychologically healthy allows you to handle challenges effectively and make the most of your college—and life—experiences.

This chapter will describe the core components of psychological health. We will cover a variety of psychological problems—from everyday challenges like shyness to serious disorders like schizophrenia—along with strategies for treating them. We will also discuss self-care techniques for promoting psychological health, and provide advice about how to get help for any psychological issues you are experiencing.

So what does it mean to have "good" psychological health? We discuss that next.

What Is Psychological Health?

Psychological health is the broad measure of well-being that encompasses the mental, emotional, and spiritual dimensions of health. **Mental health** can be described as the "thinking" component of psychological health. The term describes your ability to perceive reality accurately and respond to its challenges rationally and effectively. Good mental health is characterized by the intellectual capacity to process information, analyze choices, and respond appropriately. **Emotional health** refers to the subjective side of psychological health, including your feelings and moods. It describes how you react emotionally to the ups and downs of life. While we all experience difficult feelings and bad moods, people with good emotional health are better able to modulate their highs and lows and keep less happy times in perspective. Emotional health also has an impact on how you behave in society and with others. Certain feelings and emotional reactions can cause you to engage socially or withdraw, and can also affect the motivation of others to interact with you. **Spiritual health** contributes to psychological health by providing a sense of connection to a larger purpose coupled with a system of core values that provide direction and meaning in life. For some, that connection takes the form of religion, either through an organized group or through personal faith and prayer. For others, spirituality focuses more on nature, other people, or altruistic causes. For many, spirituality is a

psychological health The broad measure of well-being that encompasses the mental, emotional, and spiritual dimensions of health.

mental health The "thinking" component of psychological health that allows you to perceive reality accurately and respond rationally and effectively.

emotional health The subjective side of psychological health, including your feelings and moods.

spiritual health A component of psychological health that provides a sense of connection to a larger purpose coupled with a system of core values that provide direction and meaning in life.

Autonomy and assertiveness
Making informed, un-coerced decisions and clearly indicating desires to others

Optimism
Interpreting life's events positively

Communication and intimacy
Expressing thoughts and feelings to others; having close relationships

Self-esteem
Holding a positive self-regard

Realism
Perceiving life as it really is

Emotional intelligence
Accurately perceiving, assessing, and regulating emotions

Prioritizing needs
Taking care of physiological and psychological needs in accordance with their urgencies

Spirituality
Feeling connection to something larger than oneself

Figure 2.1 Characteristics of psychological health. Each of these characteristics contributes to your psychological health.

lifelong quest for the answers to life's biggest questions such as "What is my purpose in this life?", "Where did I come from?", and "What happens when I die?"

Psychological health isn't always easy to measure, but people in good psychological health usually:

- Express feelings in ways that are honest, self-accepting, and not harmful to others.
- Prevent and manage conflict and stress in ways that lead to optimal health.
- Seek help for troublesome or disruptive feelings.
- Focus on positive activities, rather than those that are harmful or self-destructive.
- Use self-control and impulse-control strategies for their own well-being.
- Are empathetic toward others.
- Understand and fulfill personal responsibilities.
- Establish and maintain relationships that are fulfilling, supportive, and based on mutual respect.

There are a number of personal characteristics that promote psychological health **(Figure 2.1)**. Let's look at each one.

Autonomy and Assertiveness

How much weight do you give to the opinions of others? Do they get more or less consideration

than your own ideas? That depends on your level of **autonomy.** Autonomy is your capacity to make informed, un-coerced decisions. People that embrace higher levels of autonomy are more likely to make decisions and take actions based on their own judgment rather than the influence of others. They are also more likely to take responsibility for the results of their decisions and actions. Autonomy does not devalue the opinions of others. It simply keeps them in perspective.

As a college student, you may find yourself with more autonomy than you have experienced before. Although it may be daunting, this is a good thing overall. Making choices for yourself now will pave the way for you to make even bigger decisions once you've graduated.[1]

Autonomy usually requires some degree of **assertiveness,** or making your needs and wants clear to others. Unlike being angry or aggressive, when you are assertive you express yourself calmly and clearly in ways that respect yourself and others. Together, your sense of autonomy and your ability to assert yourself contribute to psychological health by giving you independence and control over your life.

Realism

Another foundation of psychological health is **realism,** or perceiving life as it really is so that you can rationally respond to its demands. This means acknowledging the people, institutions, and other forces around you for what they are, realizing what you want from others, knowing your own strengths and weaknesses, and perceiving how much you can actually change in your environment or relationships. Realism can help you focus on things in your life that you can control and learn to accept those things that are beyond your influence.

Realism can be a positive force. Many of us spend time dwelling on our problems and flaws, while ignoring our unique strengths and gifts. A realistic view of yourself can focus on the strengths that enhance your life instead of the weaknesses that hold you back.

Self-Esteem

Self-esteem is a sense of positive self-regard, producing feelings of self-respect, self-worth, self-confidence, and self-satisfaction. People with high self-esteem tend to feel good about themselves and their lives, respond to challenges in resilient ways, have optimistic outlooks on life, capitalize on opportunities, and even enjoy better physical health.[2] Self-esteem also promotes healthy, fulfilling relationships with others.

Self-esteem is largely developed in childhood as a result of the relationships we have with our parents, peers, and caregivers. A child who feels loved, valued, and listened to is more likely to have higher self-esteem later in life. Alternately, if a child is abused or feels unloved or ignored, that child may develop poor self-esteem that continues into adulthood.

However, it is never too late to build up self-esteem. See **Practical Strategies for Change: Building Self-Esteem** on page 22.

autonomy The capacity to make informed, un-coerced decisions.

assertiveness The ability to clearly express your needs and wants to others in an appropriate way.

realism The ability to perceive life as it really is so that you can rationally respond to its demands.

self-esteem A sense of positive self-regard, resulting in elevated levels of self-respect, self-worth, self-confidence, and self-satisfaction.

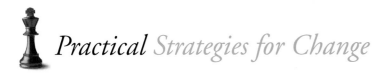

Practical Strategies for Change

Building Self-Esteem

- **Take good care of yourself.** Eat healthfully, exercise, and make sure you leave time in your schedule for fun. Don't wait for others to take care of you—you are your own best caretaker.

- **Pat yourself on the back.** Notice when something you've done turns out well, and take a moment to congratulate yourself.

- **Practice positive "self-talk."** If you criticize yourself in your head, stop. Instead, make a habit of complimenting yourself, or repeating positive affirmations.

- **Stretch your abilities.** Decide to learn something new, whether it's a school subject that seems intimidating or a sport you've never tried. Give yourself time to learn your new skill piece by piece, and then watch your talents grow.

- **Tackle your "to do" list.** Think about tasks you've been putting off, like calling a relative you haven't spoken with in a while or cleaning out your closet. Get a couple of them done each week. You'll be reminded of how much you can accomplish, and feel less distracted by loose ends.

- **Listen to yourself.** What do you really want, need, and value? If you want others to listen to you, you need to understand and respect your own thoughts and feelings first.

- **Reach out.** There is no simpler, or more generous, way to build self-esteem than doing something nice for someone else. You'll both benefit.

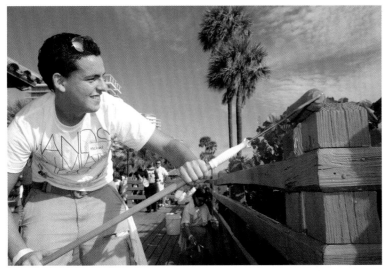

Participating in volunteer activities is a great way to boost self-esteem.

Optimism

Optimism is the psychological tendency to have a positive interpretation of life's events. Optimistic people embrace the belief that positive outcomes are more likely to occur than negative ones. People with optimistic outlooks do not ignore negative situations when they occur, but instead balance the negative with the positive. They are motivated to action by the belief that most problems have solutions.

Optimism helps us in a broad range of situations. Studies of U.S. Olympic champions show that elite athletes share high levels of opti-

mism.[3] On the other end of the spectrum, optimism also helps patients fighting serious diseases maintain a positive outlook during treatment and cope better with the ups and downs of illness.[4] The effect of optimism on health is well documented, and is part of the *mind-body connection*. For more about the mind-body connection, see the **Spotlight** on page 24.

As with self-esteem, people tend to develop an optimistic view of life at a young age from their families and caregivers, but you can cultivate optimism at any age. See **Practical Strategies for Change: Building Optimism** for tips.

Prioritizing Needs

You have a variety of physiological, mental, emotional, and spiritual needs. You cannot ignore physiological needs and be healthy and happy, but at the same time, you have to address your psychological needs if you are to live a life that is fulfilling. How do you prioritize all these needs? Psychologist Abraham Maslow theorized that humans have an innate drive to meet inner needs, and that drive motivates them to achieve higher levels of psychological health. He created a *hierarchy of needs pyramid* that illustrates how psychologically healthy people prioritize their physiological and psychological needs. Your most basic, urgent needs are positioned at the base of the pyramid, while progressively less urgent but more enlightening needs appear toward the top **(Figure 2.2).** Maslow hypothesized that we all seek to have the physiological needs at the base of the pyramid met first, and once they are, we focus on our next set of unmet needs. As you move up the pyramid, you begin to address higher and higher psychological needs. When you finally reach the top of the pyramid, you realize **self-actualization,** or truly fulfilling your potential. In later work, Maslow added one higher goal—selfless actualization, or working toward a values-driven goal larger than yourself.[5]

Communication and Intimacy

There are probably times when you disagree with someone you are close to or have something weighing on your mind that you are afraid to express. Although these situations may be difficult, they can often be resolved through communication.

Communication is a cornerstone of psychological health because it allows you to fully participate in relationships. Expressing your thoughts and feelings to others lets your true self interact with the world, and listening to the thoughts and feelings people communicate to you broadens your perspective and shows others that you value them. Chapter 9 covers specific communication skills that can help you communicate in healthful ways.

Communication is an essential part of intimacy. **Intimacy,** or close relationships with others, is a key part of human happiness. True intimacy, in friendships, families, or romantic relationships, occurs only with honest communication. If you take a chance and communicate your feelings about a difficult topic, you may clear the air, find shared values, or become closer to others. If

optimism The psychological tendency to have a positive interpretation of life's events.

self-actualization The pinnacle of Maslow's hierarchy of needs pyramid, which indicates truly fulfilling your potential.

intimacy A close relationship with another person.

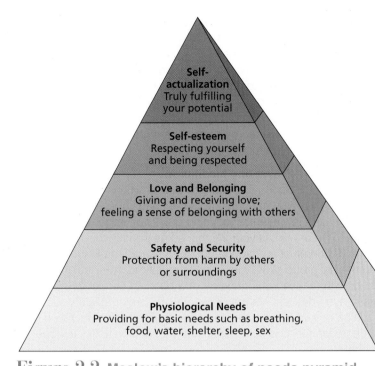

Figure 2.2 Maslow's hierarchy of needs pyramid.
Basic, physiological needs appear at the base of the pyramid. As you move upward, you address needs that are less urgent to satisfy, but develop greater and greater psychological health, until you realize self-actualization.

Source: Maslow, A. (1997). *Motivation and personality* (3rd ed.). New York: Harper Collins College Publishers.

you find that your values don't mesh well with someone, you may decide to focus on other relationships where stronger connections and greater intimacy are more likely.

Emotional Intelligence

Emotional intelligence is the ability to accurately sense, assess, and manage emotions. Emotional intelligence allows you to process information of an emotional nature and use it to guide your thoughts, actions, and reactions to others.[6,7] For example, imagine you want to dispute a grade you received on a test. As you approach your professor's office, you hear her arguing with someone on the phone. Emotional intelligence may prompt you to delay your visit. People with higher levels of emotional intelligence tend to conduct themselves in a balanced way, neither denying their emotions nor letting them fly out of control. They also tend to be more productive, less prone to stress, and happier overall than those with lower emotional intelligence.[8] Emotional intelligence can be increased by consciously recognizing and naming your emotions when you feel them, thinking about other people's feelings and motivations in relation to specific situations or actions, and accepting your emotions without allowing them to overrule other desires and priorities.

Spirituality

You may have a healthy sense of self-esteem, strong connections with others, and a balanced, optimistic view of life. But do you have a higher purpose? For many people, happiness and con-

emotional intelligence The ability to accurately monitor, assess, and manage your emotions and those of others.

spirituality A sense of connection to something larger than yourself.

Building Optimism

- **Notice when things go right.** When something works out for the better, take note. Recognizing when things go well will show you the likelihood of positive outcomes.

- **Learn from mistakes.** Everybody fails to reach a goal at some point. That doesn't mean it will happen again next time. Learn from what happened, and decide what you'll do differently in the future.

- **Challenge negative thoughts.** Are you really that hopeless at something? Is there truly no way to fix a problem? Chances are that things are not as bad as they seem.

- **Avoid absolutes.** Thinking about yourself or the challenges you face in black and white terms usually isn't helpful or realistic. Few things in life are all good or all bad.

- **Give yourself time.** When you are first hit with a disappointment, it's not always easy to step back and be optimistic. Take time to feel the way you feel. Then, gradually, start to modify negative thoughts and feelings.

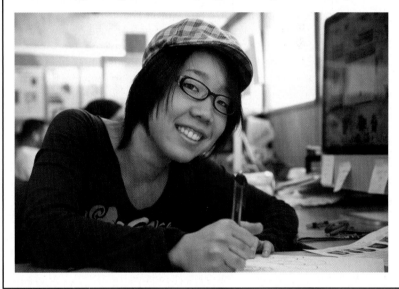

tentment also require another element—a sense of connection to something larger than yourself.

The search for that connection, or **spirituality,** takes many forms. For some people, it means religion, either through an organized group, such as a church, or through personal exploration of faith and prayer. For others, spiritual connections focus more on helping others, having a closer connection to nature, or striving toward a goal that feels meaningful. Although spirituality is deeply individual and highly complex, it usually encompasses four main themes of personal development:

- **Everyday values.** Putting personal beliefs and spiritual values into practice in small ways each day.

- **Mindfulness.** Being fully present in each moment, rather than simply going through the motions of life while your thoughts are elsewhere.

- **Connectedness.** Seeking a sense of connection and harmony with yourself, others, and a higher purpose.
- **Community.** Living in values-centered and humanistic ways that ultimately put us in greater harmony with others.

Before turning outward to search for larger meaning, spiritual health usually starts by turning inward, to see what matters most to you.

Clarifying Values

We all have **values,** our internal guidelines we use to make decisions and evaluate the world around us. Values help you form your opinions and ultimately guide your behavior. Building your spirituality starts with knowing your values and putting them into practice. The answers to the following questions will help indicate your values.

- What is important to me in my life?
- What principles do I want to live by?
- What do I want to stand for?

Developing and understanding your values evolves over the course of your lifetime. The values you learned in childhood from parents and caregivers may have changed when you reached your teenage years and started learning more from your peers. For example, many college students arrive on campus with political views very similar to those of their parents. However, because of new and profound influences and experiences during the college years, some reexamine and change their political beliefs because they have actually changed what they value. In adult life, a wide array of influences and circumstances puts your values to the test, requiring you to refine your values time and time again.

When you truly have values, you implement them when you make every decision in your life. Depending on your spiritual philosophy,

values Internal guidelines used to make decisions and evaluate the world around you.

you can implement your values in a variety of ways. For example, if you value the dignity of all human beings you may be compelled to take action to stop homelessness. If you are religious, this might lead you to join the homeless outreach program run by your place of worship. If you prefer non-religious action, you might choose to volunteer at a soup kitchen. And if you opt for political expression of your values, you might campaign for candidates who back stronger actions to fight homelessness—or even run for office yourself.

Prayer and Meditation

Spiritual health also thrives when you withdraw your thoughts from the chaos of everyday life and spend at least a few minutes focusing quietly on larger forces you perceive to be at work in your life. For some people, this focus takes the form of prayer, or a dialogue with a higher power. Prayer can be a personal or group activity in which you seek spiritual insights, personal growth, or even guidance on how best to conduct different aspects of everyday life. For many people who prefer religious spirituality, prayer offers a way to gather their thoughts, focus on values, decrease feelings of loneliness, and boost the ability to cope with challenges.

Prayer can have powerful effects on the body. Prayer triggers the *relaxation response,* a state of relaxation defined by slowed metabolism, reduced blood pressure, slower breathing, decreased heart rate, and less active brain waves.[9] Evidence also suggests that prayer is associated with positive health outcomes in sick people.[10]

Another form of quiet contemplation practiced by both religious and non-religious people is meditation. Meditation produces a deep state of relaxation and calms the mind.[11] Meditation can have different intended purposes, such as reaching higher states of conscious-

SPOTLIGHT

The Mind-Body Connection

It's finals week, you've been cramming for days, you're stressed and anxious, and now, to top it all off, you're starting to get a vicious cold. If this sounds familiar, you are probably experiencing the mind-body connection at work.

The mind-body connection describes how mental and emotional factors can affect you physically. Some everyday examples of the mind-body connection are your heart beating faster when you are excited, blushing when you get embarrassed, or trembling when you are

nervous. Numerous research studies link mental attitudes and emotional balance to how long you live, and how well.[1] Recent studies have shown:

- People who are happier, carry less anger, and are more optimistic are more likely to live longer. They are also less likely to get sick with minor illnesses, such as the flu, or more serious ones, such as heart disease or cancer.[2, 3]
- People who take better care of themselves mentally and physically,

or use physical stress reduction techniques such as relaxation exercises, usually see reductions in physical health problems.[4]

- Men who are under high levels of psychological distress have double the risk of developing diabetes.[5]

You can also use the mind-body connection to your benefit. The next time you are feeling stressed, upset, or anxious, try doing half an hour of physical activity to help calm your mind.

References: **1.** Fredrickson, B. (2000). Cultivating positive emotions to optimize health and well-being. *Prevention & Treatment, 3,* 1–24. **2.** Korvumaa-Honkanen, H., Hodkanen, R., Viinamaki, H., Heikkila, K., Kaprio, J., & Koskenvuo, M. (2000). Self-reported life and 20-year mortality in healthy Finnish adults. *American Journal of Epidemiology, 152,* 983–991. **3.** Siahpush, M., Spittal, M. & Singh, G. (2008). Happiness and life satisfaction prospectively predict self-rated health, and the presence of limiting, long term conditions. *American Journal of Health Promotion, 23*(1), 18–26. **4.** Astin, J., Shapiro, S., Eisenberg, D., & Forys, K. (2003). Mind-body medicine: State of the science, implications for practice. *The Journal of the American Board of Family Medicine, 16*(2), 131–147. **5.** Eriksson, A. K., Ekbom, A., Granath, F., Hilding, A., Efendic, S., & Ostenson, C. G. (2008). Psychological distress and risk of pre-diabetes and Type 2 diabetes in a prospective study of Swedish middle-aged men and women. *25*(7), 834–842.

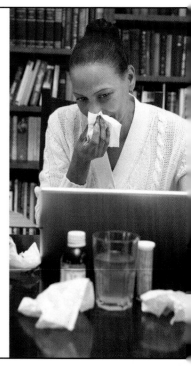

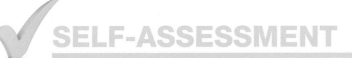

SELF-ASSESSMENT

Satisfaction with Life Scale

Instructions: Answer each question on a scale of 1–7 to determine your overall satisfaction with life.

1 = Strongly disagree
2 = Disagree
3 = Slightly disagree
4 = Neither agree nor disagree
5 = Slightly agree
6 = Agree
7 = Strongly agree

1. In most ways, my life is close to my ideal. _____
2. The conditions of my life are excellent. _____
3. I am satisfied with my life. _____
4. So far I have gotten the important things I want in life. _____
5. If I could live my life over, I would change almost nothing. _____

Total: _____

HOW TO INTERPRET YOUR SCORE

31–35: You are very satisfied with your life
26–30: Satisfied
21–25: Slightly satisfied
20: You are neither satisfied nor dissatisfied
15–19: Slightly dissatisfied
10–14: Dissatisfied
5–9: Very dissatisfied

Source: Diener, E., Larson, R. A., & Griffin, S. (1985). The satisfaction with life scale. *Journal of Personality Assessment, 49:* 71–75.

To complete this self-assessment online, visit **www.pearsonhighered.com/ choosinghealth.**

ness, developing creativity and self-awareness, or simply achieving a more relaxed and peaceful state of mind. For some, the practice of meditation is as simple as sitting quietly and focusing attention on a single idea, word, or symbol. Others find meditative contemplation in nature, drawing on their connection to the outside world to shake off daily hassles and quiet their mind. This might mean a solitary walk through the park or finding peace in the twists and turns of a challenging mountain bike ride.

Don't know how to meditate? Try one of these tools: **www.mayoclinic .com/health/meditation/MM00623** or **http://health.howstuffworks.com/ wellness/stress-management/how-to-relieve-stress-in-daily-life2.htm.**

Gratitude and Altruism

Just as it is easy to focus on your flaws, it is also convenient to gripe about all the ways the world lets you down. However, spiritual growth flourishes when you can see everything that is worth being grateful for. College may be tough, but at least you have the chance to attend. A few generations ago, that might not have been the case. You may have caught a bad flu a couple of weeks back, but you had the chance to recover, unlike people in other parts of the world where more serious diseases are far more common.

Adopting a mental attitude focused on gratitude, rather than complaints, can brighten your outlook on life. This, in turn, can lead to **altruism,** the practice of helping and giving to others out of genuine

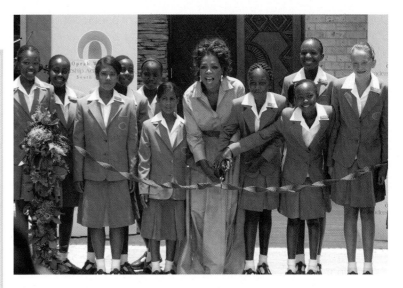

Oprah Winfrey acted altruistically when she started the Leadership Academy for Girls in South Africa.

concern for their well-being. Altruism can be a means of acting on your values. These acts of giving will, in turn, bring you their own benefits: Helping others can put your own life in perspective, build self-esteem, and even help you manage stress.[12]

Handling Common Psychological Problems

There may come times when you face challenges to your psychological well-being, just as you do to your physical health. This vulnerability does not mean there is something "wrong" with you. These challenges are common, and all of us grapple with them to some degree at various points in our lives. In almost every instance, there are steps you can take to feel more positive and in control.

Shyness

Shyness is characterized by a feeling of apprehension or intimidation in social situations, especially in reaction to unfamiliar people or new environments. Shyness can vary in severity from a slight feeling of discomfort to a social phobia that is completely inhibiting. Many people experience some degree of shyness, and an estimated 40–50% of college students consider themselves shy.[13]

Unlike introverts, who prefer to keep to themselves, shy people want to participate in social interactions, but feel they can't due to excessive self-consciousness, fear of embarrassment, or negative self-image. Shyness can be confined to one type of situation, such as being in large groups or interacting with an authority figure, or it can be more general, materializing during all types of social events. Shyness can limit personal and professional advancement if shy people hesitate to speak up for themselves or

altruism The practice of helping and giving to others out of genuine concern for their well-being.

shyness The feeling of apprehension or intimidation in social situations, especially in reaction to unfamiliar people or new environments.

avoid situations where they need to be leaders or speak publicly.[14] Shyness can also lead to *social isolation,* a general withdrawal or avoidance of social contact or communication.

A common misperception is that you are "born" shy, but that's not necessarily true. There is some evidence that genes can contribute to shyness. In particular, one variation of a gene that helps regulate brain chemistry has been linked to some cases of being shy.[15] But this "shy" gene appears to be more significant when someone has been exposed to uncomfortable social pressures that also encourage shyness.[16] In other words, the gene doesn't work alone. And for some people, life experiences alone are enough to make them shy.

Shyness can be a life-long personality trait, or it may diminish with age. However, even grown adults can develop shyness, especially during difficult transitions such as a divorce or getting laid off.[17]

Mild forms of shyness can usually be overcome with practice. Try making small talk with someone you'll never see again, like a person in line at the bookstore, then slowly push yourself out of your comfort zone. In addition, stress management techniques (discussed in Chapter 3) can help reduce your anxiety in social situations.

For some, intense shyness causes such severe anxiety that it impairs functioning in at least one area of daily life, resulting in a mental disorder called *social anxiety disorder,* discussed on pages 32–33.

Loneliness

Loneliness can do more than make you feel blue. It has been linked to higher levels of depression and general health problems.[18] As we age, connections with others are essential for overall health—studies of older people have found that those who are unmarried and lonely may have shorter life expectancy than those in meaningful relationships.[19]

If you feel as though you need more meaningful connections in your life, you have many options:

- **Take advantage of the social opportunities offered on college campuses or community centers.** Seek out groups that share your interests, such as sports organizations, civic organizations, or religious gatherings. By focusing on activities of genuine interest to you, you are more likely to meet others who share your passions and values—and more likely to form meaningful relationships.

- **Express yourself openly and honestly.** Sharing your true feelings with someone can encourage a feeling of connection for both of you that merely socializing in a superficial way does not.

- **Look into college counseling center resources.** Campus counseling centers usually offer a variety of resources that can help you build your social skills and increase your capacity for developing more meaningful relationships.

Anger

Anger is a completely normal and even healthy human emotion. Recognizing factors that make you angry can help you understand your values and help you assert yourself. Expressing anger is an important facet of the communication process.

However, anger that is out of control can be destructive. It can damage your relationships and may make it difficult for you to hold jobs or participate in group activities. One study of anger found that people prone to irritability and aggressiveness were more likely to display hostility even when they weren't provoked.[20] Anger can even damage your health. The exploding rage you feel when you get really angry raises your blood pressure and appears to be associated with risk factors for heart disease.[21] In fact, studies suggest that the cardiovascular effects of anger can still be detected even a week after the angry outburst, if the person continues to dwell on the event.[22]

Anger that remains bottled up can also be harmful; it raises your levels of tension and stress and darkens your view of the world.[23] Harboring anger may also leave you feeling defensive, assuming you are being attacked more often than may actually be the case.

The key is to express your anger in a way that releases your emotions but doesn't damage your relationships. When you find yourself getting angry or defensive, take a step back and assess the situation objectively. Try to relax—a few deep breaths can often

Handling Homesickness

"Hi, I'm Chase. I'm in my first year at a college, about a three-hour drive away from home. I was so excited about starting college and getting some freedom. Now it's a month into the semester, and I am shocked at how much work my classes are. Plus, all my dorm-mates seem to have a ton of friends already and I don't feel like I've connected with anyone. I never thought I'd say this, but I'm feeling pretty homesick. I miss my family, I miss my best friend, and I miss my old routine. I feel embarrassed that things are so hard for me, so instead of going out with my dorm-mates in the evenings, I just sit in my room and surf the Internet. I don't know, I thought I was prepared for college, but now I wonder if it may not be right for me."

1: What psychological and environmental factors do you think are contributing to Chase's homesickness?

2: What could Chase do to feel better?

3: What characteristics of psychological health could Chase build to help him manage situations like this in the future?

Do you have a story similar to Chase's? Share your story at **www.pearsonhighered.com/choosinghealth.**

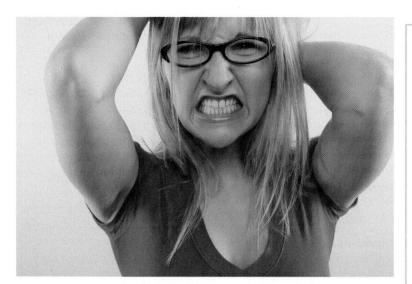

Although it may not feel like it, you can modify **anger** and **bad moods**.

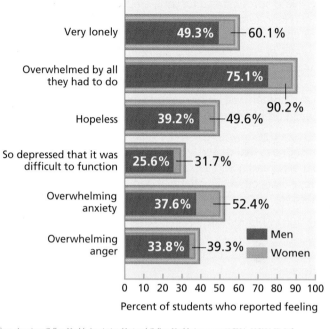

STUDENT STATS

Mental Health on Campus

Students reported feeling the following within the last 12 months:

	Men	Women
Very lonely	49.3%	60.1%
Overwhelmed by all they had to do	75.1%	90.2%
Hopeless	39.2%	49.6%
So depressed that it was difficult to function	25.6%	31.7%
Overwhelming anxiety	37.6%	52.4%
Overwhelming anger	33.8%	39.3%

0 10 20 30 40 50 60 70 80 90 100
Percent of students who reported feeling

Data from *American College Health Association National College Health Assessment (ACHA- NCHA II) Reference Group Executive Summary, Fall 2009* by the American College Health Association, 2009, retrieved from http://www.acha-ncha.org/reports_ACHA-NCHAII.html

do the trick. Then express what's upsetting you while avoiding criticism, blame, or threats. Once you're calmer, you may see solutions to the problem that you didn't notice before.

Bad Mood

Prolonged emotional states, or **moods,** can shape your view of the world for hours or days at a time. Although moods may often feel like they are caused by outside factors—a good or a bad grade on a paper, a fight with a friend—you have the ability to influence your moods. If you are in a bad mood, here are some strategies for breaking out of it:

- **Change what has upset you.** If you have to miss a night out with friends in order to study, plan another one for a time you know you will be free. Taking action can reshape your mood.
- **Don't drink or use drugs to cope.** Don't try to drown out your feelings with alcohol or drugs. You may feel better temporarily, but the circumstances that dragged down your mood will still be there after you have a couple of beers.
- **Act, don't stew.** Dwelling on a problem or bad mood without taking action is unproductive and increases the chances you will misdirect your frustrations at an innocent person later on.[24]
- **If you can't change one thing, change another.** If a fight with a friend has put you in a bad mood, and there is no way to resolve the dispute right now, focus on calming yourself down. You can work on resolving the fight when the time is right.

Mental Disorders

Everyone occasionally feels sad, worried, angry, or moody for a short period of time. We usually get over it and move on with our lives. But some people can develop serious psychological problems called **mental disorders.** Mental disorders are significant behavioral and psychological disorders that disrupt thoughts and feelings, impair ability to function, and increase risk of pain, disability, or even

death. The American Psychiatric Association classifies and defines all the mental disorders currently recognized in the U.S. in the *Diagnostic and Statistical Manual of Mental Disorders* (DSM).

Mental disorders can be caused by past or current experiences, extreme stress, illnesses, or trauma. In addition, chemical imbalances, genetic factors, and even alcohol or drugs can disrupt and impair your mental health.

Mental disorders are common, affecting more than 1 in 4 Americans over the age of 18 every year—a figure that translates to almost 60 million people.[25] Many people suffer from more than one mental disorder at a given time; 45% of those with any mental disorder meet the criteria for two or more disorders.[25] College students, facing distinct academic and social pressures, are not immune. In 2008, almost 20% of college students in the U.S. reported being treated for or diagnosed with at least one mental disorder in the past year.[26]

moods Prolonged emotional states.

mental disorders Significant behavioral and psychological disorders that disrupt thoughts and feelings, impair ability to function, and increase risk of pain, disability, or even death.

> **This National Public Radio program discusses mental health on campus:** www.npr.org/templates/story/story.php?storyId=113835383.

Depressive Disorders

The term *depression* refers to a mood state most commonly characterized by sadness. Though we have all felt depressed or lost interest in things that normally engage us, these feelings are usually temporary and in reaction to a sad event or loss. However, when a person is diagnosed with a **depressive disorder,** these feelings are more profound and long-term, and interfere with daily life and normal functioning. Approximately 18 million or about 8% of adult Americans suffer from a depressive disorder every year.[25] The World Health Organization estimates that by the year 2020, depressive disorders will be the second most common health problem in the world.[27]

The most basic symptom of depressive disorders is sadness that doesn't go away. But in addition to feeling sad and discouraged for long periods of time, other symptoms of depressive disorders are:

- A feeling of being slowed down or lacking energy.
- Feelings of helplessness, hopelessness, meaninglessness, or "emptiness."
- Feelings of worthlessness or guilt.
- Loss of interest in school, work, or activities you once enjoyed.
- Social withdrawal.
- Difficulty thinking clearly or making decisions.
- Sleep disturbances.
- Changes in eating habits, eating more or less than you used to.
- Restlessness, irritability.
- In the most severe cases, recurring thoughts of death or suicide.

Depressive disorders also often occur in conjunction with anxiety disorders and substance abuse.[25]

Types of Depressive Disorders

Two of the most common forms of depressive disorder are major depressive disorder and dysthymic disorder.

Major Depressive Disorder. **Major depressive disorder,** also called *major depression*, is diagnosed if someone consistently experiences five or more depressive symptoms, including either depressed mood or loss of interest or pleasure, for at least two weeks straight.[28] In those cases, the person is said to be experiencing a "major depressive episode." These prolonged and severe symptoms prevent normal functioning. They can interfere with or completely impair a person's ability to study, work, eat, sleep, maintain relationships, and feel pleasure or joy. A major depressive episode may happen only once, but more often occurs several times throughout a person's life. More than 6% of American adults experience this form of depression in a given year.[25]

Dysthymic Disorder. **Dysthymic disorder,** or *dysthymia,* is characterized by milder chronic depressive symptoms. Symptoms of dysthymic disorder must persist for at least two years in adults (one year in children) to meet criteria for the diagnosis. Those with dysthymia are more likely to suffer a major depressive illness in their

depressive disorder A mental disorder usually characterized by profound, long-term sadness or loss of interest that interferes with daily life and normal functioning.

major depressive disorder (major depression) A type of depressive disorder characterized by experiencing five or more symptoms of depression, including either depressed mood or loss of interest or pleasure, for at least two weeks straight.

dysthymic disorder (dysthymia) A milder, chronic type of depressive disorder that lasts two years or more.

seasonal affective disorder (SAD) A type of depressive disorder caused by fewer hours of daylight during the winter months.

lifetime. This type of depression is less common, affecting about 1.5% of American adults in a given year.[25]

Causes of Depressive Disorders

Depressive disorders can strike for a variety of reasons. The causes of depression tend to be complex and interrelated; it is often not possible to attribute a depressive disorder to a single source.

When depressive disorders run in families, it can be due to genetics or to certain learned behaviors family members pass from one generation to the next or to a mix of both. We don't yet understand how or to what extent genes influence depression, but it is likely that whatever role they play, it is due to the interaction of several genes along with external influences or other factors.[29] Genetics alone will not cause depression.

There are several ways physical or biochemical problems can lead to depressive disorders as well. Many people with serious depression experience an imbalance in the brain chemicals that affect mood, mainly the neurotransmitters (chemicals that transmit information in the brain) serotonin, dopamine, and norepinephrine. However, the cause of these imbalances may vary from person to person. Some people are biologically prone to an imbalance, whereas others may have an imbalance resulting from extreme trauma or distress. Irregular hormone levels can also cause depression, which is why doctors will often test a patient's thyroid, a gland that regulates and secretes hormones, before diagnosing a depressive disorder. Prolonged illness, chronic pain, and even certain medications can also contribute to feelings of depression and sadness.

At the same time, external influences can be powerful factors in depression too. Traumatic events, grief, financial problems, school pressures, and substance abuse can all knock thoughts and emotions off balance. People with low self-esteem or a pessimistic view of the world are more prone to depression. If a person's network of emotional support is limited, or changes due to the loss of a loved one, he or she may be especially vulnerable to depression when stress or trauma strikes.

Experiencing fewer hours of daylight during the winter months can lead to depression as well, a condition known as **seasonal affective disorder (SAD).** SAD is normally worse in winter months and improves in the summer, and it is more common for women and those living in higher latitudes, where winter days are shorter and darker. Treatment for SAD usually involves *light therapy*— sitting near a special lamp that mimics sunlight (not a sun-tanning lamp)—for a certain length of time each day.

Students and teachers talk about how the pressures of college can lead to depression: www.depressioncenter.org/video/TheViewFromHere/default.asp.

Depression in Men and Women

Approximately 6 million men and 12 million women suffer from depressive disorders in any given year.[30] The causes and symptoms of depression may vary between sexes.

Mental Health
Through the Lenses of Ethnicity and Sexuality

A deeply personal issue, mental health is shaped by our individual life experiences. As a result, race, ethnicity, and sexual orientation often have an effect on whether someone develops depression or other mental disorders and on the treatment that person receives.

Although there are not many large-scale studies on mental health in minority populations, it is known that in the U.S. many people of minority racial, ethnic, or sexuality status appear to be at greater risk for mental health problems than their Caucasian, heterosexual counterparts.[1,2] A recent national survey shows that 8% of African Americans and 6.3% of Mexican Americans suffer from depression, compared to 4.8% of Caucasians.[3]

The tendency toward depression and other mental illness is no more inborn in minorities than in heterosexual Caucasians, but appears to be related to the obstacles and challenges that African Americans, Hispanics, Asian Americans, Pacific Islanders, Native Americans, and homosexuals face in society. Many minority groups experience higher rates of certain social factors that can contribute to mental illness, such as poverty, homelessness, incarceration, exposure to violence or trauma, refugee status, and childhood placement in foster care.[1] In addition, feelings of discrimination can exacerbate mental health issues. A recent study found that the increased likelihood of mental disorders in Latinos adapting to U.S.

society is at least partially due to feelings that they are members of a group that is devalued and discriminated against.[4]

To make matters worse, minorities often lack access to culturally or linguistically appropriate mental health services. Only 2% of psychologists and psychiatrists in the United States are African American, most mental health providers in the U.S. speak only English, and the majority of mental health practitioners are not trained in the particular needs of homosexual clients.[1,2] Minority groups are also less likely to have health insurance that would cover the cost of such services—for example, only 41% of Hispanics have private health insurance, compared to 75% of Caucasions.[5] Even when care is available, misdiagnosis of mental health disorders is more common in minorities than in Caucasians, and cultural stigmas against mental illnesses or distrust of mental health care can lead to underreporting of mental health problems or reliance on less-effective traditional remedies rather than medical treatment.

If you are interested in learning more about culturally compatible mental health services on your campus, contact your student health center or ask your health instructor.

Sources: 1. U.S. Department of Health and Human Services. (2001). *Mental health: Culture, race, and ethnicity.; A supplement to Mental health: A report of the surgeon general.* retrieved from http://www.surgeongeneral.gov/library/mentalhealth/cre/sma-01-3613.pdf 2. National Alliance on Mental Illness, NAMI Multicultural Action Center. (2007). *Mental Health Fact Sheets.* 3. U.S. Department of Health and Human Services. (2008). *Depression in the United States Household Population 2005–2006*, NCHS Data Brief, No. 7. 4. Torres, L. (2009). Attributions to discrimination among Latino/as: The mediating role of competence. *American Journal of Orthopsychiatry, 79*(1), 118–124. 5. The Henry J. Kaiser Family Foundation. (2007). *The uninsured: a primer. Key facts about Americans without health insurance.* Retrieved from http://www.kff.org/uninsured/upload/7451-03.pdf.

Listen to a radio story on mental health in the African American community: www.npr.org/templates/story/story.php?storyId=87952114&ft=1&f=88201937.

Women and Depression. Until adolescence, girls and boys experience depressive disorders at about the same rate.[30] But after puberty, women's rates of both major depressive disorder and dysthymia rise relative to men. Women are more likely to experience depression at younger ages, for longer periods of time, and with more reoccurrences than men are. Women are also more likely to have feelings of guilt when they are depressed, and depressive disorders in women are more likely to be associated with anxiety disorders and eating disorders than in men.[31]

Scientists continue to examine why there is an increased rate of depressive disorders in women, but there are no definitive answers yet. Women's greater risk may be partially attributed to physical factors.

Women experience hormonal changes in connection with monthly periods, pregnancy, childbirth, the postpartum period, the years just before menopause, and menopause. Many of these hormonal shifts increase the risk of either short-term or long-term depression.

In addition, there are a number of social and interpersonal factors that increase the risk for depression in women. Because women still tend to play a larger role in child care, especially if they are single parents, they juggle the dual duties of professional careers as well as raising children, a situation that increases their stress levels and may lead to depression. On a whole, women also experience higher rates of poverty and sexual abuse, and lower socioeconomic status, than men do, all of which are risk factors for depression. A few studies have also noted a tendency among women to pay more attention to difficulties and negative feelings, which can increase the risk of depression.[32] However, research in this area is not conclusive, and it remains to be seen how changing gender roles will affect this theory over time.

For women who have just had a baby, the combination of wildly shifting hormonal and physical changes, a radical change in lifestyle, the potentially overwhelming responsibility of a new baby, and a lack of sleep may contribute to *postpartum depression*. This is a depressive disorder that can make it difficult for a mother to bond with her new baby, or in the most serious cases, can promote thoughts of harming herself or the newborn. Women who have previously experienced depression or postpartum depression are more likely to suffer from it. When left untreated, postpartum depression can last up to a year. A recent report by the Centers for Disease Control estimates that about 12–20% of new mothers experience postpartum depression.[33]

Men and Depression. Depressive disorders in men are often under-diagnosed and under-treated. Because of that, the disparity in rates of depressive disorders between men and women may not actually be as large as reported. Some of the lack of recognition may arise from the different ways men express their depression. Rather than appearing sad, men with depression may be irritable, fatigued, or extremely cynical. Men with depression may also be especially prone to physical effects like digestive problems, sleep disturbances, sexual problems, and headaches. Men may also have a hard time accepting their depression out of fear of social stigmatization, feeling that "true men" should be tough and not subject to feeling sad.

But though men's depression may be harder to recognize than women's depression, treating it is equally important. One study found that men with depression are not only more likely to contract heart disease than other men, but also to die from it.[32] Depressed men are also more likely than women to self-medicate through destructive be-

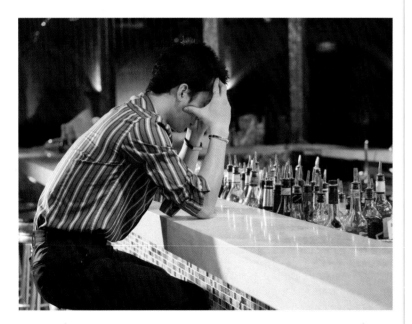

Depressed men are more likely than women to self-medicate through alcohol or drug abuse.

haviors such as drug and alcohol abuse, or engage in reckless, risky behavior.[30] Depression is also a risk factor for suicide, and suicide is the seventh leading cause of death for males in the U.S.[34]

Treating Depressive Disorders

Depressive disorders are among the most treatable mental disorders, with successful treatment outcomes in more than 80% of cases.[31] Yet only about half the people with depressive disorders seek treatment.

One of the first steps in getting treatment should be an evaluation by a medical doctor, to check for any physical causes of depression. If physical sources have been ruled out, several types of treatments can help depressed people get their lives back on track.

Talk Therapies. Talking with a trained counselor or psychologist can make all the difference for many people with depression. Talk therapies such as cognitive therapy or psychodynamic therapy (discussed on pages 37 and 38) encourage depressed people to open up about their thoughts, feelings, relationships, and experiences in order to recognize problems that underlie their depression and work to improve them. Talk therapy may be the best treatment option for mild to moderate depressive disorders.[30]

Antidepressants. For many people, especially those who are severely depressed or suicidal, medication is a helpful or necessary addition to talk therapies. Antidepressants are the class of drugs designed to adjust the chemical imbalances in the brain that accompany depression. They work by normalizing the levels of the neurotransmitters serotonin, norepinephrine, or dopamine. The most prescribed types of antidepressants are called selective serotonin reuptake inhibitors (SSRIs) and include drugs like fluoxetine (Prozac), citalopram (Celexa) and sertraline (Zoloft). Antidepressants do not relieve symptoms immediately, and patients must take regular doses for at least three to four weeks before experiencing the full therapeutic effect. These medications are not addictive, but abruptly stopping them can cause withdrawal symptoms or lead to a relapse of depressive symptoms. Occasionally, people taking an antidepressant will stop the medication once they begin feeling better, believing that they no longer need it, only to be hit by withdrawal symptoms and a devastating return of depressive feelings. Antidepressants should only be discontinued under a medical provider's supervision.

Although many depressed people have been helped by antidepressants, these medications do come with uncertainties and risks. The same drug that helps one person may provide no benefit for another. If one medication does not work, it may be necessary to try another or couple two medications together. Most antidepressants also have side effects that range from mild (headache, dry mouth) to severe (suicidal thoughts). Despite the relative safety and popularity of SSRIs, in recent years the media has highlighted the increased risk of teenage suicides after starting antidepressants. In 2005, the FDA required all antidepressant labels to carry a warning that alerts consumers about the suicide risk among this population. In 2007, this warning was extended to include young adults up to the age of 24. Despite these concerns, studies have shown that the benefits of antidepressants outweigh their risk to children, adolescents, and young adults with major depression.[35]

Currently, 25–50% of college students seen in counseling and student health centers are taking an antidepressant.[36] If your doctor suggests an antidepressant, see **Practical Strategies for Health: Questions to Ask Before Starting an Antidepressant** for questions to ask before accepting a prescription.

Bipolar Disorder

Bipolar disorder, also known as *manic-depressive disorder,* is characterized by occurrences of abnormally elevated mood (or mania) alternating with depressive episodes, with periods of normal mood in between. Mania can cause increased energy and decreased need for sleep, an expansive or irritable mood, impulsive behavior, and unrealistic beliefs or expectations. Manic people's thoughts race, their speech is rapid, their attention span is low, and their judgment is poor. Extreme manic episodes can sometime lead to aggression or psychotic symptoms such as delusions and hallucinations. The alternating depressive episodes can be terrible, leading to thoughts of suicide. Many people with bipolar disorder abuse alcohol or drugs, which can make their symptoms worse and also make it harder to identify that they are bipolar. A psychotic break can be the first sign of bipolar disorder in some people.

Bipolar disorder affects approximately 5.7 million American adults (approximately 2.6% of the population).[25] It occurs equally among both sexes and occurs in all races and ethnic groups.[37] Bipolar disorder usually develops in the late teens or early adult years and at least half of all cases start before the age of 25. The disorder has a tendency to run in families, and because of this scientists are looking for genes that may increase a person's likelihood of developing the illness. However, most agree there is no single gene but many different genes acting together, along with external factors, to produce the illness. Bipolar disorder is usually a lifelong condition, but with treatment people with the disorder can lead fulfilling lives. If left untreated, bipolar disorder can worsen over time, resulting in increasingly frequent and severe episodes. The most common treatments for bipolar disorder are mood stabilizers such as lithium, and anticonvulsant medications, which can also help to control mood.

Hear people with bipolar disorder discuss their condition: **www.webmd .com/bipolar-disorder/bipolar-tv/default.htm.**

Attention Disorders

Attention disorders create difficulty with jobs that require sustained concentration, such as completing a single task over a long period of time or sitting still for extended periods. One study of children with attention disorders also found that they had difficulty forming social connections and durable friendships.[38] The most common form of attention disorder is **attention-deficit/hyperactivity disorder (ADHD),** which causes inattention, hyperactive behavior, fidgeting, and a tendency toward impulsive behavior.

Attention disorders are most commonly diagnosed in young children. National surveys estimate that almost 9% of children and teenagers have attention disorders.[39] Boys are more than twice as likely as girls to have attention disorders. Although attention disorders had been considered a disease of childhood, it is now thought that up to 60% of cases continue into adult life, and it is diagnosed in about 4.5% of adults.[40] Among college students in the United States, 3.5% reported that they were diagnosed or

Practical Strategies for Health

Questions to Ask Before Starting an Antidepressant

If your doctor thinks you might benefit from an antidepressant, ask the following questions to make sure it's right for you:

- How will I know if the antidepressant is working?
- When will I feel its effects? What should I do while I wait for it to work?
- What are the side effects? Am I at risk for them?
- Why is this the best antidepressant for me?
- How will you follow up on the drug's effects?
- How and when do I stop taking it?

If an antidepressant doesn't seem to be helping or has side effects, let your doctor know right away. You may be able to find a different medication that proves more helpful to you, or discuss other treatment options.

treated for ADHD in the past year.[26] Because these disorders make it difficult to complete complex tasks such as school assignments, college students with ADHD are at high risk for poor academic performance, and it is important that they receive treatment.[41] Adults with attention disorders may also have problems in work and personal relationships. They can have difficulty following directions, remembering information, and making deadlines; they may be chronically late, anxious, unorganized, or irritable. One study of adults with ADHD found that they could readily detect a problem, but preferred impulsive decisions over planning when trying to resolve it.[42]

Attention disorders sometimes occur in conjunction with other mental disorders such as anxiety or depression, and physical health risk factors such as being overweight.[39] People with attention disorders are also at higher risk for tobacco use and substance abuse.

Options for treating attention disorders include behavioral and cognitive therapies (discussed on page 37) and prescription medications. The medications often used to treat ADHD are amphetamines such as methylphenidate (Ritalin or Concerta) or amphetamine/dextroamphetamine (Adderall). Although these drugs are stimulants, they have the opposite effect in people with ADHD. Chapter 7 discusses unprescribed use of ADHD drugs, a growing problem on college campuses.

bipolar disorder (manic-depressive disorder) A mental disorder characterized by occurrences of abnormally elevated mood (or mania), often alternating with depressive episodes, with periods of normal mood in between.

attention disorders A category of mental disorders characterized by problems with mental focus.

attention-deficit/hyperactivity disorder (ADHD) A type of attention disorder characterized by inattention, hyperactive behavior, fidgeting, and a tendency toward impulsive behavior.

anxiety disorders A category of mental disorders characterized by persistent feelings of fear, dread, and worry.

generalized anxiety disorder (GAD) An anxiety disorder characterized by chronic worry and pessimism about everyday events that lasts at least six months and may be accompanied by physical symptoms.

panic attacks Episodes of sudden terror that strike without warning.

panic disorder A mental disorder characterized both by recurring panic attacks and the fear of a panic attack occurring.

social anxiety disorder (social phobia) An anxiety disorder characterized by an intense fear of being judged by others and of being humiliated by your own actions, which may be accompanied by physical symptoms.

Anxiety Disorders

Anxiety disorders cover a wide range of conditions characterized by persistent feelings of fear, dread, and worry. They are the most common mental health problems among American adults, affecting over 40 million people each year.[25] Anxiety disorders frequently occur in conjunction with depressive disorders or substance abuse problems.[25]

Generalized Anxiety Disorder (GAD)

People who suffer from **generalized anxiety disorder (GAD)** feel chronic anxiety, exaggerated worry, and pessimism, even when there is little or nothing to provoke it or they know they are overreacting. People with GAD develop a continuous cycle of worrying that can be extremely difficult to break. They worry about common things and even when the concerns are valid, they worry to excess. GAD can be diagnosed when this excessive worry lasts at least six months. Physical symptoms that often accompany the anxiety include fatigue, headaches, muscle tension, muscle aches, difficulty swallowing, trembling, and nausea. GAD affects about 6.8 million adult Americans and about twice as many women as men.[25] It usually develops gradually, with the highest risk of onset between childhood and middle age. It is often accompanied by depression, other anxiety disorders, or substance abuse.

Panic Attacks and Panic Disorder

Panic attacks are sudden feelings of terror that strike without warning. Symptoms include chest pain, shortness of breath, dizziness, weakness, and nausea. Panic attacks usually induce a sense of unreality and fears of impending doom, losing control, or dying. Panic attacks usually go away on their own in less than 10 minutes, and are sometimes much shorter. Although people experiencing panic attacks often truly fear that they might die, panic attacks will not kill you. Many people have just one panic attack and never have another, but those experiencing repeated panic attacks may have **panic disorder.** Panic disorder affects about 6 million adults in the U.S. and is twice as common in women as men.[43] It often begins in late adolescence or early adulthood, and the susceptibility to panic attacks appears to be inherited.

A debilitating symptom of panic disorder is the dread of the next panic attack. People with panic disorder may begin to fear or avoid places where they have suffered a panic attack in the past, which can progressively restrict their mobility and even make it difficult for them to seek and receive treatment. This avoidance causes about a third of the people who suffer from panic disorder to develop *agoraphobia,* the fear of being places where they cannot quickly leave or where they cannot quickly receive help should they have a panic attack. Agoraphobia can eventually leave victims virtually housebound.[43]

Social Anxiety Disorder

Social anxiety disorder, also called *social phobia,* typically involves an intense fear of being judged by others and of being humiliated by your own actions. It can be accompanied by physical symptoms such as sweating, blushing, increased heart rate, trembling, and stuttering. It may strike only in certain situations, for instance speaking in public or eating in front of others, but in its most severe form a person might experience the symptoms anytime he or she is around other people.[44] Social anxiety disorder affects about 15 million adults in the United States, and women and men are equally likely to develop it.[44]

This condition can be debilitating—leading people to avoid social situations even if doing so negatively impacts them professionally or

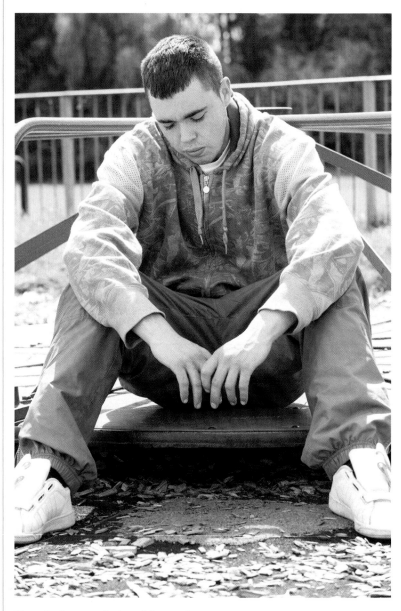

Social anxiety disorder can cause people to isolate themselves from others.

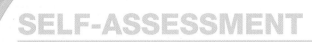

Anxiety Assessment

Instructions: How has each of these symptoms disturbed or worried you during the last seven days? Circle the most appropriate score relating to your state.

0 = Never   1 = A little   2 = Moderately   3 = A lot   4 = Extremely

1. Nervousness or shaking inside.   0 1 2 3 4
2. Nausea, stomach pain or discomfort.   0 1 2 3 4
3. Feeling scared suddenly and without any reason.   0 1 2 3 4
4. Palpitations or feeling that your heart is beating faster.   0 1 2 3 4
5. Significant difficulty falling asleep.   0 1 2 3 4
6. Difficulty relaxing.   0 1 2 3 4
7. Tendency to startle easily.   0 1 2 3 4
8. Tendency to be easily irritable or bothered.   0 1 2 3 4
9. Inability to free yourself of obsessive thoughts.   0 1 2 3 4
10. Tendency to awaken early in the morning and not go back to sleep.   0 1 2 3 4
11. Feeling nervous when alone.   0 1 2 3 4

HOW TO INTERPRET YOUR SCORE

If you indicated scores of 3 or 4 to 5 or 6 questions, your anxiety level is significant and you should consider different strategies such as better health practices, or adding relaxation techniques or physical exercise to your daily routine. If you indicated scores of 3 or 4 in all your answers, your level of anxiety is critical and you should consult your doctor.

Source: "Anxiety Self-assessment Questionnaire" used by permission of the Mental Illness Foundation, Montreal.

To complete this self-assessment online, visit www.pearsonhighered.com/ choosinghealth.

personally. In one survey of people with social anxiety disorder, 87% said their condition had a negative effect on personal relationships, 75% said it harmed their ability to perform normal daily activities, and 73% said it impaired their satisfaction with work.[45] Some sufferers try to self-medicate to reduce the anxiety, leading to drug and alcohol abuse. Here are some signs that may indicate social anxiety disorder:

- Cancelling social engagements at the last moment.
- Having few good friends who really know you.
- Avoidance of activities that are enjoyable but require social interaction.
- Pessimism and low self-esteem, especially in regard to social situations or skills.
- Excessive computer use that is not social in nature and that takes the place of direct contact with other people.

In rare instances, people with social anxiety eventually blend their feelings of isolation and withdrawal with anger. This resulting mix, a phenomenon psychologists call *cynical shyness,* is more common in boys and men, and may be a factor in some episodes of violence at schools and other social environments.[46]

If you experience social anxiety or isolation at a level that feels debilitating or makes you angry, seek professional help. Many campus health centers offer support services and psychotherapy. You may also benefit from medication, which has helped some people with social anxiety disorders live happier, more connected lives.[47]

Phobias

A **phobia** is an extreme, disabling, irrational fear of something that poses little or no actual danger. Phobias are the most common types of anxiety disorder, and the usual age of onset is childhood to late adolescence. Women are twice as likely to suffer from phobias as men, and African Americans are more likely to suffer from phobias than Caucasians.[48] The American Psychiatric Association classifies simple phobias into five categories:[28]

- **Animal phobias.** Triggered by animals or insects such as cats (ailurophobia) or spiders (arachnophobia).
- **Natural environment phobias.** Triggered by objects in the environment such as heights (acrophobia) or water (hydrophobia).
- **Situational phobias.** Triggered by being in specific situations such as on bridges (gephyrophobia) or in small confined spaces (claustrophobia) or in the dark (nyctophobia).
- **Blood, injection, or injury phobias.** Triggered by witnessing an invasive medical procedure such as an injection (trypanophobia) or by witnessing an injury or blood.
- **Other phobias.** Triggered by some other stimuli such as the number 13 (triskaidekaphobia) or clowns (coulrophobia).

Fear of **spiders** is a common phobia.

Obsessive-Compulsive Disorder (OCD)

People with **obsessive-compulsive disorder (OCD)** have repeated and unwanted thoughts (obsessions), which causes them to develop rituals (compulsions) in an attempt to control the anxiety produced by these thoughts. The obsessions tend to be overblown or unrealistic worries, such as extreme concern about contamination by germs, fear of home intruders, or even fear of certain numbers, letters, or colors. The rituals provide brief relief from anxiety, even though the sufferer often knows they are meaningless. In many cases the rituals end up controlling their lives, and although sufferers might be distressed or embarrassed by their situation, they cannot resist completing them. For example, a student obsessed with germs and sickness may develop hand-washing rituals that are so extensive that he is unable to leave his apartment to get to class on time. Other common rituals include the compulsion to repeatedly check things, touch things (in a certain order or a certain number of times), horde unnecessary items, or count things. Occurring equally in men and women, OCD affects 2.2 million adults in the U.S.[25] First symptoms of OCD frequently appear in childhood or adolescence, and it is often diagnosed concurrently with eating disorders, other anxiety disorders, or depression.

phobia An extreme, disabling, irrational fear of something that poses little or no actual danger.

obsessive-compulsive disorder (OCD) An anxiety disorder characterized by repeated and unwanted thoughts (obsessions) that lead to rituals (compulsions) in an attempt to control the anxiety.

Sufferers of OCD tell their stories: www.nytimes.com/interactive/2009/09/24/health/healthguide/TE_OCD.html?ref=health.

Post-Traumatic Stress Disorder (PTSD)

After a traumatic event, people sometimes feel recurrent fear, anger, and depression, a condition known as **post-traumatic stress disorder (PTSD)**. Events that commonly cause PTSD are war, child abuse, natural disasters, automobile accidents, or being the victim of a violent crime. People with PTSD often startle easily, feel numb emotionally, and can become irritable or even violent. They tend to obsessively relive the trauma in flashbacks or dreams, or they will avoid places or experiences that might remind them of the traumatic event. PTSD can be accompanied by depression, other anxiety disorders, and substance abuse.

About 7.7 million adults in the U.S. experience PTSD each year, but it can strike children as well.[25] The condition strikes women more than men. Factors that increase the likelihood of developing PTSD are how intense the trauma was, how long it lasted, how close to the event the victim was, whether the victim was injured or someone they were close to died, how in control of events the victim felt, and how much help or support the victim received after the event.[49]

> Listen to soldiers talk about PTSD in their own words: www.youtube.com/watch?v=bsFg8wZuI-4 and www.pbs.org/wgbh/pages/frontline/shows/heart/view.

Treating Anxiety Disorders

Cognitive and behavioral therapies (discussed on page 37) are effective at teaching people with anxiety to recognize and redirect anxiety-producing thought patterns. One effective treatment, called *exposure therapy* or *systematic desensitization,* encourages patients to face their fears head-on. For instance, if a student with OCD fears dirt and germs, part of his therapy might involve getting his hands dirty and waiting progressively longer amounts of time before washing them. The therapist will help him work through his anxiety while his hands are dirty, and eventually his reaction will become less severe.

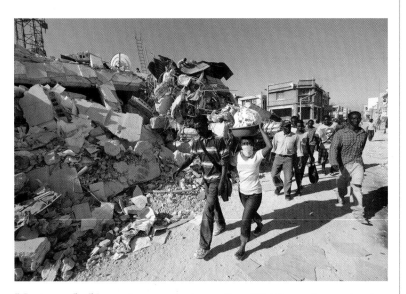

Natural disasters, such as the 2010 earthquake in Haiti, can cause PTSD.

Schizophrenia

Schizophrenia is a severe, chronic, and disabling mental disorder that is the most common type of *psychotic disorder,* or disorder marked by abnormal thinking and detachment from reality. It affects about 1% of adults in the U.S., but it occurs in 10% of people who have a first-degree relative (parent or sibling) with the disorder.[25,50] Although there is a genetic risk for schizophrenia, researchers conclude that it is doubtful that genetics alone are sufficient to cause the disorder. Interactions between genetics, brain chemistry, and environment are thought to be necessary for the disease to develop.

People with schizophrenia often suffer from incorrect perceptions of reality, an altered sense of self, and radical changes in emotions, movements, and behaviors. They often have difficulty distinguishing what is real from what is imaginary, and have trouble functioning in society. Primary symptoms of schizophrenia include:[50]

- **Delusions.** False beliefs, such as thinking you possess unusual powers or believing that others are plotting against you.
- **Hallucinations.** False perceptions of reality, such as hearing or seeing things that are not there, most often voices.
- **Thought disorders.** Often called *disorganized thinking*—problems with thinking or speaking clearly or maintaining focus.
- **Movement disorders.** Agitated or repetitive body movements, or in some extreme cases becoming catatonic (immobile).
- **Reduction in professional and social functioning.** Social withdrawal, unpredictable behavior, poor hygiene, or paranoia can all impair social and professional function.
- **Inappropriate emotions.** Aloof or flat emotions or inappropriate or bizarre reactions to events.

Psychotic symptoms such as these usually appear in men in the late teens and early 20s and in women about a decade later. Research has shown that schizophrenia affects both sexes equally and occurs in similar rates in all ethnic groups.[50]

Schizophrenia cannot be cured; however, many of its symptoms can be controlled with antipsychotic medication. Once symptoms are controlled, talk therapy can help those suffering from schizophrenia lead meaningful lives. Expert help is usually essential in controlling schizophrenia.

Suicide and Self-Injury

For some people, the mental disorders or traumas they've experienced produce deep anguish that causes them to harm themselves. Two common areas of self-harm are suicide and self-injury.

Self-Injury

Self-injury occurs in the form of intentional, self-inflicted cuts, burns, bruises, or other injuries, without suicidal intent. Self-injury is often

post-traumatic stress disorder (PTSD) An anxiety disorder characterized by recurrent fear, anger, and depression occurring after a traumatic event.

schizophrenia A severe mental disorder characterized by incorrect perceptions of reality, an altered sense of self, and radical changes in emotions, movements, and behaviors.

performed in an effort to deal with negative or overwhelming feelings. Although it provides the injurer with a moment of calm, it is usually followed by feelings of guilt and shame. Once largely hidden from public view, self-injury has become more prominent and may even be increasing due to discussion of the practice on websites and in online forums. One study of online self-injury discussions found hundreds of message boards and forums on the topic with thousands of members.[51] More than 5% of college students in the U.S. admit to performing self-injury in the past year, but the reliability of these statistics is questionable because most who do injure themselves conceal it.[26]

Self-injury often begins or occurs in adolescence and during the teen years. Although early research suggested that women were more likely than men to self-injure, more recent research has shown that rates are similar across sexes.[52] No one racial or ethnic group is more or less likely to self-injure than others. Therapy and medications can help self-injurers learn to deal with their difficult feelings more appropriately and stop their self-abuse.

Suicide

More than 32,000 people in the U.S. take their own lives every year, and for every death there are at least another eight attempted suicides.[53] College students are more likely than the general population to try to take their own lives, and some, unfortunately, succeed. Suicide is the second leading cause of death on college campuses, and more than 6% of students said they had seriously considered attempting suicide in the past year.[26] Although women attempt suicide two to three times more often than men, men are four times more likely to actually die by suicide, possibly because they choose more lethal means in their attempts. Native Americans and Alaska Natives are the ethnic groups with the highest overall suicide rates.[53] Caucasians are also at high risk, whereas Hispanics, Asians, and Pacific Islanders all have lower than average suicide rates.[53] Historically, African American teens and young adults have had lower suicide rates than their Caucasian counterparts, but their suicide rates have increased dramatically in recent decades. Now researchers predict that before the age of 17, 7% of African American females will attempt suicide.[54] Another group that is at high risk for suicide is older adults, with Caucasian males over the age of 85 having the highest suicide rate of any group in the U.S.[53]

Causes and Warning Signs of Suicide

Several factors clearly play a role in driving up suicide risk. More than 90% of people who commit suicide in the U.S. have a diagnosable mental health or substance abuse problem.[25] In addition, financial problems, serious illness, and the loss of a loved one are frequently cited as catalysts. A family history of suicide, previous suicide attempts, having access to guns in the home, and a history of substance abuse also increase suicide risk. Ultimately, it seems that suicide becomes appealing to people when they feel hopeless about the direction of their life and helpless to change it. Signs that a person may be considering suicide include:

- Statements that indirectly imply suicidal thoughts such as "I don't have much to live for" or "You won't have to worry about me much longer."
- An inability to let go of grief.

- Changes in behavior and personality that focus on hopeless, negative thoughts and feelings.
- A noticeable downturn in mood within the first few weeks of starting a new antidepressant medication.
- Loss of interest in classes, work, hobbies, or spending time with friends and loved ones.
- Expressions of self-hatred, excessive risk taking, or apathy toward one's own well-being.
- Disregard for personal appearance.
- Changes in sleep patterns or eating habits.
- A preoccupation with thoughts or themes of death.

Preventing Suicide

Most suicide attempts are expressions of extreme distress. Don't assume that a person who talks of suicide is just having a bad day or seeking attention. Instead, take steps to help them move through this crisis until longer-term solutions can be found. If you think someone is suicidal let the person know you care and that you are there to help. Offer to call a crisis hotline together, go to a counseling center, or head to the nearest emergency room **(Figure 2.3)**.

NATIONAL SUICIDE PREVENTION LIFELINE™

1-800-273-TALK

www.suicidepreventionlifeline.org

Figure 2.3 National suicide prevention lifeline.

Source: U.S. Department of Health and Human Services, Substance Abuse and Mental Health Services Administration.

Subscribe to National Public Radio's mental health podcasts at www.npr.org/templates/rss/podlayer.php?id=88201937.

Getting Help

If you or someone you know is ready to seek help for a psychological problem, you'll find many resources available. The first place to start is with your own self-care.

Self-Care

When you are under mental or emotional distress, the basic tasks of daily life can feel overwhelming. Self-care becomes more important than ever. If you are feeling mentally or emotionally on edge, be sure to:

- **Eat well.** Don't skip meals or binge on junk food. Calming your mind and emotions will be easier if your body isn't nutritionally stressed.
- **Get the right amount of sleep.** A regular sleep schedule that includes 7–9 hours of quality sleep every night is important to both your physical and mental well-being. In your busy schedule as a college student, make sure you make sleep a priority. If you are depressed and having trouble getting out of bed, convince yourself to get up and move around during the day. Light and air will help improve your mood. If you are having trouble sleeping, create a restful environment for yourself without lights, loud music, computers, or TV. Daytime exercise will also help make you tired and make it easier to sleep.

- **Get some exercise.** Exercise releases endorphins, body chemicals that boost mood. Even a half-hour walk will probably improve your mood, clear your head, and make you feel better.
- **Set realistic goals.** If you don't feel well, don't expect yourself to function at your regular level. Set smaller goals, and break big jobs up into small ones.
- **Seek company and support.** Mental and emotional concerns are common. Talk to a supportive friend or see if your campus counseling center offers a support group that is right for you. Support groups are often free or low-cost, and are usually led by a trained professional who can steer the group's conversations and interactions in positive ways.

Find online support at one of these websites: www.patientslikeme.com/mood/community, www.dailystrength.org, www.wellsphere.com/communities.

Professional Help

Most campuses offer a range of counseling and mental health services to help address the mental and emotional pressures students face. Most of these services are provided for free or at low cost, or are covered by your campus insurance plan if you have one—so your campus health or counseling center is a good place to start looking for help. Your health education instructor should also know about services available on campus or in the community.

Types of Mental Health Professionals

In seeking care, you will most likely work with one of the following types of licensed professionals:

- **Counselors.** Counselors have a master's degree in counseling and focus on talk therapy. Counselors may lead group or individual therapy sessions.

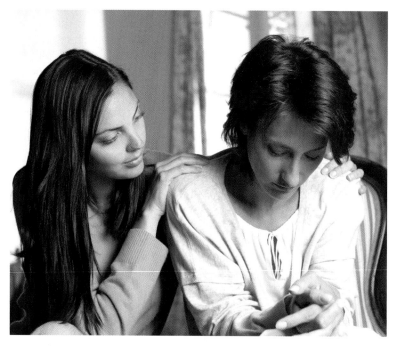

Speaking with a supportive friend can help you work through mental and emotional problems.

- **Psychologists.** Psychologists have a doctoral degree and focus on talk therapy. Many have particular specialties, and they may lead group or individual therapy sessions.
- **Psychiatrists.** Psychiatrists have a medical degree and usually focus on the medical aspects of psychological issues. Unlike counselors or psychologists, psychiatrists can prescribe medication and may have admitting privileges at local hospitals. Psychiatrists and talk therapy professionals often work together to provide a person a full range of care if needed.

See **Consumer Corner: Choosing a Therapist Who's Right for You** for information about the things you should discuss before picking a therapist.

Once you have found a mental health professional, the real work begins. Your treatment can succeed only if you are open and honest about your thoughts, emotions, and what is going on in your life. Therapy can sometimes bring up sad or uncomfortable feelings, but that isn't necessarily a bad thing—it can be a sign that you are working through issues. However, if at any point something happens in therapy that you don't like, say so. Therapists should be eager to work with you to resolve any problems that come up.

Types of Therapy
The type of therapy you choose should depend on your specific condition and your preferences. Some people benefit from a combination of several types of therapy. For example, cognitive and behavioral therapies are often used together to treat depression.

Cognitive Therapy. **Cognitive therapy** focuses on thoughts and beliefs, and how they influence a person's mood and actions. Its premise is that consistent dysfunctional thinking, sometimes called *cognitive distortions,* results in unwanted feelings and behaviors. See **Practical Strategies for Change: Spotting Destructive Thoughts** on page 38 for tips on how to notice cognitive distortions that you may have.

In cognitive therapy, the therapist and patient work collaboratively to identify distorted, negative thinking and replace it with more positive, reinforcing thinking. Gradually, the patient is able to think and behave in more healthful ways. Cognitive therapy is most effective in treating depressive disorders and anxiety disorders but can also be helpful—along with medication—for bipolar disorder and schizophrenia.

Behavioral Therapy. **Behavioral therapy** focuses on changing learned behaviors, with the idea that once the behavior changes, our thoughts, feelings, attitudes, and moods will follow. Common behavioral therapy techniques include exposure therapy, which is gradual exposure to an anxiety-provoking situation paired with relaxation techniques; positive reinforcement, which encourages desired behaviors; and aversion therapy, or negative reinforcement that discourages unwanted behaviors. Behavioral therapy is often used for anxiety and attention disorders.

---

cognitive therapy A type of therapy that focuses on thoughts and beliefs and how they influence your mood.

behavioral therapy A type of therapy that focuses on a patient's behavior and its relationship to psychological health.

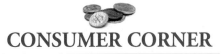

CONSUMER CORNER

Choosing a Therapist Who's Right for You

Therapy can help people with a variety of issues, but it's important to find a therapist with whom you feel comfortable and who is qualified to address your needs. Key points that you should address in your first discussion with a potential therapist are:

- Cost. Make sure you understand what the costs are and how they will be covered—whether it's low- or no-cost campus mental health care, outside care covered by an insurance plan, or paid directly out of your own pocket. If paying for care yourself, therapists will sometimes offer a sliding scale for fees, so be sure to ask.
- The therapist's credentials, education, and approach to therapy.
- Areas of specialization that the therapist has or that you would prefer. For example, specializations in bipolar disorder, childhood trauma, cognitive therapy, and so on.
- An overview of the problems you are experiencing and your goals for therapy.
- The experience the therapist has in helping people with similar problems.
- Whether or not you are taking or are interested in taking antidepressants or other medication. Keep in mind that psychologists and counselors cannot prescribe medication.
- Frequency and length of therapy session.

The information that you get from this preliminary conversation, as well as your overall impression of the therapist, will help you determine whether you would like to embark on therapy with that person. Don't be afraid to try a few different therapists or switch to someone else if you don't feel comfortable.

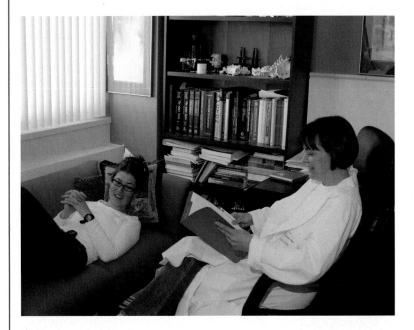

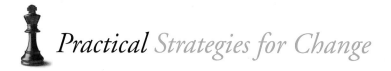
Spotting Destructive Thoughts

Do you ever find yourself thinking thoughts like, "I *never* get things right!" or "I'm such a failure!"? If so, these cognitive distortions may be the sources of a bad mood or even a serious depression. Cognitive therapy can help you learn to challenge them. Here are some thought patterns to watch out for:

- **All-or-nothing thinking.** In all-or-nothing thinking there is no middle ground. You think of situations or yourself as either perfect or a complete failure.

- **Overgeneralization.** You make a general conclusion based on a single event or experience from the past. You see one negative event as a never-ending pattern of defeat.

- **Mental filter.** You dwell excessively on a single negative detail, although everything else is positive, so that your whole outlook is darkened.

- **Disqualifying the positive.** You reject positive experiences because they "don't count" for one reason or another.

- **Jumping to conclusions.** Without any definite facts to support it, you assume that other people are thinking or feeling negatively toward you. Or, you predict that a situation will turn out badly and feel convinced that it is an already-established fact.

- **Magnification (catastrophizing) or minimization.** You exaggerate the importance of something minor (such as a poor grade on a quiz) or minimize a larger, positive event (such as acing the final exam).

- **Emotional reasoning.** You assume that your negative emotions necessarily reflect the way things really are: "I feel it, so it must be true."

- **Should statements.** You tell yourself what you "should" do, and if you don't perform, you feel guilty. This can also be applied to other people; if they don't live up to the should statement, you can feel angry, frustrated, or resentful.

- **Labeling and mislabeling.** Instead of thinking of something in a balanced way, you attach labels to yourself or others. For example, "I'm a loser," or "He's no good." Mislabeling involves describing an event with highly colored or emotionally loaded language.

- **Personalization.** You think that everything people do or say is in reaction to you; you think you are the cause of a negative external event that, in reality, you had nothing to do with.

Source: Adapted from Burns, D. D. (1989). *The feeling good handbook.* New York: William Morrow and Company, Inc.

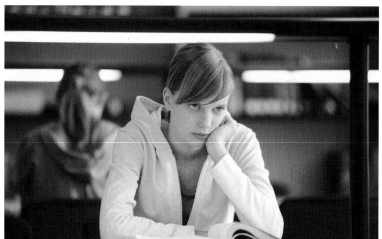

Psychodynamic Therapy. Psychodynamic therapy is founded on the idea that there are unconscious sources for a person's behavior and psychological state. In psychodynamic therapy, patients and therapists explore unresolved conflicts buried in the unconscious, often stemming from childhood experiences. The goal is to "talk through" these conflicts, understand them, and change how they affect the patient today. Psychodynamic therapy can take time, sometimes two years or more, although there are forms of psychodynamic therapy that focus on just one issue, which can be briefer. Psychodynamic therapy is often used for depressive disorders.

Positive Psychology. Positive psychology is an emerging field of psychology that focuses on increasing psychological strengths and improving happiness, rather than dwelling on psychological problems. This type of therapy aims to highlight traits such as kindness, originality, humor, optimism, generosity, and gratitude in order to help you develop a more positive outlook and foster the best parts of yourself. In positive psychology, you perform activities such as noting three good things that happen to you each day, with the goal of increasing your happiness.[55]

psychodynamic therapy A type of therapy that focuses on the unconscious sources for a patient's behavior and psychological state.

positive psychology A new field of psychology that focuses on increasing psychological strengths and improving happiness, rather than on psychological problems.

Hear prominent positive psychologist Martin Seligman explain positive psychology: www.ted.com/talks/martin_seligman_on_the_state_of_psychology.html.

On iTunes, search for Live Happy, an iPhone application that can walk you through positive psychology activities.

Watch videos of real students discussing their psychological health at: www.pearsonhighered.com/choosinghealth.

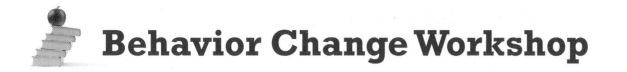

Behavior Change Workshop

To complete this workshop online, visit **www.pearsonhighered.com/choosinghealth.**

Changing long-ingrained behaviors is one of the toughest things to do. Consider the Student Stories presented throughout this chapter, and then think about your own life. How can you improve your own psychological health? What stage of behavior change are you in? (Review the stages of behavior change in Chapter 1.) Given your current stage of change, what is an appropriate goal you can set to reach the next stage?

Part I. Building the Qualities of Psychological Health

1. Take a look at Figure 2.1 on page 21. Which of the qualities of psychological health do you have? Which qualities do you think you need to work on or improve?

Have: _____

_____

Need to improve: _____

_____

2. Pick one of the qualities of psychological health that you most want to improve. Ask yourself honestly: How ready am I to commit to a change that will help me increase that quality? What stage of behavior change am I in?

Quality to improve: _____

_____

Stage of behavior change: _____

_____

3. Keeping your current stage of behavior change in mind, describe what you might do or think about as a "next step" to improve that quality of psychological health. You can use the strategies and tips presented in this chapter for ideas. Also list your timeline for making your next step.

_____

_____

_____

_____

4. In our daily lives we sometimes experience challenging situations that can put our psychological health to the test. What techniques can you use to counter roadblocks to developing your psychological health to the fullest? Again, you can refer to the information provided in this chapter.

_____

_____

_____

_____

Part II. Reducing Cognitive Distortions and Increasing Positive Thinking

Far too often we engage in negative self-talk and destructive thinking patterns. If you have thoughts that consistently weigh you down, work through the steps below to unravel that harmful pattern of thinking.

1. Take a look at the types of cognitive distortions discussed in Practical Strategies for Change: Spotting Destructive Thoughts on page 38. Do any of these thinking patterns sound familiar to you? Write down any negative thoughts you have, and list which category each fits into.

Thoughts: _____ Categories: _____

_____

_____

_____

2. Pick one of these thoughts to focus on. Do the facts of your current situation back up your negative perception? Write down all the facts that go against your current negative interpretation.

Thought: _____

Facts that go against the negative interpretation: _____

_____

_____

3. Can you think of something that has happened in the past—no matter how small—that goes against the negative self-talk you're experiencing? Write it down.

Example: I received a good grade on my last test, so although I did poorly on this test, I know I can do well at school.

_____

_____

_____

4. Imagine that a friend or a family member was thinking these things. What would you say to cheer that person up? Would things seem so bad if they weren't happening to you?

_____

_____

_____

5. Taking into account the evidence above that goes against your negative self-talk, can you think about the situation in a more optimistic way? Write down your new, more positive interpretation, and repeat it to yourself whenever your negative thought pops up.

Example: Instead of thinking "I received a bad grade on this test, I'm going to flunk out of school!" you could think "I did poorly on this test, but I've done well on tests before. Now I know to create a study plan and attend review sessions before the next test."

_____

_____

Chapter Summary

- Psychological health encompasses mental, emotional, and spiritual health.

- Psychological health allows you to express yourself effectively, manage stress and conflict, seek help for troublesome feelings when needed, focus on positive activities, use self-control, be responsible, and maintain healthy relationships.

- Autonomy and assertiveness, realism, self-esteem, optimism, prioritizing needs, communication skills, emotional intelligence, and spirituality all factor into psychological health.

- Everyone faces psychological challenges. Common concerns, such as shyness, loneliness, anger, and bad moods can often be addressed through rethinking and thoughtful self-care.

- Sometimes psychological issues become more serious mental disorders. College, with its pressures, is a high-risk time for mental health concerns.

- Depressive disorders are a serious concern for many students, arising from a mix of physical, mental, and emotional issues. Although women experience depressive disorders at higher rates than men, depressed men are more likely to suffer physical effects.

- Other mental disorders include bipolar disorder, attention disorders, anxiety disorders, and schizophrenia.

- Self-injury is the act of cutting, burning, bruising, or otherwise injuring yourself in an effort to deal with negative or overwhelming feelings.

- Suicide is an attempt to relieve overwhelming distress, not a plea for attention, and should be taken seriously. Two to three times as many women attempt suicide than men, although four times as many men actually die from suicide.

- Self-care can be a good place to start if you are having psychological problems. Self-care includes eating well, getting the right amount of sleep, exercise, realistic goals, and seeking company and support.

- Help for mental health difficulties includes a wide range of professionals offering everything from talk therapy to medication if necessary. Most campuses offer counseling and mental health services.

- There are many types of therapy including cognitive therapy, behavioral therapy, psychodynamic therapy, and positive psychology.

Test Your Knowledge

1. Psychological health refers to
   a. how your personality lets you connect with your friends.
   b. your mental health.
   c. emotional imbalance.
   d. your mental, emotional, and spiritual well-being.

2. In Maslow's hierarchy of needs pyramid
   a. basic survival needs must be met first.
   b. all of our needs can be met simultaneously.
   c. emotional needs matter relatively little.
   d. self-actualization is the first step.

3. Self-esteem is
   a. something you are born with.
   b. something that you can build throughout life.
   c. not based on childhood relationships.
   d. not important to psychological health.

4. Assertiveness is
   a. getting angry.
   b. expressing your needs and wants clearly and calmly.
   c. letting people know, up front, that they can't push you around.
   d. something you can only learn in childhood.

Get Critical

What happened:

On March 12, 2010, Matthew Zika, a junior engineering student at Cornell University died when he dropped from a bridge that crosses one of the deep gorges running through the campus. The day before, sophomore William Sinclair's body was found at the base of another bridge on campus. Matthew and William were two of six apparent student suicides at Cornell in the 2009–2010 school year, shocking the campus community and making national headlines. The university's administration responded swiftly by erecting temporary fences on six of the campus bridges, increasing the availability of appointments at the counseling center, creating a new anti-suicide website, screening all visitors to the campus's health services center for depression, and meeting with students, staff, and faculty about the importance of spotting signs of distress in students.

What do you think?

- Do you think it's the responsibility of a college to make sure its students don't commit suicide?

- How would you feel if you were screened for depression when you visited your campus health center, even if your visit was for a non-psychological illness?

- Are there any other steps Cornell could take to avoid student suicides in the future?

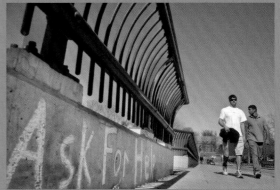

One of the bridges on the Cornell campus.

5. Spirituality matters in psychological health
   a. only if you are religious.
   b. only a little—it's a separate issue.
   c. because it connects your life to a sense of larger purpose.
   d. because it helps solve problems.

6. Depressive disorders
   a. are only a concern for women.
   b. are always driven by hormones.
   c. happen mostly in older people.
   d. none of the above

7. Antidepressants
   a. act on certain chemicals in the brain.
   b. can be stopped whenever you feel ready.
   c. usually don't have side effects.
   d. work well for everyone.

8. People who have panic attacks
   a. are usually depressed.
   b. could die.
   c. may have inherited the tendency to have them.
   d. need immediate emergency medical attention.

9. A suicidal person
   a. is not making idle threats.
   b. needs help immediately.
   c. wants relief from a situation that feels unbearable.
   d. all of the above

10. Psychiatrists
   a. specialize in group therapy.
   b. only see severe mental health cases.
   c. can prescribe medication.
   d. all of the above

Get Connected

Health Online Visit the following websites for further information about the topics in this chapter:

- American Psychological Association Help Center
  www.apa.org/helpcenter
- National Institute of Mental Health
  www.nimh.nih.gov/index.shtml
- Beliefnet
  www.beliefnet.com
- ScienceDaily: Mind & Brain
  www.sciencedaily.com/news/mind_brain/

- Anxiety Disorders Association of America
  www.adaa.org
- National Suicide Prevention Lifeline
  www.suicidepreventionlifeline.org/
- American Psychological Association Psychologist Locator
  http://locator.apa.org
- Active Minds
  www.activeminds.org/

Website links are subject to change. To access updated Web links, please visit **www.pearsonhighered.com/choosinghealth.**

References

i. National Institute of Mental Health. (2008). *The numbers count: Mental disorders in America*. Retrieved from http://www.nimh.nih.gov/health/publications/the-numbers-count-mental-disorders-in-america/index.shtml

ii. National Institute of Mental Health. (n.d.). Panic disorder. Bipolar disorder. Obsessive-compulsive disorder. Retrieved from http://www.nimh.nih.gov/health/topics/index.shtml

iii. American College Health Association. (2008). American College Health Association National College Health Assessment (ACHA-NCHA II) Reference Group Executive Summary Fall 2008. Retrieved from http://www.acha-ncha.org/docs/ACHA-NCHA_Reference_Group_ExecutiveSummary_Fall2008.pdf

iv. National Center for Injury Prevention and Control. (2009). *Suicide: Facts at a glance*. Retrieved from http://www.cdc.gov/violenceprevention/pdf/Suicide-DataSheet-a.pdf

1. Marano, H. (2004). A nation of wimps. *Psychology Today, Nov/Dec*, 58–70, 103.

2. Stinson, D., Logel, C., Zanna, M., Holmes, J., Cameron, J., Wood, J., & Spenser, S. J. (2008). The cost of lower self-esteem: Testing a self- and social-bonds model of health. *Journal of Personality and Social Psychology, 94*(3), 412–428.

3. Gould, D., Dieffenbach, K., & Moffett, A. (2002). Psychological characteristics and their development in Olympic champions. *Journal of Applied Sport Psychology, 14*, 172–204.

4. Pinquart, M., Frohlich, C., & Silbereisen, R. (2007). Optimism, pessimism, and change of psychological well-being in cancer patients. *Psychology, Health & Medicine, 12*(4), 421–432.

5. Greene, L., & Burke, G. (2007). Beyond self-actualization. *Journal of Health and Human Services Administration, Fall*, 116–128.

6. Mayer, J. D., Salovey, P., & Caruso, D. R. (2004). Emotional intelligence: Theory, findings, and implications. *Psychological Inquiry, 15* (3), 197–215. Retrieved from http://www.unh.edu/emotional_intelligence/EI%20Assets/Reprints...EI%20Proper/EI2004MayerSaloveyCarusotarget.pdf

7. Bradberry, T., & Su, L. (2003). Ability-versus skill-based assessment of emotional intelligence. *Psicothema, 18*, supl., pp. 59–66. Retrieved from http://www.psicothema.com/pdf/3277.pdf

8. Day, A., Therrien, D., & Carroll, S. (2005). Predicting psychological health: Assessing the incremental validity of emotional intelligence beyond personality, type A behavior, and daily hassles. *European Journal of Personality, 19*, 519–536.

9. Koenig, H. G., Idler, E., Kasl, S., Hays, J. C., George, L. K., Musick, M., . . . Benson, H. (1999). Religion, spirituality, and medicine: A rebuttal to skeptics. *International Journal of Psychiatry in Medicine, 29*(2), 123–131.

10. Jantos, M., & Kiat, H. (2007). Prayer as medicine: How much have we learned? *Medical Journal of Australia, 186*(10), 851–853.

11. Mayo Clinic. (2009). *Meditation: Take a stress-reduction break wherever you are.* Retrieved from http://www.mayoclinic.com/health/meditation/HQ01070

12. Milne, D. (2007). People can learn markers on road to resilience. *Psychiatric News, 42*(2), 5. Retrieved from http://www.pn.psychiatryonline.org/cgi/content/full/42/2/5

13. Saunder, P. L., & Chester, A. (2008). Shyness and the Internet: Social problem or panacea? *Computers in Human Behavior, 24*(6), 2649–2658.

14. Jones, W. H., Briggs, S. R., & Smith, T. G. (1986). Shyness: Conceptualization and measurement. *Journal of Personality and Social Psychology, 51*(3), 629–639.

15. Gonda, X., Fountoulakis, K. N., Rihmer, Z., Lazary, J., Laszik, A., & Akiskal, K. K. (2009). Towards a genetically validated new affective temperament scale: A delineation of the temperament phenotype of 5-HTTLPR using the TEMPS-A. *Journal of Affective Disorders, Jan, 112* (1–3), 19–29.

16. Arbelle, S., Benjamin, J., Golin, M., Kremer, I., Belmaker, R. H., Ebstein R. P. (2003). Relation of shyness in grade school children to the genotype for the long form of the serotonin transporter promoter region polymorphism. *American Journal of Psychiatry, 160*(4), 671–676.

17. Carducci, B. J., & Zimbardo, P. G. (1995). Are you shy? *Psychology Today, November.* Retrieved from http://www.psychologytoday.com/articles/200910/are-you-shy.

18. Swami, V., Chamorro-Premuzic, T., Sinniah, D., Maniam, T., Kannan, K., Stanistreet, D., & Furnham, A. (2007). General health mediates the relationship between loneliness, life satisfaction and depression. *Social Psychiatry and Psychiatric Epidemiology, 42,* 161–166.

19. Lin, C. C., Rogot, E., Johnson, N. J., Sorlie, P. D., & Arias, E. (2003). A further study of life expectancy by socioeconomic factors in the National Longitudinal Mortality Study. *Ethnicity and Disease, 13*(2), 240–247.

20. Bettencourt, B., Talley, A., Benjamin, A., & Valentine, J. (2006). Personality and aggressive behavior under provoking and neutral conditions: A meta-analytic review. *Psychological Bulletin, 132*(5), 751–777.

21. László, K. D., Janszky, I., & Ahnve, S. (2008). Anger expression and prognosis after a coronary event in women. *International Journal of Cardiology.* Advance online publication.

22. Vrana, S. (2007). Psychophysiology of anger: Introduction to the special issue. *International Journal of Psychophysiology, 66*(2), 93–94.

23. Kubzansky, L. D., & Kawachi, I. (2000). Going to the heart of the matter: Do negative emotions cause coronary heart disease? *Journal of Psychosomatic Research, 48,* 323–337.

24. Bushman, B., Bonacci, A., Pedersen, W., Vasquez, E., & Miller, N. (2005). Chewing on it can chew you up: Effects of rumination on triggered displaced aggression. *Journal of Personality and Social Psychology, 88*(6), 969–983.

25. National Institute of Mental Health. (2008). The numbers count: Mental disorders in America. Retrieved from http://www.nimh.nih.gov/health/publications/the-numbers-count-mental-disorders-in-america/index.shtml

26. American College Health Association. (2008). American College Health Association National College Health Assessment (ACHA-NCHA II) Reference Group Executive Summary Fall 2008. Retrieved from http://www.acha-ncha.org/reports_ACHA-NCHAII.html

27. World Health Organization. (n.d.). *Depression.* Retrieved from http://www.who.int/mental_health/management/depression/definition/en/

28. American Psychiatric Association. (2000). *Diagnostic and statistical manual of mental disorders DSM-IV-TR* (4th ed.). Arlington, VA: American Psychiatric Publishing.

29. Levinson, D. (2005). The genetics of depression: A review. *Biological Psychiatry,* 60(2), 84-92. Retrieved from http://www.journals.elsevierhealth.com/periodicals/bps/article/S0006-3223(05)01013-9/pdf

30. National Institute of Mental Health. (2009). *Depression.* Retrieved from http://www.nimh.nih.gov/health/publications/depression/index.shtml

31. WebMD. (2009). *Depression guide: Depression in women.* Retrieved from http://www.webmd.com/depression/guide/depression-women

32. Fertick, A. K.,. (2002). Depression as an antecedent to heart disease among women and men in the NHANESI study: National Health and Nutrition Examination Survey. *Archives of Internal Medicine, 160*(9). 1261–1268.

33. Centers for Disease Control and Prevention. (2008). Prevalence of self-reported postpartum depressive symptoms—17 states, 2004–2005. *Morbidity and Mortality Weekly Report, 57*(14), 361–366. Retrieved from http://www.cdc.gov/mmwr/preview/mmwrhtml/mm5714a1.htm

34. National Center for Injury Prevention and Control. (2009). *Suicide: Facts at a glance.* Retrieved from http://www.cdc.gov/violenceprevention/pdf/Suicide-DataSheet-a.pdf

35. Bridge, J. A., Iyengar, S., Salary, C. B., Barbe, R. P., Birmaher, B., Pincus, . . . Brent, D. A. (2007). Clinical response and risk for reported suicidal ideation and suicide attempts in pediatric antidepressant treatment, a meta-analysis of randomized controlled trials. *Journal of the American Medical Association, 297*(15), 1683–1696.

36. Kadison, R. (2005). Getting an edge—Use of stimulants and antidepressants in college. *New England Journal of Medicine, 353*(September 15), 1089–1091.

37. National Institute of Mental Health. (2009). *Bipolar disorder.* Retrieved from http://www.nimh.nih.gov/health/publications/bipolar-disorder/index.shtml

38. Hoza, B., Mrug, S., Gerdes, A., Hinshaw, S., Bukowski, W., Gold, J., . . . Eugene, A. L. (2005). What aspects of peer relationships are impaired in children with attention-deficit/hyperactivity disorder?. *Journal of Consulting and Clinical Psychology, 73*(3), 411–423.

39. Waring, M. E., & Lapane, K. L. (2008). Overweight in children and adolescents in relation to attention-deficit/hyperactivity disorder: Results from a national sample. *Pediatrics, 112*(1), e1–e6.

40. Gentile, J. P., Atiq, R., & Gillig, P. M. (2006). Adult ADHD: Diagnosis, differential diagnosis, and medication management. *Psychiatry* 3(8), 24–30.

41. DuPaul, G. J., & Weyandt, L. L. (2004, August). *College students with ADHD: What do we know and where do we go from here?.* Paper presented at the annual meeting of the Children and Adults With Attention-Deficit/Hyperactivity Disorder, Nashville, TN. Retrieved from http://www.allacademic.com/meta/p116618_index.html

42. Price, M. (2007). Adults with ADHD see a problem, and then lose control. *Monitor on Psychology, 38*(11), 12.

43. National Institute of Mental Health. (2009). *Panic disorder.* Retrieved from http://www.nimh.nih.gov/health/publications/anxiety-disorders/panic-disorder.shtml

44. National Institute of Mental Health. (2009). *Social phobia (social anxiety disorder).* Retrieved from http://www.nimh.nih.gov/health/topics/social-phobia-social-anxiety-disorder/index.shtml.

45. Anxiety Disorders Association of America, (2007). *The effects of social anxiety disorder on personal relationships: Survey results.* p. 1–5.

46. Carducci, B. J., & Nethery, K. T. (2007, August). *High school shooters as cynically shy: Content analysis and characteristic features.* Poster session presented at the 115th annual convention of the American Psychological Association, San Francisco, CA.

47. Rosenthal, J., Jacobs, L., Marcus, M., & Katzman, M. (2007). Beyond shy: When to suspect social anxiety disorder. *The Journal of Family Practice, 56*(5), 369–374.

48. U. S. Department of Health and Human Services, U. S. Public Health Service. (2001). *Mental health: Culture, race, and ethnicity; A supplement to Mental health: A report of the surgeon general.* Rockville, MD: U. S. Department of Health and Human Services, Substance Abuse and Mental Health Services Administration, Center for Mental Health Services. Retrieved from http://www.surgeongeneral.gov/library/mentalhealth/cre/sma-01-3613.pdf

49. U. S. Department of Veterans Affairs, National Center for PTSD. (2009). *What is PTSD?* Retrieved from http://www.ptsd.va.gov/public/pages/what-is-ptsd.asp

50. National Institute of Mental Health. (2009). *Schizophrenia.* Retrieved from http://www.nimh.nih.gov/health/publications/schizophrenia/index.shtml

51. Whitlock, J., Powers, J., & Eckenrode, J. (2006). The virtual cutting edge: The Internet and adolescent self-injury. *Developmental Psychology, 42*(3), 407–417.

52. Young, R., van Beinum, M., Sweeting H., & West, P. (2007). Young people who self-harm. *British Journal of Psychiatry, 191,* 44–49.

53. National Institute of Mental Health. (2009). *Suicide prevention in the U. S.: Statistics and prevention.* Retrieved from www.nimh.gov/health/publications/suicide-in-the-us-statistics-and-prevention.shtml

54. Baser, R. S., Neighbors, H. W., Caldwell, C. H., & Jackson, J. (2009). 12-month and lifetime prevalence of suicide attempts among black adolescents in the National Survey of American Life. *Journal of the American Academy of Child and Adolescent Psychiatry, 48*(3), 271–282.

55. Seligman, M. E. P., Steen, T. A., Park, N., & Peterson, C. (2005). Positive psychology progress. *American Psychologist, 60*(5), 410–421.

3 Stress Management

- Year after year, college students report **stress** as the number one **obstacle** to their academic achievement.[i]

- In a recent survey, **19.3%** of college students reported that **sleep difficulties** negatively affected their academic performance.[ii]

- **29%** of adults aged 18–29 report feeling **extreme stress levels** of 8, 9, or 10 on a 10-point scale.[iii]

LEARNING OBJECTIVES

DEFINE *stress, eustress,* and *distress.*

DESCRIBE the body's stress response.

EXPLAIN why chronic, long-term stress is harmful.

IDENTIFY common sources of stress.

DESCRIBE strategies for effectively managing stress.

ASSESS the sources of stress in your own life.

CREATE a personalized plan for stress management.

Health Online icons are found throughout the chapter, directing you to web links, videos, podcasts, and other useful online resources.

As a student, you live with stress every day.

Assignments, exams, relationships, worrying about the future, and financial challenges can all add up to plenty of pressure as you navigate your college years. But take heart: while you may not always be able to control the sources of stress in your life, you have a great deal of control over how you choose to *deal* with stress. In fact, how you manage stress can have a profound effect on your health.

In this chapter, we will describe the body's physical response to stress, explain why uncontrolled, long-term stress is harmful, and introduce several strategies for reducing and managing stress. By the end of the chapter, you will have the tools to analyze the sources of stress in your own life and to create a personalized action plan for better stress management. To begin, let's first examine what we mean by *stress.*

What Is Stress?

The term **stress** is often used to mean different things. It can refer to external factors—such as being stuck in a traffic jam—that create feelings of tension and anxiety. It can refer to physical or emotional responses—such as sweaty palms or a feeling of panic—that result when a person faces a challenging situation (for example, a job interview). It can even refer to the *anticipation* of discomfort that a person may feel about an impending deadline or the prospect of public speaking. For the purposes of this textbook, we will define *stress* as the collective psychobiological condition that occurs in reaction to a disruptive, unexpected, or exciting stimulus. We will use the term **stressor** to refer to any physical or psychological condition, event, or factor that causes stress.

We usually think of stress as unpleasant, but not all stressors are negative. Exciting, positive events—such as going on a first date, or winning a big game—can also be stressful. Hans Selye, a pioneering stress scientist, coined the term **eustress** ("eu" = "good"), his term for stress resulting from positive stressors. He called stress resulting from nega-

tive stressors **distress,** a reflection of the harmful effects these stressors often have on the mind and body.[1] Think about how you felt the last time your favorite athlete or sports team came from behind at the last minute to win. Then think about the last time you got a lower grade than you had hoped, or realized you had blown your budget for the month. The likely differences in your feelings—amped-up excitement in the first case, dismay and worry in the second—help illustrate the distinctions between *eustress* and *distress.* However, as we'll see next, your body's response to both types of stress is the same.

The Body's Stress Response

If *stress* is the body's state of disruption resulting from a *stressor,* then the **stress response** is the specific psychobiological changes that occur as the body attempts to cope with the stressor and return to **homeostasis,** or balance. Imagine you are walking to your car late at night in a poorly-lit parking lot. Suddenly and without warning, you feel a hand on your

stress The collective psychobiological condition that occurs in reaction to a disruptive, unexpected, or exciting stimulus.

stressor Any physical or psychological condition, event, or factor that causes positive or negative stress.

eustress Stress resulting from positive stressors.

distress Stress resulting from negative stressors.

stress response The specific psychobiological changes that occur as the body attempts to cope with a stressor and return to homeostasis.

homeostasis The body's desired state of physiological equilibrium or balance.

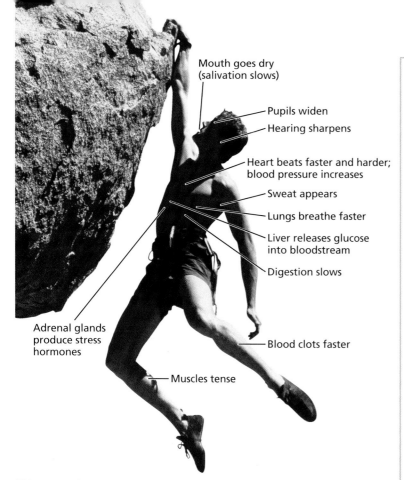

Mouth goes dry
(salivation slows)

Pupils widen

Hearing sharpens

Heart beats faster and harder;
blood pressure increases

Sweat appears

Lungs breathe faster

Liver releases glucose
into bloodstream

Digestion slows

Adrenal glands
produce stress
hormones

Blood clots faster

Muscles tense

Figure 3.1 The fight-or-flight response. The fight-or-flight response is a set of physical reactions that prepares you to deal with a perceived threat.

 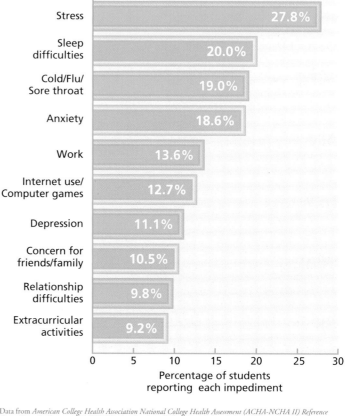
Top 10 Impediments to Academic Performance

	Percentage
Stress	27.8%
Sleep difficulties	20.0%
Cold/Flu/ Sore throat	19.0%
Anxiety	18.6%
Work	13.6%
Internet use/ Computer games	12.7%
Depression	11.1%
Concern for friends/family	10.5%
Relationship difficulties	9.8%
Extracurricular activities	9.2%

Percentage of students
reporting each impediment

Data from *American College Health Association National College Health Assessment (ACHA-NCHA II) Reference Group Executive Summary, Fall 2009* by the American College Health Association, 2009, retrieved from http://www.acha-ncha.org/reports_ACHA-NCHAII.html.

shoulder. Before you realize it's just a friend sneaking up on you, you are likely to experience the following physical reactions **(Figure 3.1)**:

- Increased heart rate
- A rush of adrenaline
- Trembling
- Sweating
- Rapid breathing

At the same time, many other physical reactions are likely occurring throughout your body:

- Your *adrenal glands*, two small organs sitting on top of your kidneys, produce stress hormones such as **cortisol** and **adrenaline** that speed up your heart rate and generally prepare your body to face the threat.
- Your blood pressure increases, in response to the release of adrenaline.
- Your pupils dilate, sharpening your vision.
- Your circulatory system, anticipating injury, starts producing blood-clotting factor.
- Your digestive system slows as blood diverts to the large muscles in your arms and legs, giving you more strength for fighting, running, or defending yourself.

- Your liver releases glucose into your bloodstream, to fuel physical action if necessary.
- Tiny hairs stand on end all over your body, a reflection of your heightened state of alarm.

cortisol Adrenal gland hormone that is secreted at higher levels during the stress response.

adrenaline Adrenal gland hormone that is secreted at higher levels during the stress response; also called *epinephrine*.

fight-or-flight response A series of physiological reactions to a stressor designed to enable the body to stand and fight or to flee.

These physical reactions comprise one of your body's most primal reactions to stress: the **fight-or-flight response.** This instantaneous set of reactions, first described by stress scientist Walter Cannon, evolved as a survival mechanism to help humans escape physical danger. Your fight-or-flight response temporarily boosts your strength and reflexes to physically enable you to dive out of the way of a fast-approaching car, or fight off a would-be mugger.

The fight-or-flight response was certainly useful to our early ancestors, who could not have survived their dangerous "eat-or-be-eaten" world without it. In modern life, however, the fight-or-

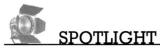

Science Discovers Stress

The science of stress studies began by accident. In the 1930s, Hans Selye, a young Hungarian-born endocrinologist, was immersed in a study of hormones at McGill University in Montreal. Selye injected lab rats with a variety of hormones and observed their responses. He found that regardless of which hormone he used, the rats all seemed to demonstrate the same basic physical re-actions each time, including enlargement of the adrenal cortex; atrophy of the thymus, spleen, and lymph nodes; and stomach ulcers. This led Selye to wonder if he could be observing something broader than merely the rats' responses to specific hormone injections. Were the rats reacting to something more general—to some other "external pressure" he was applying?

Selye decided to find out, using the simplest and cheapest method he could find. He set the hormones aside, and looked for a different external pressure to apply to the rats. He found inspiration in the frigid weather outside the walls of his laboratory. He placed a group of rats in a box and left them outside on his windowsill overnight. The next morning, the unhappy rats reacted in much the same way as those that had previously been injected with hormones. The rats' overall behavior, Selye surmised, had much more to do with external pressures—introduced hormones, freezing weather—than any one specific substance or force. In short, the rats' response reflected *stress.*

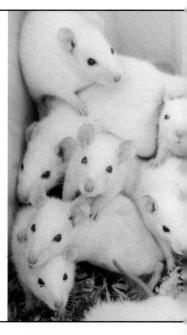

flight response can be unhelpful or even harmful. Most of our modern-day stressors are not the extreme physical threats that the fight-or-flight response is designed to resolve. Yet fight-or-flight kicks in *any* time you face a stressor—even when that stressor is mostly emotional or psychological, such as the frustration of being stuck behind a slow driver on the highway, or finding yourself standing in a long grocery line. If you experience fight-or-flight too often, this response can take a powerful toll on your body and your health.

The General Adaptation Syndrome

Our bodies are always striving to stay in physiological balance (homeostasis). But stressors disrupt this equilibrium, forcing our bodies to respond and attempt to reinstate it. One of the best-known theories explaining the biology of this **adaptive response** is the **general adaptation syndrome (GAS),** developed by Hans Selye **(Figure 3.2).** The GAS consists of three stages:[2]

- **Alarm.** When first confronted by a stressor, the body activates the fight-or-flight response, boosts levels of stress hormones, and increases heart rate. When you first realize you've completely forgotten about a quiz in class tomorrow, and haven't left much time in your evening to study, the rush of worry you may feel marks this stage.

- **Resistance.** As the stressor continues, your body continues to turn to its internal resources to deal with the stressor and try to restore balance. As you get ready to cram for the quiz, for example, you may not feel as worried, and the little jolt of adrenaline you sensed at first may subside. But as you resolve to stay up late to study, your body may continue to produce slightly elevated levels of stress hormones to help keep you awake.

adaptive response Protective physiological adaptations in response to stressors.

general adaptation syndrome (GAS) An adaptive response consisting of three stages (alarm, resistance, exhaustion) through which the body strives to maintain or restore homeostasis.

- **Exhaustion.** After long exposure to the stressor, your body's ability to adapt eventually wears out, and you cannot continue to function normally. You can probably withstand one late night cramming for a quiz, but if you repeatedly put off studying until the last minute, cutting into your sleep night after night, your entire school experience may suffer as you become sick or exhausted from too little sleep and too much worry.

If you think about how stressful situations make you feel, both mentally and physically, you may recognize these phases in some of your own experiences.

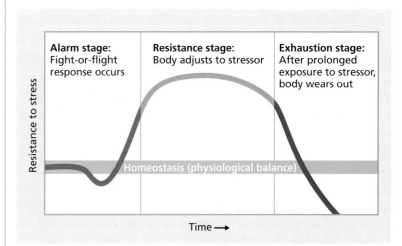

Figure 3.2 The general adaptation syndrome. The general adaptation syndrome, developed by Hans Selye, is a theory that attempts to explain the biology of stress.

Stressed Out

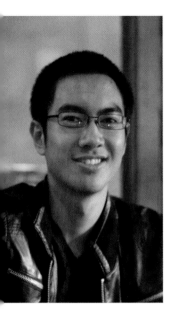

"Hi, I'm Steven. I'm pre-med, double majoring in chemistry and biology. I also volunteer at the local children's hospital and am a research assistant at one of my professor's labs. I work in the lab three days a week, and since my afternoons are busy with classes and hospital work, I wake up at 5 a.m. to take a bus to the lab by 6 a.m. I'm completely exhausted from my long mornings, and then I have to hop on another bus to get to the hospital. I try to catch up on sleep on the weekends, but I never feel completely rested. I'm really frustrated with myself because it seems like a lot of other students are able to take on similar schedules without getting so tired. I feel like I need a caffeine drip to keep me going!"

1: Identify at least three stressors that Steven is dealing with. Are these stressors caused by *eustress* or *distress*?

2: What are the long-term health risks if Steven does nothing to reduce or manage his stress load?

Do you have a story similar to Steven's? Share your story at **www.pearsonhighered.com/choosinghealth.**

Allostasis and Allostatic Overload

In recent years, scientists have concluded that the stress response itself can take a toll on our bodies. **Allostasis** refers to the short-term adaptive processes that help the body deal with the challenges of stress. It literally means "maintaining stability (homeostasis) through change." For example, the release of stress hormones such as adrenaline and cortisol is an allostatic response. While this response may be effective in addressing stress in the short term, long-term elevation of these hormones can cause harm. When allostatic responses are prolonged to the point that they cause wear and tear on the body, the condition is termed **allostatic overload.** You may recognize *allostatic overload* as the feeling of being mentally and physically stressed out. Scientists currently studying stress now believe that this overwhelmed feeling contributes to many of our major health concerns.[3]

Health Effects of Chronic Stress

Physical symptoms associated with stress include fatigue, lying awake at night, headache, upset stomach, muscle tension, change in sex drive, teeth grinding, dizziness, feeling a tightness in the chest, and change in menstrual cycle (for women). Psychological symptoms of stress include feeling angry or irritable, lacking interest or motivation in daily activities, feeling anxious or nervous, and feeling sad or depressed.[4]

When your body maintains the fight-or-flight response for extended periods of time, **chronic stress syndrome** can develop. Chronic stress syndrome is a collection of symptoms resulting from the long-term effects of prolonged exposure to the body's physiological stress responses **(Figure 3.3).** While the specific effects of chronic stress vary from person to person, they can ultimately affect nearly every system of the body.

allostasis The body's process of restoring homeostasis through short-term adaptive mechanisms.

allostatic overload The wear and tear the body experiences as the result of the continuous or repeated demands of allostasis.

chronic stress syndrome Collection of symptoms resulting from the long-term effects of prolonged exposure to the body's physiological stress responses.

Effects on the Cardiovascular System

The fight-or-flight response causes the heart to work harder and faster, raising blood pressure. Over time, high blood pressure can damage internal organs, greatly increasing the risk of heart disease or a heart attack. Stress can also indirectly affect heart disease incidence by increasing the likelihood of its risk factors. For example, those under chronic stress may overeat and exercise less, thereby increasing their risk of obesity. Obesity increases cholesterol levels and diabetes risk, and both are leading risk factors for heart disease.

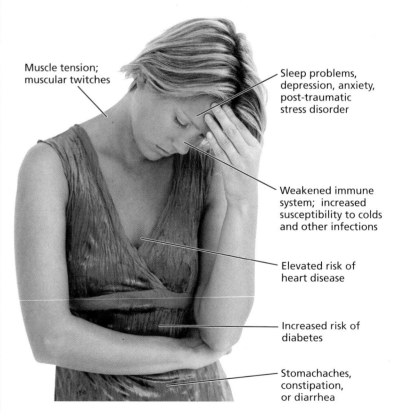

Muscle tension; muscular twitches

Sleep problems, depression, anxiety, post-traumatic stress disorder

Weakened immune system; increased susceptibility to colds and other infections

Elevated risk of heart disease

Increased risk of diabetes

Stomachaches, constipation, or diarrhea

Figure 3.3 **Health effects of long-term stress.** Chronic stress can have long-term health effects, ranging from stomachaches to increased risk of disease.

Effects on the Digestive System

When the fight-or-flight response constantly directs blood away from the stomach and intestines, the digestive system doesn't get the fuel it needs to do its job. This can result in stomachache, constipation, or diarrhea. Stress hormones can also affect the body's ability to regulate blood sugar levels, which may increase the risk of diabetes.

Effects on the Immune System

Do you always seem to get sick during finals week? At the end of the term, a quarter or semester's worth of stress may weaken your body's ability to fight off viruses.

Psychoneuroimmunology is the study of interactions among psychological processes, the nervous system, hormones, and the immune system.[5] When acute stress activates the fight-or-flight response, your body releases cortisol and other stress hormones. In the short term, these hormones enable you to effectively respond to stressors and may actually strengthen your immune system. However, long-term overproduction of these hormones due to chronic stressors can suppress the immune system, reducing your ability to fight off infection.[6] Long-term exposure to cortisol can cause immune cells to decrease, promote weight gain, lead to the breakdown of muscle, increase fluid retention, and decrease inflammatory response. In addition, the fear, tension, anxiety, or depression that accompany stress may also increase heart rate or blood pressure, which can compromise your immune system further.

Even stress caused by relatively minor events such as academic exams can cause temporary increases in white blood cell counts.[7] Such demands on the immune system may leave you vulnerable to colds, trigger flare-ups of asthma or cold sores, and put you at risk of developing more serious diseases.

psychoneuroimmunology The study of the interactions among psychological processes, the nervous system, hormones, and the immune system.

Effects on Mood, Mind, and Mental Health

Chronic stress is an important risk factor for many mental health problems. Stress contributes to the development of depression, panic attacks, anxiety disorders, eating disorders, and post-traumatic stress disorder (PTSD). Unfortunately, stress and these mental health problems often form a vicious cycle where one feeds

☺ *Practical Strategies For Health*

Recognizing the Signs of Stress Overload

It's important to be able to recognize the warning signs of too much stress before they add up to a serious health problem. While many people find the following symptoms common, keep in mind that stress affects different individuals in different ways. You may have less typical signs of stress, but they still merit the same attention.

Emotional warning signs

- Anxiety
- Sleep disruption
- Anger and agitation
- Trouble concentrating
- Unproductive worry
- Frequent mood swings
- Depression

Physical warning signs

- Stooped posture
- Sweaty palms

- Chronic fatigue
- Weight loss or weight gain
- Migraine or tension headaches
- Neck aches
- Digestive problems
- Asthma attacks
- Physical symptoms that your doctor can't attribute to another condition

Behavioral warning signs

- Overreacting to problems or difficult situations
- Increased use of alcohol, tobacco, or drugs
- Unusually impulsive behavior
- Withdrawing from relationships or contact with others
- Feeling "burned out" on school or work
- Frequent bouts of crying
- Feelings of anxiety or panic

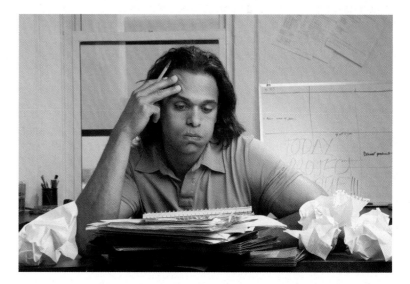

If you are experiencing the warning signs of stress overload, be proactive and seek the solutions that are right for you. Use the stress management techniques outlined in this chapter to help you manage your stress load. Also, consult your college health center, which may offer classes, workshops, or individual and group counseling to further help you cope with stress.

the other, complicating treatment. People experiencing severe long-term stress may develop depression, for example, only to have their condition create more stress in their lives.[8] (For more information on other mental health concerns, see Chapter 2.)

Common Causes of Stress

You have assignments to complete, tests to take, and papers to write. You may be juggling school and work, or facing loans and credit card debt. First-year students and sophomores, newer to the pressures of undergraduate academics, often face more schoolwork stress than juniors or seniors.[9] Meanwhile, seniors close to getting their diploma need to grapple with the question of what to do after graduation.

As we've mentioned, any event that triggers your stress response is called a *stressor*. In today's world, many stressors are psychological, emotional, or biological. A looming deadline, angry parents, or a nasty case of food poisoning all count as potential stressors with the ability to throw your body into a state of heightened alarm. Some stressors come and go fairly quickly, such as getting called on in class or taking a big exam. Others may have effects that linger much longer, such as a bad breakup or the death of someone you love. Chronic stressors reflect long-term, life-changing events, such as the struggle to recover from a serious injury. And some stressors, such as childhood abuse, can continue to haunt a person's emotions and psyche long after the actual event itself has passed.[6]

Financial Stressors

The economy's in a slump. Perhaps one or both of your parents are out of a job, and you are starting to worry about how you will pay for tuition next term—not to mention your student loans after you graduate. Maybe you already have credit card debt. Almost everyone must deal with some form of financial stress in their lifetime. **Practical Strategies for Change: Coping with Financial Stress** provides some tips for relieving money-related stress.

Daily Hassles

The school registration office says they can't find the check you sent to cover your tuition this term, even though your bank says the check has been cashed. You've completely gone over your limit of cell phone minutes for the month, and you can't find the research material you need for a class paper because your Internet connection has crashed. These problems may sound small, but daily hassles can add up to a significant source of stress.

Academic Pressure

College represents a great opportunity—and a big responsibility. To graduate, get good internships, and land a fantastic job, you need to perform. As a student, you probably worry about doing well in school. But studies have shown that too much anxiety about grades, exams, papers, and deadlines can actually prevent you from being successful in college.[10]

Practical Strategies for Change

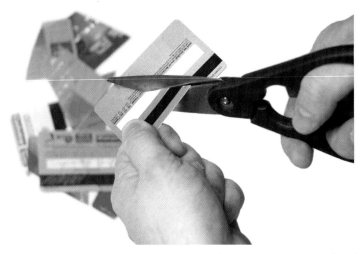

Managing Financial Stress

"Hi, I'm Will. I'm halfway through my freshman year. I took out a large student loan to pay for school, but after paying tuition and room and board, I'm realizing there is not a whole lot left to pay for everything else—like my books, car, and groceries. My mom also just lost her job, so I don't want to ask my family for money. On top of everything else, tuition is supposed to go up next year! I'm just not sure how I'll ever pay all of my bills—not to mention that student loan when I graduate. Sometimes I feel pretty overwhelmed."

1: Based on what you've read in this chapter, what advice would you give Will to better manage his financial stressors?

2: Think about the financial stressors in your life. To address them, ask yourself: Do you have a plan for how to carefully track your spending? How much of what you spend money on is truly essential (versus a luxury)? What can you do to lessen your expenses? What can you do to increase your income?

Do you have a story similar to Will's? Share your story at www.pearsonhighered.com/choosinghealth.

Job-Related Stressors

Show up to work on time, excel at your job to get that raise—and try not to think about all the school assignments you have hanging over your head at the same time! Many college students work to ease the financial pressure of school, but earning money brings stress of its own when it cuts into your time for classwork.

Social Stressors

Friends, relationships, and the opinions of others all carry the potential to trigger or reduce stress. Strong, supportive social networks can do a great deal to help carry you through tough times. Researchers have discovered, for instance, that the perceived emotional support college students experience using a social networking site like Facebook can lower their stress levels.[11] Social interactions that aren't supportive, on the other hand, increase stress. In addition, members of minority groups may perceive discrimination or isolation to be a source of stress on campuses.[12] The box **Diversity & Health: Stress Through the Lenses of Sex, Race, Age, and Geography** on page 52 examines the differences in how men, women, and members of different demographic groups perceive the stress in their lives.

Major Life Events

Traumas such as a bad breakup or a death in the family are obvious stressors. But positive, exhilarating events such as starting college, graduating, or getting married can also bring heavy doses of stress. In 1967, psychiatrists Thomas Holmes and Richard Rahe published what has come to be known as Holmes and Rahe's Social Readjustment Rating Scale (SRRS), an inventory of 43 stressful life events that can increase the risk of illness.[13] The scale assigns "life change units" from 1–100 for each stressful event, such as the death of a spouse (100 units), divorce (73 units), imprisonment (63 units), death of a close family member (63 units), personal injury or illness (53 units), marriage (50 units), and job loss (47 units). The scale also includes more minor stressors, such as Christmas (12 units), a change in sleeping habits (16 units), and a change in living conditions (25 units). According to this scale, the higher the number of "life change units" that a person accumulates over a given year, the greater that person's risk of illness.

An adaptation of Holmes and Rahe's scale is the College Undergraduate Stress Scale developed by Michael Renner and R. Scott Mackin.[14] You can use this scale in the **Self-Assessment** on page 53 to assign ratings to common stressors encountered by college students and gauge the stress load in your own life.

Environmental Stressors

Environmental stressors are factors in your living or working environments that you find disruptive. Examples of environmental stressors include poor air quality, pollution, noise, toxic chemicals, and severe weather—as well as living in an unsafe neighborhood, having an annoying roommate, and dealing with a long commute. Digital technologies (such as cell phones or other mobile hand-held devices) that beep at you every few minutes to alert you to text messages or voicemails can also be a source of environmental stress.

Internal Stressors

Worries, critical thoughts, and the demands we place on ourselves represent some of our most constant stressors. One study of university honors students, for example, found that those highly critical of themselves were more prone to feelings of stress, depression, and hopelessness.[15]

In an era where fewer of our stressors are physical, we assign increasing value to psychological or emotional stressors, and our bodies' stress response kicks in accordingly.[16] Do you find yourself overreacting to small problems? Do you view every task as critical when many of them really aren't? Are you often imagining horrific consequences for your actions that will probably, in reality, never come to pass? Do you procrastinate? These are all examples of situations you have the power to control or minimize, and thereby reduce your stress level.

To be sure, at some point in our lives, we all face stressors inflicted on us by events beyond our control. But often, many of us suffer from stress brought about by our own thoughts and actions. The good news is that if we are the creators of our own stress, we can also find ways to lessen and manage that stress, as we will discuss shortly.

Stress Through the Lenses of

Sex, Race, Age, and Geography

In 2009, the American Psychological Association conducted a national survey of how Americans perceived the stress in their lives. Among the survey's findings:

Stress

- Stress levels for Americans on a whole seemed to peak in 2008 but are still high. 24% of respondents rated their stress levels as an 8, 9, or 10 on a 10-point scale.

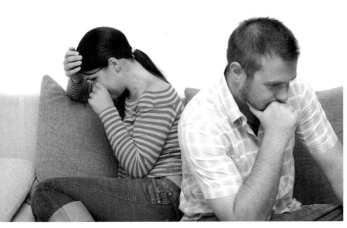

Women, in general, report higher levels of stress than men.

Sex

- Women reported higher levels of stress than men, across all categories. A greater percentage of women than men cited the economy, money, family health problems, and housing costs as significant stressors.

- Significantly more women than men reported experiencing headaches, depression, sadness, nervousness, anxiety, and a lack of energy and motivation as symptoms of stress.

Race

- Hispanics are more likely than Caucasians or African Americans to cite money as a significant source of stress. African Americans are more likely than Caucasians or Hispanics to cite personal health concerns and family concerns as sources of stress. Caucasians are the group most likely to cite work as a source of significant stress.

Age

- 18–30 year-olds see money as their most significant stressor. 31–63 year-olds see work as their most significant stressor. People aged 64 and older are less likely to feel significant stress about most areas except personal and family health concerns.

Geography

- Americans living in the South reported the highest levels of stress related to the economy and family responsibilities.

- Although stress levels are similar across the country, Americans living in the Midwest reported slightly higher stress levels overall.

- Adults in the East and West most commonly use exercise or walking as a stress management technique. Adults in the Midwest and South most commonly use listening to music as a stress management technique.

Data from *Stress in America 2009* by the American Psychological Association. 2009.

View the results of the complete Stress in America survey at **www.apa.org/news/press/releases/stress/index.aspx.**

> **"If we are the creators of our own stress, we can also find ways to lessen and manage that stress."**

Strategies for Reducing Stressors and Managing Your Stress

When you face too much pressure, effective stress management techniques can help you relax, step back from stressful situations, and face your challenges with renewed energy and confidence. Some of these techniques involve making changes to your lifestyle and cultivating habits that strengthen your resilience and energy. Some give you ways to reframe situations in your mind, gain perspective about your stressors, and quiet your fight-or-flight response. If you face truly overwhelming stress, you can seek out the help of mental health professionals.

✓ **SELF-ASSESSMENT**

To complete this self-assessment online, visit www.pearsonhighered.com/choosinghealth.

The College Undergraduate Stress Scale

Below is a list of stressful events commonly experienced by college students. For each event that you have personally experienced over the past 12 months, note the corresponding "stress rating" and record this number in the "Your Items" column. Add up your total.

Event	Stress Rating	Your Items
Being raped	100	_____
Finding out that you are HIV positive	100	_____
Being accused of rape	98	_____
Death of a close friend	97	_____
Death of a close family member	96	_____
Contracting a sexually transmitted disease (other than AIDS)	94	_____
Concerns about being pregnant	91	_____
Finals week	90	_____
Concerns about your partner being pregnant	90	_____
Oversleeping for an exam	89	_____
Flunking a class	89	_____
Having a boyfriend or girlfriend cheat on you	85	_____
Ending a steady dating relationship	85	_____
Serious illness in a close friend or family member	85	_____
Financial difficulties	84	_____
Writing a major term paper	83	_____
Being caught cheating on a test	83	_____
Drunk driving	82	_____
Sense of overload in school or work	82	_____
Two exams in one day	80	_____
Cheating on your boyfriend or girlfriend	77	_____
Getting married	76	_____
Negative consequences of drinking or drug use	75	_____

Event	Stress Rating	Your Items
Depression or crisis in your best friend	73	_____
Difficulties with parents	73	_____
Talking in front of a class	72	_____
Lack of sleep	69	_____
Change in housing situation (hassles, moves)	69	_____
Competing or performing in public	69	_____
Getting in a physical fight	66	_____
Difficulties with a roommate	66	_____
Job changes (applying, new job, work hassles)	65	_____
Declaring a major or concerns about future plans	65	_____
A class you hate	62	_____
Drinking or use of drugs	61	_____
Confrontations with professors	60	_____
Starting a new semester	58	_____
Going on a first date	57	_____
Registration	55	_____
Maintaining a steady dating relationship	55	_____
Commuting to campus or work, or both	54	_____
Peer pressures	53	_____
Being away from home for the first time	53	_____
Getting sick	52	_____
Concerns about your appearance	52	_____
Getting straight A's	51	_____
A difficult class that you love	48	_____
Making new friends; getting along with friends	47	_____
Fraternity or sorority rush	47	_____
Falling asleep in class	40	_____
Attending an athletic event	20	_____
Your Total:		_____

HOW TO INTERPRET YOUR SCORE

- When this scale was administered by its authors to a sample group of undergraduate college students, the mean total stress rating was 1247. Individual scores ranged from as low as 182 to as high as 2571. How does your rating compare?
- How does your rating compare to those of your classmates? Is your stress rating higher or lower than most of your classmates?

- Remember that higher stress is correlated with a higher risk of health problems—so if your rating is on the higher end, take steps now to actively reduce and manage the stress in your life.

Source: Renner, Michael J., & Mackin, R. Scott. (1998). A life stress instrument for college use. *Teaching of Psychology 25 (1).* 46–48. Published by Routledge. Used by permission of Taylor & Francis Group. http://www.informaworld.com.

Several studies of college students show that with a few changes, life on campus can be more fun, and less stressful.[17] These changes, though, take some effort and time. You can't expect to eliminate stress overnight. But by making changes to your daily routine, giving yourself opportunities to relax, and thinking about stress in useful ways, you can reduce and better manage the stressors in your life.

Live a Healthier Lifestyle

You can go a long way toward reducing your stress level by practicing the following basic wellness habits:

- **Manage your time effectively.** For many students, a 24-hour day seems about 10 hours too short. You may feel like you can't cram your classes, studying, assignments, job, friends, significant others, hobbies, physical activity, chores, and even basic survival needs (remember eating and sleeping?) into a typical day. Better time management can often result in better stress management.

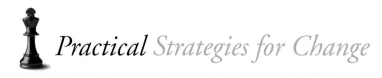
Effective Time Management

Unless you are a remarkably organized and efficient person, chances are that you can benefit from time management techniques. The **Behavior Change Workshop** at the end of this chapter offers one way to evaluate where your time goes. The following are additional strategies you can employ for better time management:

- **Plan, even just a little.** Use a daily scheduler or planner to remind you of big events and track your to-do list. Even a simple paper-based scheduler can keep important tasks from sneaking up on you.

- **Stay prepared.** When you find out the dates of big assignments and tests at the start of the term, make note of them in your planner so you can prepare ahead of time. Read assignments before class, and review your class notes shortly after class ends. Both strategies will help you get more out of class, and make big study sessions a lot easier.

- **Break down big jobs.** Remember that a forest consists of individual trees. When a task feels overwhelming, write down all the steps required to get it done, and then tackle them one at a time.

- **Hate it? Do it first.** If you can get the task you like the least out of the way, everything that follows will feel much easier.

- **Leave time for surprises.** Your car breaks down, and you need a couple of hours to get it to the shop, for example. If every hour of your schedule is always booked, you won't have room to deal with the unexpected turns life takes.

- **Reward yourself.** Been wrestling with an impossible assignment for half an hour? Take a break. Finish a paper early for a change? Let your laundry slide, and watch a movie. And leave time in your schedule to relax. If you are working hard in college, you've more than earned a reward.

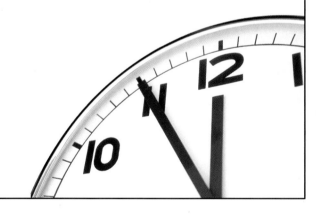

For specific strategies for managing your time, see **Practical Strategies for Change: Effective Time Management.** Also, complete Part II of the **Behavior Change Workshop** at the end of this chapter.

- **Get enough sleep.** Sleep is a naturally restorative process that is essential for healthy physical and psychological functioning. See the special feature on sleep on page 56.

- **Eat well.** Food and stress have a reciprocal relationship. On the one hand, a nutritious diet allows your body to function smoothly and helps keep your stress responses in balance. On the other hand, chronic stress can lead to unhealthful eating habits. When they are stressed, many people turn to foods with sugar to increase their energy level. Sugar may satisfy in the short term, but after an hour or two, it actually leaves you with less energy and craving more food. People under stress may also turn to caffeine to help them keep going, but too much caffeine can cause sleep problems and add to the physiological effects of stress.[18] Weight gain is also associated with the too-busy-to-exercise lives of those with chronic stress.

- **Exercise.** Exercise, especially activities such as walking, cycling, weight training, or running that work your large muscles and build sustained strength, is a very effective stress-reducer.[3] Scientists theorize that physical activity allows the body to complete the fight-or-flight response by actually doing what it has been prepared to do. After all, whether you are running around a track or running from a bear, you are still "fleeing" and thereby helping your body return to homeostasis. As little as 20 minutes a day can help.[19] Even one exercise session can generate postexercise euphoria that can last anywhere from 90 to 120 minutes.[20]

- **Strengthen your support network.** Call your family. Ask your professors for help. Make time for your friends, especially old friends from high school who may now be far away. They know you well, and can help you keep the stress in your life in perspective. At the same time, building a new network of college friends through your dorm life or social clubs will let you find and give support in a group that knows the pressures you face first-hand.

- **Communicate.** Don't be afraid to express your feelings. Let your roommates know that you have a big test in a couple of days and need them to wear headphones when the TV is on, for example. Talk with supportive friends and family about the pressures you face and how they can help you cope. One study of university students found that those who talked about their stressors and sought support suffered less depression from academic stress.[21]

- **Take time for hobbies and leisure.** It probably feels like you have no time at all right now for hiking, dance class, mountain biking, scrapbooking, or helping design t-shirts for friends' bands. But even small amounts of time spent away from school and work will reduce your stress and give you new energy to face the main tasks at hand. Research backs up this commonsense advice—one study of undergraduates found that those who valued their leisure time enjoyed better health and mental well-being.[22]

- **Keep a journal.** Make time to write down the events in your life. Keeping a journal may seem like a low priority amid all your schoolwork, but recording your activities and thoughts has actually been linked to improved moods for students and higher GPAs.[23] If you don't feel like toting around a traditional diary, online blogs and personal Web pages (with privacy controls) are also good ways to keep a journal.

Improve Your Test-Taking Skills

These steps can help reduce the stress of test taking.

- **Learn test taking skills.** Many colleges offer courses on test taking skills. Sign up for one!
- **Learn about the test ahead of time.** Find out what topics the test will cover and what format it will be in. If your instructor provides practice tests or preparation materials, use them.
- **Schedule your study time.** Study over a series of days or weeks; avoid cramming at the last minute or "all nighters."
- **Talk with your instructor.** Tell your instructor in advance that you experience test anxiety. He or she may be able to offer suggestions or help.
- **Read your syllabus.** Syllabi and course web sites often contain information about tests and how to succeed in the course.
- **Prepare yourself mentally.** Think positively. In the days leading up to the test, visualize yourself calmly taking the test and knowing the answers.
- **Prepare yourself physically.** Get enough sleep the night before. Eat a light meal so you are not hungry. Arrive early to avoid having to rush, and once in the testing room, sit in a location that is comfortable for you.
- **Do not talk with other students right before the test.** They might confuse you or reduce your confidence.
- **Stay calm.** If you find yourself getting anxious during the test: (1) relax, remind yourself that you are in control and are well-prepared for this test; (2) take slow, deep breaths; (3) concentrate on the questions, not on your fear; (4) remind yourself that some anxiety is natural.
- **Answer the easy questions first.** This will give you confidence and allow you to budget your remaining time on the more difficult questions.
- **If you get stuck, move on.** You can turn back to the question later.
- **Even if you don't know the final answer, show your work.** Graders may give you partial credit.
- **Don't be alarmed if students turn in their tests before you.** Use all the time you need.
- **When you have finished, check your work.** However, do not second-guess yourself or change an answer unless you have remembered new information.

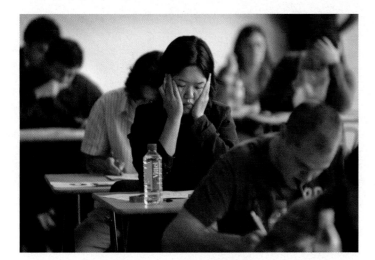

Exercising for Stress Management

Having trouble getting moving? Consider the following tips:

- Think of exercise as "recess"—not as a chore, but as a chance to break up an otherwise routine day with a fun, active, recreational activity.
- Vary your exercise activity. You might go swimming one day and bicycling another day. This way, you will have more options to choose from depending on your mood on any given day.
- Pick activities you genuinely enjoy. If you hate jogging but love to dance, by all means, dance!
- Remember that any activity that gets your body moving can ease stress. If you're not into sports, consider walking around campus just for fun, walking your dog, or even walking in a shopping center. Any physical activity is better than none!
- Consider exercise classes such as yoga or tai chi that focus on breathing and relaxation.
- Enlist a friend as an exercise partner. You can keep each other encouraged and have more fun while you exercise.
- Make exercise a regular part of your schedule. Prioritize it the same way you would prioritize your schoolwork or a job.
- Exercise releases endorphins in the body, which makes you feel good. So the next time you find yourself resisting the thought of getting up and moving, remind yourself of how great you will feel afterward!

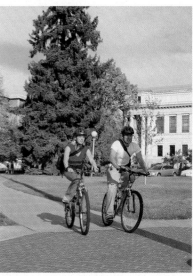

"*As little as 20 minutes of exercise per day can help you better manage your stress.*"

GETTING enough SLEEP

The stress-sleep connection is a reciprocal one: sleep deprivation adds stress to your life, and stress affects the quality of your sleep. Few things jangle your nerves, upset your internal balance, and leave you more prone to getting stressed out than sleep deprivation. Even short-changing your sleep an hour or two, if done on a regular basis, can affect how alert you feel during the day. Although most people require 7 to 9 hours of sleep each night, a third of Americans sleep only 6 hours. A study conducted at Cornell University found that college students, on average, sleep only 6 hours nightly. Less than 1% of students report that they can stay fully alert during the entire day.

Poor quality or inadequate periods of sleep affect all domains of health. During the deepest stages of sleep, called *rapid eye movement (REM) sleep*, your body undergoes normal growth and repair of body tissues. Those processes are diminished when you don't get enough sleep. Emotional and social health suffer due to heightened irritability, frustration, and nervousness caused by inadequate sleep. Sleep deprivation also affects mental health by reducing the capacity to learn new material, reducing reaction time, and impairing coordination and judgment.

It may be difficult for college students to adopt healthful sleep practices because the parties, stress, and work of college life, coupled with communal living arrangements in dormitories and other student-focused housing, provide many challenges to turning in early. Additionally, a recent study of college undergraduates found that certain risky behaviors appear to be associated with poor sleep quality, including alcohol and marijuana use, smoking, fighting and thoughts of suicide.

College students are particularly prone to developing **sleep debt,** a condition caused by getting less sleep than you need. While it may sound logical to reduce sleep debt by sleeping late on weekends, in fact, it may actually increase sleep problems by disrupting your sleep schedule. Sleep debt cannot be made up; instead you must avoid accumulating debt by getting sufficient amounts of quality sleep each night.

Just as the negative affects of poor sleep can add stress to your life, stress can be one of the causes of poor sleep. We have all had the experience of intrusive thoughts about some stressor in our lives preventing us from falling asleep at night. It is a vicious circle: the stressor keeps us awake and the resulting lack of sleep impairs our ability to deal with that same stressor during the day. So what should you do to keep your stressors out of your bed? See **Practical Strategies for Change: Settle Into a Better Night's Sleep** for tactics to get enough shut eye.

References: 1. Maas, J.B., Wherry, M.L., Axelrod, D.J., Hogan, B.R., & Bloom, J. (1998). *Power sleep: the revolutionary program that prepares your mind for peak performance.* New York, NY: Random House and HarperCollins. 2. Vail-Smith, K., Felts W., and Becker, C. (2009). Relationship between sleep quality and health risk behaviors in undergraduate college students. *College Student Journal,* 43(3) 715–725.

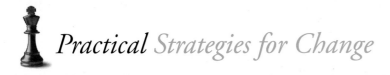

Settle Into a Better Night's Sleep

In college, sleep may feel like the last thing you can fit into your schedule. But investing in sufficient, regular sleep will pay off with better performance in school, better health, and a happier you. Here are some general tips for a better night's sleep:

- **Go to bed on the earlier side.** You need to go to bed early enough to get a full night's sleep—usually about 7 to 9 hours for most students.

- **Be regular about what time you go to sleep and what time you wake up.** Try going to bed at roughly the same time each night, and be consistent about the hour you rise as well. This helps your body get into a regular sleep pattern.

- **Don't stare at the ceiling.** If you've gone to bed and can't fall asleep within 20 minutes, get up and do something relaxing until you feel sleepy again and can head back to bed.

- **Think of your bedroom as your "sleep cave."** Make your bedroom dark, quiet, and a little cool. These conditions help your body know that it's time to sleep.

- **Cut caffeine.** Try to avoid caffeinated drinks after lunchtime, as caffeine can stay in your system for hours and interfere with sleep.

- **Avoid alcohol and cigarettes before bedtime.** A drink or a smoke might seem relaxing, but both can interfere with sleep.

- **Hit the gym earlier in the day.** Avoid tough exercise within a few hours of bedtime, as the activity can make it hard to wind down later.

- **Set stress aside until morning.** Try to deal with or put aside things that make you worried when you go to bed. Sleep is your chance to rest and recover.

- **Try not to nap.** You may feel like crashing in the late afternoon, but you'll cut into your ability to sleep later. If you do need to nap, keep it to less than an hour and do it before 3 p.m.

- **Avoid all-nighters.** Studying all night will obviously leave you exhausted and unrested, as well as throw off your normal sleep routine for days afterward. Plan study time in advance to make all-nighters unnecessary.

- **Try not to work in bed.** If you read, study or work on your laptop in bed, you may associate your bed with these activities instead of as a place for rest. Try to reserve your bed only for sleep.

- **Give yourself time to wind down.** You'll get a better night's sleep if you take some time to step away from your laptop, turn off the TV, and relax before you settle in to bed.

- **Try not to sleep-in on weekends.** Try to get up within two to three hours of your usual wakeup time. That will help your body keep its regular sleep rhythms and make Monday easier.

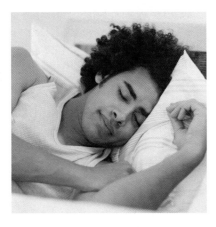

References: 1. Centers for Disease Control and Prevention. (2007). *Sleep Hygiene Tips.* Retrieved from http://www.cdc.gov/sleep/hygiene.htm 2. American Academy of Sleep Medicine. (2009). *Sleep Hygiene – The Healthy Habits of Good Sleep.* Retrieved from http://www.sleepeducation.com/Hygiene.aspx 3.American Academy of Sleep Medicine. (2007). *Sleep Tips for Students.* Retrieved from http://www.sleepeducation.com/Topic.aspx?id=53

Practice Relaxation Techniques

Just as stressors drive your heart rate up, other influences can soothe your fight-or-flight response. You can develop your body's **relaxation response** to slow your breathing and metabolism, quiet your mind, and greatly reduce stress. To activate your own relaxation response, try the following:

- **Listen to music.** Taking a break can be as close as your MP3 player. Music can help lower blood pressure and quiet your mind. Choose calming music. One study found that classical music can be effective at lowering blood pressure after a stressful situation.[24] Make time to listen—it doesn't count if you merely put on headphones while cramming for a test.

- **Meditation or prayer.** Reflective thought, done regularly at a peaceful time and place, can help reduce stress and quiet your mind. Studies conclude that meditation can help protect against stress and improve the ability to learn.[25] Many fitness centers and yoga studios, along with campus gyms and student health centers, offer classes on meditation. If you belong to a particular religious group and prefer prayer, check to see if your organization offers quiet, reflective prayer groups or meetings.

- **Progressive muscle relaxation.** This technique helps you relax each major muscle group in your body, one by one, adding up to a powerful reduction in physical tension. Start by choosing one part of your body, such as your left foot. Inhale as you flex and tense it. Then exhale as you relax it. Repeat this once or twice. Then move on to your left leg and repeat the same process. Slowly move through all the major muscle groups of your body, deliberately tensing and relaxing each one, until your whole body relaxes.

- **Visualization and guided imagery.** Stressed out by your surroundings? Imagine you are somewhere you find relaxing. Close your eyes and visualize yourself lying on a beach, resting under a tree on a warm day, or napping on your favorite couch. If you are nervous about an upcoming event, such as giving a presentation in front of a class, imagine yourself giving the talk and getting a standing ovation at the end. Athletes often use visualization techniques to handle the pressures of competitive events.

- **Massage.** A professional massage therapist uses pressure, stretching, and rubbing to manipulate skin and muscles in order to relieve tension. Some studies have shown that massage can be helpful in reducing anxiety, decreasing pain, relieving sports-related soreness, and boosting the immune system.[26] Check with your campus wellness center to see if it offers reduced-price massages on campus.

- **Biofeedback.** In biofeedback, a device monitors your physiological stress responses, alerting you to stress symptoms such as increased heart rate or a rise in skin temperature. By becoming more aware of when your body exhibits signs of a stress response, you can take steps to actively reduce that response, such as implementing relaxation techniques.

sleep debt A condition occurring when the amount of sleep you attain is less than the amount you need for optimal functioning.

relaxation response The physiological opposite response to fight-or-flight that can be activated through relaxation techniques.

Change Your Thinking

Changing the way you think about the pressures in your life can help hold stress at bay. To keep your everyday stressors from turning into mountains of tension, consider the following:

- **Rewrite internal messages.** How do you talk to yourself? When you have a test coming up, do you tell yourself you can ace it with a little work ahead of time? Or do you tell yourself that you'll probably fail, so why bother studying? If you tend to tell yourself negative messages, actively try to change your thoughts and tell yourself positive, solution-oriented, constructive messages.

- **Set realistic expectations.** College brings new challenges—and a whole new level of competition. Do you feel disappointed if you don't ace every single course you take? Or do you give yourself permission to feel that your best effort is reward enough? Regardless of how ambitious you are, be honest with yourself and try to set realistic goals in order to keep your stress level manageable.

- **Build your self-esteem.** Increasing your self-worth through positive affirmations and self-talk, replaying compliments in your head, and the other self-esteem boosting tips we discussed in Chapter 2 can help you build the inner strength and confidence to handle stressful situations when they come along.

- **Be proactive.** Do you have a professor who enjoys pop quizzes, and does this make you think about skipping class some days? Unfortunately, avoidance is a poor strategy for stress management. Studies have found that trying to avoid stressful scenes ahead of time will only worsen your stress later.[27] If you have a class with a professor who likes surprises, be prepared by keeping up with your studies. A little planning now will mean less stress later on.

- **Tackle problems head-on.** When confronted by a difficult task or situation, do you believe in your ability to find a creative, effective solution? Or do you automatically assume you'll fail from the start? Strong problem-solving skills are closely linked to better health and fewer feelings of stress in college students.[28] If a problem seems overwhelming, try breaking it into pieces and tackling one bit at a time. Ask your professors, classmates, and friends for help. Taking active steps to solve a problem can reduce your feelings of stress, whereas doing nothing but worrying has the opposite effect.

- **Have a sense of humor.** A little laughter can go a long way toward reducing stress. Watch a funny movie, check out a humorous website, or talk to your most hilarious friend. Humor can help you get a better perspective on which stressors are really important and which ones are overblown.

- **Take the long view.** Are most of the stressors in your life right now going to matter to you in a few years? Cultivating patience and a sense of what matters in the long term can help you keep problems in perspective.

- **Accept that you cannot control everything.** If you play college baseball, will winning this weekend's game really be up to only you? If you need to do laundry, but all the machines at the laundromat are already full, do you get angry or do you just come back later? Being able to accept that you can't control everything—and being adaptable to less-than-ideal situations—can make a big difference in how well you deal with stress.

CONSUMER CORNER

Can Video Games Help Reduce Stress?

Can playing video games help relieve stress? The answer depends on the type of game. Some games involve exercise and movement—and as you've learned in this chapter, physical activity is a proven stress reducer. Other games require calm, focused concentration, a type of activity that also helps many people reduce stress. In one study, people suffering from PTSD (post-traumatic stress disorder) experienced fewer symptoms if they played a relatively quiet, systematic video game such as Tetris for 30 minutes a week.[1] On the other hand, studies have shown that games that simulate violence may actually increase players' levels of stress by triggering the body's fight-or-flight response.[2]

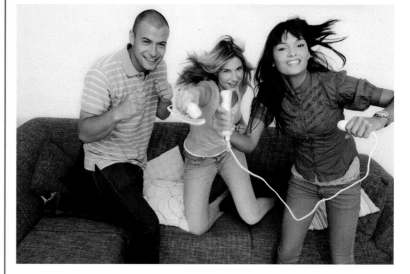

References: 1. Holmes, E. A., James, E. L., Coode-Bate, T., & Deeprose, C. (2009). Can playing the computer game "Tetris" reduce the build-up of flashbacks for trauma? A proposal from cognitive science. *PLoS ONE, 4*(1), e4153. doi:10.1371/journal.pone.0004153. 2. Sharm, R., Kera. S., Mohan, A., Gupta, S., & Ray, R. (2006). Assessment of computer game as a psychological stressor. *Indian Journal of Physiology and Pharmacology, 50*(4), 367–374.

- **Share your feelings.** When you feel stressed out on campus, look around and you'll realize very quickly that you aren't alone. Talk to your friends, classmates, and roommates about how you are feeling. Many student organizations and student health centers also offer support groups where you can vent about stress, hear what others are going through, and swap suggestions for coping.

Seek Help from Health Professionals

Sometimes we face stress that feels truly overwhelming. If you find yourself having trouble managing stress on your own, trained professionals can help.

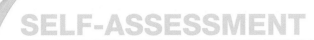
Perceived Stress Scale

Instructions: The questions in this scale ask you about your feelings and thoughts during the last month. In each case, please indicate with a check how often you felt or thought a certain way.

1. In the last month, how often have you been upset because of something that happened unexpectedly?

- ☐ 0=never
- ☐ 1=almost never
- ☐ 2=sometimes
- ☐ 3=fairly often
- ☐ 4=very often

2. In the last month, how often have you felt that you were unable to control the important things in your life?

- ☐ 0=never
- ☐ 1=almost never
- ☐ 2=sometimes
- ☐ 3=fairly often
- ☐ 4=very often

3. In the last month, how often have you felt nervous and "stressed"?

- ☐ 0=never
- ☐ 1=almost never
- ☐ 2=sometimes
- ☐ 3=fairly often
- ☐ 4=very often

4. In the last month, how often have you felt confident about your ability to handle your personal problems?

- ☐ 0=never
- ☐ 1=almost never
- ☐ 2=sometimes
- ☐ 3=fairly often
- ☐ 4=very often

5. In the last month, how often have you felt that things were going your way?

- ☐ 0=never
- ☐ 1=almost never
- ☐ 2=sometimes
- ☐ 3=fairly often
- ☐ 4=very often

6. In the last month, how often have you found that you could not cope with all the things that you had to do?

- ☐ 0=never
- ☐ 1=almost never
- ☐ 2=sometimes
- ☐ 3=fairly often
- ☐ 4=very often

7. In the last month, how often have you been able to control irritations in your life?

- ☐ 0=never
- ☐ 1=almost never
- ☐ 2=sometimes
- ☐ 3=fairly often
- ☐ 4=very often

8. In the last month, how often have you felt that you were on top of things?

- ☐ 0=never
- ☐ 1=almost never
- ☐ 2=sometimes
- ☐ 3=fairly often
- ☐ 4=very often

9. In the last month, how often have you been angered because of things that were outside of your control?

- ☐ 0=never
- ☐ 1=almost never
- ☐ 2=sometimes
- ☐ 3=fairly often
- ☐ 4=very often

10. In the last month, how often have you felt difficulties were piling up so high that you could not overcome them?

- ☐ 0=never
- ☐ 1=almost never
- ☐ 2=sometimes
- ☐ 3=fairly often
- ☐ 4=very often

HOW TO INTERPRET YOUR SCORE

- For items 4, 5, 7, and 8, give yourself the following points: Never = 4 points; almost never = 3 points; sometimes = 2 points; fairly often = 1 point; very often = 0 points
- For items 1, 2, 3, 6, 9, and 10, give yourself the following points: Never = 0 points; almost never = 1 point; sometimes = 2 points; fairly often = 3 points; very often = 4 points
- The higher your score, the greater your perceived stress. If your PSS score is 20 or greater, you should take additional steps to manage your stress.

Source: Cohen, S., & Williamson, G. (1988). Perceived stress in a probability sample of the United States. In S. Spacapam & S. Oskamp (Eds.), *The social psychology of health: Claremont symposium on applied social psychology.* Newbury Park, CA: Sage. Used by permission of Dr. Sheldon Cohen and ASA (American Sociological Association).

- **Consider counseling.** Talking with a mental health professional, either in group therapy or an individual setting, can help you manage the stressors in your life and reframe how you confront them. Talk to a health professional at your student health center about free or low-cost group and individual counseling.

- **Talk with a doctor.** If you are experiencing a serious stress-related condition such as depression or severe anxiety, a doctor may recommend prescription medication to help you get your symptoms under control.

- **Use caution with alternative remedies.** Many herbal supplement and vitamin companies sell products that promise to reduce stress or ease its symptoms. Before you try any of these products, however, talk to a health professional and ask whether these supplements have proven benefits, side effects, or dangers. Some supplements can mix badly with other medications you may be taking, so be sure to also ask about possible drug interactions before taking any supplement.

- **Avoid caffeine, alcohol, tobacco, or other drugs.** Coffee and energy drinks might seem like harmless substances that keep you going. Likewise, drinking, smoking, and recreational drugs can seem to offer a brief vacation from stress. But numerous studies have shown that too much caffeine can cause physical symptoms such as jitteriness, and that the long-term health risks of smoking, drugs, or excess drinking far outweigh the few moments of relief they offer. If you find yourself drawn to potentially addictive substances to relieve stress, seek help from your doctor or from a health professional at your student health center.

View videos of stress management techniques at: **http://health .howstuffworks.com/wellness/stress-management.**

Creating a Personalized Stress Management Plan

As we have discussed in this chapter, many common stressors are either emotional or psychological in nature. Nonetheless, these stressors still trigger a physical stress response, and over time, the stress response itself can negatively affect your health. A growing number of researchers believe that managing stress effectively is an important aspect of staying healthy. You can start creating your own stress management plan by first identifying and examining the stressors in your own life. By writing them down and spelling them out, you can then think about ways to reduce their occurrence, or to mentally reframe them in ways that can lessen your stress response.

Assessing Stressors

Assess the stressors in your own life by completing the following:

- Complete the **Self-Assessments** on pages 53 and 59 to assess your current level of perceived stress.
- Complete the **Behavior Change Workshop** found at the end of this chapter to identify the top sources of stress in your life, evaluate your readiness for behavior change, and take steps to reduce the controllable stressors.

Once you have done everything you can to minimize the controllable stressors in your life, it's time to think about how you can better respond to (and manage) the stress that remains. Review the section on strategies for managing stress. Which techniques seem like the best fit for your life and personality? Select the options you find the most comfortable and natural for you. Keep the following guidelines in mind:

- Remember that not all stress is harmful. You may find one of your classes tough, for example, but intellectually fun and challenging. Focus on changing your response to stressors that leave you exhausted, irritable, anxious, or sick.
- If the stress management technique that you pick requires adjustments to your schedule, take action to make room for it. For example, if school stress leaves you feeling anxious, and you've resolved to shake some of that stress through more exercise, prioritize time for workouts in your schedule.
- Decide how long you will try the stress management technique to see if it is working. Remember that managing stress is a long-term commitment. Tackle your stressors little by little, rather than trying to eliminate all of your stress at once.

Watch videos of real students discussing stress management at **www.pearsonhighered.com/choosinghealth.**

MYTH OR FACT?

Can Stress Give You an Ulcer?

You've got a huge set of lab problems to solve for class, and you're way behind on getting it done. After a quick dinner of extremely cold, old pizza, you head for the library. Your stomach is killing you — again.

Yes, the pizza was kind of nasty. But you still can't help but wonder if all the pressure this term is giving you an ulcer.

Ulcers are lesions in the lining of the stomach or small intestine that can cause pain, bloating, and nausea. But while all the stress you face could indeed be making you feel terrible, it probably isn't causing an ulcer. Researchers have found that most ulcers are caused by bacteria called *Helicobacter pylori*. The small numbers of ulcers not triggered by bacterial infection are often due to the overuse of painkillers, such as aspirin or ibuprofen, or alcohol.

By diverting blood away from your digestive system, stress can definitely cause stomachaches and other digestive problems. Some studies have also shown that stress can make the symptoms of an ulcer worse. If you suffer from ongoing stomach pain, visit your campus health center or personal doctor.

Reference: Mayo Clinic. (2009). *Peptic ulcer: Causes.* Retrieved from http://www.mayoclinic.com/health/peptic-ulcer/DS00242/DSECTION=causes.

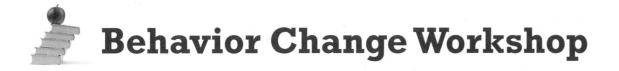

Behavior Change Workshop

To complete this workshop online, visit www.pearsonhighered.com/choosinghealth.

Changing long-ingrained behaviors is one of the toughest things to do. Consider the student case studies presented throughout this chapter, and then think about your own life. What stressors can you reduce or eliminate? How can you change the way you respond to the stressors that remain? What stage of behavior change are you in? Given your current stage of change, what is an appropriate goal you can set to reach the next stage?

Part I. Assessing the Stressors in Your Life

1. What are the main sources of stress in your own life? List the top five.

_____

_____

_____

_____

_____

2. Mark one of the stressors above that you want to target. Ask yourself honestly: How ready are you to commit to a behavior change that will help you reduce or eliminate that stressor? What stage of behavior change are you in?

Target stressor: _____

_____

Current stage of behavior change: _____

_____

3. Keeping your current stage of behavior change in mind, describe what you might do or think about as a "next step" to reduce or eliminate that stressor in your life. Also list your timeline for making your next step.

Next step: _____

_____

Deadline for next step: _____

_____

4. Consider the stressors that you have some control over. Now consider the stress management techniques introduced in this chapter. Which techniques can you try to better respond to and manage the stress you feel over those stressors?

_____

_____

_____

_____

Chapter 3 • Stress Management 61

Part II. Effective Time Management

Got too much to do, and not enough time to do it all? You can reduce some of your stress, and handle the pressures in your life more effectively, by rethinking how you use your time. Start by taking a closer look at your schedule. Using the following chart, fill in your activities every day for a week.

Time	Monday	Tuesday	Wednesday	Thursday	Friday	Saturday	Sunday
5:00 a.m.							
6:00 a.m.							
7:00 a.m.							
8:00 a.m.							
9:00 a.m.							
10:00 a.m.							
11:00 a.m.							
12:00 p.m.							
1:00 p.m.							
2:00 p.m.							
3:00 p.m.							
4:00 p.m.							
5:00 p.m.							
6:00 p.m.							
7:00 p.m.							
8:00 p.m.							
9:00 p.m.							
10:00 p.m.							
11:00 p.m.							
12:00 a.m.							
12 a.m.–5 a.m.							

Now, examine the chart and consider the following: Which tasks are most important to your goals in school and in your personal life? Which tasks are needed to keep you healthy, such as eating, sleeping, and making time to relax? Which tasks are unnecessary time-busters—that is, activities that eat away at your time, or waste it (be honest). Decide how you can kick a time-buster or two out of your schedule. Mark these areas with red pencil, and see how much more time you have for important tasks.

Chapter Summary

- *Stress* is the collective psychobiological condition that occurs in reaction to a disruptive, unexpected, or exciting stimulus.

- *Eustress* is stress resulting from positive stressors; *distress* is stress resulting from negative stressors.

- The *stress response* is the set of specific psychobiological changes that occurs as the body attempts to cope with a stressor and return to *homeostasis* (a balanced state).

- The *fight-or-flight response* is a component of the stress response. It is an instantaneous set of reactions that temporarily boosts strength and reflexes to physically prepare the body to deal with a stressor.

- The *general adaptation syndrome (GAS)* is a theory developed by Hans Selye that attempts to explain the biology of the stress response. It consists of three stages: alarm, resistance, and exhaustion.

- *Allostatic overload* is the long-term wear and tear experienced by the body as a result of continuous or repeated reactions to stressors.

- Chronic stress can increase your risk of heart disease, result in digestive problems, weaken your immune system, and compromise your mental health.

- Common sources of stress include daily hassles, academic pressure, job-related issues, social stressors, major life changes, environmental stressors, and internal stressors.

- How you view, think about, respond to, and manage your stress can have a critical impact on how stress affects your health.

- General strategies for reducing stress include getting enough sleep, eating well, exercising, strengthening your support network, communicating, taking time for hobbies, keeping a journal, practicing relaxation techniques, changing your thinking, and seeking help from health professionals.

Test Your Knowledge

1. The stress that results from positive experiences (such as graduating from college or getting married) is called
   a. eustress.
   b. distress.
   c. homeostasis.
   d. allostasis.

2. The fight-or-flight response
   a. is a physical reaction to stress.
   b. governs your body's reaction to stress.
   c. can take a toll on your body.
   d. All of the above are correct.

3. In the "alarm" phase of the general adaptation syndrome, the body
   a. activates its fight-or-flight response.
   b. boosts levels of stress hormones.
   c. increases heart rate.
   d. All of the above are correct.

4. The long-term wear and tear on the body that results from continuous or repeated responses to stress is termed
   a. homeostasis.
   b. allostasis.
   c. allostatic overload.
   d. eustress.

5. The effects of chronic stress can include
   a. increased risk of heart disease.
   b. stomachache, constipation, or diarrhea.
   c. a weakened immune system.
   d. All of the above are correct.

6. Worries, critical thoughts, and the demands we place upon ourselves are examples of
   a. environmental stressors.
   b. internal stressors.
   c. social stressors.
   d. post-traumatic stress disorder.

7. An example of an ideal exercise program for stress reduction consists of
   a. 1 hour of high-intensity cardiovascular activity per month.
   b. 20 to 30 minutes of walking at a brisk pace 5 days a week.
   c. 45 minutes of strength training every weekend.
   d. light activity such as shopping or cleaning your room.

8. Keeping a journal
   a. has been found to increase GPA.
   b. can be an effective way to reduce stress.
   c. can improve mood.
   d. All of the above are correct.

9. Progressive muscle relaxation involves
   a. systematically contracting and relaxing muscle groups.
   b. taking naps of longer and longer lengths.
   c. working on relaxing a little more each day.
   d. sitting quietly and meditating.

10. The average college student
    a. has a sleep debt of 1 hour or more per night.
    b. sleeps more than the recommended hours each night.
    c. is always alert during waking hours.
    d. receives the recommended hours of sleep.

Get Critical

What happened:

On January 15, 2009, Chesley B. "Sully" Sullenberger was piloting US Airways flight 1549 from New York's LaGuardia airport to Charlotte, North Carolina, when at least one of the plane's engines failed after being struck by birds upon takeoff. All of the passengers and crew on the flight survived the plane's amazing landing in the Hudson River. The experience of Sullenberger and his crew appeared to have prepared them for the dangerous and unexpected situation. "There was no panic, no hysterics," an official said. "It was professional, it was calm, it was methodical. It was everything you hoped it could be."

What do you think?

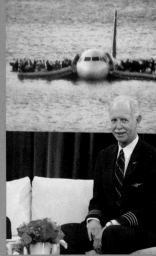

- Using what you've learned from this chapter, apply the fight-or-flight response to Captain Sullenberger's situation. When do you think the fight-or-flight response kicked in? What would Sullenberger have been likely to experience as events unfolded?

- How do you think Sullenberger may have used stress management techniques such as visualization, guided imagery, and effective thinking to respond to his highly stressful situation?

Get Connected

References

i - iii. American College Health Association. (2008). ACHA–NCHA II: Reference group executive summary. Retrieved from http://www.acha-ncha.org/reports_ACHA-NCHAII.html. Also, The American Psychological Association. (2008, October 7). Stress in America. Retrieved from http://apahelpcenter.mediaroom.com/index.php?s=pageC.

1. Selye, H. (1980). *Selye's guide to stress research* (Vol. 1). New York: Van Nostrand Reinhold.

2. Selye, H. (1974). *Stress without distress.* New York: Lippincott.

3. Flatow, I. (2004). [Interview] Dr. Robert Sapolsky discusses physiological and psychological ways stress affects the body. *Talk of the Nation/Science, Friday (NPR).*

4. American Psychological Association. (2008). Stress in America. Retrieved from http://www.apa.org/releases/women-stress1008.html.

5. Friedman, H., Herman, T.W., & Friedman, A.L., Eds. (1995). *Psychoneuroimmunology, stress, and infection.* Florida: CRC Press.

6. Segerstrom, S. C., & Miller, G. E. (2004). Psychological stress and the human immune system: A meta-analytic study of 30 years of inquiry. *Psychological Bulletin, 130*(4), 601–630.

7. Nemade, R., Reiss, N. S., & Dombeck, M. (Jul 20, 2007). Biology of depression: Psychoneuroimmunology. Retrieved from http://www.mentalhelp.net.

8. Joiner, Jr., T. E., Wingate, L. R., Gencoz, T., & Gencoz, F. (2005). Stress generation in depression: Three studies on its resilience, possible mechanism, and symptom specificity. *Journal of Social and Clinical Psychology, (24)*2, 236–253.

9. Misra, R., McKean, M., West, S., & Russo, T. (2000). Academic stress of college students: Comparison of student and faculty perceptions. *College Student Journal, 34*(2), 236–246.

10. Murff, S. H. (2005, Sept./Oct.). The impact of stress on academic success in college students. *The Association of Black Nursing Faculty Journal*, 102–104.

11. Wright, K. B., Craig, E. A., Cunningham, C. B., and Igiel, M. (2007). Emotional support and perceived stress among college students using facebook.com: An exploration of the relationship between source perceptions and emotional support. Paper presented at the annual meeting of the NCA 93rd Annual Convention, TBA, Chicago, IL.

12. King, K. (2005). Why is discrimination stressful? The mediating role of cognitive appraisal. *Cultural Diversity and Ethnic Minority Psychology, 11*(3), 202–212.

13. Holmes, T.H., & Rahe, R.H. (1967). The social readjustment rating scale. *Journal of Psychosomatic Research, 11*, 213–218.

14. Renner, Michael J., & Mackin, R. Scott. A life stress instrument for college use. (1998). *Teaching of Psychology 25 (1),*. 46–48.

15. Rice, K.G., Leever, B. A., Christopher, J., & Porter, J. D. (2006). Perfectionism, stress, and social (dis)connection: A short-term study of hopelessness, depression, and academic adjustment among honors students. *Journal of Counseling Psychology, 33*(4), 524–534.

16. Lazarus, R. S., & Folkman, S. (1984). *Stress, appraisal, and coping.* New York: Springer.

17. Deckro, G. R., Ballinger, K. M., Hoyt, M., Wilcher, M., Dusek, J., Myers, P., et al. (2002). The evaluation of a mind/body intervention to reduce psychological distress and perceived stress in college students. *Journal of American College Health, 50*(6), 281–287; Iglesias, S. E., Azzara, S., Squillace, M., Jeifetz, M., Lores Arnais, M. R., Desimone, M. R., et al. (2005). A study on the effectiveness of a stress management program for college students. *Pharmacy Education, 5*(1), 27–31.

18. Lande, R. G. (2009). Caffeine-related psychiatric disorders. *eMedicine from WebMD.* Retrieved from http://emedicine.medscape.com/article/290113-overview.

19. Vorvick, Linda. (2009). *Exercise and stress reduction.* National Institutes of Health. Retrieved from http://www.nlm.nih.gov/medlineplus/ency/article/002081.htm.

20. American Council on Exercise. (2009). *Exercise can help control stress.* Retrieved from http://www.acefitness.org/FITFACTS/fitfacts_display.aspx?itemid=51

21. MacGeorge, E. L., Samter, W., & Gillihan, S. (2005). Academic stress, supportive communication, and health. *Communication Education, 54*(4), 365–372.

22. Iwasaki, Y. (2003). Roles of leisure in coping with stress among university students: A repeated-assessment field study. *Anxiety, Stress, and Coping, 16*(1), 31–57.

23. Lumley, M. A., & Provenzano, K. M. (2003). Stress management through written emotional disclosure improves academic performance among college students with physical symptoms. *Journal of Educational Psychology, 95*(3), 641–649.

24. Chafin, S., Roy, M., Gerin, W., & Christenfeld, N. (2004). Music can facilitate blood pressure recovery from stress. *British Journal of Health Psychology, 9*, 393–403.

25. Travis, F., Haaga, D. A. F., Hagelin, J., Tanner, M., Nidich, S., Gaylord-King, C., Grosswld, S., & Schneider, R. H. (2009). Effects of transcendental meditation practice on brain functioning and stress reactivity in college students. *International Journal of Psychophysiology, 71*, 170–176.

26. Zeitlin, D., Keller, S. E., Shiflett, S. C., Schleifer, S. J., & Bartlett, J. A. (2000). Immunological effects of massage therapy during academic stress. *Psychosomatic Medicine, 83*–84.

27. Snow, D. L., Swan, S. C., Ragavan, C., Connell, C. M., & Klein, I. (2003). The relationship of work stressors, coping, and social support to psychological symptoms among female secretarial employees. *Work and Stress, 17*(3), 241–263.

28. Largo-Wright, E., Peterson, P. M., & Chen, W.W. (2005). Perceived problem solving, stress, and health among college students. *American Journal of Health Behavior, 29*(4), 360–370.

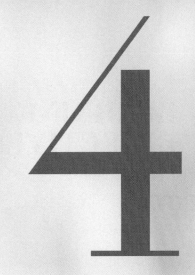

4

The average person in the U.S. consumes the equivalent of 30 teaspoons of added sugar each day.[i]

A meal consisting of a McDonald's Big Mac, extra large fries, and apple pie contains 1,430 calories, 47% of which is fat.[ii]

Eight foods cause more than 90% of all food allergies: milk, eggs, peanuts, tree nuts, soy, wheat, fish, and shellfish.[iii]

Nutrition and You

IDENTIFY the six classes of nutrients and explain their functions in the body.

DESCRIBE how to use Dietary Reference Intakes, food labels, the Dietary Guidelines for Americans, and MyPyramid to design a healthful diet.

EXPLAIN how nutrition guidelines can vary depending on a person's age, gender, activity level, and dietary preferences or needs.

IDENTIFY strategies for handling food safely.

ANALYZE your current diet and create a personalized plan for improving your nutrition.

Health Online icons are found throughout the chapter, directing you to web links, videos, podcasts, and other useful online resources.

Why is orange juice more nutritious than orange soda?

Why does a baked potato beat French fries? Why is fat from a fish better than fat from a cow? In short, what foods should you limit, and what foods should you try to consume more of? Most importantly, why should you care?

The science of **nutrition** examines how the foods you eat affect your body and health. Nutritious **diets** provide you with energy, help you stay healthy, and allow you to function at your best. Diets lacking in nutrition not only can drain your energy and decrease your sense of well-being, but also can make you more likely to develop chronic health problems such as high blood pressure, heart disease, type 2 diabetes, and obesity.

In this chapter, we'll discuss what nutrients are, explain how they function in the body, and identify foods that are good nutrient sources. We'll share national guidelines for eating right, and show you how to use tools like food labels to improve your nutrition. You'll also learn how to handle food safely and make sense of news stories debating the safety of the U.S. food supply. Finally, we'll help you evaluate your current nutrition habits so that you can develop a personalized plan to improve your diet. Whether you're in a grocery store, in line at the dining hall, or in front of a vending machine after a late-night study session, knowing the basic principles of good nutrition will help you make choices that will benefit your health.

What Are Nutrients?

Your body relies on food to provide chemical compounds called **nutrients.** In a process called digestion, the food you eat is broken down into nutrients that are small enough to be absorbed into your bloodstream **(Figure 4.1).** Once in your body, nutrients work together to provide energy; support growth, repair, and maintenance of body tissues; and regulate body processes.

Six major classes of nutrients are found in food:

- carbohydrates
- fats (more appropriately called *lipids*)
- proteins
- vitamins
- minerals
- water

Within these six classes are about 45 specific nutrients that your body is unable to make or can't make in needed quantities to support health. These are called **essential nutrients.** You must obtain essential nutrients from food, beverages, and/or supplements.

Nutrients your body needs in relatively large quantities are called *macronutrients* (*macro* means large). These are carbohydrates, fats, proteins, and water. Nutrients you need in relatively small quantities are

nutrition The scientific study of food and its physiological functions.

diet The food you regularly consume.

nutrients Chemical substances in food that you need for energy, growth, and survival.

essential nutrients Nutrients you must obtain from food or supplements because your body either cannot produce them or cannot make them in sufficient quantities to maintain health.

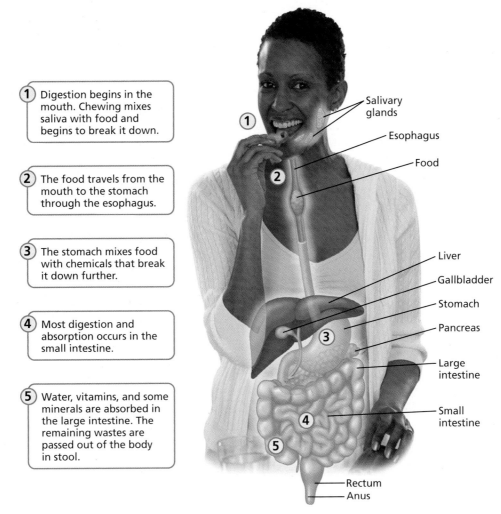

1 Digestion begins in the mouth. Chewing mixes saliva with food and begins to break it down.

2 The food travels from the mouth to the stomach through the esophagus.

3 The stomach mixes food with chemicals that break it down further.

4 Most digestion and absorption occurs in the small intestine.

5 Water, vitamins, and some minerals are absorbed in the large intestine. The remaining wastes are passed out of the body in stool.

Salivary glands
Esophagus
Food
Liver
Gallbladder
Stomach
Pancreas
Large intestine
Small intestine
Rectum
Anus

Figure 4.1 The digestive process. Digestion is the process of breaking food down into nutrients that can be used by the body for energy.

called *micronutrients* (*micro* means small). These are vitamins and minerals.

Three of the four macronutrients—carbohydrates, fats, and proteins—are also known as *energy-yielding nutrients* because they help provide you with the energy you need to move, to think, and simply to survive. The amount of energy in food is measured as kilocalories (kcals). You're probably more familiar with the word **calorie,** which is used in the media and on food labels, so we'll use that term instead of kilocalorie throughout this chapter as well.

The energy nutrients differ in their calorie content. Carbohydrates and proteins each provide 4 calories per gram. (A gram is a very small amount; for instance, a standard packet of sugar contains about 3 grams!) Fats provide 9 calories per gram—more than twice the amount in carbohydrates or proteins. Alcohol is not a nutrient because it doesn't provide any substance you need to grow or survive. However, alcohol does provide energy, 7 calories per gram, which explains why consuming alcohol regularly can pack on the pounds. Regardless of their source, calories consumed in excess of energy needs are converted to fat and stored in the body.

calorie Also called *kilocalorie.* A unit of measure that indicates the amount of energy that food provides, specifically, the amount of energy required to raise the temperature of one kilogram of water by one degree Celsius.

carbohydrates A macronutrient that is the body's universal energy source, supplying sugar to all body cells.

Vitamins, minerals, and water provide no energy. However, vitamins and minerals serve as structural components, help regulate body processes, and assist the body in breaking down the energy in foods into nutrients that can be absorbed. Water is calorie-free, but regulates body temperature and provides a medium in which chemical reactions can occur.

Food also provides non-nutrient components with potential health benefits. In the following sections, we'll examine each nutrient class and other healthful substances in more detail.

Carbohydrates

Carbohydrates are the body's universal energy source because most body cells, whether during high-, medium-, or low-intensity activities, can use carbohydrates for energy. Some body cells, such as brain cells and blood cells, can use only carbohydrates for fuel.

There are two categories of carbohydrates: *simple carbohydrates* and *complex carbohydrates.* The basic building blocks of carbohydrates are sugar molecules, whose names usually end in "ose."

Simple Carbohydrates

Simple carbohydrates are constructed from just one or two sugar molecules. That means they are easily digested. We commonly refer to simple carbohydrates as *sugars*, and six are important in nutrition: glucose, fructose (fruit sugar), galactose, maltose (malt sugar), sucrose (table sugar), and lactose (milk sugar). Sugars provide much of the sweetness found naturally in fruits, some vegetables, honey, and milk. They are also added to beverages, candies, and desserts. In fact, studies indicate that people in the United States consume an average of 30 teaspoons of added sugars a day.[1]

As it breaks down, absorbs, burns, or stores the simple carbohydrates you eat, your body is unable to distinguish between those that came naturally from whole foods and those that were added to foods as sweeteners. Chemically, they are the same. This doesn't mean, however, that drinking orange juice is the same as drinking orange soda! Foods with naturally occurring sugars contain many vitamins, minerals, and other substances that promote health. Foods high in added sugars generally provide empty calories and few, if any, health-promoting benefits.

Complex Carbohydrates

Complex carbohydrates are made up of chains of multiple sugar molecules (three or more); therefore, they take longer to digest. Just as we commonly refer to simple carbohydrates as sugars, complex carbohydrates are commonly called *starches*. However, there are two non-starch forms of complex carbohydrate. These are *glycogen*, a storage form of glucose in animal tissues, and *fiber*, a non-digestible component of plants that we'll discuss in more detail later. Starches make up the majority of complex carbohydrates in foods, and are found in a variety of plants, especially grains (barley, buckwheat, millet, oats, quinoa, rice, rye, wheat), legumes (dried beans, lentils, peas), most vegetables, and some fruits. Processed foods from grains, such as breads, pasta, and cereals, also are good sources of starch.

Choose Whole Grains

Unrefined grains, or **whole grains,** include three parts—bran, germ, and endosperm—and generally can be sprouted **(Figure 4.2).** Common examples are rolled or whole oats, hulled barley, popcorn, brown rice, whole wheat, rye, millet, and quinoa. Whole grains are especially nutritious because the bran and germ contain valuable vitamins, minerals, fiber, phytochemicals, and antioxidants (all discussed in later sections), which help maintain body functions and may reduce the risk of certain diseases. In addition, whole grains are bulky, and the body digests them slowly, allowing people to feel full sooner and for a longer time, so fewer calories are consumed. Because nutrients from whole grains enter the bloodstream at a slow, steady pace, the body is able to use the energy they provide more efficiently.

In contrast, refined grains are stripped of their bran and germ during processing. Only the starchy endosperm is retained. By removing fiber, some nutrients, and other healthful substances, refinement turns whole grains into less nutritious foods such as white bread, most pasta, white rice, pretzels, crackers, some cereals, and most baked goods such as cakes, cookies, and pastries. De-

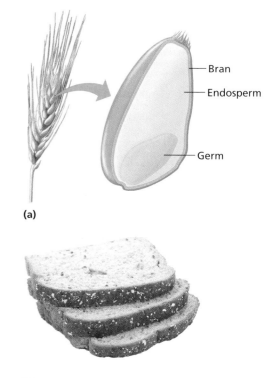

(a)

(b)

Figure 4.2 **Whole grains.** (a) A whole grain includes the bran, endosperm, and germ. (b) Whole wheat bread is an excellent source of whole grain.

spite having fewer nutrients, these products usually retain all the calories of their unrefined counterparts.

Many refined carbohydrates are "enriched" after processing, meaning that some of the lost nutrients such as iron and some B vitamins are replaced. However, many other important nutrients and healthful non-nutrient substances are not replaced.

Most people in the U.S. eat less than one serving of whole grains a day.[2] If you're one of them, you may be missing out on essential nutrients and other healthful substances, while over-consuming calories. So the next time you're debating between the plain bagel or the whole grain toast, go for the whole grain.

Recommended Carbohydrate Intake

You should aim to consume at least 130 grams of carbohydrates, including simple and complex, each day.[3] That said, if your diet only meets this minimum requirement for carbohydrates, then it's likely to be inadequate in other nutrients as well as fiber and other healthful substances, and may be high in fat. For these reasons, experts recommend that adults consume about half (45–65%) of their total daily calories as carbohydrate, roughly 225 to 325 grams for someone consuming 2,000 calories per day. The actual amount you need depends on the total calories you require per day. Focus on consuming foods rich in whole grains and other complex carbohydrates. **Practical Strategies for Health: Choosing Complex Carbohydrates** shows you how.

simple carbohydrates The most basic unit of carbohydrates, consisting of one or two sugar molecules.

complex carbohydrates Contain chains of multiple sugar molecules; commonly called *starches* but also come in two non-starch forms: *glycogen* and *fiber*.

whole grains Unrefined grains that contain bran, germ, and endosperm.

😊 *Practical Strategies for Health*

Choosing Complex Carbohydrates

A diet high in complex carbohydrates provides a wide variety of essential nutrients. It's also rich in fiber, a non-nutrient substance that keeps your digestive tract running smoothly. Maintaining a high complex-carbohydrate diet also reduces your risk of obesity, heart disease, and type 2 diabetes. So how can you choose more complex carbohydrates? Here are some tips:

- Start your day with whole grain cereal and a piece of fresh fruit.

- Switch to whole grain bread for morning toast and lunchtime sandwiches.

- Instead of a side of french fries or potato chips, choose a small salad, carrot sticks, or slices of sweet red pepper.

- For an afternoon snack, mix dried fruits with nuts, sunflower seeds, and pieces of whole grain cereal.

- If dinner includes rice, pasta, pizza crust, or tortillas, choose whole grain versions.

- Include a side of beans, peas, or lentils with dinner, along with a leafy green vegetable, sweet potato, or vegetable soup.

- For an evening snack, choose popcorn, popcorn cakes, a whole grain toaster pastry, low-fat oatmeal cookies, or a bowl of whole grain cereal with milk.

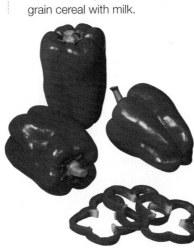

Fats

Lipids are a group of substances that share one important characteristic: They are not soluble in water. Olive oil will float to the top of your salad dressing because it's a lipid. In moderate amounts, certain lipids are important for good nutrition and health. They help your body absorb fat-soluble vitamins, cushion and insulate your organs, and add flavor and tenderness to foods. They are also the most concentrated energy source in your diet, supplying 9 calories per gram. In fact, lipids supply your body with energy both while you are active and while you sleep.

Fats are the type of lipid found most abundantly in your diet, in a wide variety of plant and animal foods. However, two other lipids are also present in a few foods. *Sterols,* such as cholesterol, are found in animal-based foods, including meats, eggs, shellfish, and whole milk. Because the liver can make cholesterol from fats, you don't need to consume it in your diet. *Phospholipids* are the third type of food lipid. They are present in peanuts, egg yolk, and a few processed foods such as salad dressing. Like cholesterol, phospholipids can be made by the body, so you don't need to consume them. Throughout the rest of this section, we'll focus on fats because of the critical role they play in human health.

Dietary fats are more precisely known as *triglycerides*, compounds that contain a chemical called glycerol (a type of alcohol) attached to three fatty acid chains. Depending on the structure of the fatty acid chains, one of three different types of fats is formed: saturated, monounsaturated, or polyunsaturated. Most fatty foods, from butter to meat to olive oil, contain a combination of these three types of fats, but one usually predominates. For example, butter consists mostly of saturated fat, whereas olive oil contains mostly monounsaturated fat. As we explain next, each type of dietary fat has different characteristics and different effects on your health.

fats (lipids) A major source of energy that helps the body absorb fat-soluble vitamins, cushions and insulates organs, and adds flavor and tenderness to foods.

saturated fats Fats that typically are solid at room temperature; generally found in animal products, dairy products, and tropical oils.

unsaturated fats (oils) Fats that typically are liquid at room temperature; generally come from plant sources.

Saturated Fats

Saturated fats got their name because their fatty acid chains are "saturated" with hydrogen. This makes them solid at room temperature, and stable; that is, they aren't easily altered, and they tend to have a long shelf life. Saturated fats generally are found in animal products such as meat, cream, whole milk, cheese, lard, shortening, and butter. Palm, palm kernel, and coconut oils, although derived from plants, also are highly saturated.

We've described saturated fats as <u>s</u>table and <u>s</u>olid, but there's one more "S" word that applies to them: They are <u>s</u>ickening to your heart. Saturated fats can increase the level of LDL (low-density lipoprotein) cholesterol in your blood. A high LDL and/or total blood cholesterol level is a major risk factor for heart disease, increases the risk of stroke, and can lead to a heart attack.[4]

Unsaturated Fats

Unsaturated fats got their name because their fatty acid chains have one or more areas that are not "saturated" with hydrogen. This makes them more flexible, and they are typically liquid at room temperature. In fact, we commonly refer to them as *oils*. These heart-healthy fats generally come from plant sources. The two types of unsaturated fats are monounsaturated and polyunsaturated.

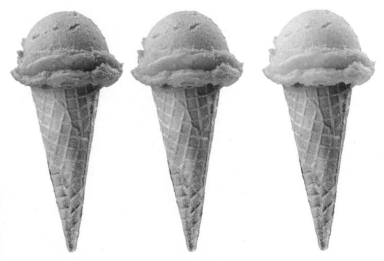

Ice cream, unfortunately, is loaded with saturated fat.

Monounsaturated fats have fatty acid chains with one unsaturated region (*mono* means one). Although liquid at room temperature, they start to solidify at refrigerator temperatures. They are less stable than saturated fats so they become rancid more quickly. Consuming monounsaturated fats triggers less total cholesterol production and decreases your blood levels of LDL cholesterol. What's more, when used in place of saturated fats, monounsaturated fats may increase your blood levels of a beneficial type of cholesterol called HDL (high-density lipoprotein) cholesterol and may help protect you against some cancers.[5] You might remind yourself that **L**DL cholesterol is "lousy" for you, whereas **H**DL cholesterol is "healthful." Sources of monounsaturated fats include canola oil, olive oil, peanut oil, nuts, avocado, and sesame seeds.

Polyunsaturated fats have fatty acid chains with two or more unsaturated regions (*poly* means many). They usually are liquid both at room temperature and in the refrigerator, and easily become rancid. Thus, they have a relatively short shelf life. Polyunsaturated fats tend to help your body get rid of newly formed cholesterol, thereby lowering your blood cholesterol levels and reducing deposits in artery walls.[4] Sources of polyunsaturated fats include corn oil, soybean oil, safflower oil, non-hydrogenated margarines, salad dressings, mayonnaise, nuts, and seeds.

Two polyunsaturated fats have been getting a lot of media attention lately. These are *omega-6 fatty acid* (also known as linoleic acid) and *omega-3 fatty acid* (also known as alpha-linolenic acid). Both are essential to your body's functioning and are thought to provide some protection against heart disease. Since they cannot be assembled by your body and must be obtained from your diet or from supplements, they are also known as the *essential fatty acids* (EFAs). Most people in the U.S. get plenty of omega-6 fatty acids from plant oils, seeds, and nuts. However, most people here need to increase significantly their consumption of omega-3 fatty acids, which are found in fatty fish (like salmon and mackerel), walnuts, flaxseed, canola oil, and dark green, leafy vegetables.

Next time you're debating between beef and salmon, keep in mind that beef is higher in saturated fat and cholesterol, whereas

trans fats Fats that are produced when liquid fat (oil) is turned into solid fat during food processing.

salmon is rich in omega-3 fatty acids. Now which will you choose?

Avoid *Trans* Fats

So far, we've been discussing fats that occur naturally in foods. Now let's turn our attention to a particularly harmful form of fat that occurs almost exclusively in processed foods: ***trans* fats.**

During food processing, unsaturated fats may undergo a chemical process called *hydrogenation.* To "hydrogenate" means to saturate with hydrogen, so as you've probably guessed, hydrogenation changes unstable, unsaturated oils into more stable, saturated, solid fats that are less likely to spoil. The greater the degree of hydrogenation, the more solid the fat becomes. For instance, canola oil can be hydrogenated to various degrees, forming a liquid (squeeze bottle), soft tub, or stick margarine.

Hydrogenation creates a unique type of fatty acid chain called a *trans* fat. Most *trans* fats in your diet come from vegetable shortenings, some margarines, commercially prepared baked goods, snack foods, processed foods, and other foods made with or fried in partially hydrogenated oils. A small amount of *trans* fats occurs naturally in beef, lamb, and dairy products. You can find out the *trans* fat content of any packaged food by reading the label. However, foods containing half a gram of *trans* fat or less per serving can claim to be "*trans* fat free," so look for the words "hydrogenated" or "partially hydrogenated vegetable oil" in the ingredients list. If they're present, the food contains *trans* fats.[5]

Trans fats are worse for blood cholesterol levels than saturated fats because they not only raise LDL cholesterol, they lower HDL cholesterol, increasing the risk of heart disease. They also increase the risk of inflammation, an immune system response that has been implicated in heart disease, stroke, diabetes, and other chronic conditions.[6] Even small amounts of *trans* fats—anything greater than 2 grams per 2,000 calories—can have harmful health effects.[7] The average person in the U.S. eats about 6 grams of *trans* fats a day. For every 2% increase of calories from *trans* fats daily, the risk of heart disease increases by 23%.[7]

Recommended Fat Intake

Dietary recommendations for fats have changed in recent years, shifting the emphasis from lowering total fat to limiting saturated and *trans* fats. Current recommendations suggest carefully replacing the saturated fats with monounsaturated and polyunsaturated fats and enjoying them in moderation.[8] Here are some specific recommendations:

- In general, fats should make up between 20% and 35% of your total calories to meet daily energy and nutrition needs while minimizing your risk for chronic disease.

- *Trans* fat intake should be kept to an absolute minimum.

- Saturated fats should be less than 7% of calories, or less than 16 grams (about 140 calories) for someone consuming 2,000 calories per day.

- Omega-6 fatty acid intake should be about 14 to 17 grams per day for men and about 11 to 12 grams per day for women.

- Omega-3 fatty acid intake should be about 1.6 grams per day for men and about 1.1 grams per day for women.

Since most college students don't monitor their diets closely every day, a good habit is to choose unsaturated fats over saturated

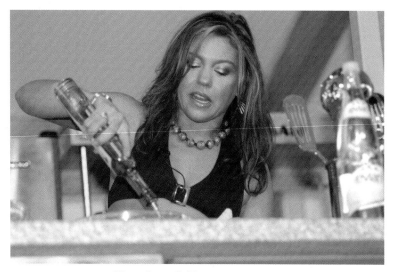

Celebrity cook **Rachael Ray** popularized the use of "EVOO": extra virgin olive oil, a monounsaturated fat.

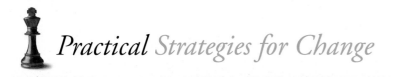
Choosing Healthful Fats

To choose healthful fats, start by sorting the good guys from the bad guys. Make it a standard practice to pick foods with zero *trans* fats, and keep your intake of saturated fats as low as possible. Replace saturated fats with unsaturated fats. In particular, consume small amounts of vegetable oils, walnuts, flaxseed, leafy green vegetables, and/or fish daily to meet your essential fatty acid needs. Here are some additional tips:

- Instead of butter or a margarine made with hydrogenated oils, spread your toast with a non-*trans* fat margarine or peanut, almond, cashew, or walnut butter.

- If you normally eat two eggs for breakfast, discard the yolk from one. Do the same when making egg dishes such as quiche or casseroles, and in baking.

- Make low-fat foods a priority at each meal. Choose whole grain foods, legumes, fruits, vegetables, non-fat or low-fat dairy products, lean red meats (rump, round, loin, and flank), skinless poultry, and fish.

- Trim all visible fat from red meat and poultry. Instead of choosing fried meats, poultry, or fish, choose baked or broiled. Finally, remove the skin from poultry before eating it.

- Skip the french fries. Opt for a baked potato or side salad instead.

- Make sure that any cookies or other baked goods you buy are *trans*-fat free.

- Instead of ice cream, which is high in saturated fat, choose ice milk, sorbet, or low-fat or non-fat frozen yogurt.

- When the munchies hit, go for air-popped popcorn, pretzels, rice cakes, or dried fruit instead of potato chips.

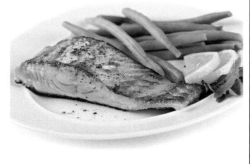

and *trans* fats whenever possible. You can do this by adopting the habits described in **Practical Strategies for Change: Choosing Healthful Fats.**

Proteins

Dietary **protein** is a macronutrient available from both animal and plant sources. Although it's one of the energy nutrients, the body uses protein primarily to build other compounds, cells, and tissues and only secondarily for fuel. Some misconceptions surround the roles of protein in the diet and in the body. For instance, people who associate meat with protein and protein with strength may eat meat to build muscle. Such thinking is only partly correct. Whenever you consume proteins, whether they come from animal or plant sources, your body digests them into smaller molecules known as **amino acids,** the building blocks of protein. So proteins in foods do not di-

protein A macronutrient that helps build many body parts, including muscle, bone, skin, and blood; key component of enzymes, hormones, transport proteins, and antibodies.

amino acids The building blocks of protein; 20 common amino acids are found in food.

rectly become body proteins; instead, they supply the amino acids from which the body assembles its own proteins.

Of the common amino acids, 20 are found in food; 11 of these can also be produced by the body, so it's not essential that you consume them. The other 9 are called *essential amino acids* because your body either cannot make them or cannot make sufficient quantities to maintain health. Thus, they must be included in your diet.

Dietary proteins are considered *complete proteins* if they supply all nine essential amino acids in adequate amounts. In contrast, *incomplete proteins* are lacking one or more of the essential amino acids. Meat, fish, poultry, dairy products, soy, and quinoa provide complete proteins. Most plant sources such as legumes, grains, vegetables, and seeds provide incomplete proteins. However, combinations of plant proteins—peanut butter on whole grain bread, for instance, or brown rice with lentils or beans—can complement each other in such a way that the essential amino acids missing from one are supplied by the other. The combination yields complete proteins.

Once absorbed, amino acids enter the bloodstream and become part of the amino acid pool. Just as you might go to an auto parts store to buy an air filter or some spark plugs for your car, your body cells draw from the amino acid pool the precise amino acids they need to build or repair a wide variety of body proteins. These include:

- **Antibodies,** which protect you from disease.
- **Enzymes,** which speed up chemical reactions.
- **Hormones,** which regulate body temperature, use of nutrients, and many other body functions.
- **Transport proteins,** which help carry substances into and out of cells.
- **Buffers,** which help maintain a healthy balance of acids and bases in your blood.

Of course, your body also uses the amino acids from dietary proteins to grow, repair, and maintain body tissues. In short, you consume dietary protein primarily to gain amino acids for your body cells to generate whatever proteins they need.

Recommended Protein Intake

For good health, experts recommend that adults consume between 10% and 35% of their calories as protein. Staying within this range can provide adequate protein and other nutrients while reducing the risk of chronic diseases such as type 2 diabetes, heart disease, and cancer. When an individual's protein intake falls above or below this range, the risk for development of chronic diseases appears to increase.[3]

How much protein do *you* need? Healthy adults typically need 0.36 grams of protein per pound (0.8 grams per kilogram) of body weight, equaling 54 grams per day for a 150-pound person. Athletes can require twice as much protein, depending on the strength and endurance requirements for their sport. Athlete or not, few people in the U.S. suffer from protein deficiencies. Surveys indicate that protein makes up about 15% of most Americans' diets.[9]

Unfortunately, many animal sources of protein are high in cholesterol and saturated fat. Follow these tips to go lean with protein:

- Avoid fried meats. Choose baked, broiled, or grilled.
- Choose lean cuts of meats such as rump, round, loin, and flank. Better yet, choose poultry (remove the skin). Best of all, choose fish.
- Vary your protein sources by consuming vegetarian meals several times a week.

Fish is a great source of protein, but the mercury levels in some kinds of fish can be harmful to women or young children. The Monterey Bay Aquarium has a handy guide for making safe and sustainable seafood choices at www.montereybayaquarium.org/cr/cr_seafoodwatch/sfw_health.aspx.

Vitamins

Vitamins are carbon-containing compounds required in small amounts to regulate body processes such as blood-cell production, nerve function, digestion, and skin and bone maintenance. They also help chemical reactions take place. For example, although not an energy nutrient, vitamins do help your body to break down carbohydrates, fats, and proteins for energy.

Humans need 13 vitamins **(Table 4.1).** Four of these—vitamins A, D, E, and K—are *fat soluble*, meaning they dissolve in fat and can be stored in your body's fatty tissues. Because your body can store them, consuming the fat-soluble vitamins two to three times a week is adequate. Nine vitamins—vitamin C and the eight B-complex vitamins (thiamin, riboflavin, niacin, pantothenic acid, B_6, biotin, folic acid, and B_{12}) are *water soluble*. They dissolve in water, and excesses are generally excreted from the body in urine. Because your body can't readily store them, it's important that you consume adequate water-soluble vitamins daily.

Your body is able to manufacture vitamin D in your skin if you have adequate exposure to sunlight. If not, vitamin D, like other vitamins, must be ingested.

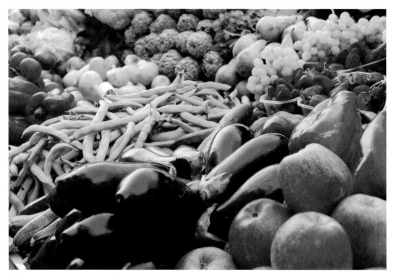

Vitamins and minerals are abundant in fruits and vegetables.

Vitamins are abundant in fruits, vegetables, and whole grains. Meat and dairy products also contain some vitamins. Food manufacturers commonly add or replace vitamins during processing, providing more dietary options for meeting needs. Because vitamins are readily available from the U.S. food supply, deficiencies among people in the United States are rare.

The likelihood of consuming too much of any vitamin from food is also remote. However, excesses of vitamins from supplements can reach toxic levels, causing side effects such as nausea, diarrhea, vomiting, skin rash, numbness of hands and feet, nosebleeds, hair loss, and pain. For this reason, vitamin supplementation is recommended only for certain populations. For example, women of childbearing age, especially if they intend to become pregnant, should consume 400 micrograms of folic acid daily either from a supplement or from fortified foods. And anyone who does not receive adequate sun exposure should

---

vitamins Substances, with no energy value of their own, needed by the body in small amounts for normal growth and function.

Table 4.1: **Key Facts About Vitamins**

Vitamin	Functions	Sample Food Source	Food Sources
Fat-soluble			
A	Required for vision, cell differentiation, reproduction; contributes to healthy bones and a healthy immune system		Beef, chicken liver, egg yolk, milk, spinach, carrots, mango, apricots, cantaloupe, pumpkin, yams
D	Regulates blood calcium levels; maintains bone health; assists in cell differentiation		Canned salmon and mackerel, fortified milk or orange juice, fortified cereals
E	Protects white blood cells, enhances immune function, improves absorption of vitamin A; protects cell membranes, fatty acids and vitamin A from oxidation		Sunflower seeds, almonds, vegetable oils, fortified cereals

Table 4.1: **Key Facts About Vitamins** (continued)

Vitamin	Functions	Sample Food Source	Food Sources
Fat-soluble (continued)			
K	Needed for the production of proteins that assist in blood coagulation and bone metabolism		Kale, spinach, turnip greens, brussels sprouts
Water-soluble			
B$_1$ (Thiamin)	Needed for carbohydrate and amino acid metabolism		Pork, fortified cereals, enriched rice and pasta, peas, tuna, beans
B$_2$ (Riboflavin)	Needed for carbohydrate and fat metabolism		Beef liver, shrimp, dairy products, fortified cereals, enriched bread and grains
B$_6$	Needed for carbohydrate and amino acid metabolism; synthesis of blood cells		Chickpeas (garbanzo beans), red meat/fish/poultry, fortified cereals, potatoes
B$_{12}$	Assists with formation of blood; required for healthy nervous system		Shellfish, red meat/fish/poultry, dairy products, fortified cereals
Niacin	Needed for carbohydrate and fat metabolism; assists in DNA replication and repair; assists in cell differentiation		Beef liver, red meat/fish/poultry, fortified cereals, enriched breads and grains, canned tomato products
Pantothenic acid	Assists with fat metabolism		Red meat/fish/poultry, mushrooms, fortified cereals, egg yolk
Biotin	Involved in carbohydrate, fat, and protein metabolism		Nuts, egg yolk
Folate (Folic acid)	Needed for amino acid metabolism and DNA synthesis		Fortified cereals, enriched breads and grains, legumes (lentils, chickpeas, pinto beans), spinach, romaine lettuce, asparagus, liver
C	Antioxidant; regenerates oxidized vitamin E; enhances immune function; assists in synthesis of hormones, neurotransmitters, and DNA; enhances iron absorption		Sweet peppers, citrus fruits and juices, broccoli, strawberries, kiwi

Source: Adapted from Thompson, J., & Manore, M. (2010). *Nutrition for life* (2nd ed.). San Francisco, CA: Pearson Education.

consume supplemental vitamin D. As a general rule, though, a vitamin supplement should never substitute for healthful eating habits.

For more detailed information on specific vitamins and minerals, visit Oregon State University's Micronutrient Information Center at http://lpi.oregonstate.edu/infocenter/vitamins.html.

Minerals

Minerals are elements that originate in the Earth and cannot be made by living organisms. They also cannot be broken down. Plants obtain minerals from the soil, and most of the minerals in your diet come directly from plants or indirectly from animal sources. Minerals also may be present in the water you drink.

> **minerals** Elements, with no energy value of their own, that regulate body processes and provide structure; constituents of all cells.
>
> **water** A liquid necessary for life.

Your body relies on more than a dozen essential minerals each day to regulate body processes and provide structure. Minerals adjust fluid balance, aid in muscle contraction and nerve transmission, help release energy, and provide structure for bones and teeth. The *major minerals* are those your body needs in amounts greater than 100 milligrams daily. These include sodium, potassium, chloride, calcium, phosphorus, sulfur, and magnesium. You need *trace minerals* in much smaller amounts, typically less than 10 milligrams daily. The trace minerals include iron, fluoride, iodine, selenium, zinc, copper, manganese, and chromium. See **Table 4.2** for more information about selected minerals.

A varied and balanced diet provides most people with all the minerals they need in adequate amounts—not too low or too high. Mineral supplements are not recommended for most healthy people and should be used only under medical supervision. Side effects of mineral toxicity can include seizures, muscle cramps or weakness, confusion, and other problems. However, supplements of individual minerals may be recommended for certain populations. For example, pregnant women and women who experience excessive menstrual bleeding may need supplemental iron. And both growing children and older adults may need supplemental calcium to maintain healthy bones. For more about the nutrients essential to bone health, see the **Spotlight** on the next page.

Water

You may be able to survive for weeks or even months without food, but you can live for only a few days without water. **Water** is dispersed throughout your body and is vital to nutrient digestion, absorption, and transportation. It serves as a lubricant, regulates body temperature, reduces fluid retention, helps prevent constipation, provides moisture to skin and other tissues, carries wastes out of the body, is the medium in which most chemical reactions take place, and gives the feeling of fullness when consumed with a meal.

Nearly all foods, particularly fruits and vegetables, contain water. On average, foods provide about 19% of an adult's total water intake. Beverages provide the remaining 81% of total water intake. Because normal hydration can be maintained by consuming a wide variety of foods and beverages, not just water, recommendations for water intake have not been established. Most adults can maintain an adequate water intake by consuming water-containing foods and drinking 9 to 13 cups (72–104 ounces) of beverages daily.[10] If you are physically active or live in a very hot climate, you may require more total water.

Table 4.2: **Key Facts About Selected Minerals**

Mineral	Functions	Sample Food Source	Other Food Sources
Calcium	Primary component of bone; needed for acid-base balance, transmission of nerve impulses, and muscle contraction		Dairy products, fortified juices, fish with bones (such as sardines or salmon), broccoli, kale, collard greens
Iron	Component of hemoglobin in blood cells; component of myoglobin in muscle cells; assists many enzyme systems		Clams, chicken, turkey, fish, ham
Magnesium	Component of bone; aids in muscle contraction; assists more than 300 enzyme systems		Oysters, beef, pork, chicken, turkey, tuna, lobster, shrimp, salmon, milk, yogurt, whole-grain cereals, almonds, walnuts, sunflower seeds, beans
Potassium	Needed for fluid balance, transmission of nerve impulses, and muscle contraction		Fruits (bananas, oranges, grapefruit, plums), vegetables (spinach, beans)
Zinc	Assists more than 100 enzyme systems; aids in immune system function, growth and sexual maturation, and gene regulation		Red meat, poultry, seafood (oysters, tuna, lobster)

Source: Adapted from Thompson, J., & Manore, M. (2010). *Nutrition for life* (2nd ed.). San Francisco, CA: Pearson Education.

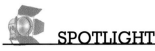

Feeding Your Bones

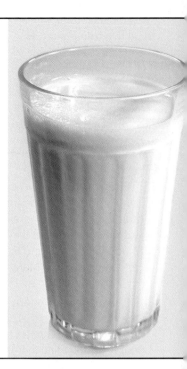

Osteoporosis is a disease characterized by brittle bones and decreased bone mass. You probably think of osteoporosis as a disease of the elderly, but even young adults can start to develop this disorder if they fail to properly nourish their bones.

Calcium is the main component of the mineral crystals that make up healthy bone. As you age from childhood to adulthood, your bones are not only lengthening, they're increasing in density. They do this by de-positing calcium-containing crystals on a protein "scaffold" in the bone interior. If you don't consume enough calcium during these critical years, the supply will run short, and your bones won't be able to increase their density. From age 9 to 18, you should try to consume 1,300 milligrams of calcium a day. After the age of 18, you should try to consume at least 1,000 milligrams per day. Some people, such as pregnant women, nursing mothers, or those over the age of 50, should con-sume more. Calcium is available in dairy foods such as milk, yogurt, and cheese; in green, leafy vegetables; and in fortified soy milk, rice milk, juices, and other beverages.

Vitamin D is another important nutrient for bone health. Your body can absorb only a small fraction of the calcium you consume if your level of vitamin D is inadequate. Recall that you synthesize vitamin D in your skin if you have adequate exposure to sunlight. If you do not spend much time in the sun, you will need to obtain vitamin D through your diet or supplements. Food sources of vitamin D include fatty fish and milk and other fortified foods.

What else can you do to keep your bones strong? Stay active. Any weight-bearing activity, from jogging to carrying textbooks up a flight of stairs, places positive stress on your skeleton and encourages your bones to increase their density.

Other Healthful Substances in Foods

Today, people are increasingly interested in consuming *functional foods*; that is, foods that confer some kind of health benefit in addition to the benefits provided by their basic nutrients. For example, researchers are studying non-nutrient substances in food that may improve your body's gastrointestinal functioning, boost your immunity, slow memory loss, delay aging, or prevent heart disease or cancer. Although many such non-nutrient substances are currently under investigation, we'll limit our discussion to those you're most likely to hear about in the news or in food advertisements—these are fiber, phytochemicals, antioxidants, and probiotics.

Fiber
Fiber is a non-nutrient, non-digestible complex carbohydrate. Whereas starch is readily digested and its components absorbed, fiber passes through the intestinal tract undigested, and provides bulk for feces. Because it absorbs water along the way, it also softens feces, making stools easier to pass.

Fiber has many health benefits. It helps promote bowel regularity, easing conditions such as hemorrhoids, constipation, and other digestive disorders. Because it makes foods bulky, it can aid in weight management. It also lowers blood cholesterol, reducing your risk for heart disease. By slowing the transit of food—including sugars and starches—through your intestinal tract, fiber also promotes a more gradual release of glucose into your blood and can help in managing diabetes.

Fiber is found naturally in grains, legumes, fruits, vegetables, nuts, and seeds. Recall that the refining process can remove fiber from grains. So be sure to consume foods made from whole grains daily.

It's recommended that men consume 38 grams of fiber per day. Women need 25 grams per day. For men and women 50 years or older, the recom-mendations are 30 and 21 grams, respectively.[3] Remember we said that fiber absorbs water, so a high-fiber diet should be accompanied by plenty of fluids to keep the fiber moving along the intestinal tract.

Phytochemicals
Phytochemicals are naturally occurring chemicals in plants (*phyto* means plant) that may have health effects, but are not considered essential nutrients.[11] Sources of phytochemicals include fruits, vegetables, legumes (including soy), nuts, seeds, and grains. Phytochemicals include:

- **Carotenoids,** which may help reduce the risk of cardiovascular disease, certain cancers, and age-related eye diseases. Carotenoids are found in red, orange, and deep-green foods such as carrots, cantaloupe, kale, spinach, pumpkin, and tomatoes.

- **Flavonoids,** which may help reduce the risk of cardiovascular disease, cancer, blood clotting, and high blood pressure. They are found in foods like berries, black and green tea, chocolate, and soy products.

- **Organosulfur compounds,** which may help protect against cancer. They are found in foods like garlic, leeks, onions, chives, broccoli, cauliflower, and cabbage.

It is likely that the health benefits of phytochemicals are the result of many of them working together along with other substances in foods.[12] Phytochemical supplements (that is, those found in pill form) can't begin to imitate the qualities of natural foods, and have not been shown to be beneficial. What's more, studies suggest that certain phytochemical supplements in high concentrations can be dangerous.

Antioxidants
As part of your day-to-day body functioning, a variety of chemical reactions called *oxidation reactions* continually occur. Although normal, oxidation reactions sometimes produce harmful chemicals

fiber A non-digestible complex carbohydrate that aids in digestion.

phytochemicals Naturally occurring plant substances thought to have disease-preventing qualities and health-promoting properties.

antioxidants Compounds in food that help protect the body from harmful molecules called free radicals.

probiotics Living, beneficial microbes that develop naturally in food and that help maintain digestive functions.

called *free radicals*, which start chain reactions that can damage cells. Environmental factors such as pollution, sunlight, strenuous exercise, cigarette smoke, and stress also contribute to free-radical production. Damage from free radicals has been linked to cancer, heart disease, Alzheimer's dementia, Parkinson's disease, arthritis, and simply aging.

It is impossible for you to avoid damage by free radicals; however, certain components of foods can help neutralize them. These substances are generally referred to as **antioxidants** because they work against oxidation. Some antioxidants are nutrients: These include vitamins C and E, beta-carotene (a form of vitamin A), and the mineral selenium. Many other antioxidants are non-nutrients; these include phytochemicals and certain other substances in foods.

Antioxidants work by stabilizing free radicals, thereby stopping the chain reaction that damages cells. In doing so, antioxidants are depleted, so you need to replenish them daily. Fortunately, antioxidants are plentiful in fruits and vegetables, whole grains, nuts, and legumes. In general, fresh and uncooked foods contain more antioxidants than processed ones. Although you have numerous choices for antioxidant-rich foods, the United States Department of Agriculture (USDA) has found the following 20 foods, in descending order, to be highest in antioxidants: small red beans, wild blueberries, red kidney beans, pinto beans, cultivated blueberries, cranberries, artichokes, blackberries, prunes, raspberries, strawberries, Red Delicious apples, Granny Smith apples, pecans, sweet cherries, black plums, Russet potatoes, black beans, plums, and Gala apples.[13] A varied diet with at least five servings of fruits and vegetables daily and beans several times a week should provide ample antioxidants.

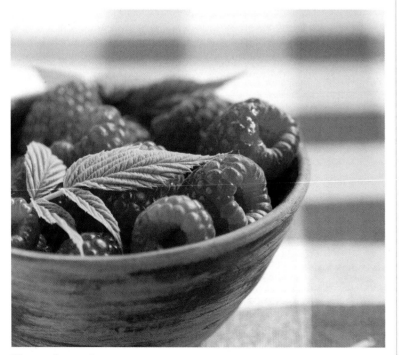

Raspberries are a rich source of antioxidants.

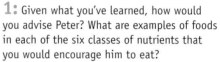
Probiotics

Probiotics are living, beneficial microbes that develop naturally in fermented dairy foods such as yogurt, buttermilk, and sour cream, as well as in fermented vegetable foods such as sauerkraut, miso, and tempeh (fermented tofu). The most common are types of bacteria. If deliberately consuming foods full of live bacteria sounds less than appealing to you, consider that *probiotic* means "pro-life"—the particular strains of bacteria in these foods help maintain your digestive functions and your health. Probiotics are thought to promote good health by crowding out harmful bacteria, viruses, and yeasts; by producing nutrients; and by assisting your immune system.

Strategies for Eating Right

You've learned how nutrients and other health-promoting substances function in your body. But how much of each nutrient do you need each day, and how do you choose real foods to meet those nutrient needs? In this section, you'll learn how to use four tools to help you eat right.

Learn About the Dietary Reference Intakes (DRIs)

Determining the amounts of energy, nutrients, and other dietary components that best support health is a huge task. For more than 50 years, scientists have provided consumers with a set of energy and nutrient standards to protect against nutrient deficiencies, support healthy functioning, and prevent chronic diseases. These recommendations are called the **Dietary Reference Intakes (DRI).**

The DRIs include four groups of recommendations:[3]

- **Recommended Dietary Allowances (RDA).** Nutrient intakes proposed to meet the needs of 98% of all healthy people of similar age and gender.
- **Adequate Intakes (AI).** Average amounts of nutrients that appear sufficient to maintain health. These values are used as a guide for nutrient intake when an RDA cannot be determined. In other words, a nutrient has either an RDA or an AI, but not both.
- **Tolerable Upper Intake Levels (UL).** The maximum amount of nutrients that appear safe for most healthy people.
- **Estimated Average Requirements (EAR).** The amounts of nutrients that meet the needs of half the people of a given age and gender. EARs are the basis for calculating RDAs.

As an example, for vitamin A, adult men have an EAR of 625 micrograms per day, RDA of 900 micrograms per day, and UL of 3000 micrograms per day.

> You can access DRI tables online at the USDA's Food and Nutrition Information Center at **http://fnic.nal.usda.gov.**

Do all these values seem confusing? For most people, they are. That's why many government agencies have developed tools that present the DRIs in more meaningful ways. One such tool is the food label found on nearly all packaged foods sold in the U.S.

Read Food Labels

Food labels provide a lot of helpful information—if you read them! In addition to identifying the product and manufacturer, they include a list of all ingredients in the food in descending order by weight. So if you're considering buying a carton of yogurt and notice that sugar is the third ingredient on the list, you might want to choose another brand.

Another helpful part of food labels is the *Nutrition Facts panel*, which provides nutrient information required by the U.S. Food and Drug Administration **(Figure 4.3).** For instance, on the panel you'll find the recommended serving size for this food, as well as the number of servings per package, the calories, and the calories from fat per serving. If you're watching your calorie intake, you should know that a food that has about 40 calories per serving is considered low in calories; 100 is considered moderate, and 400 or more is high.[14]

Beneath this line, the panel identifies the macronutrients, sodium, and fiber found in a serving of the food. Notice that both saturated fat and *trans* fat are listed separately to inform you of the quantity of these unhealthful fats provided by this food.

If you wanted to track the total grams of fiber you were eating each day, all you'd need to note would be the number of grams per serving. But let's say you wanted to know what *percentage* a serving of this food would con-

Dietary Reference Intakes (DRIs) A set of energy and nutrient recommendations for supporting good health.

percent Daily Value (% DV) Nutrient standards that estimate how much a serving of a given food contributes to the overall intake of nutrients listed on the food label.

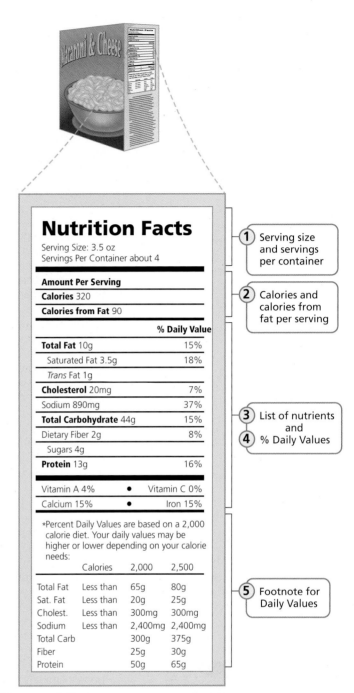

Figure 4.3 Read food labels wisely. When reading a Nutrition Facts panel, note the serving size, calories (and calories from fat) per serving, and the nutrients contained per serving.

tribute toward your daily need for fiber. For that, you'd look at the right-hand column of the panel to find the **percent Daily Value (% DV).** These nutrient standards, which were developed specifically for use on the Nutrition Facts panel, give you a rough estimate of how much a serving of the food contributes to the overall intake of nutrients in a "typical" 2,000-calorie diet.[14]

Even if your daily calorie needs are higher or lower than 2,000, you can still use the % DV to help you judge the nutritional quality of a food: 5% DV or less is a low level for that nutrient, whereas 20% or more is high. So if a frozen veggie burger provides 5% of the DV for

A Blueprint for Better Nutrition

The Dietary Guidelines for Americans is a set of nine strategies for maintaining or improving your health. The following is a brief summary of each.

Obtain Adequate Nutrients Within Calorie Needs

Be careful that you don't take in more calories than you need each day. Choosing fresh fruits, vegetables, whole grains, and low-fat or fat-free dairy products will help you stay within your calorie allowance. That's because these foods are *nutrient-dense,* meaning they provide generous amounts of vitamins, minerals, fiber, and other health-promoting substances but contain relatively few calories.

Focus on Healthful Foods

Build meals and snacks around four food groups: fruits, vegetables, whole grains, and low-fat or fat-free dairy products. These foods are low in saturated and *trans* fats, cholesterol, added sugars, and salt, but rich in essential nutrients as well as fiber and phytochemicals. They are also lower in calories, so choosing them will help you stay within your calorie allowance each day.

Watch Your Intake of Fats

The type and amount of fat you consume can make a big difference to the health of your heart. To reduce your risk of heart disease, keep your intake of saturated and *trans* fats as low as possible. Replace these with unsaturated fats from fish, nuts, and plant oils. When selecting red meat, poultry, and dairy products, make choices that are lean, low-fat, or fat-free. Also keep your total fat intake between 20% and 35% of your total calorie intake.

Choose Carbohydrates Wisely

Fresh fruits, vegetables, and whole grains promote health and reduce your risk of chronic disease. Eat more of these and less of foods containing refined carbohydrates, such as pastries, white bread, white rice, crackers, and candies. Also avoid sweetened beverages, from soft drinks to sweetened flavored waters, as these contain huge amounts of simple sugars. Drink more low-fat or non-fat milk. It contains many essential nutrients. If you're not sure whether a food or beverage has added sweeteners, look for these terms on the food label: sugars (brown, invert, raw, beet, or cane), corn sweetener, corn syrup, high fructose corn syrup, fruit juice concentrates, honey, malt syrup, molasses, glucose, fructose, maltose, sucrose, lactose, and dextrose.

Maintain Proper Levels of Sodium and Potassium

If you're like most Americans, you consume substantially more salt (sodium chloride) than you need. On average, as sodium intake rises, so does blood pressure, so by reducing your sodium intake, you help keep your blood pressure down. Keeping your blood pressure in the normal range, approximately 120 over 80 millimeters of mercury (120/80 mm Hg), reduces your risk for heart disease and stroke. Surprisingly, hiding the salt shaker is not the most important strategy for controlling your sodium intake. That's because most of us get far more sodium every day from the processed foods we eat. So read the Nutrition Facts panel on food labels to check the amount of sodium in the food. Less than 140 milligrams (mg) or 5% of the Daily Value is low in salt. At the same time, make sure you're getting enough potassium, which helps blunt the effects of sodium on blood pressure. The best potassium sources are fruits and vegetables, especially apricots, bananas, broccoli, cantaloupe, carrots, dates, mushrooms, oranges, potatoes, prunes, raisins, spinach, sweet potato, watermelon, and winter squash. Other good potassium sources are milk products, legumes, peanuts, and almonds.

Manage Your Body Weight

Achieve and maintain a healthful body weight by balancing the calories you consume in foods and beverages with the calories you burn in physical activity. For help in maintaining a body weight that's right for you, see Chapter 6.

Engage in Regular Physical Activity

Regular physical activity improves physical fitness, promotes psychological well-being, and helps manage weight. It also reduces the risk of many chronic diseases. Adults should be moderately active for at least 30 minutes most days of the week. For help in getting and staying fit, see Chapter 5.

Use Alcohol Moderately or Not at All

Alcoholic beverages supply 7 calories per gram—that's 150 calories for a 12-ounce beer! No wonder drinking a lot of alcohol can make it hard to maintain a healthy weight. Moderate alcohol intake—defined as up to one drink per day for women and up to two drinks per day for men—is associated with mortality reduction in middle-aged and older adults. But among younger people, alcohol consumption provides little, if any, health benefit, and it is harmful for women who are or may become pregnant or are breastfeeding, anyone taking medications, people with certain medical conditions, and anyone who will be driving or using machinery. For more on alcohol, see Chapter 8.

Be Food Safe

Every year about 76 million people in the U.S. experience foodborne illness. Simple measures such as washing your hands and food-contact surfaces; separating raw, cooked, and ready-to-eat foods while shopping, preparing, or storing them; cooking foods to the proper temperature; and keeping cold foods cold will reduce your risk of foodborne illness. We discuss food safety in more detail later in this chapter.

As this textbook went to press, the 2010 Dietary Guidelines had not yet been released. For updates, visit **www.health.gov/dietaryguidelines.**

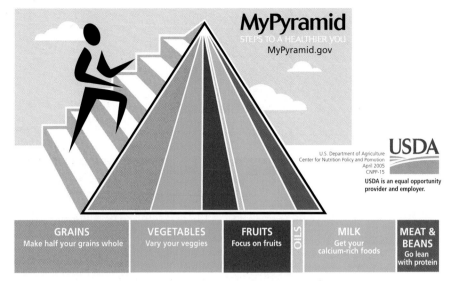

Figure 4.4 **The USDA's MyPyramid.** To generate your personalized MyPyramid recommendations, visit www.MyPyramid.gov.

saturated fat, 0% for cholesterol, and 24% for protein, you can assume that it's a nutritious choice.

Use the % DV whenever possible. Consider not only the serving size, but also how many servings you will actually consume. If you will eat double the serving size listed on the package, then you must also double the calories, nutrients, and % DV.

Follow the Dietary Guidelines for Americans

The *Dietary Guidelines for Americans* has been published jointly every five years since 1980 by the U.S. Department of Health and Human Services (HHS) and the U.S. Department of Agriculture (USDA). The Guidelines provide expert advice for reducing risk of chronic disease and promoting health. The message to Americans is clear and concise: Consume fewer calories, be more active, and make wiser choices within and among food groups. Check out the details on the facing page.

Food Guide Pyramid (MyPyramid) A graphic representation of the Dietary Guidelines for Americans, which encourage intake of complex carbohydrates and discourage intake of fats and sweets.

Log Onto MyPyramid

The **Food Guide Pyramid,** commonly known as MyPyramid, is a simple pictographic representation of the Dietary Guidelines for Americans **(Figure 4.4),** as well as a starting point for assessing and improving your eating habits.

When you visit www.MyPyramid.gov, you'll be guided to develop an eating plan tailored to your specific gender, age, current weight, and level of activity. Using a feature called MyPyramid Tracker, you can enter the foods you've eaten over one or more days and find out how closely your diet corresponds to the Dietary Guidelines for Americans.

Two additional components of MyPyramid can provide help in planning your daily diet. You can use MyPyramid's calorie table to help you estimate your daily calorie needs **(Table 4.3).** The recommended calorie level for each sex and age is based on physical activity level, from sedentary to active. Once you've figured out

Table 4.3: **MyPyramid Estimated Daily Calorie Needs**

	Calorie Range		
Age (years)	*Sedentary*[a]	*Moderately Active*[b]	*Active*[c]
Children			
2–3	1000	1000–1400	1000–1400
Females			
4–8	1200–1400	1400–1600	1400–1800
9–13	1400–1600	1600–2000	1800–2200
14–18	1800	2000	2400
19–30	1800–2000	2000–2200	2400
31–50	1800	2000	2200
51+	1600	1800	2000–2200
Males			
4–8	1200–1400	1400–1600	1600–2000
9–13	1600–2000	1800–2200	2000–2600
14–18	2000–2400	2400–2800	2800–3200
19–30	2400–2600	2600–2800	3000
31–51	2200–2400	2400–2600	2800–3000
51+	2000–2200	2200–2400	2600–2800

[a]Sedentary: A lifestyle that includes only light activity associated with normal daily routine.

[b]Moderately active: A lifestyle that includes physical activity equivalent to walking 1.5 to 3 miles per day at 3 to 4 miles per hour (30–60 minutes a day) in addition to normal daily routine.

[c]Active: A lifestyle that includes physical activity equivalent to walking more than 3 miles per day at 3 to 4 miles per hour (60 or more minutes a day) in addition to normal daily routine.

Source: U.S. Department of Agriculture, Center for Nutrition Policy and Promotion. (2005). MyPyramid food intake pattern calorie levels. Retrieved from http://www.mypyramid.gov/downloads/mypyramid_calorie_levels.pdf

Energy intake	Grains	Vegetables	Fruits	Oils	Milk	Meat & Beans	Discretionary calorie allowance
1,000 kcal/day	3 oz-equivalent	1 cup	1 cup	3 tsp.	2 cups	2 oz-equivalent	165
1,800 kcal/day	6 oz-equivalent	2.5 cups	1.5 cups	5 tsp.	3 cups	5 oz-equivalent	195
2,600 kcal/day	9 oz-equivalent	3.5 cups	2 cups	8 tsp.	3 cups	6.5 oz-equivalent	410
3,200 kcal/day	10 oz-equivalent	4 cups	2.5 cups	11 tsp.	3 cups	7 oz-equivalent	648

Figure 4.5 **How much should you consume from each food group?** Here are sample recommendations based on four different levels of energy intake.

about how many calories you should take in each day, check out **Figure 4.5,** which identifies the amounts of foods in each food group that you need to consume to meet your calorie and nutrient needs. It also shows you how many discretionary calories can be consumed at each calorie level. These are calories "left over" after you have met all your nutrient needs. You can use them for an occasional treat or for an additional healthful food. People who want to lose weight may simply choose not to use their discretionary calories.

Understanding serving size is fundamental to success using the MyPyramid plan. A *serving* isn't what you happen to put on your plate. It is a recommended amount of food defined by common measurements such as cups, ounces, or pieces. An unusual term used in MyPyramid to define a serving size in the grains and the meat and beans groups is *ounce-equivalent*. As you might guess, it

The Harvard Healthy Eating Pyramid, developed by scientists at the Harvard School of Public Health, offers a popular alternative to MyPyramid. To find out more, visit **www.hsph.harvard.edu/nutritionsource/what-you-should-eat/pyramid.**

identifies an amount that's about equivalent to an ounce. For instance, 1/2 cup of cooked rice is about an ounce. **Figure 4.6** shows other examples of "ounce-equivalents." Figure 6.6 in Chapter 6 shows additional ways for estimating serving sizes.

Eat Smart When You're Eating Out

If you're like most college students, you get most of your meals from the campus dining hall, food kiosks, restaurants, or fast food restaurants. But you can still make smart choices when you're eating out. For instance, consider two sample fast food meals: (1) a McDonald's Big Mac, extra large fries, and an apple pie and (2) a Subway 6-inch Cold Cut Combo sandwich, a granola bar, and an apple. The McDonald's meal contains about 1,430 calories and a whopping 47% of its total energy as fat. The Subway lunch contains about 610 calories and 31% of its energy as fat.[15] In short, simple choices you make every day can make a difference in your nutrition, weight, and health. For some tips for eating at fast food restaurants, see **Practical Strategies for Change: Eating Right While on the Run.**

This site compares serving sizes, calories, saturated fat, *trans* fat, and sodium content for several popular fast foods: **www.acaloriecounter.com/fast-food.php.**

How Do Nutrition Guidelines Vary for Different Groups?

The Dietary Guidelines for Americans provide expert advice for lowering risk of chronic disease and promoting health. However, some population groups, based on their age, sex, level of physical activity, or diet preferences may have special dietary needs.

Nutrition Needs Change Over Time

Whatever his or her age, everyone needs the same nutrients, only in different amounts. Here are key ways the DRI amounts differ throughout the lifecycle:[14]

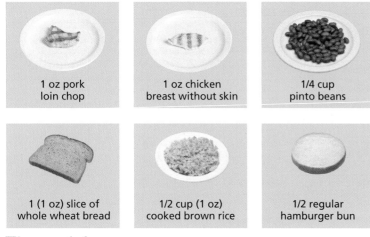

| 1 oz pork loin chop | 1 oz chicken breast without skin | 1/4 cup pinto beans |
| 1 (1 oz) slice of whole wheat bread | 1/2 cup (1 oz) cooked brown rice | 1/2 regular hamburger bun |

Figure 4.6 **What's an "ounce-equivalent"?** Here are sample 1 "ounce-equivalent" servings of various meats, beans, and grains.

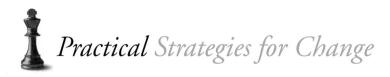

Eating Right While on the Run

You're a college student, right? So almost by definition, you eat lots of your meals on the run. Fortunately, healthful choices are available, even from fast food restaurants. Here are some tips:

- Order a vegetarian version of popular fast foods, such as burgers, pizzas, tacos, burritos, or subs.
- When ordering meat, choose chicken, turkey, or fish instead of beef or pork.
- Order your burger or sub without cheese.
- Don't super-size it! Instead, order the smallest size of burger or sandwich available, or cut it in half and share it with a friend.
- Order a side salad instead of a side of fries.
- If you crave fries, order the smallest serving size.
- Order a carton of low-fat or skim milk, a bottle of water, or a diet soda instead of a regular soda or a milkshake.
- Skip dessert or order a piece of fruit instead. Watch out for those "yogurt parfaits" now offered at many fast food restaurants. They're typically loaded with saturated fat, added sugars, and calories.
- Monitor your sensations of fullness as you eat, and stop as soon as you're full.

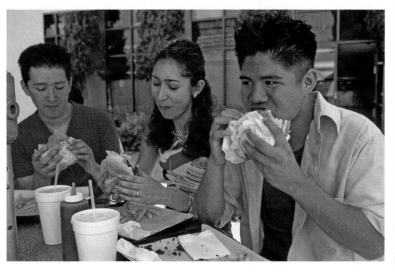

- Children and teens need a greater amount of calcium, potassium, fiber, magnesium, and vitamin E than adults.
- College students and other adults should make an extra effort to consume recommended amounts of calcium, potassium, fiber, magnesium, and vitamins A, C, and E.
- Mature adults over 50 years old need to consume more calcium, vitamin B_6, vitamin B_{12}, and vitamin D. They have slightly decreased needs for iron and fiber. Why the differences? One reason is that physical changes with aging affect how your body digests food, absorbs nutrients, and excretes wastes. For instance, many mature adults have a reduced ability to absorb naturally occurring vitamin B_{12}, but are able to absorb the synthetic

form. For this reason, all mature adults are encouraged to eat foods with added vitamin B_{12} or take the vitamin as a supplement.

With a little effort, older Americans can consume adequate amounts of these nutrients. Fruits, vegetables, whole grains, and low-fat or fat-free dairy products should be the focus of an older adult's diet. Nuts, seeds, or a small amount of vegetable oil should be consumed daily to meet vitamin E needs. Consuming some foods from animal sources will improve vitamin B_{12} intake.

Nutrition Needs Differ for Men and Women

Men and women have slightly different nutrient needs. Because most men are larger, taller, and have more muscle mass (lean muscle tissue) than most women, they require more calories—as many as 600 to 800 more per day.[3] Eating more means it's easier for men to obtain the nutrients they need even if their food choices aren't the wisest.

Unless men shift their physical activity level, their nutrition needs don't change much over a lifetime. That's not true for women. Complexities of the reproductive system, hormone shifts, pregnancy, and breastfeeding all affect nutrition needs. During childbearing years, women's nutrition requirements for iron and folic acid increase. Iron, found mostly in the blood, is lost during menstruation and is used by the developing fetus during pregnancy. Folic acid helps to make new cells and DNA, the blueprint of the body. Adequate amounts are critical in the first few weeks after conception, before most women even know they are pregnant, to reduce the risk of fetal spinal cord defects. And as we discussed in the Spotlight on page 75, later in life, with the onset of menopause and depletion of the hormone estrogen, women's needs for calcium and vitamin D to ward off osteoporosis become greater. However, this recommendation increases for older males, too.

Athletes May Have Increased Nutrition Needs

Whether you train for competitive sports, work out for the health of it, or are physically active for fun, nutrition is fundamental to peak physical performance. Athletes require the same nutrients as nonathletes, but need to pay more attention to meeting energy needs and consuming fluids.[16]

An athlete's diet should provide enough carbohydrates (45–65% of calories) and fats (10–35% of calories) for weight maintenance and energy production. Athletes also need adequate protein to build, repair, and maintain body tissues—approximately 0.5 to 0.8 grams of protein per pound of body weight. Note, however, that extra protein will not make muscles larger and may hinder performance.[15] Athletes should consume fruits or vegetables with every meal and as snacks to gain essential vitamins and minerals. They are naturally low in fat, convenient, economical, and provide carbohydrates for energy. A multivitamin/mineral supplement may be appropriate if an athlete is dieting, regularly eliminating foods or food groups, or is ill or recovering from injury. Single-nutrient supplements may be appropriate for a specific medical or nutrition reason (for example, iron supplements to correct iron deficiency anemia).

Fluids, especially water, are important to health and athletic performance. Dehydration of as little as 2% can keep even the finest athletes from performing their best. Drink plenty of fluids, early and often—about eight ounces (1 cup) every 15 minutes during exercise.

Vegetarian Options

STUDENT STORY

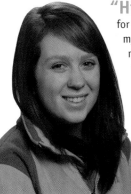

"Hi, I'm Alexandra. I'm a vegetarian. I do it for my own personal reasons. I'm not trying to impose my beliefs on anyone else. To fellow students who might be interested in vegetarianism, I would say there are a lot of good options. There are things like tofu ice cream, as well as "meat" products made out of tofu like tofu bacon, tofu sausage, and tofu chicken breast. They all taste really good!"

1: Review what you read earlier in this chapter about proteins. What can vegetarians like Alexandra do to ensure they consume all the amino acids they need?

2: What other nutrients should Alexandra be sure she consumes enough of? What are good non-animal sources for those nutrients?

Do you have a story similar to Alexandra's? Share your story at **www.pearsonhighered.com/choosinghealth**.

vegetarian A person who avoids some or all foods from animal sources: red meat, poultry, seafood, eggs, and dairy products.

foodborne illness (food poisoning) Illness caused by pathogenic microorganisms consumed through food or beverages.

Athletes should be counseled regarding the appropriate use of ergogenic aids (performance enhancers). Most are a waste of money and some are dangerous. Such products should only be used after careful evaluation for safety, effectiveness, strength, and legality.

Vegetarians Have Unique Nutrition Concerns

A plant-based diet isn't new. For years, people have chosen vegetarianism for religious, personal, health, ethical, environmental, or economic reasons. Today, **vegetarian** foods and eating styles are gaining more attention among consumers, health professionals, environmentalists, restaurant owners, and the food industry. See **Diversity & Health: Vegetarian Diets** for more details.

The MyPyramid site provides some tips and resources for vegetarians: **www.mypyramid.gov/tips_resources/vegetarian_diets.html**.

Is Our Food Supply Safe?

In early 2009, a nationwide outbreak of foodborne illness caused by contaminated peanut products killed nine people in the United States and sickened over 700 more.[17] In response to this and other outbreaks, the U.S. House of Representatives in July 2009 passed legislation that would require more frequent inspections of food pro-

cessing plants and would give the Food and Drug Administration (FDA) the authority to order the recall of tainted food. These measures are important, yet most of the 76 million cases of foodborne illness that occur in the U.S. each year are not associated with outbreaks, but occur in isolation.[18] By taking a few basic precautions, you can significantly reduce your risk of becoming sick.

Foodborne Illness

Foodborne illness, which most people call "food poisoning," generally refers to illnesses caused by microbes consumed through food or beverages. The most common causes of foodborne illness are bacteria and the toxins that certain bacteria can release into foods. Generally, bacteria spread easily and rapidly, requiring only nourishment, moisture, a favorable temperature, and time to multiply. Animal protein foods—red meat, poultry, eggs, and seafood—are common hosts for foodborne bacteria. So are sponges, dish towels, cutting boards, wooden utensils, and human hands.

The three types of bacteria responsible for most foodborne illnesses are *Campylobacter, Salmonella,* and *E. coli. Campylobacter* is most commonly found in raw or undercooked red meat, poultry, or shellfish, cake icing, untreated water, and unpasteurized milk. *Salmonella* is a risk in raw or undercooked eggs, undercooked red meat and poultry, raw milk and dairy products, seafood, fruits, and vegetables. Meanwhile, *E.coli* can be found in contaminated water, raw milk, raw or rare ground beef, unpasteurized juice or cider, and uncooked fruits and vegetables. The effects of foodborne illness can range from relatively minor discomfort to more serious symptoms such as fever, diarrhea, vomiting, dehydration, and even death. Children, pregnant women, the elderly, and those with weakened immune systems are more at risk for severe complications.

So what steps can you take to handle food safely at home? The USDA and the Partnership for Food Safety Education recommend four basic steps to "Be Food Safe."[19] They are:

1. **Clean.** Make sure you wash your hands, utensils, and cutting boards with warm water and soap before and after contact with raw red meat, poultry, seafood, and eggs.
2. **Separate.** Use different cutting boards for raw meat and foods that won't be cooked.
3. **Cook.** When cooking meat, use a food thermometer to make sure the meat is cooked to a temperature that is safe for eating.
4. **Chill.** Refrigerate leftover food within two hours at a temperature of 40°F.

If you're not sure whether a food has been prepared, served, and/or stored safely, don't risk it. Heed the advice, "When in doubt, throw it out!"

Learn more about food safety at **www.foodsafety.gov/keep/basics/index.html**.

Food Allergies and Intolerances

Another food safety concern for millions of people in the U.S. is food allergies and intolerances. Although allergies to pollen, grass, or other environmental sources typically cause discomfort during spring and fall, food allergies know no season. Approximately 12 million people in the U.S.—4% of adults and 6–8% of children under age three—have a food allergy.[20] Food intolerances are even more common.

DIVERSITY & HEALTH

Vegetarian Diets

What does it mean to be a vegetarian? For some it's an eating style, for others a lifestyle. In its broadest description, vegetarian means avoiding foods from animal sources: red meat, poultry, seafood, eggs, and dairy products. But the term has many subcategories:

- The strictest vegetarians are *vegans.* They consume no animal products—no red meat, poultry, seafood, eggs, milk, cheese, or other dairy products. Many vegans also avoid products made from or tested on animals.

- More moderate vegetarians are *lacto-ovo-vegetarians.* They avoid red meat, poultry, and seafood but will consume dairy products and eggs. *Lacto-vegetarians* avoid red meat, poultry, seafood, and eggs but consume dairy products, whereas *ovo-vegetarians* avoid red meat, poultry, seafood, and milk but will eat eggs.

- *Pesco-vegetarians* avoid red meat and chicken but will eat seafood (*pesce* means fish), dairy products, and eggs.

- *Semivegetarians* (also called *flexitarians*) may avoid only red meat, or may eat animal-based foods only once or twice a week.

Can vegetarians get enough protein without consuming red meat, poultry, or seafood? Yes, they can. Except for fruit, every edible plant contains protein—grains, vegetables, legumes, nuts, and seeds. When meals and snacks contain a variety of plant-based foods and caloric intake is sufficient to meet energy needs, protein needs can be met easily.

Vegetarians who consume dairy products and eggs don't have different nutrient needs from their non-vegetarian counterparts. But for vegans, nutrition requires special attention. Because vegans consume no products of animal origin, they may find consuming enough calories to maintain a healthy weight challenging. They also may not get enough vitamin B_{12}, which is available only from animal sources or fortified foods or supplements. Other nutrients of concern include riboflavin, vitamin D, vitamin A, calcium, iron, and zinc. Even so, planned wisely, a vegan diet can provide adequate nutrients for overall good health.

Vegetarian diets tend to be lower in saturated fat and cholesterol, and higher in carbohydrates, fiber, magnesium, folate, potassium, and antioxidants than the typical American diet. Studies show that a vegetarian diet can reduce the risk for obesity as well as several chronic, degenerative diseases including coronary artery disease, high blood pressure, diabetes, and some forms of cancer.[1]

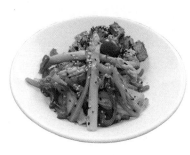

Reference: **1.** Mangels, A.R., Messina, V., & Melina, V. (2003). Position of the American dietetic association and dietitians of Canada: Vegetarian diets. *Journal of the American Dietetic Association,* 103(11), 748–765.

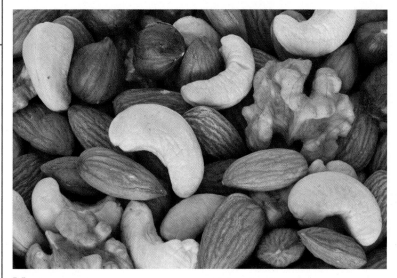

Nuts are a common source of food allergies.

testinal cramps, vomiting or diarrhea, skin hives or rashes, and wheezing, coughing, or breathing problems. The most severe response, called *anaphylaxis,* causes most of these symptoms within minutes of exposure to the allergen. If not treated quickly, it can progress to anaphylactic shock, which is usually fatal.

Eight foods cause more than 90% of all food allergies: milk, eggs, peanuts, tree nuts (such as almonds, Brazil nuts, cashews, hazelnuts, pine nuts, and walnuts), soy, wheat, fish, and shellfish (such as lobster, crab, and shrimp).[20] Food labels are required to clearly identify below the ingredient list the presence of any of these eight allergens.

Adverse food reactions that don't involve the immune system are known as *food intolerances.* These reactions generally develop over a prolonged time (within a half hour to a couple of days after eating the offending food). The most common example is *lactose intolerance,* an inability to properly digest the milk sugar lactose. Symptoms, which occur within about 30 minutes of consuming dairy products, include abdominal bloating, painful intestinal cramps, and diarrhea.

Food Additives

Food additives are substances that manufacturers add to foods to preserve, blend, flavor, color, or thicken them, or to add or replace essential nutrients. Of the more than 3,000 substances intentionally added to food, the most common are flavorings (spices, salt, vinegar, and artificial flavors) and sweeteners (sucrose, corn syrup, fructose, dextrose).[21] Preservatives are also common additives, and help ensure the availability of safe, convenient, and affordable foods year-round.

A **food allergy** is an adverse reaction of the body's immune system to a food or food component, usually a dietary protein. The body's immune system recognizes a food allergen as foreign and produces antibodies and inflammatory chemicals to combat the "invasion." As the battle ensues, symptoms of inflammation appear, sometimes in just one region, and other times throughout the body. These may include swelling of the lips or throat, digestive upset, in-

For decades, consumers have been questioning whether food additives are safe. All food additives are regulated carefully by federal authorities to ensure that they are safe to consume and are accurately labeled. When an additive is approved for use, the FDA regulates the types of foods

food allergy An adverse reaction of the body's immune system to a food or food component.

food additive A substance added to foods during processing to improve color, texture, flavor, aroma, nutrition content, or shelf life.

in which it can be used and the maximum amounts to be used. If new evidence suggests that a product being used may be unsafe, federal authorities can stop its use or conduct further studies to determine its continued safety.[22]

If you are concerned about food additives, read the ingredient list on food labels and choose products with fewer chemicals, colorants, and preservatives. Food additives usually are the long, unfamiliar names in the ingredient list. Another way to detect food additives is by the length of the ingredient list. Generally, the longer the list, the more additives a food contains.

Food Residues

Food residues are chemicals that are not naturally part of the food, but remain in the food despite cleaning and processing. Two residues of concern to consumers are pollutants and pesticides.

Many different chemicals are released into the air, soil, and water as a result of industry, agriculture, automobile emissions, and improper waste disposal. If a pollutant gets into the soil, a plant can absorb it, and then you can ingest it when you eat the plant. The plant can also pass it on to food animals that feed on it. Fish and land animals can also absorb pollutants directly into their tissues as well as ingest them when they eat other animals that are contaminated. Pollution residues have been found in virtually all categories of foods, including baked goods, fruits, vegetables, red meat, poultry, seafood, and dairy products.

Pesticides are chemicals used in the field and in storage areas to help protect crops from weeds, insects, fungus, and birds and mammals. When pesticide residues are not effectively removed, they can build up and damage body tissues. The health effects depend on the type of pesticide. Some cause disorders of nerves, others affect glands, and still others can potentially cause cancer.

The U.S. Environmental Protection Agency (EPA) provides the following tips to reduce your exposure to pesticides:[22]

- Scrub all fresh fruits and vegetables thoroughly under running water.
- Peel fruits and vegetables whenever possible and discard the outer leaves of leafy vegetables such as cabbage and lettuce.
- Trim the fat from meat and remove the skin from poultry and fish because some pesticide residues collect in the fat.
- Eat a variety of foods from various sources, as this can reduce the risk of exposure to a single pesticide.

Considering the health effects of pesticides, are organic foods better? See **Consumer Corner: Are Organic Foods Better?** to find out.

Genetically Modified Foods

Scientists create genetically modified fruits and vegetables by altering the genetic material inside the cells of plants, then cultivating their seeds for agricultural production. For example, the process is used to produce food plants that resist heat or pests, tolerate poor soils, or have a

genetic modification Altering a plant's or animal's genetic material in order to produce desirable traits such as resistance to pests, poor soil tolerance, or lower fat.

CONSUMER CORNER

Are Organic Foods Better?

You're at the deli, waiting for your sandwich, so you go to the cooler to look for a beverage. You spy a bottle of apple juice with an enticing label showing an apple orchard and the words "100% organic" beside an organic seal. You're about to select it when you notice beside it a bottle of a commercial brand of apple juice, apparently not organic, costing about $1 less. Which should you buy?

Organic foods are grown without the use of synthetic pesticides. Red meat, poultry, eggs, and dairy products certified organic come from animals fed only organic feed and not given growth hormones or antibiotics. To earn the USDA organic seal, a food must contain 95% organically produced ingredients by weight, excluding water and salt. Farms must be certified as organic by the USDA, and any companies that handle the food after it leaves the farm must also be certified.

Does this mean that organic foods are safer choices than foods grown with pesticides? That depends. If a conventionally grown fruit or vegetable can be thoroughly scrubbed or peeled, or if it tends to have a low pesticide residue anyway, then its safety is probably comparable to that of organically grown versions. Foods that don't tend to absorb pesticides include onions, corn, peas, broccoli, asparagus, tomatoes, and eggplant. Foods that have tended to show a high level of pesticides include peaches, nectarines, apples, strawberries, cherries, imported grapes, celery, sweet bell peppers, and carrots, among others.[1]

Are organic foods more nutritious? To date, research does not support this. Keep in mind that the term "organic" refers only to how food has been farmed and produced. It is not synonymous with "nutritionally better for you." As a consumer, it is up to you to weigh the pros and cons of organic versus conventional produce and then decide for yourself what is right for you.

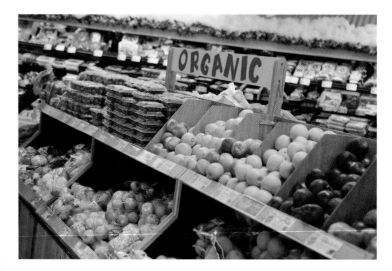

Reference: **1.** Environmental Working Group. Shopper's Guide to Pesticides. Based on USDA food consumption data 1994–1996. Retrieved from http://www.foodnews.org/walletguide.php.

---

higher yield. **Genetic modification** is also used on animals, to produce meat or poultry products with lower fat, for instance.

Supporters of genetically modified foods say that their use increases agricultural productivity, decreases the level of pesticides used, and can improve nutrient content. Opponents express concern about environmental hazards, such as loss of biodiversity, or unin-

Using MyPyramid to Analyze Your Nutrition

1. Log on to www.mypyramidtracker.gov.
2. Click "Assess Your Food Intake."
3. If you are accessing this site for the first time, click the link for new users to set up your personalized user ID and password. When prompted, enter your age, gender, height, and weight. When you're done, click "Proceed to Food Intake."

4. Enter all of the food items you have eaten today. (It's best to complete this at the end of the day, when you are done with all of your meals.) Enter each food individually by entering the name of the food in the search field, clicking "Search," and then clicking "Add." If you cannot find the exact food you are looking for, select the food that is the most similar. After you have added a food, it should pop up on the right side of the screen. Click "Select Quantity" and select a serving size from the drop-down menu. Enter the number of servings you consumed. Click "Enter Foods" to enter additional foods. Repeat until you have entered all of the foods you consumed today. (Don't forget to include snacks and beverages!)

5. When your list of foods consumed is complete, click "Save and Analyze" or "Analyze Your Food Intake."

6. You will see a screen with several links to analyzed data. Click "Calculate Nutrient Intakes from Foods." This screen will illustrate how your nutrient intake compares to the recommended or acceptable range. Print this page.

- Does your intake of any nutrient fall short of the "recommended or acceptable" range? If so, which nutrient(s)?
- Does your intake of any nutrient exceed the "recommended or acceptable" range? If so, which nutrient(s)?

7. Click "Analyze Your Food Intake" to return to the main screen containing links to analyzed data. This time, click "MyPyramid Recommendation." Print this page.

- How does your food intake compare to the MyPyramid recommendations?

NOTE:

For more accurate results, record your intake for at least three consecutive days and then analyze your data again.

> For more information on genetically modified foods, check out this special report from PBS *Nova/Frontline,* which presents both sides of the debate, along with interactive activities and a video: **www.pbs.org/wgbh/harvest**.

tended transfer of modified genes to other crops when pollen is spread on the wind or by bees or birds. The debate continues to this day.

Creating a Personalized Nutrition Plan

Maintaining a healthy diet is easier than you might believe. Start by visiting MyPyramid.gov for a step-by-step guide to healthful eating and physical activity that's tailored to your age, sex, body type, lifestyle, and calorie needs. Then use MyPyramid Tracker to analyze a day's or week's food choices. What food groups do you need to eat more of? What do you need to decrease? Are you eating too many calories overall, or too few? To assess your diet using MyPyramid Tracker, see the **Self-Assessment** above.

Once you've identified your dietary drawbacks, you're ready to create a practical plan for improving your nutritional health. The **Behavior Change Workshop** at the end of this chapter will help you generate a plan that fits your food preferences, your goals—your life! But even with a plan in place, how do you put it into action? Follow these guidelines:

- **Be realistic.** Make small changes consistently over time—they often work better than giant leaps. If your fruit intake is lacking, try adding a serving to one of your meals each day or as a snack. You don't have to add fruits to all meals right away. Or if you need to increase your calcium intake, start replacing soda with milk every day at lunch, or choose a cup of yogurt every day as your afternoon snack.

- **Be sensible.** Enjoy food, but in moderation. Pay attention to portion sizes and discretionary calories. Remember that if you're physically active, you can consume more calories than if you are sedentary. Plan a diet that makes sense for your energy needs.

- **Be adventurous.** Expand your tastes to include a variety of fruits, vegetables, and grains. Make it your goal to try a new whole grain once a month.

- **Be flexible.** If there is no way to avoid eating at a fast food restaurant, select the most healthful option you can find on the menu. If you happen to overeat for one meal, let it go. Get back on track the next meal. Overeating or indulging for one meal, one occasion, or one day does not make you unhealthy or overweight. Don't let yourself get stressed out about it.

- **Be active.** As we'll discuss in Chapter 5, you don't need to run 10 miles a day. You just need to be physically active. Consistently choose the stairs instead of the elevator or escalator. Park farther away from a building rather than circling the parking lot until the space closest to the building becomes available. Walk over to your friends' dorm room rather than calling them on your cell phone. Every step counts—just get moving.

Stay on the pathway to good health every day. Make smart food choices, watch portion sizes, and find your balance between food and activity. Over time, these little changes can have an enormous impact on your health and well-being.

> Watch videos of real students discussing their nutrition at: **www.pearsonhighered.com/choosinghealth**.

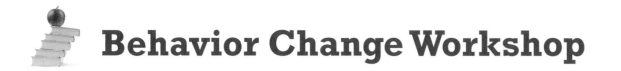

Behavior Change Workshop

To complete this workshop online, visit **www.pearsonhighered.com/choosinghealth**.

First, complete the Self-Assessment on the previous page. After you've printed out your personalized data from MyPyramid Tracker, you're ready to create a personalized nutrition plan that fits your unique eating habits and food preferences.

1. Let's start with the Comparison of Your Intake with MyPyramid Recommendations. Below, list the food groups for which your intake didn't meet recommendations. Beside the group name, identify one action you'll take tomorrow to increase your intake from this group. The first line provides an example.

Milk group—Have milk instead of soda with lunch.

_____

_____

_____

2. Next, look at how your intake of total fat, saturated fat, cholesterol, and sodium compare to the recommendations. Below, list those you exceeded. Beside the entry, identify one action you'll take tomorrow to reduce your intake of this nutrient. The first line provides an example.

Sodium—Instead of buying regular peanuts, choose the ones that say "lightly salted."

_____

_____

_____

3. Next, jot down a more long-term goal for *increasing* your intake of one of the food groups you listed in step 1, and for *decreasing* your intake of one of the less healthful nutrients you listed in step 2. Remember to give yourself a reasonable amount of time to achieve the goal! An example is provided.

By the end of this semester, I'll be consuming at least three servings of dairy every day.

_____

_____

_____

4. Finally, journal below about any obstacles you see that might interfere with your ability to meet your goal. For instance, are you concerned that you won't have enough money to purchase fresh fruits and vegetables? Or that your lunch break is so short that you have no time for anything but fast food? For each obstacle you identify, jot down a strategy to get around it.

_____

_____

_____

Chapter Summary

- The science of nutrition explores how the foods you eat and the beverages you drink affect your body and your health.

- There are six major classes of nutrients found in foods: carbohydrates, proteins, fats, vitamins, minerals, and water. Within these classes are essential nutrients, or substances that must be obtained from foods, drinks, and/or supplements because the body either cannot make them or cannot make sufficient quantities to support health.

- Carbohydrates and proteins contain 4 calories per gram. Fats contain 9 calories per gram. Alcohol contains 7 calories per gram. Vitamins, minerals, and water are calorie-free.

- Carbohydrates are the body's universal energy source because most body cells can use carbohydrates for energy.

- Fats are the most concentrated energy source. Each type of dietary fat—saturated, unsaturated, and *trans*—has different characteristics and effects on your health.

- Proteins are made up of different combinations of 20 different building blocks called amino acids. Nine are essential and the other 11 can be made by the body.

- Vitamins regulate blood cell production, nerve function, digestion, and skin and bone maintenance. They help chemical reactions take place.

- Minerals regulate body processes and provide structure to the body.

- Water is vital to life.

- Fiber, phytochemicals, antioxidants, and probiotics are thought to have disease-preventing qualities and health-promoting properties.

- Strategies for eating right include learning about the Dietary Reference Intakes, reading food labels, following the Dietary Guidelines, and using MyPyramid to help you evaluate your current diet and develop and follow a personalized diet plan that's right for you.

- Your age, sex, level of physical activity, participation in sports, and many other factors influence the way you eat.

- Vegetarians who include eggs and dairy products in their diet typically have no nutritional concerns different from those of meat-eaters. However, strict vegetarians, called *vegans*, need to plan their diet carefully to ensure they are getting enough calories, vitamin B_{12}, riboflavin, vitamin D, vitamin A, calcium, iron, and zinc.

- Foodborne illness, food allergies and intolerances, food additives, and food residues pose potential risks to health and wellness.

- The benefits and risks of genetically modified foods are the subject of considerable debate.

- Creating a personalized nutrition plan that includes smart food choices, finding your balance between food and physical activity, and getting the most nutrition out of your calories can improve your health and well-being.

Test Your Knowledge

1. Which of the following substances is most fattening to the body?
   a. alcohol
   b. proteins
   c. carbohydrates
   d. vitamins

2. Which of the following is true of MyPyramid?
   a. It recommends that you consume no more than 2,000 calories a day.
   b. It recommends that you use your discretionary calories for treats.
   c. It recommends that you participate in physical activity most days of the week.
   d. It recommends that you drink alcohol in moderation most days of the week.

3. Fiber is
   a. a type of starch.
   b. a nutrient.
   c. a simple carbohydrate.
   d. a complex carbohydrate.

4. Which of the following is characteristic of an essential nutrient?
   a. It cannot be found in food.
   b. It cannot be degraded by the body.
   c. It cannot be made in sufficient quantities by the body.
   d. It cannot be used to manufacture other compounds in the body.

Get Critical

What happened:

International soccer star and celebrity David Beckham is featured in Pepsi advertisements in which he presents the soft drink as a choice for strong, physically fit people. The leading medical journal in Great Britain responded to these ads by urging Beckham to drop the campaign, arguing that he was helping to create a false impression about the nutritional effects of soft drinks. What do you think?

What do you think?

- Do ad campaigns featuring athletes promoting foods, beverages, or supplements create the impression that these products are healthful?

- Do athletes have an ethical responsibility to promote products that boost health, or should they be able to profit from their celebrity to promote anything?

- Imagine that you were at a friend or relative's house and saw a group of children watching a TV ad showing

Beckham and other soccer stars enjoying Pepsi after a demanding game. What might you explain to them about the product—and about the ad itself?

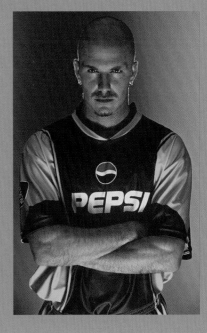

5. What type of carbohydrate is found primarily in milk?
   a. maltose
   b. lactose
   c. fructose
   d. sucrose

6. The acronym DRI represents which words?
   a. Daily Recommended Intakes
   b. Dietary Reference Intakes
   c. Daily Reference Intakes
   d. Dietary Recommended Intakes

7. Approximately how many different amino acids are used to manufacture body proteins?
   a. 5
   b. 11
   c. 20
   d. 29

8. Which of the following fats is most "heart healthy"?
   a. unsaturated
   b. saturated
   c. *trans*
   d. hydrogenated

9. Most foodborne illnesses
   a. are deadly.
   b. are due to viruses.
   c. occur in outbreaks.
   d. occur in isolated cases.

10. Which of the following would be considered a food residue?
   a. phytochemicals
   b. probiotics
   c. preservatives
   d. pesticides

Get Connected

Health Online Visit the following websites for further information about the topics in this chapter:

- Food and Drug Administration: For Consumers
  www.fda.gov/ForConsumers/default.htm

- Northwestern Nutrition
  www.preventivemedicine.northwestern.edu/Divisions/nutrition/index.htm

- American Dietetic Association
  www.eatright.org

- The International Food Information Council (IFIC) Foundation FoodInsight
  www.foodinsight.org

- The Center for Science in the Public Interest
  www.cspinet.org

Website links are subject to change. To access updated Web links, please visit **www.pearsonhighered.com/choosinghealth**.

References

i. Putnam, J., & Haley, S. (2003). Estimating consumption of caloric sweeteners. *Amber Waves: April 2003*. Economic Research Service, USDA. Retrieved from: http://www.ers.usda.gov/AmberWaves/April03/Indicators/behinddata.htm.

ii. Thompson, J., & Manore, M. (2010). *Nutrition for life* (2nd ed.). San Francisco, CA: Pearson Education.

iii. Sicherer, S. H., & Sampson, H. A. (2006). Food allergy. *Journal of Allergy and Clinical Immunology, 117*(2 supplemental mini-primer), S470–475.

1. Putnam, J., & Haley, S. (2003). Estimating consumption of caloric sweeteners. *Amber Waves: April 2003*. Economic Research Service, USDA. Retrieved from: http://www.ers.usda.gov/AmberWaves/April03/Indicators/behinddata.htm.

2. Liebman, B., & Jurley, J. (2006). Whole grains: The inside story. *Nutrition Action Health Letter,* May, 3–7; Liebman, B. (1997). The whole grain guide. *Nutrition Action Health Letter,* March. Retrieved from http://www.cspinet.org/nah/wwheat.html.

3. Food and Nutrition Board, Institute of Medicine of the National Academies. (2005). *Dietary reference intakes for energy, carbohydrate, fiber, fat, fatty acids, cholesterol, protein, and amino acids.* Washington, D.C.: The National Academies Press. Retrieved from: http://www.nap.edu/openbook.php?record_id=10490.

4. American Heart Association. (2010). Fat. Retrieved from http://www.americanheart.org/presenter.jhtml?identifier=4582.

5. U.S. Food and Drug Administration, Center for Food Safety and Applied Nutrition. (2006). Questions and answers about trans fat nutrition labeling. Retrieved from http://www.cfsan.fda.gov/~dms/qatrans2.html.

6. Harvard School of Public Health. (2010). Fats and cholesterol: Out with the bad, in with the good. Retrieved from http://www.hsph.harvard.edu/nutritionsource/what-should-you-eat/fats-full-story/index.html.

7. Mozaffarian, D., Katan, M. B., Ascherio, A., Stampfer, M. J., & Willett, W. C. (2006). Trans fatty acids and cardiovascular disease. *New England Journal of Medicine, 354,* 1601–1613.

8. National Cholesterol Education Program Expert Panel on Detection, Evaluation, and Treatment of High Blood Cholesterol in Adults (Adult Treatment Panel III). (2002). Third report of the national cholesterol education program (NCEP) expert panel on detection, evaluation, and treatment of high blood cholesterol in adults (adult treatment panel III) final report. *Circulation 106* (25): 3143.

9. Wright, J. D., Kennedy-Stephenson, J., Wang, C.Y., McDowell, M.A., & Johnson, C.L. (2004). Trends in intake of energy and macronutrients–United States, 1971-2000.

MMWR Weekly 53 (04), 80-82. Retrieved from http://www.cdc.gov/mmwr/preview/mmwrhtml/mm5304a3.htm.

10. U.S. Department of Health and Human Services & U.S. Department of Agriculture. (2005). *Dietary Guidelines for Americans* (6th ed.). Washington, DC: U.S. Government Printing Office.

11. Linus Pauling Institute. (2010). Micronutrient Information Center: Phytochemicals. Retrieved from http://lpi.oregonstate.edu/infocenter/phytochemicals.html.

12. Magee, E. (2007). *Food synergy: Unleash hundreds of powerful healing food combinations to fight disease and live well.* New York, NY: Rodale.

13. Prior, R.L., Wu, X., Beecher, G., Holden, J., Haytowitz, D., & Gebhardt, S. E. (2004). Lipophilic and hydrophilic antioxidant capacities of common foods in the United States. *Journal of Agricultural and Food Chemistry, 52*(12), 4026–4037.

14. U.S. Food and Drug Administration. (2004). How to understand and use the Nutrition Facts label. Retrieved from http://www.fda.gov/Food/LabelingNutrition/ConsumerInformation/UCM078889.htm.

15. Thompson, J., & Manore, M. (2010). *Nutrition for life* (2nd ed.). San Francisco, CA: Pearson Education.

16. Rodriguez, N., DiMarco, N., & Langley, S. (2009). Position of the American Dietetic Association, Dietitians of Canada, and the American College of Sports Medicine: Nutrition and athletic performance. *Journal of the American Dietetic Association, 109*(31), 509–527.

17. Centers for Disease Control and Prevention. (2005). Foodborne illness. Retrieved from http://www.cdc.gov/ncidod/dbmd/diseaseinfo/foodborneinfections_g.htm.

18. Centers for Disease Control and Prevention. (2005). Foodborne illness. Retrieved from http://www.cdc.gov/ncidod/dbmd/diseaseinfo/foodborneinfections_g.htm.

19. U.S. Department of Health & Human Services. (2010). The basics: Clean, separate, cook, and chill. Retrieved from http://www.foodsafety.gov/keep/basics/index.html.

20. Sicherer, S. H., & Sampson, H. A. (2006). Food allergy. *Journal of Allergy and Clinical Immunology, 117*(2 supplemental mini-primer), S470–475.

21. Lagasse, P. (2000). *The Columbia encyclopedia* (6th ed.). New York, NY: Columbia University Press.

22. U.S. Environmental Protection Agency. (2006). Pesticides and food: Healthy, sensible food practices. Retrieved from http://www.epa.gov/pesticides/food/tips.htm.

Physical Activity for Fitness and Health 5

- People who are physically active for about 7 hours a week have a 40% lower risk of dying early than those who are active for less than 30 minutes a week.[i]

- Young adults 18 to 30 years old with low cardiovascular fitness levels are two to three times more likely to develop diabetes in 20 years than those who are fit.[ii]

- In a recent study, women who performed one year of strength training significantly improved their ability to maintain mental focus and resolve conflicts.[iii]

Health Online icons are found throughout the chapter, directing you to web links, videos, podcasts, and other useful online resources.

As a society, we are chronically out of shape.

Many of our daily activities no longer require significant physical effort, and busy schedules cut into our time for exercise—an especially critical problem for students, who often see their physical activity levels decline in college. Even when we do have time for recreation, hours that could be spent getting exercise or playing sports are instead too often spent in the car, in front of the TV, or on the computer. The result: People who aren't physically active tend to experience more long-term health problems, such as overweight and obesity, diabetes, heart disease, lower energy levels, and even reduced mental health.

The good news is that in recent years the percentage of people in the United States who report getting at least some regular physical activity has grown from 43% to 46.7% among women and from 48% to 49.7% among men, a small but hopeful sign that more people are aware of the benefits of fitness.[1] And if given the chance to be more active, our bodies thrive. Even small changes in physical activity levels can make a significant difference in your fitness and health, both in school now and in the years ahead.

In this chapter, we will describe physical fitness and its health benefits, explain how to create a fitness program, discuss the various types of exercise that contribute to fitness, and list guidelines for how much physical activity and exercise you need. We will also provide tips for how to stick with a physical fitness program once you've started and explain how you can be sure you're exercising safely. Let's begin by looking at what makes a person physically fit.

What Is Physical Fitness?

Most of us equate fitness with appearance. We assume that those of us with trim builds or visible muscles are more fit, while those of us with a bit of a belly or flabby triceps are less fit. But physical fitness is not that simplistic. **Physical fitness** is the ability to perform moderate to vigorous levels of activity, and to respond to physical demands without excessive fatigue. Physical fitness can be built up through physical activity or exercise. **Physical activity** is bodily movement that substantially increases energy expenditure. Taking the stairs instead of the elevator, walking or biking to class instead of driving, gardening, and walking the dog all count as types of physical activity. **Exercise** is physical activity that is carried out in a planned and structured format. Any type of activity will provide health benefits, but optimal physical fitness can only be achieved through regular exercise. Team sports, aerobic classes, and working out at the gym all count as exercise.

There are two types of physical fitness: **skills-related fitness** and **health-related fitness.** In this chapter, we will focus on health-related fitness. The five key components of health-related fitness are cardiorespiratory fitness, muscular strength, muscular endurance, flexibility, and body composition.

Cardiorespiratory Fitness

Put together "cardio" for heart and "respiratory" for breath, and you've got a good idea of what this com-

physical fitness The ability to perform moderate to vigorous levels of activity and to respond to physical demands without excessive fatigue.

physical activity Bodily movement that substantially increases energy expenditure.

exercise A type of physical activity that is planned and structured.

skills-related fitness The capacity to perform specific physical skills related to a sport or other physically demanding activity.

health-related fitness The ability to perform activities of daily living with vigor.

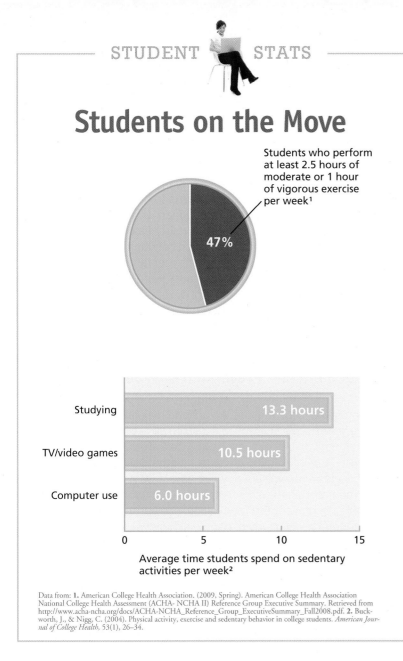
Students on the Move

Students who perform at least 2.5 hours of moderate or 1 hour of vigorous exercise per week[1]

47%

Studying — 13.3 hours

TV/video games — 10.5 hours

Computer use — 6.0 hours

Average time students spend on sedentary activities per week[2]

Data from: **1.** American College Health Association. (2009, Spring). American College Health Association National College Health Assessment (ACHA- NCHA II) Reference Group Executive Summary. Retrieved from http://www.acha-ncha.org/docs/ACHA-NCHA_Reference_Group_ExecutiveSummary_Fall2008.pdf. **2.** Buckworth, J., & Nigg, C. (2004). Physical activity, exercise and sedentary behavior in college students. *American Journal of College Health*, 53(1), 26–34.

muscular strength by performing strength training exercises using machines, free weights, resistance bands, or simply the weight of your own body (as in push-ups, for example).

Muscular Endurance

Muscular endurance is the capacity of your muscles to repeatedly exert force, or to maintain force, over a period of time without tiring. Muscular endurance is measured in two ways–*static muscular endurance,* or how long you can hold a force that is motionless, and *dynamic muscular endurance,* or how long you can sustain a force in motion. A sustained sit-up, where you contract your abdominal muscles and do not move until they fatigue, is an example of static muscle endurance. Repeated sit-ups, done until you can't contract your abdominals any more, rely on dynamic muscle endurance. Muscular endurance is important for posture and for performing extended activities. Muscular endurance can be improved by gradually increasing the duration that your muscles work in each bout of strength exercises, such as slowly increasing the number of push-ups you perform each time you exercise.

Flexibility

Flexibility refers to the ability of your joints to move through their full ranges of motion, such as how far you can bend your trunk from side to side or how far you can bend forward from the hips toward your toes. Flexibility does not only pertain to the movement of muscle, but also depends on connective tissues such as your ligaments and tendons. Benefits of flexibility include the relief of muscle tension, reduction of joint pain, reduction of back pain, and improved posture. Flexibility can be improved through stretching exercises and activities such as yoga, Pilates, and tai chi.

Body Composition

Body composition refers to the relative proportions of fat tissue and lean tissue (muscle, bone, water, organs) in your body. A low ratio of fat to lean tissue is optimal. As we'll discuss in Chapter 6, many of us carry more body fat than is healthful. Excessive body fat, especially in the abdominal area, increases the risk of three of the four leading causes of death in the U.S.: heart disease, cancer, and stroke. It is also related to other serious conditions including osteoarthritis, diabetes, hypertension (high blood pressure), hyperlipidemia (high cholesterol), and sleep apnea. The newest research indicates that even if you are healthy in other ways, having too much body fat will still negatively impact your health.[4] Body composition affects your level of fitness, but the reverse is also true—as you become more physically fit, your body composition will usually improve.

ponent of fitness covers. **Cardiorespiratory fitness** refers to the ability of your heart and lungs to effectively deliver oxygen to your muscles during prolonged physical activity. Experts agree that cardiorespiratory fitness should be the foundation upon which all the other areas of fitness are built. It is the fitness component that is the best indicator of overall physical fitness and in addition it helps lower risk of premature death and disease.[2] You can boost your cardiorespiratory fitness by any continuous, rhythmic exercise that works your large muscle groups and increases your heart rate, such as brisk walking, swimming, or cycling.

Muscular Strength

Muscular strength is the maximum force your muscles can apply in a single effort of lifting, pushing, or pressing. Building stronger muscles will help keep your skeleton properly aligned, aid balance, protect your back, boost your athletic performance, and increase your metabolic rate. Building muscular strength also results in much higher bone mineral density and stronger bones.[3] You can build

cardiorespiratory fitness The ability of your heart and lungs to effectively deliver oxygen to your muscles during prolonged physical activity.

muscular strength The maximum force your muscles can apply in a single maximum effort of lifting, pushing, or pressing.

muscular endurance The capacity of muscles to repeatedly exert force, or to maintain a force, over a period of time.

flexibility The ability of joints to move through their full ranges of motion.

body composition The relative proportions of the body's lean tissue and fat tissue.

What Are the Benefits of Physical Activity?

Physical activity is one of the best things you can do for yourself. It benefits every aspect of your health, at every stage of your life. Some of these benefits are purely physical, such as a stronger heart and healthier lungs. But physical activity can also put you in a better mood and help you to manage stress. Physical activity lowers your risk of premature death, and as you age it will help postpone physical decline and many of the diseases that can reduce quality of life in your later years.

Figure 5.1 summarizes the major benefits of physical activity; we'll discuss each one next.

Stronger Heart and Lungs

As the organs that pump your blood and deliver oxygen throughout your body, your heart, lungs, and entire circulatory system literally keep you going. By increasing your body's demand for oxygen, physical activity pushes these systems to work harder, which helps keep them strong and efficient, even as you age. As your body adapts to physical activity, your heart becomes stronger and pumps a greater volume of blood with each beat. Your lungs become able to inhale more air and absorb more oxygen. Physical activity also appears to help by stabilizing the parts of your brain that control the function of these vital systems.[5]

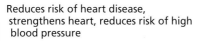

Reduces risk of heart disease, strengthens heart, reduces risk of high blood pressure

Increases lung efficiency and capacity

Reduces risk of type 2 diabetes

Reduces risk of colorectal, breast, and ovarian cancers

Strengthens immune system

Strengthens bones

Reduces risk of bone, muscle, and joint injuries

Promotes healthful body composition and weight management

Benefits psychological health and stress management

Figure 5.1 Health benefits of physical activity.

Participating in physical activity and exercise can reduce your risk of heart disease by half through their positive effect on several major risk factors for heart disease: They lower LDL (bad) cholesterol, raise HDL (good) cholesterol, help prevent or control diabetes, and help you lose excess weight.[6] Physical activity also keeps your blood vessels healthier and lowers your risk of related illnesses, such as high blood pressure.

Cardiorespiratory fitness is, by definition, the fitness component that most relates to your heart and lungs. Research has noted just how essential cardiorespiratory fitness is to health and longevity. One study followed more than 20,000 men who weren't overweight, but had differing levels of cardiorespiratory fitness.[7] The researchers found that just being thin isn't enough to protect your health—fitness is also key. In the eight-year-long study, thin men with low rates of cardiorespiratory fitness were twice as likely to die from any cause as thin men with higher rates of cardiorespiratory fitness. Those greater risks included a higher risk of dying from heart disease. (See Chapter 12 for a more detailed discussion of heart disease.)

Management and Prevention of Type 2 Diabetes

Exercise can control your blood sugar (blood glucose level) and blood pressure, help you lose weight and maintain weight loss, and improve your body's ability to use insulin, all of which help control or prevent type 2 diabetes. If you have type 2 diabetes, any daily physical activity is helpful. If you are at risk for the disease, even as little as 30 minutes of exercise a day five days a week can help lower your risk.[8] When combined with a healthful diet, exercise proves more powerful than prescription medication in lowering type 2 diabetes risk. A federal health study of people at high risk for diabetes showed that daily exercise and a healthful diet lowered risk by 58%, compared to a 31% reduction in risk for a common prescription diabetes drug.[8–10] (We'll discuss diabetes in more detail in Chapter 12.)

Reduced Risk of Some Cancers

Inactivity is one of the most significant risk factors for cancer that you can control. Physical activity lowers the long-term risks of developing colorectal cancer in men and women and breast and ovarian cancers in women.[11, 12] One long-term study of more than 110,000 women found that those who performed at least five hours of moderate to strenuous exercise a week cut their risk of breast cancer by at least half.[13] Activity appears to help in part by controlling weight, a risk factor for certain cancers. It may also help by regulating certain hormones which are factors in some types of cancers and by encouraging your body to process and remove substances—including potential toxins that might cause cancer—more quickly.

Increased Immune Function

Do you want to lower your risk of getting sick during the next cold and flu season? Physical activity can help you fend off common illnesses by boosting your immune system. In one study, 60–90% of active individuals felt that they experienced fewer colds than their non-active counterparts.[14] Scientists still aren't entirely sure how physical activity helps build immunity, but exercise's role in flushing impurities from the body, along with regulating hormones related to immune function, may play a part.[15] (For more information on infectious diseases and immunity, see Chapter 11.)

Stronger Bones

Physical activity builds and protects your bones.[16] Weight-bearing exercise such as walking, running, or lifting weights stimulates the bone tissue to create new bone cells, making your bones bigger and stronger. Non–weight-bearing exercise, such as swimming, is healthful in other ways but does not strengthen bones. Bone strength helps protect your skeleton from injury, so it is important for everyone, but it is especially important for those at risk for **osteoporosis,** a serious condition that mostly affects older women, in which reduced bone mineral density causes the bones to become weak and brittle. Although many college-aged students don't think they need to worry about osteoporosis, the young-adult years are an important time to build the bone strength that prevents the disease's onset later.

Reduced Risk of Injury

The stronger bones, muscles, tendons, and ligaments that result from physical activity can help protect you from injury. A strong back, for example, is much less likely to get strained and sore the next time you lift boxes while moving to a new dorm or apartment. Strong muscles can help you keep your balance and avoid falls, and strong joint-supporting muscles can help reduce the risk of a variety of injuries including sprains, tendonitis, runner's knee, and shin splints.

Healthful Weight Management

Physical activity helps you lose and control weight in more ways than one. Not only does it burn calories, but it also boosts your *metabolism,* or the rate at which your body uses calories in order to function. This boost in metabolism occurs both during and after workouts. Consistent exercise can slowly lower your overall percentage of body fat and help build and maintain muscle, whereas if you try to lose weight by dieting alone, you risk burning muscle mass along with body fat. Having more muscle also increases your metabolism and helps you maintain your weight long-term. (We'll look more closely at metabolism and weight loss in Chapter 6.)

Benefits to Psychological Health and Stress Management

When people say they work out to "blow off steam," they are describing the effect physical activity has on their stress levels. Physical activity reduces stress and anxiety, and also helps boost concentration. These benefits appear to hold true no matter what type of physical activity you enjoy. Some may go for a long hike to help reduce stress and recharge, other people might prefer a spin class, 30 minutes on the rock wall at a climbing gym, or a pickup game of hoops. Any activity can help, especially if you participate in it regularly. In one study of the Chinese movement and meditation discipline called qigong, participants saw a significant decrease in stress, anxiety, and fatigue.[17]

Certain studies have shown that exercise can be just as effective in relieving depression as antidepressant medication.[18] And the latest research concludes that exercise can prevent depression in the first place.[19] Any type of physical activity is considered helpful, but in one study of college women with signs of depression, vigorous-intensity exercise classes led to the most significant decrease in symptoms.[20] (You can learn more about depression and its treatments in Chapter 2.)

In addition, active lifestyles may be associated with higher levels of alertness and mental ability, including the ability to learn and achieve academically.[5, 21] Exercise also keeps your mind sharp as you age. Physical activity reduces the risk of dementia and Alzheimer's disease in later life.[22]

How Do You Design a Fitness Program?

Participating in regular exercise and physical activity is one of the most healthful habits you can maintain throughout your life. In order to design an effective fitness program, you should first understand the basic principles of fitness training.

Principles of Fitness Training

To be effective, a fitness-building program should follow the principles of fitness training. These principles are *overload, specificity, reversibility,* and *individuality.*

Overload

The **overload** principle is the idea that in order to increase fitness level, you must increase the stress placed on your body through exercise, creating a greater demand than your body is accustomed to meeting, which forces it to adapt and become more fit. In other words, you improve fitness by exercising beyond your comfort zone. **Progressive overload** is gradually increasing the demands on your body over time in order to avoid injury. Your body will adapt to slowly increasing levels of overload, but if you push yourself too intensely too quickly, you will risk injury.

osteoporosis A condition in which reduced bone mineral density causes the bones to become weak and brittle.

overload Increasing the stress placed on your body through exercise, which results in an improved fitness level.

progressive overload Gradually overloading the body over time in order to avoid injury.

FITT Exercise variables that can be modified in order to accomplish progressive overload: frequency, intensity, time, and type.

You can achieve progressive overload by modifying one or more of the exercise variables collectively known as **FITT.** FITT stands for:

- **Frequency.** The number of times you engage in a particular exercise each week.
- **Intensity.** The level of effort at which you exercise. For cardiorespiratory fitness, intensity is usually measured in terms of how fast you get your heart beating (your heart rate). For muscular strength and endurance training, intensity depends on the amount of resistance and number of repetitions. For flexibility, intensity is measured by the depth of the stretch.
- **Time (duration).** The amount of time you spend on a particular exercise.
- **Type.** The kind of exercise you choose to do.

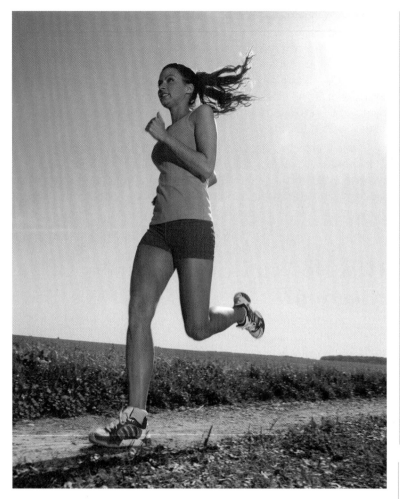

Using the FITT principle will help you achieve progressive overload.

Specificity

The **specificity** principle means that in order to improve a specific component of fitness, you must perform exercises specifically designed to address that component. Many exercises will improve some components of fitness but not others. Cycling, for example, is great for cardiorespiratory fitness, but doesn't build upper body strength or increase your flexibility. You should take into account the principle of specificity when deciding which activities you choose to perform.

Reversibility

The **reversibility** principle states that your fitness level will decline if you don't maintain your physical activity. Just as your body adapts to overload to increase your fitness, if you stop or reduce your exercise routine your body will adapt to the reduced demand and your fitness will suffer. Fitness declines can happen quickly, sometimes in as little as 10 days.[23] Therefore, it is important to maintain a consistent exercise routine to avoid reversing your fitness gains.

Individuality

The principle of **individuality** means that you will respond to the demands you place on your body in your own unique way. We each react differently to

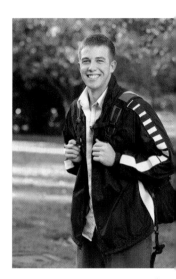
specific exercises, with some people gaining more benefit from a particular exercise than others. These individual responses are shaped, in part, by genetics. Identifying the exercises best suited to you is a key part of designing an effective fitness program.

What Types of Physical Activity Should You Consider?

Any type of regular, sustained physical activity is beneficial, especially if you have been inactive for a while. However, in order to increase your overall health and fitness, you should look into activities that increase your cardiorespiratory fitness, muscular strength and endurance, and flexibility. Whatever activities you choose, be sure they are ones you truly enjoy, which will help you stick with them over the long-term.

Exercises for Improving Cardiorespiratory Fitness

You can build cardiorespiratory fitness through **aerobic exercise,** which is any prolonged physical activity that raises your heart rate and works the large muscle groups. Aerobic exercise makes your heart, lungs, and entire circulatory system stronger by requiring them to work harder to deliver adequate oxygen to your muscles.

There are numerous forms of popular aerobic exercise, including:

- Running and jogging
- Hiking or brisk walking for extended periods of time

---

specificity The principle that a fitness component is improved only by exercises that address that specific component.

reversibility The principle that fitness levels decline when the demand placed on the body is decreased.

individuality The principle that individuals will respond to fitness training in their own unique ways.

aerobic exercise Prolonged physical activity that raises the heart rate and works the large muscle groups.

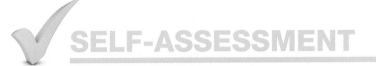
Determining Your Maximum Heart Rate and Target Heart Rate Range

During aerobic exercise, the rate at which your heart is working lets you know if you are exercising effectively. You will gain the most cardiorespiratory benefit if you exercise within your target heart rate range.

MAXIMUM HEART RATE

To start, you need to know your maximum heart rate. The American College of Sports Medicine (ACSM) has found the most accurate way to determine your maximum heart rate is through the following equation:[1]

$$206.9 - (0.67 \times age) = \text{maximum heart rate}$$

Step 1: _____ × 0.67 = _____
(your age)

Step 2: 206.9 − _____ = _____ = maximum heart rate
(answer from Step 1)

TARGET HEART RATE RANGE

You can narrow down the ACSM's target heart rate range of 64–91% of your maximum heart rate based on your current activity level.[2]

- If you perform only minimal physical activity right now, aim for a target heart rate of about 64–74% of your maximum heart rate. Use the following formulas to determine your target heart rate range:

  Low-end of target heart rate range: _____ × 0.64 = _____
  (maximum heart rate)

  High-end of target heart rate range: _____ × 0.74 = _____
  (maximum heart rate)

- If you perform sporadic physical activity right now, aim for a target heart rate of about 74–84% of your maximum heart rate. Use the following formulas to determine your target heart rate range:

  Low-end of target heart rate range: _____ × 0.74 = _____
  (maximal heart rate)

  High-end of target heart rate range: _____ × 0.84 = _____
  (maximal heart rate)

- If you perform regular physical activity right now, aim for a target heart rate of about 80–91% of your maximum heart rate. Use the following formulas to determine your target heart rate range:

  Low-end of target heart rate range: _____ × 0.80 = _____
  (maximal heart rate)

  High-end of target heart rate range: _____ × 0.91 = _____
  (maximal heart rate)

MEASURING YOUR HEART RATE

While you exercise, take your pulse by placing your first two fingers (not your thumb) on the side of your neck next to your windpipe. Using a clock or watch, take your pulse for six seconds and then multiply that number by 10. The result will be your number of heartbeats per minute, which is your heart rate.

HOW TO INTERPRET YOUR SCORE

- Some cardiorespiratory equipment in gyms, such as stair climbers, offer real time heart rate calculators. But you can easily track your heart rate using the measurement method above.
- If your heart rate is below your target heart rate range, increase your intensity until you are in your target range; if your heart rate is above your target heart rate range, reduce your intensity.

- There are several methods for calculating maximum heart rate and target heart rate ranges. The formula presented above is the ACSM's most accurate method; some organizations or online calculators may calculate your target heart rate range differently.

References: **1.** American College of Sports Medicine. (2010). *ACSM's guidelines for exercise testing and prescription* (8th edition, p. 155). Baltimore, MD: Wolters Kluwer/Lippincott Williams & Wilkins. **2.** American College of Sports Medicine. (2010). *ACSM's guidelines* (pp. 166–167).

- Cycling and "spinning" (a structured workout on a stationary bicycle)
- Swimming
- Rowing
- Cardio classes, including aerobic dance and step aerobics training
- Vigorous martial arts, such as karate or cardio kickboxing
- Jumping rope
- Stair-climbing

Aerobic intensity is usually measured by heart rate because increased heart rate indicates that your cardiorespiratory system is working harder. In order to achieve the maximum cardiorespiratory benefit, you should aim to raise your heart rate so that it falls within your **target heart rate range.** For healthy adults who are not entirely sedentary or exceptionally active, the American College of Sports Medicine (ACSM) recommends a target heart rate range of anywhere from 64% to 91% of your maximum heart rate.[24] See **Self-Assessment: Determining Your Maximum Heart Rate and Target Heart Rate Range** for how to determine these indicators.

target heart rate range The heart rate range to aim for during exercise. A target heart rate range of 64–91% of your maximum heart rate is recommended.

Aerobic exercises are often categorized as lifestyle/light-intensity, moderate-intensity, or vigorous-intensity activities. According to the Centers for Disease Control and Prevention, light-intensity activity gets you moving but raises your heart rate to less than 50% of your maximum heart rate, moderate-intensity activities will raise your heart rate to 50–70% of your maximum heart rate, and vigorous-intensity activities raise your heart rate to 70–85% of your maximum heart rate.[25] **Table 5.1** shows the examples and benefits of these three categories of aerobic activities.

The best way to begin an aerobic exercise program is to start by performing exercises at intensities near the low end of your target heart rate range, or even lower if you have not exercised in a while. Start with a minimum of 10 minutes of activity at a time, more if you are able. Slowly increase the duration of your exercise by 5–10 minutes every 1–2 weeks for the first 4–6 weeks of your program.[24] After that, you can build fitness by gradually increasing the duration, frequency, or intensity of exercises. Always be sure to warm up before and cool down after an aerobic session, and to follow other safety pre-

Table 5.1: **Physical Activity Intensities**

Activity Intensity Level	Heart Rate Range	Examples	Health Benefits
Lifestyle/light	Less than 50% maximum heart rate	Light yard work and housework, leisurely walking, self-care and bathing, light stretching, light occupational activity	A moderate increase in health and wellness in those who are completely sedentary; reduced risk of some chronic diseases
Moderate	50–70% maximum heart rate	Walking 3–4.5 miles per hour on a level surface, resistance training, hiking, climbing stairs, bicycling 5–9 miles per hour on a level surface, dancing, doubles tennis, using a manual wheelchair, softball, recreational swimming, water aerobics, moderate yard work and housework	Increased cardiorespiratory endurance, lower body fat levels, improved blood cholesterol and pressure, better blood sugar management, decreased risk of disease, increased overall physical fitness
Vigorous	70–85% maximum heart rate	Jogging, running, basketball, soccer, circuit training, backpacking, aerobic classes, competitive sports, swimming laps, martial arts, singles tennis, heavy yard work or housework, hard physical labor/construction, bicycling 10 miles per hour or faster up steep terrain	Increased overall physical fitness, decreased risk of disease, further improvements in overall strength and muscular endurance

Data from: 1. Centers for Disease Control and Prevention. (2009). *Physical activity for everyone: Target heart rate and estimated maximum heart rate.* Retrieved from http://www.cdc.gov/physicalactivity/everyone/measuring/heartrate.html. 2. Hopson, J., Donatelle. R., & Littrell, T. (2009). *Get fit, stay well!* (brief edition, fig. 2.1, p. 31). San Francisco: Pearson Benjamin Cummings.

cautions for exercise. See pages 104–108 for more about warming up, cooling down, and safety.

Some full-body exercises don't increase cardiorespiratory fitness. Short, intense activities, such as sprint running, sprint swimming, or heavy weight lifting, usually require more oxygen than the body can take in and deliver quickly, consequently the muscles develop an oxygen deficit and you tire in a short amount of time. These **anaerobic exercises** build your body's ability to deliver short bursts of energy rapidly and build muscular strength, which we'll look at next.

Exercises for Improving Muscular Strength and Endurance
Many people think building muscle means increasing the amount of weight you can lift—in other words, building strength. But endurance is also an important component of muscular fitness. Strength allows you to lift that heavy box when you move to your next apartment, but muscular endurance will let you carry it all the way out to the moving truck without straining your shoulders or wrenching your back.

anaerobic exercise Short, intense exercise that causes an oxygen deficit in the muscles.

isometric exercise Exercise where the muscle contracts but the body does not move.

isotonic exercise Exercise where the muscle contraction causes body movement.

In order to build muscle, the muscle must work against some form of resistance—this is called *resistance training* or *strength training*. There are several ways to create resistance that your muscles can work against: free weights (such as dumbbells or barbells), weight machines, resistance bands, or even using your own body weight. You can perform a variety of different exercises with free weights, resistance bands, and your own body weight, whereas weight machines are usually designed for only one or two specific exercises. Weight machines, however, promote correct movement and safe lifting and allow you to easily change the amount of resistance or pinpoint specific muscles.

You can do several different types of exercises while your muscles work against resistance. In **isometric exercise,** the muscle contracts but there is no visible movement. This is accomplished by working against some immovable form of resistance such as your body's own muscle (pressing the palms together) or a structural item (pushing against a door frame). It is most helpful to hold isometric contractions for 6–8 seconds and to perform each exercise 5–10 times. During **isotonic exercise,** muscle force is able to cause

repetitions The number of times you perform an exercise repeatedly.

sets Separate groups of repetitions.

recovery The period necessary for the body to recover from exercise demands and adapt to higher levels of fitness.

static flexibility The ability to reach and hold a stretch at one endpoint of a joint's range of motion.

dynamic flexibility The ability to move quickly and fluidly through a joint's entire range of motion with little resistance.

static stretching Gradually lengthening a muscle to an elongated position and sustaining that position.

movement. The tension in the muscle remains unchanged, but the muscle length changes. Performing a bicep curl with a free weight, walking up stairs, and punching a punching bag are examples of isotonic exercises.

When developing your resistance training program, you should decide on the numbers of sets and repetitions that you will do for each exercise. **Repetitions** are the number of times you perform the exercise continuously. **Sets** are separate groups of repetitions. The numbers of sets and repetitions to do depends on whether you are trying to build strength or endurance. Strength develops best when you do a few repetitions (approximately 8–12) with heavier weights or more resistance. Endurance develops best when you do more repetitions (approximately 15–25) with lighter weights or less resistance. Increase the amount of resistance once you can easily perform the desired number of repetitions.

Resistance Training Tips When participating in a resistance training program, be sure to follow these guidelines:

- It's important to use proper technique when performing weight-lifting exercises. See **Practical Strategies for Health: Safe Weight Lifting.**
- Because resistance exercises are specific to the particular muscles they are designed for, be sure to include exercises for all the major muscle groups.
- Rest for 2–3 minutes between sets. If you are building muscular endurance you can slightly shorten the time between sets.[24]

- Vary your resistance training routine from time to time to lessen the risk of injury and keep your workouts from getting dull. You'll also want to revisit a maintenance program as you age. You may need different levels or types of resistance training to preserve fitness and muscle mass as you get older.

Figure 5.2 on pages 98–99 shows examples of some simple resistance exercises you can perform.

Recovery Once you've begun a resistance program, be sure to allow overloaded muscle at least 48 hours for repair and **recovery** before another exercise bout. However, because muscles begin to atrophy after about 96 hours, don't let too much time pass without another training session. If different muscle groups are worked on different days (for example, lower body versus upper body), it is acceptable to perform resistance exercise on consecutive days as long as each muscle group receives the recommended 48 hours of recovery time.

> 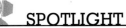 Keep a log of your workouts so you can be sure to allow each muscle group adequate recovery time. Try these online logs: www.tweetyourhealth.com, www.wellsphere.com/wellPhoneLogProgress.s, www.sparkpeople.com, www.mypyramidtracker.gov.

Exercises for Improving Flexibility

There are two major types of flexibility. **Static flexibility** is the ability to reach and hold a stretch at one endpoint of a joint's range of motion. **Dynamic flexibility** is the ability to move quickly and fluidly through a joint's entire range of motion with little resistance. Static flexibility determines whether a martial artist can reach her leg as high as her opponent's head, but it is dynamic flexibility that would enable her to kick her leg that high in one fast, fluid motion. Flexibility can vary a lot among individuals, but everyone can increase his or her flexibility through consistent stretching exercises.

Stretching applies gentle, elongating force to both a muscle and its connective tissue. **Static stretching,** the most common and

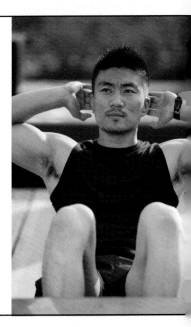

SPOTLIGHT

Core Concerns: Why You Should Strengthen Your Core

Your core muscles run the entire length of your torso, stabilizing the spine, pelvis, and shoulders. They also provide a solid foundation for movement of the arms and legs and make it possible for you to stand upright, move on two feet, balance, and shift movement in any

direction. Standing upright and walking around on two feet is not easy on your body. A strong core distributes the stresses of bearing your weight and protects the back.

Weak core muscles can compromise the appropriate

curvature of your spine, often resulting in low back pain and other injuries. The greatest benefit of core strength is increased functional fitness—the fitness that is essential to both daily living and regular activities. Core strength can be built through exercises

such as abdominal curls, planks, back extensions, Pilates, and any other exercises that work core muscles.

> Watch a video about core training at www.webmd.com/video/core-strengthening-tips.

(a) Squat

Stand with feet shoulder-width apart, toes pointing forward, hips and shoulders aligned, abdominals pulled in. Bend your knees and lower until you have between a 45- and 90-degree angle. Keep your knees behind the front of your toes. Contract your abdominals while coming up.

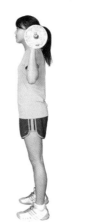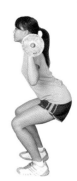

(b) Lunge

Stand with feet shoulder-width apart. As you step forward, keep your front knee in line with your ankle; make sure the front knee does not extend over your toes. Distribute your weight evenly between the front and back leg.

(c) Hip Abduction

Connect a resistance band to a stable object and loop around your outside leg. Stand with good posture and hold onto something stable. Slowly extend your leg out and return.

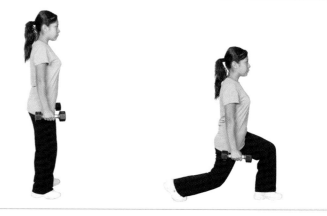

(d) Biceps Curl

Place the center of the resistance band under one foot and grab the free ends of the band with a straight arm on the same side. Keep your hips and shoulders in-line and your abdominals pulled in. Lift your arm toward your shoulder until your arm is fully contracted, and slowly return.

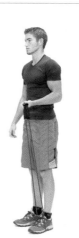

Figure 5.2 Simple resistance exercises. Be sure to perform exercises equally on both sides.

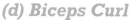

(e) Hip Adduction

Lie on your back with an exercise ball pressed between your knees. Squeeze the ball with your knees for 3–10 seconds and release.

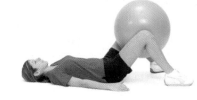

(f) Abdominal Curl

Lie back with the exercise ball placed at your low to mid-back region. Place your feet shoulder-width apart with your knees bent at about 90-degrees. Cross your hands at your chest or place lightly behind your head. Contract your abdominals, pulling them in, while you raise your upper torso. Slowly return to starting position.

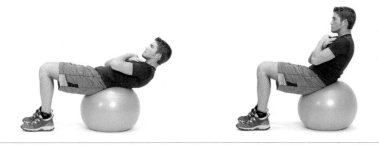

(g) Reverse Curl

Lie on your back and lift your legs to 90-degrees from the floor. Your knees may be bent or straight. Contract your abdominals, pulling them in, while you lift your hips off the floor. Slowly return hips to floor. Be careful not to rock back and forth.

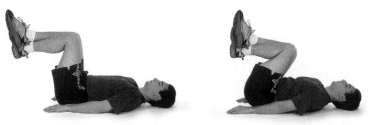

(h) Back Extension

Start lying on your stomach with your arms and legs extended, forehead on the floor. Lift and further extend your arms and legs using your back muscles. Hold for 3–5 seconds and slowly lower back down.

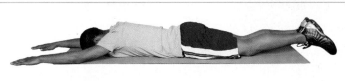

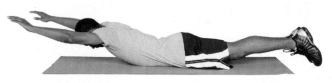

(i) Plank

Support yourself in plank position (from the forearms or hands) by contracting your trunk muscles so that your neck, back, and hips are completely straight. Hold for 5–60 seconds, increasing time as you become stronger. Your forearms should be slightly wider than your shoulders.

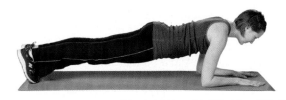

(j) Modified Push-Ups

Support yourself in push-up position as shown by contracting your trunk muscles. Place hands slightly wider than your shoulders. Keep your neck, back, and hips completely straight; do not let your trunk sag in the middle or raise your hips. Slowly lower your body down toward the floor, being careful to keep a straight body position. Your elbows will press out and back as you lower to a 90-degree elbow joint. Press yourself back up to start position.

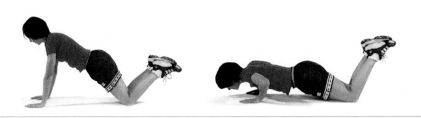

Practical Strategies for Health

Safe Weight Lifting

- If you are just beginning to use weights, make an appointment with a fitness specialist who can teach you the proper techniques that reduce the risk of injury and maximize the benefits you receive.

- Always warm up before weight lifting.

- Take your time and lift mindfully.

- Breathe out as you lift the weight and in as you release the weight—don't hold your breath, it can cause dangerous increases in blood pressure.

- Focus on the muscle you're trying to work. Feel the effort in the muscle, not in the joint.

- Equally train opposing muscle groups, such as the lower back and abdomen or the biceps and triceps.

- Use only the amount of weights that your body can handle without having to cheat by using other muscles or momentum.

- When using free weights, always have a partner who can check your form and "spot" for you.

legs). Also, stretching cold muscles is not a good idea. Instead, warm up muscles by walking or jogging or some other low intensity activity for at least 5 minutes prior to stretching or stretch at the end of your workout. The following tips will help you create a flexibility program for yourself:[24]

- A stretching session should last at least 10 minutes.
- Hold static stretches for 15–60 seconds.
- Perform four or more repetitions of each stretch.
- Stretch at least 2–3 days per week.
- Stretch until your muscle feels tight but not to the point of discomfort.
- Do not hold your breath while stretching. Try to relax and breathe deeply.
- Do not lock your joints while stretching.

In addition to regular stretching exercises, there are several other types of activities that increase flexibility. Three of the most popular are yoga, Pilates, and tai chi:

- **Yoga.** Yoga moves you through a set of carefully constructed poses designed to increase flexibility and strengthen your body. Yoga also focuses on mood and thought, using techniques such as breathing exercises to encourage reduced stress and anxiety. Many people start yoga in a class setting, gradually developing their own personal yoga practices.

- **Pilates.** Pilates combines stretching and resistance exercises to create a sequence of precise, controlled movements that focuses on flexibility, joint mobility, and core strength. Many movements in Pilates are performed on an exercise mat, but some require a machine called a Reformer, which can be found at many gyms. Because Pilates movements are so precise, it is recommended to begin Pilates in a group or private class rather than on your own.

- **Tai chi.** Tai chi is a Chinese practice designed to work the entire body gently through a series of quiet, fluid motions. The discipline also focuses on your energy, referred to in Chinese as "chi" (sometimes spelled "qi") or life force. The practice aims to keep a participant's body and chi in balance, requiring a focus on mood and thought.

easiest form of stretching, involves a gradual stretch and then hold of the stretched position for a certain amount of time. **Passive stretching,** on the other hand, is performed with a partner who gently applies pressure to your body in a stretched position to deepen the stretch. Passive stretching provides a more intense flexibility workout but also increases the risk of injury because you are not controlling the stretch yourself. In **ballistic stretching** you gently bounce once you are in a stretch. If ballistic stretching is performed improperly, it can increase the risk of injury, so it is best for recreational exercisers to avoid this form of stretching.[26]

Flexibility varies for each joint, and flexibility exercises are specific to the joint they're designed for, so when creating a flexibility program, be sure to stretch all the major muscle and joint areas of the body (neck, shoulders, upper and lower back, pelvis, hips, and

passive stretching Stretching performed with a partner who increases the intensity of the stretch by gently applying pressure to your body as it stretches.

ballistic stretching Performing rhythmic bouncing movements in a stretch to increase the intensity of the stretch.

You can find classes for yoga, Pilates, tai chi, and other flexibility-improving programs through private studios, community centers, and campus wellness centers. **Figure 5.3** on pages 101–102 shows simple flexibility exercises you can easily perform on your own as well.

> Visit the iTunes store, click on the podcasts tab, and look for podcasts on topics like running, action sports, yoga, or activities in the great outdoors.

How Much Physical Activity Do You Need?

Creating a fitness program is more than determining what types of exercise to do; you'll also want to decide how often to be active so that you can move from overload to recovery and back again in an effective, consistent way.

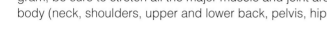

(a) Pectoral and Bicep Stretch

Stand arm's length away from a wall. Reach your arm to the side, place your palm flat on the wall, and turn your body away until you feel a comfortable stretch.

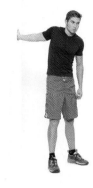

(b) Upper-Back Stretch

Reach your arms in front of you and clasp your hands while rounding your back and lowering your head.

(c) Shoulder Stretch

Reach one arm across your chest and hold it above or below the elbow with the other hand.

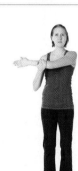

(d) Tricep Stretch

Lift your arm overhead, reaching the elbow toward the ceiling. Press the arm back from the front or reach your other arm over your head and gently pull the elbow toward your head.

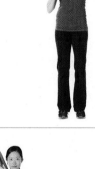

(e) Torso Twist

Sit with your legs straight out in front of you. Bend one knee and cross it over your other leg. Turn your body toward the bent knee and twist to look behind you. Place the opposite arm on the bent leg to gently press the stretch further.

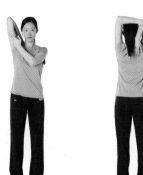

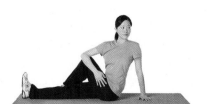

Figure 5.3 Simple stretching exercises. Be sure to perform exercises equally on both sides.

(f) Hip Stretch

While lying on your back, bend both knees and cross one over the other. Gently lower your legs sideways toward the knee that is closest to you.

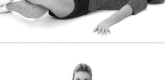

(g) Inner-Thigh Butterfly Stretch

Bring the bottoms of your feet together and pull your feet gently toward you. Actively contract your hip muscles to lower your knees closer to the ground.

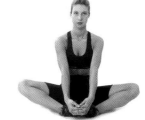

(h) Hip Flexor Stretch

Lunge forward and gently place the back knee on a mat and release your back foot. Lean forward into the hip. Make sure your front ankle is directly under your front knee and not in front of it.

(i) Quadriceps Stretch

Grab your foot from behind and pull it back toward your rear until you feel a stretch in the front of your thighs. Maintain straight body alignment and keep your thighs parallel. Assist your balance by holding onto a stable object.

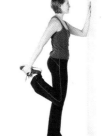

(j) Hamstrings Stretch

Sit with one leg extended and the other leg bent with the knee facing sideways. Keeping your back as straight as possible, lean your body forward, moving your chest closer to your extended leg. If you are moderately flexible, you can reach for and hold your foot but only if this does not cause pain.

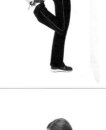
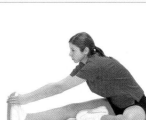

(k) Shin Stretch

Reach one leg behind you and place the tips of your toes on the ground. Bend both knees and lower the body slightly as you press the top of your back foot toward the ground. Use a wall for support if needed.

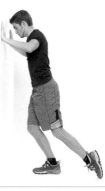

Figure 5.3 Simple stretching exercises (continued).

The *Physical Activity Guidelines for Americans* from the Centers for Disease Control and Prevention recommends the following activity levels for the creation and maintenance of health-related fitness in healthy adults:[27]

- At least 2 hours and 30 minutes (150 minutes) of moderate-intensity aerobic activity each week.

OR

- At least 1 hour and 15 minutes (75 minutes) of vigorous-intensity aerobic activity each week.

OR

- An equivalent mix of moderate- and vigorous-intensity aerobic activity each week.

AND

- Resistance exercise 2 days a week or more, for all major muscle groups, in sets of at least 8–12 repetitions.

You should also perform flexibility exercises twice a week or more and take part in lifestyle/light-intensity physical activity daily.[24] **Figure 5.4** summarizes these exercise recommendations.

A good way to meet the aerobic guidelines is to perform 30 minutes of moderate-intensity activity 5 days a week. For greater health benefits, increase your weekly aerobic activity to 300 minutes (5 hours) of moderate-intensity activity or 150 minutes (2 hours and 30 minutes) of high-intensity activity.[27] If weight loss or maintenance of weight loss is one of your fitness goals, aim for at least 60–90 minutes of moderate-intensity physical activity a day.[28]

The following tips can help you increase your activity levels and meet the recommendations.

If You Aren't Active Now

If you usually get little or no regular physical activity, start by doing what you can, and then look for ways to add more. If you tire easily you can work out in as little as 10 minute intervals.[29] Below are a couple easy ways you can add activity into your life:

- Park your car at the far end of the parking lot to extend the amount of walking you do.
- Walk briskly or ride your bike to class.
- Take the stairs instead of the elevator.
- Begin an active new hobby like in-line skating, yoga, or dance classes.
- Get an exercise buddy: You can be social as you exercise and it will help keep you motivated.
- Don't forget to include resistance and flexibility exercises at least 2 days per week.

If You Get Some Physical Activity Now

If you engage in some physical activity on a regular basis, focus on increasing your activity level:[29]

- Increase the intensity of your aerobic exercise by replacing moderate- with vigorous-intensity activities.
- Be active for longer; instead of walking for 30 minutes, try walking for 50 minutes.
- Be active more often; if you work out 2 days a week, try building up to 4 days a week.

MYTH OR FACT?
Does Stretching Prevent Injury?

Many exercisers like to stretch because they believe it substantially reduces injury rates, but is that actually the case? The latest research says no.[1–3]

Researchers are finding that stretching is ineffective at preventing injuries unless it is in preparation for an activity that demands a wide range of flexibility, such as gymnastics. Stretching also seems to be ineffective at preventing muscle soreness. Static stretching may even be linked to decreased muscle strength and endurance, although other types of stretching may not have this effect.[4]

However, stretching is still an important component of your exercise routine. Stretching helps you maintain the flexibility necessary for a full range of motion for activities like swinging, throwing, reaching, or swimming. If you are performing an activity where there is a high demand for muscle strength or endurance, stretch after the activity rather than before, but do not forego this important fitness exercise.

References: **1.** Hart, L. (2008). Which interventions prevent sport injuries? A review. *Clinical Review of Sports Medicine, 18*(5), 471–472. **2.** Herbert, R. D., & Gabriel, M. (2002). Effects of stretching before and after exercising on muscle soreness and risk of injury: Systematic review. *BMJ, 325,* 468. **3.** Fradkin, A. J., Gabbe, B. J., & Cameron, P. A. (2006). Does warming up prevent injury in sport? The evidence from randomized controlled trials. *Journal of Sports Science and Medicine, 9,* 214–220. **4.** Yamaguchi, T., & Ishii, K. (2005). Effects of static stretching for 30 seconds and dynamic stretching on leg extension power. *Journal of Strength & Conditioning Research, 19,* 677–683.

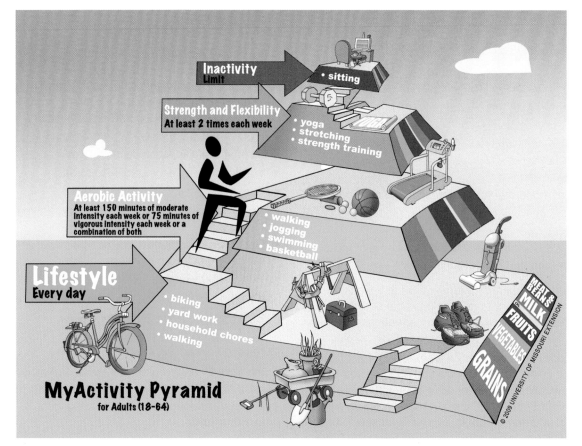

Figure 5.4 MyActivityPyramid. This pyramid summarizes the physical activity recommendations for adults.

Source: "MyActivity Pyramid" from University of Missouri Extension website. http://extension.missouri.edu. Used by permission of University of Missouri Extension.

- If you already perform resistance exercises, try adding an extra day of resistance exercises to your fitness program.
- Incorporate a variety of activities into your fitness program to avoid boredom.
- If you already meet the minimum recommendations for activity, strive for the elevated recommendations of 300 minutes of moderate-intensity or 150 minutes of vigorous-intensity activity per week.

If You Are Overweight

Many people who are overweight or obese feel that they can't start an activity program, but that isn't true. If you are overweight, it is especially important to introduce activity into your life because being overweight is a risk factor for many health problems. To get started with an activity program, try the following:

- Seek out environments in which you feel supported. Some fitness clubs are gender-specific; others are geared toward those who are overweight.
- If your current weight puts stress on your joints choose non–weight-bearing exercise. Swimming and water-based exercise classes can get you moving without stressing your joints.
- Remember that everyday activities, such as light housework or gardening, walking the dog, or washing the car, can get you moving. Any activity that puts your body in motion helps. Try increasing your physical activity slightly each day.
- If you haven't worked out in a while, begin with light-intensity (40–50% of your maximum heart rate) aerobic activity that gets

your whole body moving. This will provide health benefits, expend energy to help with weight loss, and set the foundation for progression to higher intensities.

> Watch videos about the Physical Activity Guidelines for Americans at **www.cdc.gov/physicalactivity/everyone/videos/index.html**.

How Do You Exercise Safely?

Exercising safely is not difficult, if you keep a few basic guidelines in mind.

Get Medical Clearance

Before you begin any exercise program, make sure you are medically healthy enough to exercise. Complete the **Self-Assessment** on page 105, or make an appointment with a doctor to make sure you do not have any health conditions that should be taken into account before you begin an exercise program.

Warm Up and Cool Down

Before you start any moderate- to vigorous-intensity exercise, give yourself about 15 minutes to warm up. Warming up slowly moves your body from a less active state to a more active one. Warming up is not the same as stretching; effective warm-up involves gentle overall motion or a slowed-down version of the activity you are about to pursue, which increases your heart rate and blood flow to

Do I Need to See a Doctor Before I Exercise?

Do you have any of the following risk factors that might affect your ability to exercise?

- Do you have a chronic disease or have risk factors for a chronic disease, such as asthma or diabetes?   __ yes __ no
- Do you have high blood pressure, high cholesterol, or a personal or family history of heart disease?   __ yes __ no
- Are you pregnant?   __ yes __ no
- Are you a smoker?   __ yes __ no
- Are you unsure of your health status or have any concerns that exercise might be unsafe for you?   __ yes __ no

HOW TO INTERPRET YOUR SCORE

If you answered "Yes" to any of the above questions, talk with your doctor or campus health service about creating a safe and effective personal exercise program.

To complete this self-assessment online, visit www.pearsonhighered.com/choosinghealth.

the muscles needed for exercise. When you are finished with your workout, give yourself another 15 minutes to cool down by performing slower and less intense movements, slowly returning your body to a less active state.

Get Training

Take the time to seek out training from fitness experts for any new activities or exercises. Learning the proper techniques from a qualified instructor will help prevent injury and increase your success at the activity. When you are choosing a trainer or fitness instructor, look for certifications from nonprofit organizations like the American College of Sports Medicine. Trainers and instructors should be knowledgeable in CPR and first aid; they should also undergo ongoing professional training on new techniques. Before settling on a fitness instructor, make sure that person makes you feel comfortable and provides helpful feedback to you during your workout.

Wear Suitable Clothes

Clothes made of lightweight, breathable fabrics such as 100% cotton will help keep you comfortable as you exercise and allow for full range of movement. Clothing marketed as moisture wicking will pull sweat away from your body to increase comfort as well. If you exercise outside, choose clothing that indicates that it is made of material that offers sun protection. Use sunscreen and a hat if you will be outside, even if it is overcast. Wear a helmet, pads, and other protective gear when cycling, skateboarding, or participating in any other activities where a fall is possible. It's also important to wear the proper athletic shoes for the activity you are pursuing. See **Consumer Corner: Choosing Athletic Shoes** for more information on how to pick a proper shoe for exercise.

Stay Hydrated

Adequate water consumption is a critical part of any workout. Studies show that dehydration limits strength, power, and endurance.[30] It is most effective to keep drinking water before, during, and after exercise as opposed to gulping down water all at once at the end of your workout. If you find yourself feeling thirsty, fatigued, with weak muscles and a minor headache, you may need to rehydrate.

To stay hydrated, fitness specialists say that water is your best choice. If, however, activity is prolonged and performed at a high intensity level, you may consider commercial sports drinks. These are beverages that combine water with sugars, flavoring, carbohydrates that provide energy, or *electrolytes,* salts that help your body function properly. Sports drinks are often expensive, provide little essential nutrition, and contain unnecessary levels of sugar. A few also contain caffeine, which may give you a quick surge of energy but does nothing to build your fitness long-term. If you prefer the taste of sports drinks to plain water but aren't performing vigorous-intensity, prolonged exercise, try mixing just a little sports drink, juice, or a few slices of lemon or lime into a bottle of water.

Prepare for Hot or Cold Weather

If you exercise outside, always check the weather report before you go out. In cold weather you need gear that keeps you warm and wicks sweat away from your body, but lets you move at the same time. Opt for layers of clothing that will keep your body temperature from dropping too low but can also be adjusted as your body heats up during exercise. Wear a hat, since much of your body heat is lost through your head, and protect your fingers and toes from the cold. If you start shivering, stop your workout, add more layers of clothing, and head inside. Constant shivering is an early sign of **hypothermia,** a potentially fatal condition in which your core body temperature dips too low. If your core temperature isn't raised you will become uncoordinated, drowsy, and confused and will have difficulty speaking. If anyone you work out with develops these symptoms, he or she should be warmed up and taken to a hospital.

If you are working out in the heat, try to exercise in early morning or evening, when the weather tends to be cooler and less humid. Hot weather requires special attention to both gear and hydration. If you get too dehydrated in hot weather, you put yourself at risk for **heat exhaustion,** a mild form of heat-related illness. Symptoms of heat exhaustion include nausea, headache, fatigue, and faintness, and mean you need to slow down, drink water, and head for a cooler spot.

If your overheating worsens, you face the possibility of **heatstroke,** a potentially fatal condition. In heatstroke, your overheated core body temperature overwhelms your body's cooling capabilities, causing dry, hot skin and rapid heart rate. Brain damage and death can follow. If you experience any of the symptoms, you need rest, a cooler location, and lots of cool fluids to drink immediately. Outdoor sports that require heavy pads, such as football, make it tough for your body to regulate its temperature effectively on hot days and put you at higher risk for heatstroke. If you participate in gear-heavy sports that leave you feeling

hypothermia A potentially fatal condition in which your core body temperature becomes too low.

heat exhaustion A mild form of heat-related illness that usually occurs as the result of exercising in hot weather without adequate hydration.

heatstroke A life-threatening heat-related illness that occurs when your core temperature rises above 105 degrees Fahrenheit.

CONSUMER CORNER

Choosing Athletic Shoes

When shopping for athletic shoes it's important to choose shoes that are made for the particular activity you are participating in, because while athletic shoes look similar on the outside, each kind is constructed differently. If you do a variety of activities, it's best to purchase shoes specifically for any activities that you participate in for more than 3 hours per week.

The following tips will help you pick the best shoe:[1, 2]

- Always go to a store that specializes in athletic shoes to find the best selection and the most knowledgeable salespeople.

- Shop for shoes at the end of the day, when your feet are at their largest.

- Wear the type of socks you plan on wearing with the shoes, in order to get the best gauge on fit.

- If your foot is wide or narrow, select a shoe made specifically for that width. If the sides of the heel, toes, or arch feel tight, it's not wide enough.

- If you have high arches, make sure to purchase a shoe or separate insoles with lots of arch support and cushioning.

- Purchase shoes made specifically for your sex. However, women with wide feet may consider trying men's or boy's shoes, which are made a bit larger throughout the heel.

- Bring your old shoes with you. Shoe professionals can give you tips based on the wear pattern on your old shoes.

- Try on both shoes, and walk, run, or perform the types of movements you will use the shoe for. The shoes should feel immediately comfortable, and your heel should fit snugly in each shoe and not slip as you walk.

- Don't assume you wear the same shoe size in athletic shoes as you do in regular shoes. Try on different sizes if the shoe feels too tight or too loose. You should have at least a half an inch—about the width of your finger—between your longest toe and the end of the shoe.

It's also important to replace shoes when they get old. Running shoes should be replaced every 300–500 miles, cross-training shoes after 5–7 months, and aerobic shoes after 100–120 hours of use.[2, 3] If your shoes are wearing through, it's time to replace them regardless of how long you've had them.

References: **1.** Mayo Clinic. (2009). *Walking shoes: Features and fit that keep you moving.* Retrieved from http://www.mayoclinic.com/health/walking/HQ00885_D. **2.** Laux, K. A. (2009). *Smart shopping for athletic shoes.* Retrieved from http://www.livestrong.com/article/353-smart-shopping-athletic-shoes. **3.** Christian, C. (2007). Selecting workout shoes: Proper sports shoes can increase pleasure and reduce pain. Retrieved from http:fitness.souite101.com/article.cfm/selecting_workout_shoes.

This interactive graphic can help you select the best walking shoes: www.mayoclinic.com/health/medical/FS00001.

overheated, such as football, talk to your coach about taking steps to make everyone cooler.

Select Facilities and Equipment Carefully

When selecting a gym, a good place to start is your campus wellness center. If looking for somewhere off campus, you should visit a few facilities before making your final choice. Take a tour of each gym and note whether the gym is clean, properly lit, adequately staffed, adequately ventilated and temperature controlled, and has an appropriate emergency response and evacuation plan.[31] Make sure the gym is at a convenient location for you, and it also helps to visit it at peak times to see how crowded it can become. Some gyms offer free trial memberships that can be helpful during your evaluation.

When buying equipment, think about what your fitness goals are and what types of exercise you are planning on performing. Think carefully about whether you will use a certain piece of equipment regularly. If you have doubts reconsider buying it. Set a budget for how much you want to spend and then buy the highest quality equipment that is within your budget. Be sure to try the equipment out before buying it; it should feel comfortable, solid, and durable. Also think about where you will store the equipment. Keeping bulky equipment in a small dorm room or apartment can be difficult.

Start Slow and Care for Injuries

It's important to start slowly when you begin an exercise program, in order to avoid injuries. However, injuries occasionally do happen when exercising. Common complaints include contusions (bruises), joint sprains, muscle strains, shin splints, and tendonitis. These injuries most often cause pain, swelling, or skin discoloration.

Another common complaint during exercise is **cramps.** These severe muscle contractions are your body's way of making you take a break. If you get a cramp, stop your activity. Drink some water and massage or apply pressure to the cramped muscle. You can also try taking a few deep breaths to give your body—and your cramped muscles—extra oxygen.

Minor injuries to the muscles and joints should be treated with the RICE protocol: rest, ice, compression, and elevation. The first step is to rest the injured area; stop exercising as soon as you feel pain. Second, ice the injured area for no more than 20 minutes at a time intermittently for the first 24–48 hours. The cold of the ice helps to decrease the swelling. After 48 hours you can apply a heating pad to the area, which improves blood flow and promotes healing. Third, compress the area with an elastic bandage, both to hold the ice in place and to decrease the swelling. If the area becomes numb or discolored loosen the bandage because you may have wrapped it too tightly. Finally, if you can elevate the injured area above your heart, do so. It will minimize the swelling and discomfort associated with your injury.

Be Wary of Performance-Enhancing Drugs

Some athletes, intent on boosting performance, look to performance-enhancing drugs. These substances are intended to increase physical strength, speed, or endurance. Some of these substances can change body composition in a way that increases overall physical power.

cramp An involuntary contracted muscle that does not relax resulting in localized intense pain.

Practical Strategies for Health

Red Flags During Exercise

If you experience any of the following symptoms while exercising, stop immediately, no matter your level of fitness. Talk with your doctor or campus health service about any of these symptoms:

- Pain, tightness, or pressure in your chest, neck, arm, or shoulder.

- Dizziness or nausea
- Cold sweats
- Severe muscle cramps
- Extreme shortness of breath
- Pain in your joints, feet, ankles, or legs

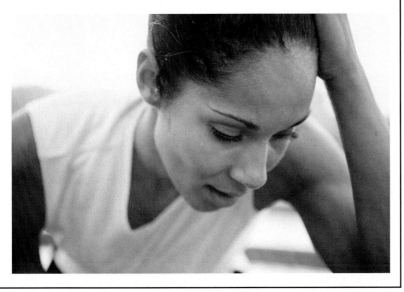

Prominent athletes, including well-known Olympic athletes, cyclists, and players in Major League Baseball, have made headlines after investigators discovered their use of performance-enhancing drugs. But use of these substances isn't confined to the top tiers of sports. According to health estimates, up to three million Americans have used performance-enhancing drugs, including an estimated 4.7% of males and 1.2% of females.[32] In a national survey, about 40% of high school seniors described these substances as "fairly easy" or "very easy" to get.[33] Although interest in improved athletics drives much of the use of these substances, some people, especially men, are motivated by appearance, hoping the drugs will help them develop more muscular bodies.[34]

Some performance-enhancing drugs are not as effective as marketers claim or carry dangerous side effects, and a few are even illegal for use or sale in the United States. Common types of performance-enhancing drugs include:

- **Anabolic steroids.** Synthetic derivatives of the male hormone testosterone, anabolic steroids can encourage muscle growth and build lean body tissue. It is illegal to use anabolic steroids to improve athletic performance, and they pose serious health risks, including liver cancer, fluid retention, high blood pressure, and severe acne. Men who use anabolic steroids may see their testicles shrink and their sperm counts drop. In women, steroid use can cause cessation of the menstrual cycle, enlargement of the clitoris, growth of facial and body hair, male-pattern baldness and deepening of the voice. Anabolic steroids can also lead to dangerous psychological side effects, including aggression, extreme mood swings, rage, and even violent behavior.

- **Creatine.** Creatine is a substance naturally produced by the body and stored in skeletal muscles. Creatine is thought to help muscles during short, high-intensity activity, but research on creatine has been inconclusive. Taking creatine may cause dehydration, reduced blood volume, and produce imbalances in blood chemistry. Federal health officials warn that creatine should only be used under a doctor's care.[35]

- **Human growth hormone.** Also known as HGH, human growth hormone is a naturally occurring compound made by the body to fuel cell growth and regeneration. Its use as an athletic supplement has been widespread because HGH is difficult to detect during athletic drug testing. But scientists warn that the long-term effects of using HGH are unknown. In the meantime, researchers have found no significant athletic benefits tied to use of the hormone. Use of HGH in athletes, for example, did not improve strength and actually appeared to worsen athletic performance. HGH users also experienced more soft tissue swelling and fatigue.[36]

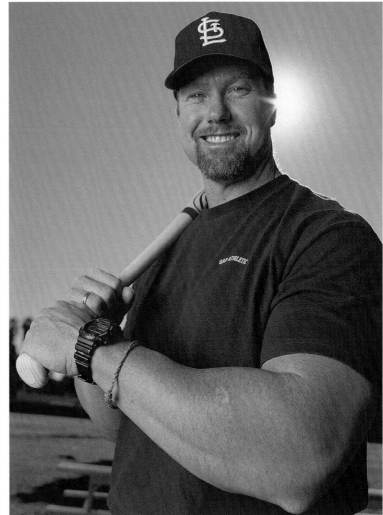

Major League Baseball player Mark McGwire recently admitted to using **anabolic steroids**.

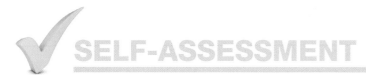

SELF-ASSESSMENT

To complete this self-assessment online, visit **www.pearsonhighered.com/choosinghealth**.

Five Simple Fitness Self-Tests

Try the following simple fitness tests to assess your current fitness level.

1. **Test Your ARM STRENGTH with Push-Ups.** Do a push-up with straight knees and keeping body in a straight line from head to ankle while you press up. Do as many in a row as you can without stopping—no time limit—and record the number.

2. **Test Your CORE STRENGTH with Crunches.** With bent knees, feet flat on the floor, chin tucked and arms crossed over your chest, bring your shoulder blades up one third of the way to sitting upright. Do as many as you can in 1 minute. Write down the number.

3. **Test Your LEG STREGTH with the Wall-Sit.** Stand with your back against a wall. Place your feet about 12 inches away from the wall and about hip-width apart. With feet planted firmly, bend your knees and slide down the wall until your knees form a 90-degree angle. (As if you are sitting in a chair.) Hold as long as you can stand it! Record your time.

4. **Test your FLEXIBILITY with the Sit-and-Reach.** You'll need a yardstick and masking tape to perform this assessment. Put the yardstick on the floor and place a 12-inch piece of tape perpendicular across the yardstick at the 15-inch mark. Sit with your legs on either side of the yardstick with your heels on the piece of masking tape. (The zero end of the yardstick should be closest to your body.) Keeping your legs extended straight in front of you, your knees straight but not locked, and your feet slightly apart, reach forward with both hands, bending at hips. What is the farthest mark on the yardstick that your fingertips can touch? If you can touch your toes, your reach is 15 inches. If you can touch 2 inches past your toes, your reach is 17 inches. Measure your reach and record the number.

5. **Test Your CARDIORESPIRATORY Fitness with the Quarter-Mile Dash.** Find a track. If you use the indoor one at your college wellness center, determine how many laps you'll need for a quarter-mile run. If you use a regulation outdoor track, one lap measures a quarter of a mile. Walk, jog, or run the distance as fast as you can. Record your time.

HOW TO INTERPRET YOUR SCORE

Record your results and set fitness goals based on what you've learned. For example, you may want to set a goal of being able to touch your toes if you currently cannot. Or, bring your scores to class and compare your results with your fellow classmates.

You may also want to track your progress by taking these assessments again after you have participated in a fitness program for 6 weeks.

- **Androstenedione.** A steroid precursor that is thought to enhance athletic performance and boost testosterone, androstenedione has been linked to many high-profile controversies among professional athletes. Androstenedione is illegal for sale or use in the United States, and its side effects include breast development and impotence in men, abnormal periods and facial hair in women, and liver disease and blood clots.

- **Ephedra.** Ephedra can be taken to boost energy and promote weight loss, but its negative effects have led lawmakers to outlaw its sale in the United States. Research has not shown ephedra to be effective in boosting energy or athletic performance, and its side effects include high blood pressure, irregular heartbeat, stroke, and gastrointestinal or psychological problems.[37]

How Do You Maintain a Fitness Program?

Scheduling regular exercise may seem daunting, but if you set goals, find activities you enjoy, think about how you will overcome obstacles, and periodically reassess your progress, you'll be able to stay motivated and enjoy the benefits of fitness.

Set Realistic Goals

One of the most important aspects of a fitness program is working at an intensity and rate that makes sense for you. Trying to reach too high a level of strength or stamina too quickly can be dangerous and discouraging. It is important to realistically assess your current fitness level (see the **Self-Assessment** above) in order to set fitness goals that are appropriate. Fitness goals can be based on a specific activity-related improvement you want to make, such as cycling 40% farther than you currently can now; a health-related goal you may have, such as reducing your blood pressure or increasing your en-ergy; or a social or lifestyle desire, like preparing for a backpacking trip with your friends. Make sure your goals are easily measurable, so you can clearly tell when you've met one.

Write down your goals and track your progress toward them. It is helpful to break down long-term goals into smaller short-term goals, and build toward your larger goal over time. For example, if your goal is to meet the Physical Activity Guidelines for Americans recommended aerobic activity levels but you haven't worked out in years, you should begin with smaller goals. Your goals could look like this:

Goal: Perform 150 minutes of moderate-intensity activity each week.

Subgoal 1: Perform 30 minutes of brisk walking twice a week for 2–3 weeks.

Subgoal 2: Add to the walking program by attending a 45-minute low-impact cardio class once a week.

Subgoal 3: After 1 month to 6 weeks of the walking and cardio class program, add 45 minutes of working out on the stationary bike at the gym each week. 150 minutes of activity attained!

If you don't make a particular goal you have set, don't get discouraged. Take that chance to reevaluate your goal and possibly break it down into smaller subgoals.

Take this self-assessment for a quick idea of how fit you are: **www.nhs.uk/Tools/Pages/Fitness.aspx.**

Find Activities You Enjoy

To exercise on a regular basis, focus on physical activities you like. Think about the types of activities you naturally enjoy, and ask yourself which of those activities will help you reach the fitness goals you have set for yourself, which ones you are most likely to stick with, which ones will fit most easily into your schedule, and which ones you can afford. Don't be afraid to mix it up—a wide range of activities can bring you all the benefits of fitness and will stave off boredom. If you can only afford to take tennis lessons twice a month, combine that with free aerobic classes at school and resistance exercises you can perform at home.

Schedule Time

One key to sticking with exercise is to schedule in exercise as you would a job or a class. If you have a set time devoted to exercise, you will be more likely to stick with it. See Part II of the **Behavior Change Workshop** at the end of this chapter for a schedule where you can plan activity.

Overcome Obstacles

You can probably come up with a long list of reasons for why you do not already have a regular fitness routine. Here are some common obstacles and solutions for overcoming them:

- **I don't have time.** Remember that only 30 minutes of moderate exercise a day can improve or maintain your fitness and that time can be broken down into 10-minute sessions. Substituting exercise for TV or computer time, even just a little, is a good place to

start. If you don't have time to make it to a gym, find activities you can do at home, such as walking, jogging, jumping rope, lifting free weights, or doing exercise videos. Another tactic is to combine exercise with social time: Get a buddy to exercise with you, or sign up for a recreational team with friends.

This podcast explains time-saving tips for weight training: www.mayoclinic.com/health/weight-training/SM00114.

- **I have kids, so I _really_ have no time.** If you are both a student and a parent, you face a tough time crunch when it comes to exercise. One study comparing students who were parents with those who weren't found that only 16% of parent-students performed enough physical activity, compared to 50% of other students.[38] If you have children, get exercise by actively playing with them. Some gyms also offer free or inexpensive child care, or, you can trade babysitting with a friend and use that time for exercise.

- **I don't know how.** If you feel like a klutz at the gym, start by walking or running on your own. If you don't know how to play a particular sport, take a class. Consider working with a personal trainer, who will build your skills with lots of one-on-one attention. Many campus wellness centers offer low-cost personal training and classes.

🌐 DIVERSITY & HEALTH

Safe Exercise
for Special Populations

Exercise can do everyone good. If you have health concerns, the key is to modify your fitness program to reduce risk and maximize the benefits you receive. The following measures can help you have a safe and effective workout.

Asthma

- If prescribed, use pre-exercise asthma inhalers before beginning exercise.

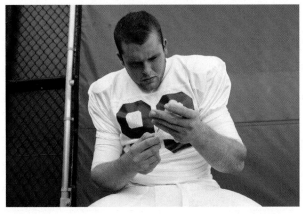

This college football player with diabetes is preparing an insulin injection for himself.

- Extend your warm-up and cool-down to help your lungs prepare for and recover from exercise.

- Check for environmental irritants that could promote an asthma attack, such as a recently mowed lawn, high pollen counts, or high levels of air pollution, and consider exercising indoors at those times. If exercising in cold weather, cover your mouth and nose with a scarf or mask.

- Try swimming. The warm, moist environment is soothing, and swimming helps build cardiorespiratory endurance.

- If you begin to cough, wheeze, have difficulty breathing, or have tightness in your chest, halt exercise and use your inhaler or other prescribed medication.

Pregnancy

- Avoid contact sports or activities that may cause trauma or a fall. Walking and swimming are great low-impact options, but you can also dance, run, or hike.

- You can still perform resistance exercises. Focus on muscular endurance ex-

ercises rather than strengthening exercises.

- Halt exercise if you experience vaginal bleeding, dizziness, headache, chest pain, calf pain or swelling, preterm labor, or decreased fetal movement.

- After the first trimester, avoid exercises where you lie on your back; they can reduce blood flow to the uterus.

Diabetes

- Monitor your blood glucose before and after exercise, especially when beginning or modifying your exercise program.

- Wear a diabetes ID bracelet during exercise.

- Carry a snack if you will be active for a few hours.

- If you begin to feel shaky, anxious, or suddenly begin to sweat more, halt exercise and consume a fast-acting carbohydrate.

- Make sure to wear well-fitting shoes and check your feet for blisters or sores before and after exercise.

- **I don't want to go to the gym.** If working out on the machines isn't your thing, try alternative exercises, like joining a dodgeball or kickball team, rock climbing, snowboarding, Ultimate Frisbee, golf, or even using video games designed for fitness, like the Wii Fit™.

- **I'm embarrassed about how I look.** If you aren't ready to hit the campus pool in a bathing suit, start with activities where you'll be comfortable in sweat pants and a T-shirt. Also, seek out exercise environments in which you feel comfortable and supported (for example, a fitness center designed for women only, or a class designed for weight-loss).

- **I don't have anywhere to exercise.** If your neighborhood and campus don't make it easy to be active, find a space in your community that does, such as a community recreation center. Remember, too, that you can exercise in the comfort of your own living room with an exercise video.

- **I don't have the money.** If you can't afford a gym membership, choose exercises that require no more than a good pair of shoes, such as walking or running. Or, purchase low-cost equipment like exercise bands, exercise balls, dumbbells, or a jump rope. Your campus or community recreation center may have free or low-cost gyms or classes. See **Consumer Corner: No-Cost Exercise Equipment** for tips on how to create equipment from everyday items.

Finding Time to Exercise

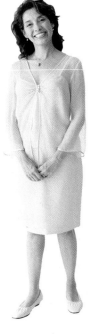

"Hi, I'm Anne. The other day the elevator was broken in my building, and I had to walk up the four flights to my apartment. I was so exhausted by the end! That really showed me that I need to work out more, but the problem is I just don't have the time. Between classes, studying, my work as a secretary at my church, and spending time with my family, I feel like I don't have a spare second. I know I need to get more fit, but I'm worried that trying to squeeze in weekly workouts will just make me feel more stressed."

1: How much daily exercise would Anne need to see improvements in her fitness?

2: How could Anne fit exercise into her week? Are there any activities she's currently doing that she could combine with exercise?

3: Do you think Anne's right that taking the time to exercise will make her more stressed?

Do you have a story similar to Anne's? Share your story at **www.pearsonhighered.com/choosinghealth.**

CONSUMER CORNER

No-Cost Exercise Equipment

Don't have the money to join a gym or buy a home exercise machine? Try improvising equipment from ordinary household items.

- **Canned goods.** Use canned goods in place of free weights when doing arm and shoulder exercises.

- **Milk or water jugs.** Fill empty jugs with water or sand and secure the tops with duct tape.

You can weigh the jugs on a scale to see how much you're lifting, and adjust the weight as you get stronger by adding more water or sand.

- **Stairs.** Are there stairs in your home or building? Try using them for calf raises, or walk up and down them for the original "stair master." Or, use the bottom stair as a step platform and choreograph a step routine.

- **Step stools.** A low, sturdy step stool can become a step platform as well.

- **Door jambs.** Stand in the middle of an open doorway and press against each side with your hands for an isometric arm workout.

Source: Adapted from MayoClinic.com. *Fitness for less: 4 low-cost ways to shape up.* 2008. http://www.mayoclinic.com/health/fitness/HQ00694_D

- **I live in a place with bad weather.** If snow, frequent rain, or high heat and humidity make exercising outside tough, look for indoor options. Consider exercise videos and free weights at home. Find a gym. If you just want to walk, check the hours at your local shopping mall. Some malls now open their doors in the early morning, long before the shops open, to give walkers a comfortable place to stroll.

Assess Your Progress

Every 4 to 6 weeks, look back and assess how far you've come. Periodically evaluating your progress can be highly motivating. Look back on all the exercise you've done, think about the positive effects on how you feel or how fit you are becoming and evaluate how close you are to the goals you set. At the beginning of an exercise program you may want to assess your progress even more often.

Watch videos of real students discussing physical activity and fitness at: **www.pearsonhighered.com/choosinghealth.**

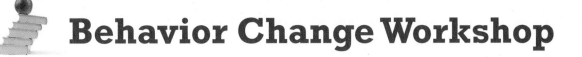

Behavior Change Workshop

To complete this workshop online, visit www.pearsonhighered.com/choosinghealth.

In order to create and maintain a fitness program you should set goals, find activities you enjoy, schedule time, overcome obstacles, and assess your progress.

Part I. Creating and Maintaining a Fitness Program

1. What are your fitness goals? Do you want to maintain a healthy lifestyle? Improve a particular component of fitness? Improve in a particular sport? Increase your energy? Something else? Make sure the goals are easily measurable, and set a realistic timeline for your goal. If your goal is large, break it down into smaller subgoals.

Goal:_____   Timeline:_____

Subgoal 1:_____   Timeline:_____

Subgoal 2:_____   Timeline:_____

Subgoal 3:_____   Timeline:_____

2. What activities do you enjoy that could help you meet your fitness goals? Think about activities that you honestly like, that you have relatively easy access to, and that you can afford. Write down all the activities that meet these criteria. Remember, participating in more than one type of activity will help you combat boredom.

_____

_____

_____

3. Think about times in your week when you can perform a minimum of 10 minutes of exercise. Factor in travel to and from your workout location. Write down all the times when exercise is possible.

_____

_____

_____

4. What obstacles might you face in adhering to a fitness program and what could you do to combat them? See pages 109–110 for tips.

Obstacle   **How to Overcome**

_____   _____

_____   _____

_____   _____

_____   _____

5. Once you have been working out for a few weeks, take some time to reflect on how your workout has affected you. Write down the improvements you see and feel.

Physical improvements:

_____

_____

_____

_____

Mental improvements:

_____

_____

_____

_____

Part II. Scheduling Time for Fitness

How do you find time to get enough exercise? One of the best ways is to write it down in a schedule as you would for any other commitment. Fill out the table below to create an exercise schedule for yourself.

Type of Activity	Monday	Tuesday	Wednesday	Thursday	Friday	Saturday	Sunday	Recommended Minimum Amount
Aerobic Exercise								150 minutes moderate-intensity OR 75 minutes vigorous-intensity OR Equivalent combination of both
Resistance Training								2 nonconsecutive days per week in sets of 8–12 reps
Flexibility Exercise								2 days per week for at least 10 minutes per session

Chapter Summary

- Physical fitness is the ability to perform moderate- to vigorous-intensity physical activity and to be able to respond to physical demands without excessive fatigue.

- The five key components of health-related fitness are cardiorespiratory fitness, muscular strength, muscular endurance, flexibility, and body composition.

- Physical activity builds the health of your heart and lungs. It also lowers your risk of certain diseases, increases immunity, helps your bones stay strong, helps protect you from injury, helps you manage your weight, and helps you cope with stress and improve mental health.

- The principles of fitness training are overload, specificity, reversibility, and individuality.

- A well-rounded fitness program should include a mix of activities that build your cardiorespiratory fitness, work your muscles, and increase your flexibility.

- You need at least 150 minutes of moderate-intensity or 75 minutes of vigorous-intensity aerobic activity each week, or an equivalent mix of the two. You also need 2–3 days of resistance training and flexibility exercise per week. Increased amounts of activity each week will promote greater health benefits and build endurance, strength, and flexibility.

- If you haven't exercised for a while, you can meet activity recommendations by starting slowly and looking for ways to build from there. If you already work out, you can meet or exceed recommendations by exercising longer, more often, or at a greater intensity. If you are overweight, it is especially important to add activity to your life.

- You can avoid injury while you exercise by taking some simple precautions, such as getting medical clearance, warming up and cooling down, getting training, wearing suitable clothes, staying hydrated, preparing for hot or cold weather, selecting facilities and equipment carefully, starting slowly, caring for your injuries, and being wary of performance-enhancing drugs.

- To maintain fitness habits, remember to set measurable goals, focus on activities you enjoy, schedule time, find ways around obstacles, and assess your progress.

Test Your Knowledge

1. Which one of the following is NOT a component of physical fitness:
    a. cardiorespiratory fitness
    b. muscular strength
    c. flexibility
    d. balance

2. Muscular strength
    a. does not help your bones.
    b. is the same thing as muscular endurance.
    c. is important for performing extended activities.
    d. is the maximum force your muscles can apply in a single effort.

3. Body composition
    a. refers to your ratio of fat to lean tissue.
    b. only matters in weight loss.
    c. can be changed by physical activity.
    d. Choices a and c are both correct.

4. People who are overweight
    a. shouldn't exercise, because it can hurt their joints.
    b. should focus on flexibility rather than cardio-vascular fitness.
    c. should begin a fitness program with light-intensity physical activity.
    d. don't need to exercise but should focus on their diets.

Get Critical

What happened:

When the 2008 U.S. Olympic Women's Swimming Team was announced, the average age of the swimmers was 22 years old, with one exception. Dara Torres, at age 41 and a mother of one, made a stir among fans and commentators alike for qualifying to the Olympic team at an age when most Olympic swimmers had long-since retired. Torres explained how she did it, "The water doesn't know how old you are. I set this crazy goal for myself, to make my fifth Olympic team as a 41-year old mother." By the end of the games, Torres had won three silvers, making her the oldest swimmer to ever win an Olympic medal.

What do you think?

- Torres has been swimming since she was a young girl. What activities would you like to participate in throughout your life?

- Setting a goal helped Torres stay motivated. What kinds of goals will help you stick with a fitness program for the long-term?

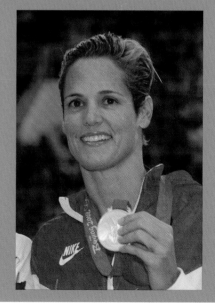

5. Students under a lot of stress
   a. shouldn't exercise, because it will just take time they don't have.
   b. can get stress relief from working out.
   c. are better off in the gym than working out on their own.
   d. won't be able to stick to an exercise program.

6. The principle of individuality means that
   a. you should only do one type of exercise during each workout.
   b. you need to do exercises in different orders each day to get the full benefit.
   c. you can improve only one component of fitness at a time.
   d. each individual adapts to exercise differently.

7. Aerobic exercise
   a. is not recommended for everyone.
   b. builds your cardiorespiratory fitness.
   c. requires expensive equipment, such as a mountain bike.
   d. can only be done in cardio classes.

8. When you get really hot during workouts
   a. stop, find a cool spot, and drink water.
   b. keep going—it means you are getting a good workout.
   c. keep going if your friends or teammates are.
   d. don't exercise outside any more until the weather changes.

9. Sports drinks
   a. should only be used with light exercise.
   b. provide the minerals you need to keep exercising.
   c. can be used during prolonged exercise.
   d. are always a good idea when working out.

10. To make exercise a habit, you should
   a. focus on physical activities that make you happy.
   b. do activities you don't like, because you need work in those areas.
   c. buy a lot of expensive equipment; it will motivate you to work out.
   d. work out at the highest possible intensity so you get fit quickly.

Get Connected ●

Health Online Visit the following websites for further information about the topics in this chapter:

- American College of Sports Medicine Public Resources
  www.acsm.org/AM/Template.cfm?Section= General_Public
- American Council on Exercise
  www.acefitness.org
- Start! Walking Program for Individuals, American Heart Association
  www.americanheart.org/presenter.jhtml?identifier= 3040791

- SparkPeople
  www.sparkpeople.com
- MyPyramid Activity Tracker
  www.mypyramidtracker.gov
- Wellsphere
  www.wellsphere.com

Website links are subject to change. To access updated Web links, please visit **www.pearsonhighered.com/choosinghealth**.

References ●

i. Centers for Disease Control and Prevention. (2008). *Physical activity for everyone: Physical activity and health.* Retrieved from http://www.cdc.gov/physicalactivity/everyone/health/index.html

ii. Aerobically unfit young adults on road to diabetes in middle age. (2009, June 20). *ScienceDaily.* Retrieved from http://www.sciencedaily.com/releases/2009/06/090618124944.htm

iii. Liu-Ambrose, T., Nagamatsu, L. S., Graf, P., Beattie, B. L., Ashe, M. C., & Handy, T. C. (2010). Resistance training and executive functions: A 12-month randomized controlled trial. *Archives of Internal Medicine, 170*(2), 170–178.

1. Centers for Disease Control and Prevention. (2007, November 23). Prevalence of regular physical activity among adults—United States, 2001 and 2005. *Morbidity and Mortality Weekly Report.* Retrieved from http://www.cdc.gov/mmwr/preview/mmwrhtml/mm5646a1.htm?s_cid=mm5646a1_e

2. William, P. T. (2008). Vigorous exercise, fitness and incident hypertension, high cho-lesterol, and diabetes. *Medicine & Science in Sport and Exercise, 40*(6), 998–1006.

3. Bushman, B., & Clark-Young, J. (2005). *Action plan for menopause.* Indianapolis, IN: American College of Sports Medicine.

4. Ärnlöv, J., Ingelsson, E., Sundström, J., & Lind, L. (2010). Impact of body mass index and the metabolic syndrome on the risk of cardiovascular disease and death in middle-aged men. *Circulation, 121*, 230–236.

5. Mueller, P. (2007). Exercise training and sympathetic nervous system activity: Evidence for physical activity dependent neural plasticity. *Clinical and Experimental Pharmacology and Physiology, 34*, 377–384.

6. Centers for Disease Control and Prevention. (1999, November 17). *Physical activity and health: A report of the Surgeon General.* Retrieved from http://www.cdc.gov/nccdphp/sgr/sgr.htm

7. Lee, C., Blair, S., & Jackson, A. (1999). Cardiorespiratory fitness, body composition, and all-cause and cardiovascular disease mortality in men. *American Journal of Clinical Nutrition, 69*(3), 373–380.

8. National Institutes of Health, National Institute of Diabetes and Digestive and Kidney Diseases. (2008, October). *Diabetes prevention program (DPP)* (NIH Publication No. 09-5099). Washington, DC: Government Printing Office.

9. Sigal, R., Kenny, G., Boulé, N., Wells, G., Prud'homme, D., Fortier, M., . . . Jaffey, J. (2007). Effects of aerobic training, resistance training, or both on glycemic control in type 2 diabetes. *American College of Physicians, 147*(6), 357–369.

10. Knowler, W., Barrett-Connor, E., Fowler, S., Hamman, R., Lachin, J., Walker, E., & Nathan, D. M. (2002). Reduction in the incidence of type 2 diabetes with lifestyle intervention or metformin. *New England Journal of Medicine, 346*(6), 393–403.

11. Slattery, M. L. (2004). Physical activity and colorectal cancer. *Sports Medicine, 34*, 239–252.

12. Clarke, C. A., Purdie, D. M., & Glaser, S. L. (2006). Population attributable risk of breast cancer in white women associated with immediately modifiable risk factors. *BMC Cancer, 6*,170.

13. Dallal, C., Sullivan-Halley, J., Ross, R., Wang, Y., Deapen, D., Horn-Ross, P., . . . Bernstein, L.. (2007). Long-term recreational physical activity and risk of invasive and in situ breast cancer: The California teachers study. *Archives of Internal Medicine, 167*(4), 408–415.

14. Nieman, D. C. (2000). Is infection risk linked to exercise workload? *Medicine & Science in Sports & Exercise,* 32(7 Suppl), S406–411.

15. Medline Plus. (2008). *Exercise and immunity.* Retrieved from http://www.nlm.nih.gov/medlineplus/ency/article/007165.htm

16. Ondrak, K., & Morgan, D. (2007). Physical activity, calcium intake and bone health in children and adolescents. *Sports Medicine, 37*(7), 587–600.

17. Johansson, M., Hassmén, P., & Jouper, J. (2008). Acute effects of qigong exercise on mood and anxiety. *International Journal of Stress Management, 15*(2), 199–207.

18. Blumenthal, J. A., Babyak, M. A., Doraiswamy, P. M., Watkins, L., Hoffman, B. M., Barbour, K. A., . . . & Sherwood, A.

(2007). Exercise and pharmacotherapy in the treatment of major depressive disorder. *Psychosomatic Medicine, 69,* 587–596.

19. Sui, X., Laditka, J. N., Church, T. S., Hardind, J. W., Chase, N., Davis, K., & Blaira, S. N. (2009). Prospective study of cardiorespiratory fitness and depressive symptoms in women and men. *Journal of Psychiatric Research, 43,*(5), 546–552.

20. Balkin, R., Tietjen-Smith, T., Caldwell, C., & Shen, Y. (2007). The utilization of exercise to decrease depressive symptoms in young adult women. *ADULTSPAN Journal, 6*(1), 30–35.

21. Åberg, M. A. I., Pedersen, N. L., Torén, K., Svartengren, M., Bäckstrand, B., Johnsson, T., . . . & Kuhn, H. G. (2009). Cardiovascular fitness is associated with cognition in young adulthood. *Proceedings of the National Academy of Sciences, 106,* 20906–20911.

22. Radak, Z. Hart, N., Sarga, L., Koltai, E., Atalay, M., Ohno, H., & Boldogh, I. (2010). Exercise plays a preventive role against Alzheimer's disease. *Journal of Alzheimer's Disease,* 10.3233/JAD-2010-091531.

23. Jespersen J. G., Nedergaard A., Andersen L. L., Schjerling P., & Andersen J. L. (2009). Myostatin expression during human muscle hypertrophy and subsequent atrophy: increased myostatin with detraining. *Scandinavian Journal of Medicine & Science in Sports.* Published online November 9, 2009.

24. American College of Sports Medicine. (2010). *ACSM's guidelines for exercise testing and prescription* (8th edition). Baltimore, MD: Wolters Kluwer/Lippincott Williams & Wilkins.

25. Centers for Disease Control and Prevention. (2009). *Physical activity for everyone: Target heart rate and estimated maximum heart rate.* Retrieved from http://www.cdc.gov/physicalactivity/everyone/measuring/heartrate.html

26. Smith, J. W. (2004). Flexibility basics: Physiology, research, and current guidelines. *ACSM's Certified News, 14*(3):7–9.

27. Centers for Disease Control and Prevention. (2008). *Physical activity guidelines for Americans.* Retrieved from http://www.health.gov/paguidelines/default.aspx

28. Ross, R., Dagnone, D., Jones, P. J. H., Smith, H., Paddags, A., Hudson, R., & Janssen, I. (2000). Reduction in obesity and related comorbid conditions after diet-induced weight loss or exercise-induced weight loss in men. *Annals of Internal Medicine, 133,* 92–103.

29. Centers for Disease Control and Prevention. (2008). *Physical activity guidelines for Americans: Be active your way: A guide for adults* (ODPHP Publication No. U0037). Retrieved from http://www.health.gov/paguidelines/adultguide/default.aspx

30. Judelson, D., Maresh, C., Anderson, J., Armstrong, L., Casa, D., Kraemer, W., . . . Volek, J. (2007). Hydration and muscular performance: Does fluid balance affect strength, power, and high-intensity endurance? *Sports Medicine, 37*(10), 907–921.

31. American College of Sports Medicine. (n.d.). Selecting and effectively using a health/fitness facility. Retrieved from http://www.acsm.org/AM/Template.cfm?Section=Brochures2&Template=/CM/ContentDisplay.cfm&ContentID=1534.

32. Hampton, Tracy. (2006). Researchers address use of performance-enhancing drugs in nonelite athletes. *Journal of the American Medical Association, 295*(6), 607.

33. U.S. House of Representatives, U.S. Government Accountability Office, Committee on Oversight and Government Reform. (2007). *Federal efforts to prevent and reduce anabolic steroid abuse among teenagers.* Washington, DC: Government Printing Office.

34. Frederick, D., Sadehgi-Azar, L., Haselton, M., Buchanan, G., Peplau, L., Berezovskaya, A., . . . Lipinski, R. (2007). Desiring the muscular ideal: Men's body satisfaction in the United States, Ukraine, and Ghana. *Psychology of Men and Masculinity, 8*(2), 103–117.

35. MedlinePlus. (n.d.). *Creatine.* Retrieved from http://www.nlm.nih.gov/medlineplus/druginfo/natural/patient-creatine.html

36. Liu, H., Bravata, D., Olkin, I., Friedlander, A., Liu, V., Roberts, B., . . . Hoffman, A. (2008). Systematic review: The effects of growth hormone on athletic performance. *Annals of Internal Medicine, 148*(10), 747–758.

37. National Center for Complementary and Alternative Medicine. (2009). *Consumer advisory: Ephedra.* Retrieved from http://nccam.nih.gov/news/alerts/ephedra/consumeradvisory.htm

38. Sabourin, S., & Irwin, J. (2008). Prevalence of sufficient physical activity among parents attending a university. *Journal of American College Health, 56*(6), 680–685.

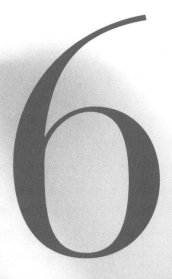

6

- An estimated 67% of Americans are overweight or obese.[i]

- Americans spend $30 billion a year on weight-loss programs and products.[ii]

- Obesity is associated with over 100,000 deaths in America each year.[iii]

- Weight gain among college students is most strongly correlated with increased alcohol consumption in men and with an increase in academic workload for women.[iv]

Weight Management

IDENTIFY health risks associated with excess weight.

DESCRIBE factors that contribute to overweight and obesity.

DISCUSS weight trends on campus, nationwide, and worldwide.

KNOW methods for assessing your weight and body fat.

COMPARE and contrast weight-management programs.

UNDERSTAND how to maintain a healthful weight.

DEFINE common eating disorders.

Health Online icons are found throughout the chapter, directing you to web links, videos, podcasts, and other useful online resources.

Excess body weight is one of our society's most pressing health concerns—so much so

that the Centers for Disease Control and Prevention has declared obesity a national epidemic. An estimated 67% of American adults over age 20 are **overweight** or **obese.**[1] Among children and teenagers, an estimated 19% of those aged 6 to 11 years and 17% of those aged 12 to 19 years are overweight.[1] The problem is also spreading globally: Between 2005 and 2015, the number of obese adults is estimated to grow from 400 million to 700 million worldwide, affecting those in both industrialized and developing nations.[2]

Why should you care? Combined with physical inactivity and poor nutrition, carrying excess weight increases your risk of many health problems, both now and later in life. Let's begin by taking a closer look at some of those risks.

The Health Risks of Excess Weight

Because overweight and obesity are common, it is easy to underestimate the health risks they pose. You could be tempted to think: How bad can a few extra pounds be, when so many people you know carry some? But just because weight concerns are common doesn't make them any less serious. Being overweight or obese is associated with many health problems, including:[3,4]

- **High blood pressure (hypertension).** High blood pressure is twice as common in obese adults because they have increased blood volume, higher heart rates, and blood vessels with a reduced capacity to transport blood.

- **Type 2 diabetes.** Excess fat makes your body resistant to insulin, a hormone that controls blood sugar (glucose) levels. If *insulin resistance* develops, blood sugar can become dangerously high and lead to a form of diabetes where insulin is produced but cells do not respond to it and don't take in glucose for energy production. More than 80% of people with diabetes are overweight or obese.

- **Abnormal levels of blood fats.** A diet high in fats and calories can lead to elevated blood levels of **low-density lipoprotein (LDL) cholesterol** ("bad" cholesterol). Obesity is also associated with low blood levels of **high-density lipoprotein (HDL) cholesterol** ("good" cholesterol) and high triglyceride levels. Triglycerides are the form in which most fat exists in food and in your body. Over time, abnormal levels of blood fats can contribute to *atherosclerosis*—a narrowing of the arteries. Atherosclerosis puts a person at risk for coronary heart disease and stroke. With increasing

overweight The condition of having a body weight that exceeds what is generally considered healthful for a particular height.

obese A weight disorder in which excess accumulations of nonessential body fat result in increased risk of health problems.

low-density lipoprotein (LDL) cholesterol Blood fats that can cause unhealthful deposits on the artery walls, resulting in increased heart disease risk.

high-density lipoprotein (HDL) cholesterol Blood fats that transport cholesterol out of arteries, reducing heart disease risk.

weight, there is a 9–18% increase in the prevalence of abnormal blood fats.[5]

- **Coronary heart disease (also called coronary artery disease).** This disease results from atherosclerosis in arteries that supply the heart. The narrowed arteries reduce the amount of blood that flows to the heart. Diminished blood flow to the heart can cause chest pain (angina). Complete blockage can lead to a heart attack.

- **Stroke.** Atherosclerosis occurs in arteries throughout the body, including those that feed the brain. If a blood clot forms in a narrowed artery leading to the brain, blood flow can be blocked, resulting in a stroke. Being obese raises your risk for having a stroke.

- **Metabolic syndrome.** This name is given to a group of obesity-related risk factors for cardiovascular disease and diabetes. A person has **metabolic syndrome** if he or she has three or more of the following risk factors:[6, 7]

  - *A large waistline.* This is a waist measurement of 40 inches or more for men and 35 inches or more for women.

  - *High triglycerides or taking medication to treat high triglycerides.* A triglyceride level of 150 mg/dL or higher is considered high.

  - *Low levels of HDL ("good") cholesterol or taking medication to treat low HDL.* Low HDL cholesterol is below 40 mg/dL for men and below 50 mg/dL for women.

  - *High blood pressure or taking medications to treat high blood pressure.* High blood pressure is 130 mmHg or higher for systolic blood pressure (top number) or 85 mmHg or higher for diastolic blood pressure (bottom number).

  - *High fasting blood glucose (sugar) or taking medication to treat high blood glucose.* This means a fasting blood glucose level of 100 mg/dL or higher.

  A person with metabolic syndrome has approximately twice the risk for coronary heart disease and five times the risk for type 2 diabetes.[6] An estimated 27% of American adults have metabolic syndrome.[8]

- **Cancer.** Being overweight may increase your risk for developing several types of cancer, including colon, rectal, esophageal, and kidney cancers. Excess weight is also linked to uterine and postmenopausal breast cancer in women and prostate cancer in men. Gaining weight during adult life increases the risk for several of these cancers, even if the weight gain does not result in overweight or obesity.

- **Osteoarthritis.** This joint disorder most often affects the knees, hips, and lower back. Excess weight places extra pressure on these joints and wears away the cartilage that protects them, resulting in joint pain and stiffness. For every 2-pound increase in weight, the risk for developing arthritis increases 9% to 13%.

- **Sleep apnea.** Sleep apnea causes a person to stop breathing for short periods during sleep. A person who has sleep apnea may suffer from daytime sleepiness, difficulty concentrating, and even heart failure. The risk for sleep apnea is higher for people who are overweight. A person who is overweight may have more fat stored around his or her neck, making the airway smaller, leading to breathing difficulty, loud snoring, or not breathing at all.

metabolic syndrome A group of obesity-related factors that increase the risk of cardiovascular disease and diabetes, including: large waistline, high triglycerides, low HDL cholesterol, high blood pressure, and high fasting blood glucose.

- **Gallbladder disease.** This disease includes inflammation or infection of the gallbladder and gallstones (solid clusters formed mostly of cholesterol). Overweight people may produce more cholesterol and/or may have an enlarged gallbladder that may not work properly. Abdominal pain, especially after consuming fatty foods, can result.

- **Fatty liver disease.** The level of stored fat often increases in the livers of overweight and obese people. When fat builds up in liver cells it can cause injury and inflammation leading to severe liver damage, cirrhosis (scar tissue that blocks proper blood flow to the liver), or even liver failure. Fatty liver disease is like alcoholic liver damage, but is not caused by alcohol and can occur in people who drink little or no alcohol.

- **Fertility problems.** Approximately 10% of women of child-bearing age experience polycystic ovary syndrome (PCOS), which is the number-one cause of female infertility. Many women with PCOS are overweight or obese.

- **Pregnancy complications.** Pregnant women who are overweight or obese raise their risk of pregnancy complications for both themselves and their child. These women are more likely to develop insulin resistance, high blood glucose, and high blood pressure. The risks associated with surgery, anesthesia, and blood loss also are increased in obese pregnant women.

Excess weight is also linked to physical discomfort, social and emotional troubles, and (in the case of obesity) lower overall life expectancy. A long-term study conducted by Oxford University found that life expectancy of severely obese individuals may be reduced by 3 to 10 years.[9] According to federal estimates, health problems caused by overweight and obesity are so pervasive, they cost our health-care systems about $117 billion each year.[10]

Figure 6.1 summarizes some of the major health risks associated with overweight and obesity.

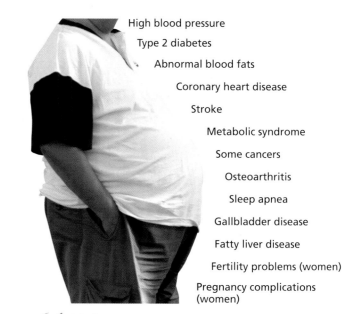

High blood pressure
Type 2 diabetes
Abnormal blood fats
Coronary heart disease
Stroke
Metabolic syndrome
Some cancers
Osteoarthritis
Sleep apnea
Gallbladder disease
Fatty liver disease
Fertility problems (women)
Pregnancy complications (women)

Figure 6.1 Major health risks associated with overweight and obesity.

Factors That Contribute to Weight Gain

Many of us watch the number on the bathroom scale rise or fall because of a simple concept: **energy balance.** The food and beverages you consume contain energy in the form of calories. Think of these calories as "energy in." Your body takes that energy and uses it to perform daily activities, from breathing and circulating your blood to studying and exercising. Think of these calorie-burning activities as "energy out." If, over time, the calories you consume match the calories you expend, then you are in energy balance and your weight will not change. If you take in fewer calories than you use, you'll lose weight. Take in more calories than you use, and you'll gain weight. It's a simple equation **(Figure 6.2).** While genes and hormones influence body weight, excess weight ultimately results from an imbalance of calories consumed and calories used.

Increased calorie consumption, physical inactivity, and environmental factors have all contributed to Americans' dramatic weight gain over recent years. We discuss each of these factors (along with less controllable factors like age, genes, gender, and differences in metabolism) in the next section.

Increased Calorie Consumption

Our diets tend to be full of calorie-dense foods high in fat (e.g., fast foods) and added sugars (e.g., soft drinks, candies, many breakfast cereals, and desserts). Large portion sizes and dining away from home also increase calorie intake. The average American ate 1,950 pounds of food in 2003, an increase from 1,675 pounds in 1970—which translates to an estimated increase of 523 calories per day.[11] Americans also consume more than the recommended servings of grains—and those grains we do eat are mostly highly processed items like pasta, tortillas, and bread rather than high-fiber whole grains. Consumption of added fats, oils, and sugar has also increased over the years.[12]

Servings of fast foods and soft drinks often are two to five times larger than when they were introduced.[12] For example, in 1954 Burger King's hamburger was 2.8 ounces and 202 calories. In 2004 it had grown to 4.3 ounces and 310 calories.[12] A serving of McDonald's French fries weighed 2.4 ounces and contained 210 calories in 1955. By 2004 the fries had reached 7 ounces and 610 calories.[12] Bottled Coca-Cola contained 6.5 fluid ounces and 79 calories in 1916. By 2004 the standard container size for the beverage reached 16 fluid ounces and 194 calories.[12] While large portions may appeal to our lifestyles, tastes, and wallets, they contribute to excess weight and can harm our health.

energy balance The state achieved when energy consumed from food is equal to energy expended, maintaining body weight.

Lack of Physical Activity

Fewer than one in three Americans get the recommended minimum of 30 minutes of moderate activity a day, most days of the week. In fact, one-fourth of Americans do not get any exercise at all.[13] *Healthy People 2010* data indicate that 70% of 12-year-olds engage in regular vigorous activity, but by the time they turn 21 only 35% do.[14]

Take the Portion Distortion Quiz to see how increasing portion sizes piles on the calories at http://hp2010.nhlbihin.net/portion.

Many people work at jobs that require sitting in front of a computer rather than actively moving and using their muscles. In 1860, the average work week was 70 hours of heavy physical labor compared to 40 hours of sedentary work today. The least physically active groups are older adolescents and adults over 60 years old who spend about 60% of their waking time in sedentary pursuits.[15] According to the Nielsen Company's "Three Screen Report" (measuring television, computer, and cell phone usage), during the first three months of 2009, Americans watched a record 153 hours per month of television, viewing over 2 hours more TV per month than in

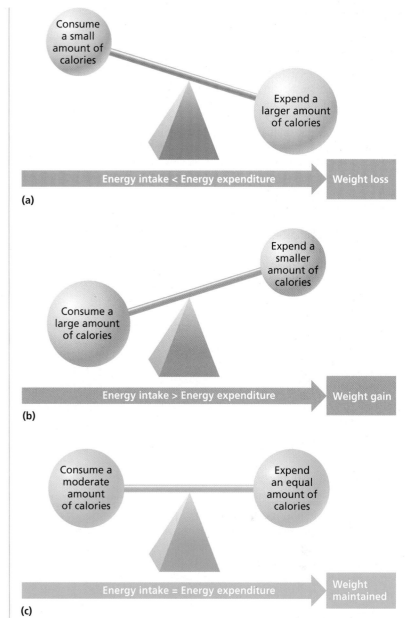

Figure 6.2 Energy balance. Energy balance is attained when the calories you consume equal the calories you expend.

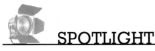

Michael Phelps's 12,000-calorie Diet

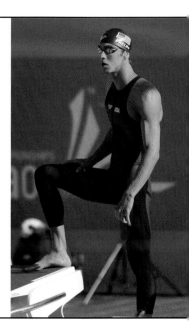

At the height of his training, Olympic swimmer Michael Phelps consumed a 12,000-calorie-per-day diet, at least four to five times the recommended calorie intake for males his age. His breakfast consisted of three fried-egg sandwiches with cheese, lettuce, tomatoes, fried onions, and mayonnaise, one five-egg omelet, one bowl of grits, three slices of French toast topped with powdered sugar, and three chocolate-chip pancakes with syrup. His other meals were just as huge, and he consumed multiple energy drinks as well. And yet, the 14-time Gold-medal winner didn't gain weight!

How did Phelps manage to eat so much and retain his athletic build? The secret is energy balance. Phelps expended so much energy during daily training sessions that all the excess calories went toward powering his laps, rather than being stored in his body as fat. In other words, he was using all the energy he was taking in, so he didn't gain weight. If Phelps hadn't eaten as much as he did, he would not have had the energy to train so intensely, and would not be the world-famous athlete he is today.

But don't count on consuming a diet like Phelps's just because you spend an extra hour at the gym. Use an online activity tracker, like the one at www.mypyramidtracker.gov, to assess how many calories you're expending on exercise and adjust your diet accordingly.

---

the previous year.[16] Americans also spent 27 hours per month on the Internet.[16]

Coupled with the fact that Americans spend more than 100 hours a year commuting to work, little time is left in the day for physical activity.[17] With less physical activity, muscle mass decreases and body fat takes its place.

Differences in Basic Energy Needs

Why can one person consume calories day after day and not gain a pound, while another person consuming a similar number of calories constantly struggles to control his or her weight? This occurs because many factors (aside from physical activity) affect a person's basic energy needs, including age, body size, body shape, body composition, gender, and a person's ability to generate heat (called *thermogenesis*).

About two-thirds of the energy a person uses each day goes toward *basal metabolism*—that is, the body's maintenance of basic physiological processes (like keeping vital organs functioning) when at complete digestive, physical, and emotional rest. The remainder of energy a person uses is for food digestion and absorption, adjusting to environmental changes such as temperature, trauma, and stress, and participating in physical activity.

The rate at which basal metabolism occurs is called **basal metabolic rate (BMR).** A similar measure of energy output, called *resting metabolic rate* (RMR), is measured when a person is awake and resting quietly. BMR and RMR may vary greatly from person to person and may vary for the same person with a change in circumstance or physical condition. In general, BMR and RMR are highest in people who are growing (children, adolescents, pregnant women), are tall (greater surface area = more heat loss = more calories burned), and in those with greater muscle mass (physically fit people and males).

basal metabolic rate (BMR) The rate at which the body expends energy for only the basic functioning of vital organs.

These people generally use more energy per day than their shorter, more softly rounded counterparts.

Regular physical activity can increase muscle mass, which increases BMR. If you increase your physical activity from light to moderate or heavy, you will reap the benefit of not only burning calories through exercise but also increasing your BMR; together those things can contribute greatly to weight loss.

Age

As people age, they tend to become less active. Also, muscle mass tends to decrease with age. Lower muscle mass leads to a decrease in basal metabolism, which in turn reduces calorie needs. BMR declines about 2% for each decade.[18] If you do not decrease your calorie intake as you age, you will likely gain weight.

Genetic Factors

Overweight and obesity tend to run in families. If one or both of your parents are overweight or obese, your chances of being overweight increase. To be sure, some of this influence may be due more to habits than genes. Families tend to share eating and exercise patterns (whether the patterns are healthful or unhealthful). However, studies have shown that genes, too, can affect the tendency to gain weight, how much fat a person stores, and where he or she carries excess weight. Scientists are also studying specific genes, such as a certain variation of a gene that is related to fat mass and obesity, known as FTO. FTO appears to increase a person's risk of obesity by 30% to 70%, depending on a specific variety of FTO and how many copies of that obesity-linked variation a person carries.[19]

Gender Differences

Men and women each have unique factors that contribute to weight gain. Men, for example, may be more prone to choosing high-calorie diets due to gender-related habits and social expectations. "Real men," according to the stereotype, eat ribs, not salad. In one study of college students, male students were less interested in making careful food choices and less inclined to scrutinize food labels. Some male students in the survey said more healthful eating was a female concern, not something men would focus on.[20]

Women, on the other hand, have health considerations that increase their risk of excess weight. Up to about age 10, energy needs for girls and boys are similar; then puberty triggers a change. When boys begin to develop more muscle, they need more calories. Their added height and size demand more energy too.[18] In contrast, women naturally keep body fat stores in reserve for pregnancy and breast-feeding. Because body fat burns less energy than muscle, fewer calories are needed to maintain body weight, and BMR goes down. In addition, pregnancy leads to necessary weight gain, and many women find that the extra pounds are difficult to lose afterward.

Environmental Factors

While our society likes to talk about weight loss, many factors in our lives encourage behaviors that run counter to healthful weight management:

- Many neighborhoods lack sidewalks, resulting in more driving and less walking. Protected bike routes are rare in many communities.
- Long work and school days, combined with commuting, leave many people little time for being physically active. One study of college students found that those with a drive time of 16 minutes or more were 64% more likely to be overweight or obese.[22]
- Most of us are stressed, and reach for food as comfort. One study found that the stresses of everyday life often trigger the urge to eat, with many people favoring less healthful food options.[22]
- Many of us also have little time to cook, turning instead to restaurants, where "super size" portions offer far more calories than we need.
- The fast food so many of us reach for could be more aptly named "fat food." Most popular fast-food choices are stuffed with calories and fat.[23]
- The food-related advertising that surrounds us usually focuses on high-calorie foods. You see a lot more ads for potato chips than you do for oranges or apples.
- In some neighborhoods, supermarkets are scarce, leaving residents to rely on smaller stores that rarely carry more healthful choices such as fresh fruits and vegetables.

Add all this up, and the recipe for our current epidemic of overweight and obesity becomes clear. We are surrounded by forces that undermine healthful weight management.

Psychological Factors

Researchers remain uncertain if there is a relationship between excess weight and psychological disorders like depression. There is no scientific evidence that overweight or obese people are any more or less likely to suffer from psychological disorders than people with a healthful weight. However, if you use food as a reward or to cope with negative emotions, you learn to eat for reasons other than satisfying hunger, making overeating and weight gain more likely.

Weight Trends: On Campus, Nationwide, and Worldwide

When you started college, you likely heard warnings about gaining 15 pounds your first year. Most students, it turns out, don't bulk up quite that much so quickly. But avoiding early weight gain and the lifestyle choices that lead to being overweight remains a challenge for many college students.

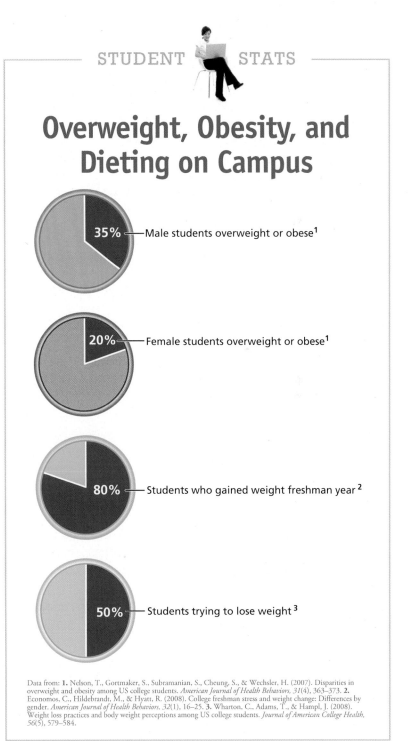

STUDENT STATS

Overweight, Obesity, and Dieting on Campus

35% — Male students overweight or obese[1]

20% — Female students overweight or obese[1]

80% — Students who gained weight freshman year[2]

50% — Students trying to lose weight[3]

Data from: **1.** Nelson, T., Gortmaker, S., Subramanian, S., Cheung, S., & Wechsler, H. (2007). Disparities in overweight and obesity among US college students. *American Journal of Health Behaviors, 31*(4), 363–373. **2.** Economos, C., Hildebrandt, M., & Hyatt, R. (2008). College freshman stress and weight change: Differences by gender. *American Journal of Health Behaviors, 32*(1), 16–25. **3.** Wharton, C., Adams, T., & Hampl, J. (2008). Weight loss practices and body weight perceptions among US college students. *Journal of American College Health, 56*(5), 579–584.

Weight Trends on Campus

Most first-year students do gain some weight once they start college—usually about 7 to 8 pounds.[24] More importantly, this weight often doesn't disappear once the first year is over. Instead, many students gain a few more pounds every year of college. One study found that 23% of students were classified as overweight their first year, and that number grew to about 28% by their fourth year.[25] Male students experienced weight gain more often—about 35% of them qualified as overweight, compared to about 20% of female students. In another survey, about 50% of college students said they were trying to lose weight.[26]

What's the big culprit behind campus weight gain? While excess calories clearly contribute, a decline in physical activity also appears to be a major factor. Female students, for example, often find that their level of physical activity drops substantially in college.[27, 28] For all students, larger amounts of time spent watching television and smaller amounts of physical activity have been closely linked with excess weight.[25]

The problem is compounded by the fact that more students are starting college at heavier weights than ever before. About 17% of American adolescents between the ages of 12 and 19 are overweight, compared to 5% in 1970.[29] Another 17% carry enough extra pounds to put them at serious risk of becoming overweight.[29] For many, these problems start during early childhood, with about 14% of children between the ages of 2 and 5 qualifying as overweight.[29] As the number of overweight children climbs, so do cases of childhood diabetes and high blood pressure, conditions once largely limited to adults. Overweight children are far more likely to carry extra pounds into adulthood.[30]

Weight Trends in the United States

With less than one-third of U.S. adults at a healthful weight, the problem touches every corner of the country. A look at adult weight statistics state by state shows the spread of the obesity epidemic over the last two decades **(Figure 6.3).**[31]

- In 1990, no state taking part in a federal weight-tracking project had an obesity rate of 15% or more. In 10 states, less than 10% of the population qualified as obese.

- By 1998, 40 states had an obesity rate of 15% or more, with 7 showing an obesity rate of 20% or more. No state had an obesity rate of less than 10%.

- By 2008, every single state had an obesity rate of at least 15% or more. Only one state had an obesity rate of less than 20%. Six states had an obesity rate of 30% or more.

If this pattern continues, researchers predict that 75% of U.S. adults will be overweight by 2015, with about 40% of those qualifying as obese.[32]

Global Obesity

Weight concerns are hardly confined to the United States. Globalization has spread Western eating and lifestyle habits—especially an affinity for high-fat, high-sugar foods and a decline in physical activity—worldwide. International health experts are now tackling overweight and obesity as global problems **(Figure 6.4).**

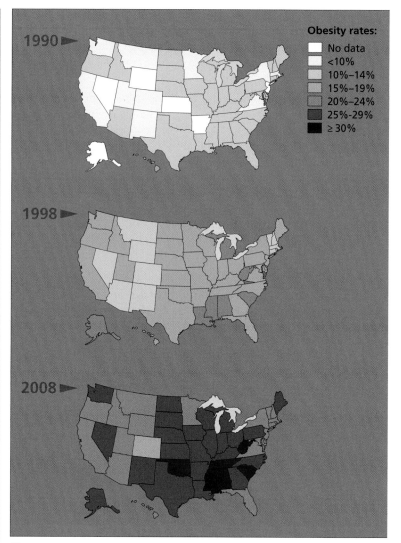

Figure 6.3 Obesity is increasing in the Unites States

Data from: **1.** Mokdad, A. H. et al. (1999). The spread of the obesity epidemic in the United States, 1991-1998. *Journal of the American Medical Association 282*(16), 1519-1522. **2.** Mokdad, A. H. et al. (2001). The continuing epidemic of obesity and diabetes in the United States. *Journal of the American Medical Association 286*(10), 1195-2000. Graphics from the Centers for Disease Control and Prevention, U.S. Obesity Trends 1985 to 2008.

According to the World Health Organization, there are more than 1 billion overweight adults globally, and at least 400 million of them are obese. Obesity rates have grown three-fold since 1980 in parts of Europe, the Middle East, the Pacific Islands, Australia, New Zealand, and China.[2]

As in the United States, an increase in serious diseases is following this rise in weight. Countries such India and China, which once had relatively low rates of heart disease and diabetes, are already seeing significant increases in these conditions. By 2020, international health experts predict that chronic conditions such as heart disease will account for more than 70% of deaths worldwide. Already, the impact of heart disease in India and China is greater than in all Western nations combined.[33] In an especially cruel twist, problems of weight and malnutrition often co-exist in some developing countries, with richer residents seeing rapid weight gains even as some of their fellow citizens suffer from a lack of adequate nutrition.

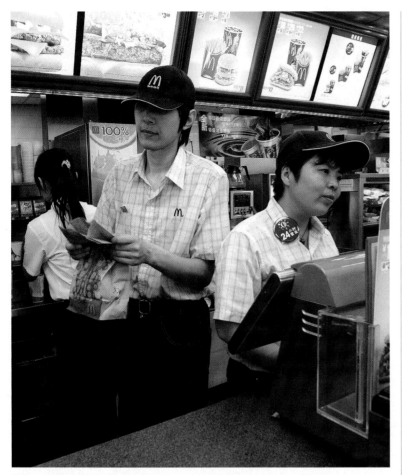

Figure 6.4 Global overweight and obesity. As developing countries adopt more Westernized diets, their rates of overweight and obesity are increasing.

Are You at a Healthful Weight?

To assess whether you are at a healthful weight, consider the following questions:

- **What is a healthful *range* of weight for you?** There is no one ideal weight that is right for all of us. Identifying a healthful range of weight is a much more practical approach. The following section will discuss several methods for determining the range of weight that's most healthful for you.

- **What's your body composition?** Your *body composition,* or the percentage of fat compared to muscle and other tissues, matters more than the number on your bathroom scale. Although it varies with age, healthful amounts of total body fat range from 8% to 24% for adult men; adult women should have a body fat range between 21% and 35%.[34]

- **How old are you?** Most of us gain weight as we age. It's not realistic to expect that you will always weigh as much as you did in high school.

- **How does gender factor in?** As we discussed on pages 120–121, men and women tend to gain and store weight in different ways.

- **What's your body type?** Some of us are naturally petite. Some of us are more stocky. Aim to look and feel like a healthy version of yourself, not someone else.

> *There is no one ideal weight that is right for all of us. Identifying a healthful range of weight is a much more practical approach.*

Methods for Assessing Healthful Weight and Body Composition

Several different methods can help you assess whether your current weight falls within a healthful range.

Body Mass Index (BMI)

Body mass index, or **BMI,** is one of the most common methods for assessing weight, as well as for defining *overweight* and *obese.* A ratio between your height and your weight, BMI is often used to predict risk factors for health problems later in life. To determine your own BMI, see **Figure 6.5** and the **Self-Assessment** on page 126.

A BMI between 18.5 and 24.9 indicates a **healthful weight.** If your BMI falls below 18.5, you are considered **underweight.** A BMI of 25–29.9 indicates **overweight,** and a BMI of 30 or above is defined as **obese.** Generally, people with a BMI between 18.5 and 24.9 have few weight-related health risks. Risks increase as BMI falls below or rises above this range, indicating that both underweight and overweight can impair health.[30]

BMI is not a reliable indicator for everyone. Athletes with large amounts of lean muscle mass may have BMIs that classify them as overweight, even though they are at a healthful weight for their build. BMI also sometimes underestimates total body fat in older people who have lost muscle. In addition, one recent study has found that measurements such as BMI are not always reliable indicators of health for young adults.[35] Thus, BMI should not be used as the sole indicator of weight-related health.

Waist Circumference and Waist-to-Hip Ratio

Other measurements used to predict weight-related health problems include *waist circumference* and *waist-to-hip ratio.* Waist circumference is an indicator of how much body fat you carry. If you carry fat mainly around your waist, you are more likely to

body mass index (BMI) A numerical measurement, calculated from height and weight measurements, that provides an indicator of health risk categories.

healthful weight The weight at which health risks are lowest for an individual; usually a weight that will result in a BMI between 18.5 and 24.9.

underweight A weight resulting in a BMI below 18.5.

overweight A weight resulting in a BMI of 25–29.9.

obese A weight resulting in a BMI of 30 or above.

	Underweight		Healthful weight							Overweight					Obese						Extreme obesity			
BMI	17	18	18.5	19	20	21	22	23	24	25	26	27	28	29	30	31	32	33	34	35	36	37	39	≥40
Height										**Weight in pounds**														
4'10"	81	86	89	91	96	100	105	110	115	119	124	129	134	138	143	148	153	158	162	167	172	177	186	191
4'11"	84	89	92	94	99	104	109	114	119	124	128	133	138	143	148	153	158	163	168	173	178	183	193	198
5'	87	92	95	97	102	107	112	118	123	128	133	138	143	148	153	158	163	158	174	179	184	189	199	204
5'1"	90	95	98	100	106	111	116	122	127	132	137	143	148	153	158	164	169	174	180	185	190	195	206	211
5'2"	93	98	101	104	109	115	120	126	131	136	142	147	153	158	164	169	175	180	186	191	196	202	213	218
5'3"	96	102	104	107	113	118	124	130	135	141	146	152	158	163	169	175	180	186	191	197	203	208	220	225
5'4"	99	105	108	110	116	122	128	134	140	145	151	157	163	169	174	180	186	192	197	204	209	215	227	232
5'5"	102	108	111	114	120	126	132	138	144	150	156	162	168	174	180	186	192	198	204	210	216	222	234	240
5'6"	105	112	115	118	124	130	136	142	148	155	161	167	173	179	186	192	198	204	210	216	223	229	241	247
5'7"	109	115	118	121	127	134	140	146	153	159	166	172	178	185	191	198	204	211	217	223	230	236	249	255
5'8"	112	118	122	125	131	138	144	151	158	164	171	177	184	190	197	203	210	216	223	230	236	243	256	262
5'9"	115	122	125	128	135	142	149	155	162	169	176	182	189	196	203	209	216	223	230	236	243	250	263	270
5'10"	119	126	129	132	139	146	153	160	167	174	181	188	195	202	209	216	222	229	236	243	250	257	271	278
5'11"	122	129	133	136	143	150	157	165	172	179	186	193	200	208	215	222	229	236	243	250	257	265	279	286
6'	125	133	136	140	147	154	162	169	177	184	191	199	206	213	221	228	235	242	250	258	265	272	287	294
6'1"	129	137	140	144	151	159	166	174	182	189	197	204	212	219	227	235	242	250	257	265	272	280	295	302
6'2"	132	140	144	148	155	163	171	179	186	194	202	210	218	225	233	241	249	256	264	272	280	287	303	311
6'3"	136	144	148	152	160	168	176	184	193	200	208	216	224	232	240	248	256	264	272	279	287	295	311	319
6'4"	140	148	152	156	164	172	180	189	197	205	213	221	230	238	246	254	263	271	279	287	295	304	320	328

Figure 6.5 Body mass index (BMI). BMI is often used to predict risk factors for health problems later in life. To determine your BMI, find your height and then scan across to find your weight. Then, scan up to find your BMI.

Source: From the National Heart, Lung, and Book Institute. http://www.nhlbi.nih.gov.

develop health problems than if you carry fat mainly in your hips and thighs. This is true even if your BMI falls within the normal range. To find out how to accurately measure your own waist, see the **Self-Assessment** on page 126. In general, a waist measuring more than 35 inches in a woman or 40 inches in a man points to greater health risks. As waist circumference increases, disease risks increase.

Waist-to-hip ratio, determined by dividing your waist circumference by your hip circumference, also can be used to predict health risks. To find out how to measure and assess your waist-to-hip ratio, see the **Self-Assessment** on page 126.

Health care professionals commonly use BMI and waist circumference measures because they are easy and inexpensive to perform. Together, these measures can be valuable in assessing a person's health risks and monitoring changes over time.[36]

Body Composition Measurements

There are a variety of ways to estimate your percent body fat using body composition measurements. Each method for measuring body composition varies in its accuracy, its cost, and its availability to the public **(Table 6.1).**

How Can You Reach a Healthful Weight?

For most people, the key to healthful weight loss lies in the ability to control "energy in" and "energy out." If you want your body to use and reduce its fat stores, you need to make sure less energy is coming in and more energy is going out. This requires consistent work.

Table 6.1: **Body Composition Analysis Methods**

Method	Procedure	Cost and Availability	Accuracy
Skinfold Measurements	The technician uses specialized calipers to pinch and measure a fold of skin and its underlying layer of fat, and repeats this process at several locations on the body.	Skinfold caliper tests are commonly available at schools, colleges, and YMCAs for free or at minimal cost.	If test is performed correctly, there is a +/−3% margin of error. The test is not ideal for those who are obese or very lean. Technical errors administering the test are common.
Underwater (Hydrostatic) Weighing	A person is first weighed while dry and then submerged in water and weighed again. Because fat has a lower density than water, it floats and reduces the weight of the person while submerged. The difference between the "dry" weight and the "wet" weight is an indicator of how much body fat the person has.	Requires specialized equipment and a trained technician Available at research institutions and colleges or universities. Test typically costs $50–$75 per assessment.	If test is performed correctly, there is a +/−1.5% margin of error.
Bod Pod®	Using a similar technique to underwater weighing, the Bod Pod® uses air instead of water. The person being measured sits in the Bod Pod chamber wearing a bathing suit, and computerized pressure sensors determine how much air has been displaced by the body.	Available only at research laboratories, professional athletic facilities, and colleges and universities. Test typically costs $40–$65 per assessment.	If test is performed correctly, there is a +/−3% margin of error. Participant must remain still and breath normally while inside the pod.
Bioelectrical Impedance Analysis (BIA)	Measures the opposition to the flow (impedance) of a very low level of electrical current through body tissues. A current will flow more slowly (be more impeded) through fat than through other body tissues. The current is passed through electrodes, measurements are recorded, and a computer calculates how lean you are from the measurement data.	Available at schools, colleges, universities, and health/fitness clubs. BIA machines can cost $100–$400 for home use. A BIA test at a school or club may be free or cost up to $30 per assessment.	If test is performed correctly, the margin of error is +/−3%. Participant must refrain from eating, drinking, or exercising in the hours prior to the test.

Data from Georgia State University (2009). The exercise and physical fitness page: Body composition, retrieved from http://www2.gsu.edu/~wwwfit/bodycomp.html.

Losing weight doesn't have to mean depriving yourself. But it does mean eating wisely and changing your lifestyle to be as physically active as possible.

Modify Your Eating Habits

You can reduce calories and eat more healthfully by following these basic guidelines.

- **Track your food intake.** Use an online tracker like the one found at www.mypyramidtracker.gov to calculate the calories you are consuming and compare them with your MyPyramid calorie intake recommendations.

- **Practice portion control. Portion control** is modifying the amount of food on your plate based on your desired servings and calorie intake level. Try gauging the higher-calorie foods you tend to choose (such as red meats, fats, and sweets), cutting their portion sizes in half, and replacing the rest with lower-calorie options **(Figure 6.6)**.

- **Drink water instead of sugary drinks filled with calories.** Approximately 20% of our total calorie consumption comes from what we drink.[37] Juices, "vitamin waters," soft drinks, and energy drinks are all extra sources of calories.

- **Use artificial sweeteners in moderation.** Artificial sweeteners are low- or no-calorie sugar substitutes. Artificial sweeteners containing aspartame (for example, Equal and Nutrasweet) have been studied extensively and

portion control A method of reducing overconsumption of calories by limiting serving sizes of food.

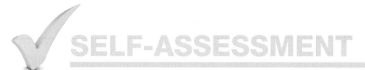

SELF-ASSESSMENT

You can skip the math and use these online calculators: www.nhlbisupport .com/bmi/ and www.healthcalculators.org/calculators/waist_hip.asp.

Assessing Your Weight-Related Health Risks

To assess your health risks related to weight, use these three key measures: BMI, waist circumference, and waist-to-hip ratio.

DETERMINE YOUR BMI

The formula for computing BMI is (your weight in pounds $\times$ 703)/your height (in)^2.

Classification of Overweight and Obesity by BMI

	BMI	Obesity Class
Underweight	<18.5	
Normal	18.5–24.9	
Overweight	25.0–29.9	
Obesity	30.0–34.9	I
	35.0–39.9	II
Extreme Obesity	≥40.0	III

MEASURE YOUR WAIST CIRCUMFERENCE

1. Place a tape measure around your bare abdomen, just above your hip bones (see photo).
2. Be sure that the tape is snug, but not pushing into your skin.
3. Breathe out, and measure the girth of your abdomen.

CALCULATE YOUR WAIST-TO-HIP RATIO

1. Measure your waist as described.
2. Use the same technique to measure your hips at the widest part.
3. Divide your waist measurement by your hip measurement.

Waist-to-Hip Ratio and Associated Health Risk Levels

Classification	Men	Women
Lower Risk	<0.90	<0.80
Moderately High Risk	0.90–1.0	0.80–0.85
High Risk	>1.0	>0.85

HOW TO INTERPRET YOUR SCORE

- BMI: Calculate your BMI and check it against the BMI table. Underweight, overweight, obesity, and extreme obesity are all associated with increased health risks.
- Waist circumference: A waist measuring more than 35 inches in a woman or 40 inches in a man points to greater health risks.
- Waist-to-hip ratio: Calculate your waist-to-hip ratio and check it against the Waist-to-Hip Ratio table. This ratio is an indicator of where you carry your excess fat; a higher ratio can mean you carry excess fat in your abdomen, a lower ratio indicates you carry more fat in your lower body.

---

have been found to be safe in moderation.[38] However, people with phenylketonuria (PKU) should avoid aspartame because it contains phenylalanine, which their bodies cannot process.

- **Eat whole foods as close to their natural state as possible.** Highly processed foods are more likely to contain extra fats, sugars, and calories. If you reach for an apple instead of a cup of processed applesauce, for example, you will avoid any sugar or calories that might have been added during the manufacturing process. You will also be consuming more fiber, which helps you feel full longer.

- **Don't rely on "diet" foods.** Food products billed as low-fat may be high in sugar or calories. "Reduced-fat" food may still be relatively high in overall calories.

- **Choose healthful fats and carbohydrates.** Healthful fats are generally from plant sources such as nuts, avocados, olives, and canola and peanut oils. Omega-3 fatty acids found in salmon and other fish are also good sources of fat. Healthful carbohydrates, such as those found in fruits, vegetables, and whole grains, provide vital nutrients, and help you feel full.

- **Change one habit at a time.** Instead of trying to overhaul all of your eating habits at once, choose one meal or snack and make small changes little by little. At lunch, for example, opt for fruit instead of dessert. Give that new habit some time to "stick" before trying another change.

Get Physically Active

Physical activity does more than burn off calories and reduce body fat. Exercise appears to help reduce feelings of hunger.[39] It also

---

STUDENT STORY

Losing Weight

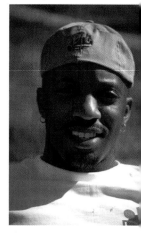

"Hi, I'm John. In high school, I was on the track and field team. My coach used to say 'eat as much as you run'—which was a lot. I ran nearly ten miles a day and also ate ten miles worth of calories. I was in great shape. Now that I'm in college, I still have the same appetite, but I don't run anymore. My schedule is packed. I'm in classes all morning and have a part-time job in the afternoon. I have a small break between my job and my night class, which is four days a week. There's never enough time to cook, so I usually pick up dinner on the run—lots of burgers and smoothies. I'm 5 feet 8 inches and I have gone from 150 pounds to 180 pounds in one year. Is this really such a big deal? I mean, I'm young, right?"

1: How has John's energy balance changed since he started college?

2: What are some of the increased health risks John faces if he does not take steps to control his weight gain?

3: What is John's BMI?

4: What advice would you give John to help him lose his extra weight?

Do you have a story similar to John's? Share your story at **www.pearsonhighered.com/choosinghealth.**

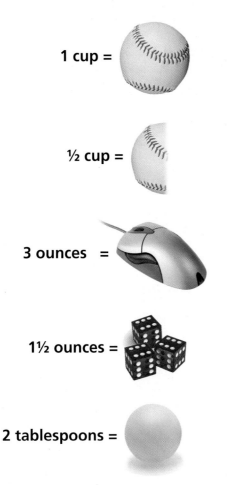

1 cup =

½ cup =

3 ounces =

1½ ounces =

2 tablespoons =

Figure 6.6 Estimating portion sizes. You can use common household items to estimate the portion sizes of your food.

builds muscle, which burns more calories than other types of tissue. Choose an activity you enjoy, whether it is dancing, skateboarding, or playing a favorite sport. If you make exercise fun, weight loss will be more enjoyable!

Keep in mind the basic exercise guidelines we discussed in Chapter 5. If you are trying to maintain weight loss or lose weight, aim for 60–90 minutes each day. At least two to three times a week, try to make sure some of that exercise focuses on building muscle. If you have time for nothing else, try to build a little more walking into your routine each day. It can make a significant difference over the long term.

Seek Support

Because weight is so closely tied to body image and self-esteem, losing weight involves emotional and psychological changes as well as physical ones. These factors can make it difficult to lose weight on your own. Reach out to friends and family. You might decide to follow a weight-loss plan with someone else, and encourage each other along the way. You also can find ideas and support online.

> There are lots of free programs that can track your diet and physical activity, such as www.mypyramidtracker.gov, www.sparkpeople.com, www. tweetyourhealth.com, and www.fitday.com.

If you'd like more formal weight-loss assistance, consider joining a support group. Commercial groups such as Weight Watchers focus on group meetings as part of their program. For those who feel like they have little control over their eating, non-profit groups such as Overeaters Anonymous provide supportive, nonjudgmental help in understanding and rethinking emotional responses to food.

> MyPyramid.gov offers multiple audio and video podcasts that provide healthful eating, activity, and snacking tips at www.mypyramid.gov/audiopoddcasts/index .html and www.mypyramid.gov/podcasts/ index.html.

hunger The physiological sensation caused by the lack of food.

appetite The psychological response to the sight, smell, thought, or taste of food that prompts or postpones eating.

satiety Physical fullness; the state in which there is no longer the desire to eat.

Can Dieting Work?

Hunger is the physiological sensation caused by a lack of food. Hunger is triggered in our brains, as a response to signals sent by the digestive tract and hormones circulating in our blood. Hunger is different from **appetite,** the psychological response to the sight, smell, thought, or taste of food that prompts or postpones eating. Appetite can prove helpful, stimulating you to eat before you get too hungry. It can also prove harmful, steering you toward too much food or toward tempting but unhealthful food choices. When we've eaten and relieved or prevented hunger, a feeling called **satiety** helps turn off the desire to eat more.

Given that both hunger and appetite compel us to eat, can dieting work? Weight-loss diets can be helpful for some people, especially those who like the support of a structured plan or program. However, dieting is a slow, steady process. You can't achieve healthful or permanent weight loss by starving yourself for a week. Diets also work best if they are accompanied by regular exercise. To keep the weight off, successful dieters must work to make their new eating and exercise habits into a way of life that they can sustain long term.

Millions of Americans participate in organized weight-loss programs each year, especially now that many are offered online. **Table 6.2** summarizes some of these popular weight-loss plans.

In a year-long study that compared four popular diets—Atkins, Ornish, The Zone, and Weight Watchers—roughly half the participants lost an average of 7 pounds and improved some of their health indicators, such as heart disease risk.[40] But in a pattern familiar to many dieters, the other half of the study's participants dropped out.

Three common dieting approaches are low-calorie diets, low-fat diets, and low-carbohydrate diets.

Low-Calorie Diets

One of the most popular dieting programs, Weight Watchers, builds its food guidelines around calorie reduction. Cutting 500 to 1,000 calories a day typically leads to a loss of 1 or 2 pounds a week. **Figure 6.7** shows a healthful way to reduce the calories in a daily diet.

But a low-calorie diet is rarely a simple matter of food math. Without a healthful eating plan in

Table 6.2: **Popular Diets**

Name	Description	Foods to Eat	Foods to Avoid	Practicality	Analysis
Atkins Diet	Claims that eating too many carbohydrates causes obesity and other health problems. Emphasizes the consumption of protein and fat over carbohydrates.	Meat, fish, poultry, eggs, cheese, low-carb vegetables, butter, oil	Carbohydrates, specifically bread, pasta, most fruits and vegetables, milk, alcohol	Difficult to eat in restaurants because only plain protein sources and limited vegetables or salads are allowed. Difficult to maintain long-term because of limited food choices.	The composition of a sample menu is 8% carbohydrate, 56% fat, and 35% protein. Initial weight loss is mostly water. Does not promote a positive attitude toward food groups. Eliminates virtually all carbohydrate foods. May encourage overly high-fat diets.
Eat Right for Your Type	Claims that blood type is the key to your immune system, which determines your diet and supplementation.	Varies based on blood type.	Varies based on blood type.	Promotes some foods, such as dairy and wheat, even if individuals experience intolerances for those foods, potentially leading to gastrointestinal discomfort and other health problems.	This diet has no scientific basis. People may use this diet to attempt to fight cancer, asthma, infections, diabetes, arthritis, hypertension, and infertility, but there is no evidence that it is effective.
Jenny Craig	This program's philosophy for successful weight loss is: (1) a healthful relationship with food, (2) an active lifestyle, and (3) a balanced approach to living. Dieters are required to have a 15-minute personal consultation weekly with Jenny Craig "counselors" (who lack formal nutrition/behavior training). A variety of online support tools are also available to strengthen dieters' motivation.	Promotes Jenny Craig–brand packaged meals, snacks, and supplements. Fruits, vegetables, and nonfat dairy foods are limited per Jenny Craig's 28-day menu planner. Vegetarian choices are available.	"Homemade" meals, commercial items (except those carrying the Jenny Craig label), sweets, and other foods that are not listed on Jenny Craig's 28-day menu planner	Eating packaged meals long-term may be difficult and not realistic.	The targeted composition of the 1,200 to 1,500-calorie menus is 60% carbohydrate, 20% fat, and 20% protein. Packaged meals are not conducive for teaching dieters how to shop, cook, and eat their own healthful, calorie-controlled meals. After completing the program, dieters who resume their usual eating habits are likely to regain weight. The cost of purchasing required ready-made meals can be expensive for some dieters.
Slim-Fast	This program promotes Slim-Fast products as staples of breakfast and noon meals; evening meal is 500 calories and nutritionally balanced. Portion control, avoidance of sugary and fatty foods, and frequent water consumption are encouraged. Dieters are expected to track food intake, physical activity, and weight changes via online Slim-Fast tools.	Promotes 3–5 servings of fruits and vegetables daily. Promotes Slim-Fast products, vegetables, fruits, whole grains, salad, lean proteins, low-fat cheese, water, and other non-calorie beverages. Snacks of 120 calories or fewer are allowed.	Regular candy, cookies, and other sweets, fried or other high-fat foods, some dairy products and snack items	Buying meal replacement products for breakfast and lunch becomes expensive over time.	The targeted composition of the 1,200 to 1,800-calorie menus is 63% carbohydrate, 15% fat, and 22% protein. The "sensible" evening meal is the most educational component of the plan because it teaches dieters about appropriate portions of a moderate-calorie meal. Dieters are expected to purchase Slim-Fast products for their breakfast and lunch meals. This requirement leads to dieters' "burnout" and limits individuals' ability to select healthful, traditional foods.
South Beach Diet	This diet advocates the intake of "good" fats and "good" carbohydrates for cardiac protection, improved nutrition, and the management of hunger, insulin resistance, and weight control. The diet is divided into three phases. Three meals plus two snacks are the eating pattern for all phases of the diet.	Mostly healthful foods are consumed. Lean proteins, some fruits, vegetables, and oils are the staples of this diet. Initially: seafood, chicken breast, lean meat, low-fat cheese, most vegetables, nuts, oils are promoted. Later: whole grains, most fruits, low-fat milk or yogurt, and beans are promoted.	Refined carbohydrates and added sugars, fatty meats, full-fat cheese, refined grains, sweets, juice, potatoes	Phase I of the diet is restrictive and may be difficult to complete. Phase II includes more foods and Phase III is maintenance.	The composition of a sample menu from Phase I of the plan is 42% carbohydrate, 43% fat, and 15% protein. Research to support this diet is very limited. The two short-term studies that were completed had a small sample size and were funded by South Beach Diet affiliates.

Popular Diets (continued)

Name	Description	Foods to Eat	Foods to Avoid	Practicality	Analysis
Volumetrics	The Volumetrics Eating Plan focuses on enhancing the feeling of fullness while simultaneously consuming fewer calories. The diet aims to maximize the amount of food available per calorie. Foods are assigned to one of four categories based on their energy (calorie) density. Category 1 foods can be enjoyed on a daily basis; Category 4 foods are portion-controlled and consumed on an occasional basis.	Focuses on fiber-rich foods with a high moisture content. Fruits, vegetables, whole-grain pasta, rice, breads and cereals, soups, salads, low-fat poultry, seafood, meats, and dairy are promoted. Moderate amounts of sugar and alcohol are permitted, too.	No foods are forbidden, but limiting fatty foods like deep-fat-fried items, sweets, and fats added at the table is recommended. Limited amount of dry foods (crackers, popcorn, pretzels, etc.) due to their high caloric value and low satiety index.	The large amount of fiber-rich foods recommended for meals and snacks may cause gastrointestinal distress for some dieters.	The composition of the diet is ≥ 55% carbohydrate, 20% to 30% fat, and 15% to 35% protein. Fiber intake is 25 to 38 grams/day. This is a sensible and nutritionally balanced eating plan developed by a nutrition researcher.
Weight Watchers	A program that uses weekly meetings and weigh-ins for motivation and behavioral support for diet and exercise changes. Clients follow a point system which they can track online.	Theoretically, all foods are allowed. Fruits, vegetables, whole grains, lean protein, low- or nonfat dairy, and 2 teaspoons of healthful oils are staples of the program.	Although there are no "forbidden" foods, limiting intake of foods high in saturated and *trans* fats, sugar, and alcohol is emphasized.	Weekly Weight Watchers meetings have been shown to significantly strengthen participants' weight-loss successes. If a dieter is unable to attend weekly meetings, his or her results could be impacted. Once clients reach their target weights, they are allowed to attend meetings for free.	The composition of the diet plan is 50% to 60% carbohydrate, 25% fat, and 15% to 25% protein. No research supports the program's effectiveness, but its sensible advice is used and supported by millions, including nutrition experts.

References: **1.** Nutrition Action Healthletter (2004, January/February). **2.** Northwestern University, Feinberg School of Medicine (2007, January). Nutrition fact sheets: fad diets, retrieved from http://www.feinberg.northwestern.edu/nutrition/fact-sheets.html. **3.** Consumer Reports (2007, June). Top diets reviewed, retrieved from http://www.ConsumerReports.org.

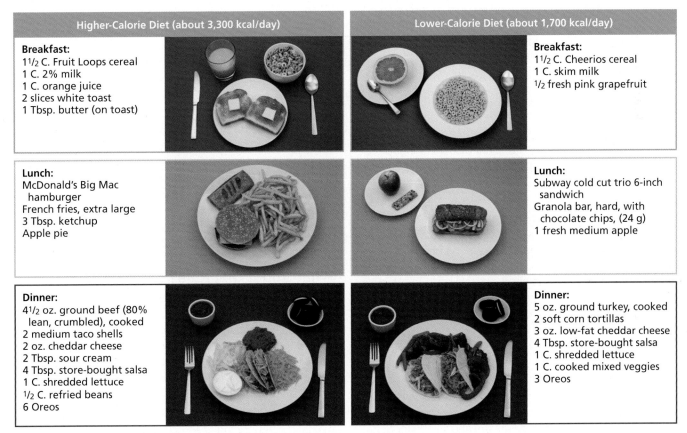

Higher-Calorie Diet (about 3,300 kcal/day)	Lower-Calorie Diet (about 1,700 kcal/day)
Breakfast: 1½ C. Fruit Loops cereal 1 C. 2% milk 1 C. orange juice 2 slices white toast 1 Tbsp. butter (on toast)	**Breakfast:** 1½ C. Cheerios cereal 1 C. skim milk ½ fresh pink grapefruit
Lunch: McDonald's Big Mac hamburger French fries, extra large 3 Tbsp. ketchup Apple pie	**Lunch:** Subway cold cut trio 6-inch sandwich Granola bar, hard, with chocolate chips, (24 g) 1 fresh medium apple
Dinner: 4½ oz. ground beef (80% lean, crumbled), cooked 2 medium taco shells 2 oz. cheddar cheese 2 Tbsp. sour cream 4 Tbsp. store-bought salsa 1 C. shredded lettuce ½ C. refried beans 6 Oreos	**Dinner:** 5 oz. ground turkey, cooked 2 soft corn tortillas 3 oz. low-fat cheddar cheese 4 Tbsp. store-bought salsa 1 C. shredded lettuce 1 C. cooked mixed veggies 3 Oreos

Figure 6.7 How to cut calories while maintaining a balanced diet. The meals on the right show healthful alternatives to the higher-calorie meals on the left.

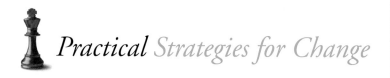

Practical *Strategies for Change*

Tips for Cutting Calories

If you're looking to cut calories, these tips can help:

- Share large portions with others.
- Avoid buying high-calorie foods that you have difficulty eating in moderate amounts.
- Don't skip meals, which can leave you overwhelmingly hungry later on. This includes breakfast, even on days you are late for class.
- Low-calorie meals do not have to be skimpy. If you fill most of your plate with vegetables alongside smaller portions of foods higher in calories, you can still have an ample meal without busting your calorie count for the day.
- If you crave snacks between meals, reach for options higher in bulk to help you feel full longer. An apple, for example, will keep your appetite at bay longer than a handful of potato chips.

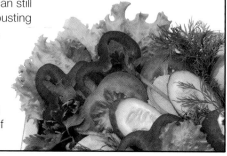

place, abruptly restricting one's daily calorie intake below recommended levels can be dangerous and deprive you of the energy you need for daily activities. You may find yourself withholding calories all day, only to lunge for a double cheeseburger at night. If you don't maintain a balanced diet while you cut calories, you will deplete your body of nutrients and possibly end up adding more calories along the way.

Low-Fat Diets

Diets that focus on reducing daily fat intake are also common. Most low-fat diets aim to cut the dieter's total fat intake to about 25% of calories or less.

Given the high-fat nature of the current American diet, most of us can benefit from some reduction in dietary fat. But fat is also essential to your health and the way your body functions. Fat is a main source of energy for your body. It regulates hormone production, and it is necessary for the absorption of vitamins A, E, D, and K. Fat can also enhance weight-loss efforts because it helps trigger feelings of satiety. For these reasons, many studies of low-fat diets show that dieters find these plans less successful in terms of weight loss and harder to maintain over the long term.

That said, we can all benefit from following these general fat intake guidelines:

- Cut *trans* fats from your diet. *Trans* fats are created when manufacturers add hydrogen to vegetable oil—a process called hydrogenation. While hydrogenation increases the shelf life of food, it raises your "bad cholesterol" (LDL) and consequently increases your risk of heart disease. Prepackaged snack and dessert foods (crackers, chips, cookies, cakes, pies, etc.) are the largest

sources of *trans* fat in our diet and account for about 40% of daily *trans* fat intake.

- Consume more "good" fats. Fats found in olive oil, walnuts, or fish can be a healthful part of your daily eating plan, when consumed in moderation.
- Make sure each meal includes some fat. This helps trigger satiety and wards off hunger longer. Good choices include lean meats, nuts, and vegetable oils.

Low-Carbohydrate Diets

Low-carbohydrate diets focus on reducing the amount of carbohydrates one consumes. First popularized by Dr. Robert Atkins, low-carbohydrate diets propose greatly reducing carbohydrate intake and eating combinations of protein and vegetables. Because protein-rich, high-fat foods such as meat and eggs are very filling and take longer to digest, some weight-loss studies have found that dieters tend to stick with low-carbohydrate approaches longer and lose slightly more weight—at first.[42,43] The diuretic effect of a low-carbohydrate diet promotes loss of water, not body fat. This offers a false sense of success that quickly disappears when water weight returns.

Most nutrition experts agree that Americans eat too many refined carbohydrates and added sugars. But removing *all* carbohydrates from your diet would mean eliminating fruit, milk, vegetables, and whole grains—all nutritious foods that are high in nutrients and fiber that your body needs. A better choice would be a *lower*-carbohydrate diet that followed these guidelines:

> *Frontline: Diet Wars* investigates popular diets and America's obesity problem. View this program online at **www.pbs.org/wgbh/pages/frontline/shows/diet.**

- Choose high-quality carbohydrates. Carbohydrates found in whole grains, fruits, and vegetables are better options than refined carbohydrates and added sugars found in highly processed foods and candy.
- Unlimited protein and fat won't help you lose weight. Total calorie consumption still matters. If you eat three cheeseburgers without the bun, you may have cut carbohydrates, but you've still eaten three cheeseburgers' worth of calories and fat. To lose weight, you need to consume fewer calories than you expend, regardless of the type of diet you are following.
- When choosing protein-rich foods, look for leaner options. Fish, skinless chicken breasts, or rump, round, flank, and loin cuts of meat are good choices. Better yet, choose plant protein, which is low in fat, high in fiber, and is nutrient dense.

What About Diet Pills?

Diet pills claim to help with weight loss in a variety of ways, from tricking your body into thinking it's full to regulating hormones that affect your desire to eat. Although many diet pills have never been proven to work, manufacturers of these products do a booming business. In 2007, Americans spent $1.4 billion on over-the-counter diet pills.[44] One study of college women at risk for eating disorders found that 32% reported having used a diet drug.[45]

Most over-the-counter diet pills are considered dietary supplements, a category that the Food and Drug Administration (FDA) only minimally regulates.[46] They do not need to be proven safe by the manufacturer unless they include a new ingredient, and are not tested by the FDA until they have already gone on the market and problems are reported. In addition, since labeling requirements remain less strict for supplements, many supplement firms downplay the risk of side effects in packaging and advertising. So, buyer beware.

Here are just some of the problems that have surfaced in recent years with over-the-counter diet pills:

- In 2009, the FDA warned consumers to immediately stop using Hydroxycut diet supplements because they were linked to serious liver injury and disease.[47]
- From December 2008 to May 2009, the FDA recalled over 70 weight-loss supplements because they were found to illegally contain prescription-drug ingredients.
- Even though the FDA prohibited the sale of weight-loss supplements containing the ingredient ephedra more than a decade ago, pills claiming to contain ephedra still appear for sale on the Internet. The ingredient has been linked to thousands of cases of side effects that include tremors, insomnia, heart palpitations, and increased risk of heart attack and stroke.[48]

Only one pill has received full clearance from the FDA for sale as an over-the-counter weight-loss medication. Alli, a lower dose of the prescription weight-loss medication Orlistat, was released to the public in 2007. The drug works by causing your body to excrete some of the fat that passes through your digestive tract, and is intended to help you lose about 5% of your body weight over time. But side effects, such as digestive discomfort and gas with oily spotting, can be unpleasant. Alli is also expensive, costing about $60 for a one-month supply of the pills.

Medical Options

For those who are dangerously obese, doctors may recommend medical treatments ranging from prescription drugs to more drastic interventions.

Prescription Drugs

Doctors may offer some prescription medications, such as Diethyl-propion, Orlistat, Phendimetrazine, Phentermine, and Sibutramine, to people who are extremely obese. Each has side effects ranging from increased blood pressure, sleepiness, nervousness, dizziness, and headaches to cramping and explosive diarrhea. These drugs only help shed a relatively small percentage of body weight, and are intended to work alongside changes in diet and exercise to promote gradual weight loss. They are usually prescribed only to patients who are obese and experiencing health problems due to their weight, and they are usually only prescribed for short-term use. While Orlistat and Sibutramine have been approved for longer-term use, their effectiveness and safety has not been established for use beyond 2 years. In fact, in August 2009, the FDA announced that it is investigating whether or not Orlistat may cause liver damage in some patients.

Surgery

A growing number of obese people—more than 205,000 in 2008 alone—are opting for surgery to alter the sizes of their stomachs.[49] This type of surgery is called **bariatric surgery,** and comprises sev-

eral different types of procedures. One subset of procedures, known as *gastric banding*, involves partitioning off part of the stomach with a removable band. The other subset, *gastric bypass*, involves permanently reducing the size of the stomach. After either type of procedure, the reshaped stomach can only hold a limited amount of food, resulting in greatly reduced calorie intake.

Some patients see significant weight loss and health improvements after undergoing these procedures. But some patients eventually gain back the weight they lost, even if all they can eat are small nibbles at a time. Others find they can no longer absorb certain nutrients properly. As with any major surgery, these procedures carry risks of complications, and may require follow-up procedures later in life.

What If You Want to Gain Weight?

If you want or need to gain weight for optimal health, you should consume more calories than you expend. As you do, use the following approaches:

- **Boost your calories, but in healthful ways.** Piling on the pizza isn't a good way to gain weight. Instead, reach for a diverse mix of foods, including fruit juices, nuts, dried fruits, peanut butter, and meal replacement drinks and bars. Keep a supply of nut-based trail mix with you, and reach for that as a snack. **Table 6.3** lists a healthful 3,000-calorie-per-day diet that can be used to gain weight.

Visit *Medline Plus* for reliable information about drugs and supplements at **www.nlm.nih.gov/medlineplus/druginformation.html.**

bariatric surgery Weight-loss surgery using various procedures to modify the stomach or other sections of the gastrointestinal tract in order to reduce calorie intake or absorption.

Table 6.3: **Healthful Weight Gain: A Sample 3,000-Calorie Diet**

Meal	Food
Breakfast	1 C. Grape Nuts 2 C. 2% milk 1 C. cranberry juice
Snack	6 Tbsp. raisins 1 C. orange juice
Lunch	8 oz. 2% milk 3 oz. tuna 2 tsp. mayonnaise 1 bun Lettuce, tomatoes, sprouts 2 oz. chips/snack food 1 C. whole baby carrots
Snack	Met-Rx fudge brownie bar 1 C. orange juice
Dinner	5 oz. chicken 1 C. instant mashed potatoes with 1/3 C. 2% dry milk powder 1 C. 2% milk 1 Tbsp. *trans*-free margarine 1 C. green beans Lettuce salad with vegetables 2 Tbsp. salad dressing
Snack	16 oz. water 16 animal crackers

How Do I Gain Weight?

"Hi, I'm Reese. My driver's license says I'm 5 feet 10 inches and 135 pounds. That was five years ago. Now I'm 5 feet 11 inches and 140 pounds. I like my height but I am tired of being skinny. I want to put on some muscle, gain weight, and look more athletic. I want the weight gain to be muscle, not fat! I've started going to the gym once in a while and doing some strength training exercises, but I'm not good about keeping up a routine. Between classes, papers, and relaxing with my friends, I just can't always find the time to get to the gym."

1: Review the stages of behavior change in Chapter 1. What stage of behavior change do you think Reese is in?

2: Why do you think Reese isn't gaining weight right now?

3: What specific things can Reese do to gain weight and build muscle?

Do you have a story similar to Reese's? Share your story at **www.pearsonhighered.com/choosinghealth.**

- **Eat smaller meals more frequently throughout the day.** If you don't have much of an appetite, try eating four or five smaller meals throughout the day, rather than two or three big ones.
- **Add calories to your favorite meals.** If you enjoy salad, for example, choose an olive oil dressing instead of a fat-free version. Add in some protein as well, such as diced chicken, cheese, avocado, or tofu. You also can add dry milk powder to mashed potatoes and meal replacement powders to milk and malt shakes.
- **Get regular exercise to build both appetite and muscle.** Participate in activities such as weightlifting to increase muscle mass and swimming to improve cardiovascular fitness.

Take a small step toward achieving your target weight. Visit **www.smallstep.gov** for tips on eating better, getting more active, and tracking your progress toward your goals.

- **Your healthful weight is a range, not a fixed number.** Sometimes you may be at the lower end of that range, and sometimes at the upper end. If you find your weight or BMI creeping up, reduce your calorie intake a bit and exercise a little more. A flexible approach lets you manage your weight and still enjoy your life.
- **Find reasons to be active.** Often, we make excuses for not exercising. Try turning that habit around. Leave your car at the far end of the parking lot and walk. Take the stairs instead of the elevator. Turn off your laptop or TV for a couple of hours a week and join an intramural sports team instead. Look for part-time work that requires being on your feet, not sitting at a desk.
- **When choosing physical activity, aim for consistency over intensity.** A half-hour brisk walk every day will do more for you in the long run than a 2-hour intense workout that is done only occasionally. In one study of college students, those with four or more low-intensity workouts a week were twice as likely to have healthful BMIs.[50]
- **Snack smarter.** Replace higher-calorie snacks such as chips and energy bars with fruits and vegetables. If you crave something more substantial, reach for whole grains or nuts before you opt for candy or a muffin. Don't leave snacks lying around, which can have you eating constantly without realizing it.
- **Don't be too hard on yourself.** If you have a few high-calorie days, don't tell yourself that you've blown your diet. Instead, follow up with a few days of lower-calorie choices.
- **Make fruits and vegetables your meal mainstays.** These healthful choices can provide the bulk of your meals, with starches and protein on the side. You'll be able to eat substantial meals, improve your nutrition, and leave the table with fewer calories under your belt.
- **Let food be one of life's pleasures.** Even if you are focused on weight maintenance, don't think about eating in terms of denial or punishment. You can indulge in foods you enjoy, and find new favorites along the way, as long as you remember that a healthful weight requires overall energy balance.
- **Take the long view.** Obtaining and maintaining a healthful weight is a lifelong commitment. You'll have ups and downs. But if you develop a plan that fits with your values and makes you happy, you'll find a balance that you can live with, and that helps keep you healthy along the way.

How Do You Maintain a Healthful Weight?

Reaching or being at a healthful weight is only one piece of the puzzle. Once you've achieved your target weight, you have to maintain it.

Long-term weight management doesn't have to mean endless days of dull meals or counting calories. Instead, look at your food habits, your level of physical activity, and your feelings about eating, and choose options that make it easy and fun to keep your weight in balance. Keep in mind:

Body Image and Unhealthful Eating Behaviors

We are constantly surrounded by conflicting messages about food and weight. In an evening spent in front of the TV, we are likely to see ads featuring delicious-looking fried chicken or cheeseburgers, followed by programs featuring models and actors so thin they look like they've never had a bite of either.

For some people, contradictions like this contribute to an unhealthful approach to eating and appearance.[51]

Body Image

When was the last time you looked at your body in a mirror and thought it could be more attractive? When did you last criticize yourself for your body shape or size? Did you use harsh terms that you'd never use to describe a friend? The way you view—and critique—your body is called **body image,** and a negative body image can affect the way you feel and the way you eat. Body image concerns affect males and females of all ages:

- Numerous studies have found that children absorb adult ideas about thinness and ideal body type, and then use these ideas to judge themselves. One study found that a desire for idealized thinness begins in girls as young as 6 years old.[52]
- Men often share women's self-criticisms of size and shape, although they may experience them more sharply at different points in their lives. One 20-year-long study found that men's dissatisfaction with their bodies went up with time and age. Women, while persistently displeased with their bodies, were often more critical when they were younger, and become more self-accepting as they grew older.[53]
- College is prime time for harsh self-judgment. In a study of college students, about 70% of female students and 35% of male students were dissatisfied with their bodies. About 70% of female students considered themselves unattractive to the opposite sex, as did about 45% of male students.[54]

Eating Disorders

Sometimes, people let negative body image or other psychological factors steer them toward unhealthful eating behaviors. When these behaviors produce drastic weight changes and put health and even life at risk, they are called **eating disorders.** Teenage girls are most at risk for eating disorders, especially if they are preoccupied with being thin, experience social or family pressure to be thin, come from more affluent families, and have tendencies toward extreme self-control and perfectionism. But young men and athletes under pressure to adhere to a particular body shape are also vulnerable.

Three dangerous eating disorders are anorexia nervosa, bulimia nervosa, and binge-eating disorder.

body image A person's perceptions, feelings, and critiques of his or her own body.

eating disorders A group of mental disorders, including anorexia nervosa, bulimia nervosa, and binge-eating disorder, that is characterized by physiological and psychological disturbances in appetite or food intake.

anorexia nervosa An eating disorder characterized by extremely low body weight, body image distortion, severe calorie restriction, and an obsessive fear of gaining weight.

Anorexia Nervosa

People with **anorexia nervosa** see food as an enemy that must be controlled. They eat as little as possible, often setting up elaborate rituals and practices to control food intake. They have an extremely unhealthful body image, seeing themselves as fat even when they fall well below a healthful weight. Cases of anorexia nervosa have increased in developed countries in recent decades, with an estimated 0.5% to 3.7% of females suffering from the condition at some point in their lifetime.[55]

Beauty in the Media: Seeing Shouldn't Be Believing

You can't miss them while you are standing in the checkout aisle at the grocery store: magazine after magazine showing perfect-looking models and celebrities on the covers.

But how realistic are those photos? The truth is, the vast majority of them have been digitally altered—boosting a curve here, shaving off a few pounds there. The result, media critics say, is a distorted representation of "the perfect body" that encourages unhealthful body perceptions in the rest of us. What's more, showcasing such unrealistic physical "ideals" can produce the desire to achieve the unattainable. Studies have shown that such images can increase body dissatisfaction in both women and men.[1, 2]

It's not always obvious where and how a photo has been changed. But every so often, original and retouched versions of the same photo appear in public. When such a photo of celebrity Kim Kardashian became public, for example, the "before" and "after" versions revealed numerous alterations, including a slimmer shape and lighter skin. When some observers called her fat, Kardashian defiantly donned a bathing suit and staged another photo session for a different magazine, promising the results would show the real her. Posting the photos on her blog, Kardashian dubbed the collection of images "My First Unretouched Photo Shoot" and asserted "I'm proud of my curves and you should be too!"

What Do You Think?

- When you see staged photos of fashion shoots, does it routinely occur to you that these images may have been altered?
- What effects do you think altered photos have on your standards of ideal body size, and your body image? Even if you know an image is altered, do you think it still affects your idea of what beauty is?
- What can you do to avoid comparing yourself unfavorably to images in magazines or advertisements? The next time you see a photo that looks a little too perfect, what will you tell yourself?

References: **1.** Murnen, S. K., Levine, M. P., Groesz, L., & Smith, J. (2007, August). Do fashion magazines promote body dissatisfaction in girls and women? A meta-analytic review. Paper presented at the 115th meeting of the American Psychology Association, San Francisco, CA. **2.** Barlett, C. P., Vowels, C. L., & Saucier, D. A. (2008). Meta-analyses of the effects of media images on men's body-image concerns. *Journal of Social and Clinical Psychology, 27*(3), 279–310.

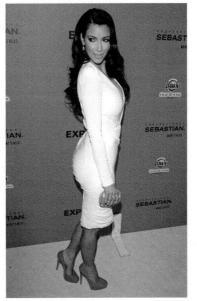

After an online magazine altered photos of her, Kim Kardashian released unretouched photos of herself to the press.

Want to see more examples of fake photos exposed? Visit www.youtube .com/watch?v=iYhCn0jf46U, and http://video.nytimes.com/video/2009/03/ 09/opinion/1194838469575/sex-lies-and-photoshop.html.

A Look at
Eating Disorders in Men

An obsession with food and body shape. Excessive exercise or calorie restriction. Feelings of low self-esteem and a drive for perfection. It sounds like a classic eating disorder, right? The difference: the victim is male.

For years, eating disorders have been thought of as "women's diseases," and it is true that the majority of those who suffer from them have been female. However, national statistics indicate that 10% of those

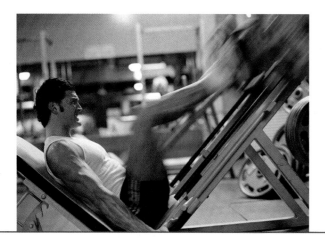

diagnosed with an eating disorder are male, and a recent Harvard study found an even higher prevalence: 25% of the people with anorexia or bulimia and 40% of the binge eaters were men.[1, 2] In addition, it is likely that the number of men with eating disorders is underdiagnosed, due to the still widespread perception among physicians and patients that eating disorders are a female concern.

Many of the factors that promote eating disorders are the same in both sexes, such as low self-esteem, depression, traumatic events or abuse in the past, or participation in a sport that values low body weight, such as gymnastics, running, or wrestling.[3] Unlike women, men who develop eating disorders are more likely to have actually been overweight in the past.[4] Men with eating disorders also tend to have higher levels of sexual anxiety than women with eating disorders.[5] There is some evidence that homosexual males may be more likely to develop eating disorders, although that could be due to higher levels of reporting among homosexual males compared to heterosexual males.[6]

Men are also much more likely than women to develop *muscle dysmorphia*, an all-consuming belief that they are not muscular enough and an obsession with building muscle.[7] These men tend to be more concerned with their percent of muscle to body fat as opposed to their weight on the scale. Men with all types of eating disorders are more likely to purge calories through compulsive exercise, rather than through vomiting or laxative abuse.[8]

A few high-profile men have spoken publicly about their battles with eating disorders, including actors Dennis Quaid and Billy Bob Thornton, and singer Elton John.[9] If you are a male and suspect you have an eating disorder, know that you are not alone—and seek help.

References: **1.** National Eating Disorders Association. (2008). Research on males and eating disorders, retrieved from www.nationaleatingdisorders.org. **2.** Hudson, J. H. (2007). The prevalence and correlates of eating disorders in the national comorbidity survey replication. *Biological Psychiatry*, 348–358. **3.** See note 1. **4.** Robb, A.S., and Dadson, M.J. (2002). Eating disorders in males. *Child Adolesc. Psychiatr. Clin. N. Am.* 11:201–218. **5-6.** See note 1. **7.** National Institute of Mental Health. (2009). Eating disorders: How are men and boys affected?, retrieved from www.nimh.nih.gov/health/publications/eating-disorders/how-are-men-and-boys-affected.shtml. **8.** Tartakovsky, M. (2008, October 7). *Eating disorders in men*, retrieved from http://psychcentral.com/blog/archives/2008/10/07/eating-disorder-in-men. **9.** Boodman, S. G. (2007, March 13). Eating disorders: Not just for women. *The Washington Post*, p. HE01.

Signs of anorexia nervosa include:

- An intense fear of gaining weight or being overweight.
- A highly distorted body image that continues to see fat where none exists.
- A refusal to maintain a normal body weight.
- A refusal to eat, or eating patterns that tightly restrict food intake.

Anorexia nervosa is classified as a serious mental disorder and can be fatal. Even if those with anorexia nervosa do not die, the disease can cause serious and sometimes irreparable damage throughout the body, especially to the bones and to the heart muscle. It is very important that anorexia nervosa be aggressively treated by a mental health professional.

Bulimia Nervosa

People who have **bulimia nervosa** have elaborate food rituals that typically start with **binge eating,** the consumption of a large amount of food in a short amount of time. After a binge, bulimics then try to remove these calories from their bodies by

bulimia nervosa An eating disorder characterized by episodes of binge eating followed by a purge behavior such as vomiting, laxative abuse, or extreme exercise.

binge eating The rapid consumption of an excessive amount of food.

purging Behaviors, such as vomiting, laxative abuse, or overexercising, intended to reduce the calories absorbed by the body.

purging through self-induced vomiting, heavy laxative use, fasting, or excessive exercise. An estimated 1% to 3% of young American teens and women develop bulimia nervosa.

Signs of bulimia nervosa include:

- Regular binge eating episodes, at a rate of at least two per week for several months.
- Binges followed by purging, strict dieting, or excessive exercise to prevent weight gain.
- Using self-induced vomiting or laxatives as part of purging.
- An obsession with weight and body shape.

Binge-Eating Disorder

Binge eaters may periodically consume thousands of calories in a matter of hours, do little to burn off those calories afterward, and then repeat that session of binge eating within a few days. As more binges lead to weight gain, many binge eaters say they begin to feel depressed, worried, and concerned about their ability to control their appetite. Those feelings lead many binge eaters to eat in private or try to hide their eating from others.

Signs of binge-eating disorder include:

- Eating large amounts of food in a relatively short period of time, whether you are hungry or not, at least twice a week.
- Eating until you feel overly full.
- Eating large amounts of food alone.
- Choosing to consume particular personal "comfort foods," such as a certain type of cookies, ice cream, or other foods you find especially pleasurable, during these concentrated sessions of heavy eating.

disordered eating A range of unhealthful eating behaviors used to deal with emotional issues that does not warrant a diagnosis of a specific eating disorder.

Other Unhealthful Eating Behaviors

There are other unhealthful eating behaviors that do not qualify as full-blown eating disorders but still have serious effects on weight, mental health, and well-being. These behaviors are classified as **disordered eating,** a range of unhealthful eating habits in which food is used primarily to deal with emotional issues. Disordered eating is common on college campuses—in one poll, about 20% of students said they had experienced some kind of disordered eating.[56]

Compulsive Overeating

Some people feel the need to eat constantly, even when they are full. They eat quickly, often snacking around the clock instead of sitting

Do you have a story similar to Beth's? Share your story at
www.pearsonhighered.com/choosinghealth.

Do I Have an Eating Disorder?

STUDENT STORY

"Hi, I'm Beth. I did competitive gymnastics in high school and there was a lot of pressure to be thin. About half of my teammates were anorexic. I was never that bad, but sometimes I would eat only one meal the whole day to make up for eating too much the day before. I'm now a college sophomore. I don't do gymnastics anymore, but I want to stay thin. I'm 5 feet 4 inches and 100 pounds. The problem is that I love to eat, and so I have this pattern where I will eat whatever I want one day and then limit myself the next. Does that mean I have an eating disorder? I think I'm still a lot healthier than some of my friends."

1: How would you describe Beth's body image?

2: Does Beth have an eating disorder?

3: If you were Beth's friend, what advice would you give her?

✓ **SELF-ASSESSMENT**

Could I Have an Eating Disorder?

To help find out, a doctor would ask you the following questions:

- Do you make yourself sick (make yourself vomit) because you feel uncomfortably full?
- Do you worry that you have lost control over how much you eat?
- Have you lost more than 14 pounds in a 3-month period?
- Do you think you are too fat, even when others say you are too thin?
- Would you say that food dominates your life?

HOW TO INTERPRET YOUR SCORE

Score 1 point for every "yes" answer. If you score 2 points or more, talk with a health professional.

Source: Morgan, J., Reid, F., & Lacey, J. H. (1999). The SCOFF questionnaire: Assessment of a new screening tool for eating disorders. *British Medical Journal, 319*, 1467–1476. Reproduced with permission from the BMJ Publishing Group.

down to eat at set meal times. They are also often embarrassed about their eating and the weight gain it brings, and may find ways to eat in private whenever possible. Compulsive overeaters, who are often women, usually turn to food as a source of comfort against feelings of self-doubt and fears of failure or abandonment.

Signs of compulsive overeating include:

- Continuing to eat, whether you are hungry or not.
- Eating quickly and often.
- A pattern of failed dieting efforts, accompanied by worries about dieting again.
- Using food as comfort or as a reward.
- Thinking and talking about food throughout the day.

Extreme Dieting

Extreme dieters, who tend to be young women, don't just watch calories or exercise often. Dieting and weight loss become obsessions focused on each bite of food taken and every pound of weight shed. While extreme dieters never lose enough weight to have anorexia nervosa, they do suffer physical effects from excessive weight loss, such as weakness from diminished muscle mass. They are also at greater risk for developing anorexia nervosa.

Signs of extreme dieting include:

- A preoccupation with eating as a source of potential weight gain.
- A preoccupation with burning off calories.
- Misconceptions about food and exercise that fuel these preoccupations. Some extreme dieters may insist, for example, that a particular type of fruit is essential to weight loss, even if little evidence supports that claim.
- Frequent use of over-the-counter pills to try to control weight, including laxatives and diet pills.

Treating Unhealthful Eating Behaviors

Any type of unhealthful eating behavior is a complex condition best addressed in a compassionate, supportive manner. Even if you don't think your eating issues are life threatening, they can still damage your health and quality of life. Seek support and treatment from trained professionals. Many people who experience eating disorders

Overweight and Obesity Through the Lenses
of Race, Ethnicity, and Socioeconomic Class

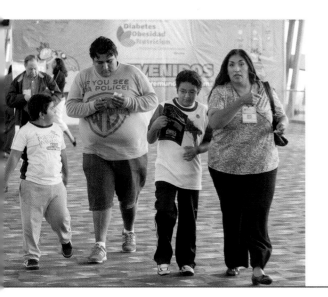

Overweight and obesity disproportionately affect certain racial, ethnic, and socioeconomic groups. According to a 2008 study conducted by the Kaiser Family Foundation, overweight and obesity are problems for:[1]

- 59.6% of Caucasian Americans
- 69.9% of African Americans
- 62.1% of Hispanic Americans
- 38.7% of Asian Americans
- 67.1% of Native Americans/Alaskan Natives
- 59.5% of other racial or ethnic groups

Another recent study reveals that college students in lower socioeconomic positions report higher rates of overweight and obesity than students in more privileged socioeconomic groups.[2] The same study also noted that in general, male students are more likely to be overweight than female students.

The reasons for these disparities are complex. Factors may include cultural differences in diet and exercise, socioeconomic differences in patterns of fast-food consumption, inequalities in access to nutritious food, and inequalities in access to education about nutrition and fitness. Regardless of whether you are in a group with higher or lower overweight and obesity rates, take heart: By enrolling in this course and reading this textbook, you will learn strategies for effective weight management.

Data from: **1.** Kaiser Family Foundation (2009). *Overweight and obesity rates for adults by race/ethnicity, 2008*, retrieved from http://www.statehealthfacts.org. **2.** Nelson, T.F., Gortmaker, S.L., Subramanian, S.V., Cheung, L., & Wechsler, H. (2007). Disparities in overweight and obesity among U.S. college students. *American Journal of Health Behavior, 31*(4), 363–373.

and disordered eating also get a great deal of help from guided support groups. In these groups, you'll not only receive help in shifting your self-perceptions and habits, but get valuable advice from others who've been in your shoes.

If you have a serious eating disorder, you may first need medical treatment to stabilize your body and stop your health from deteriorating. Once your health is stabilized, your network of social and emotional support will be an essential part of reframing your views of yourself, food, and how your eating habits have defined your life so far.

If you think someone you know has an unhealthful eating behavior:

- Locate support and treatment resources on campus or in your community.
- Once you know where to find help, have a compassionate, open conversation with the person you are concerned about. Try to listen and talk about your worries, rather than accuse or blame.

- Try not to talk with your friend or loved one about dieting, body size, or weight. Instead, focus on behaviors that worry you and how they might be unhealthful.
- Offer to direct the person to the treatment resources you've found, and offer to go along for support if desired.
- Know that one conversation may not go far. Keep trying. If you let your friend or loved one know that you are concerned, that person will know where to turn when he or she is ready to seek help.

Watch videos of real students discussing weight management at: www.pearsonhighered.com/choosinghealth.

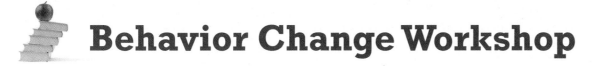

Behavior Change Workshop

To complete this workshop online, visit **www.pearsonhighered.com/choosinghealth.**

Changing long-ingrained behaviors is one of the toughest things to do. Consider the student stories presented throughout this chapter, and then think about your own life. What can you do to manage your weight? What stage of behavior change are you in? Given your current stage of change, what is an appropriate goal you can set to reach the next stage?

Part I. Creating a Weight-Management Plan

1. What does your BMI and waist-to-hip ratio tell you about the effect of your weight on your health? How do you feel about your weight when you look in the mirror? Do you want to maintain your current weight? Gain weight? Lose weight? By how many pounds? Write down exactly what you want to accomplish with your weight-management plan.

BMI and waist-to-hip ratio: _____

_____

Weight-management goal: _____

_____

_____

2. Ask yourself honestly: How ready are you to commit to a behavior change that will help you manage your weight? What stage of behavior change are you in?

_____

_____

_____

_____

3. Keeping your current stage of behavior change in mind, describe what you might do or think about as a "next step" to manage your weight. Which side of the energy balance equation do you want to change: energy in or energy out? You can also modify both.

_____

_____

_____

_____

4. Consider that a healthful prescription for weight loss is cutting 500 to 1,000 calories a day, through reduced calorie intake or increased exercise. This typically leads to a weight loss of 1 or 2 pounds a week. To gain weight, you would add a similar amount of calories daily. Now, consider the weight-management techniques introduced in this chapter. Which techniques can you try to better manage your weight? Keep in mind that you should not cut calories below the recommended MyPyramid levels shown in Table 4.3 on page 79.

_____

_____

_____

5. If you want to simply maintain your current weight, what will you do to ensure that your energy expenditure meets the energy you consume? Think about extended amounts of time when you might consistently consume more food (such as holiday breaks), or where you might be less active than usual (such as during finals). What steps can you take during those times to make sure you stay in energy balance?

_____

_____

_____

_____

Part II. How Would You Change This Meal?

Imagine that you're out with friends one night and you stop by a local diner for dinner. When your meal arrives, it contains the foods shown below. Does it surprise you to hear that there are over 1,450 calories on your plate? How would you use portion control and other diet tools to change your dinner to reduce your calorie intake?

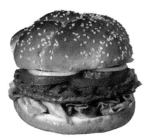

One diner hamburger: 690 calories
Reduce calories by: _____

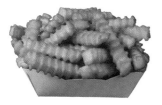

Medium French fries: 400 calories
Reduce calories by: _____

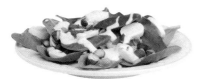

Side salad with full-fat ranch dressing: 240 calories
Reduce calories by: _____

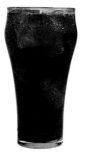

1 16-oz Coke: 150 calories
Reduce calories by: _____

See page BC-1 for sample answers to this workshop.

Chapter Summary

- Your weight affects your health, not just your appearance.

- Health risks of excess weight include high blood pressure, type 2 diabetes, abnormal blood fats, coronary heart disease, stroke, metabolic syndrome, cancer, osteoarthritis, sleep apnea, gallbladder disease, fatty liver disease, and fertility and pregnancy complications.

- Your weight is shaped by your energy balance, physical activity, basic energy needs, age, genes, gender, and environment. Ultimately, excess weight results from an imbalance of calories consumed and calories used.

- Excess body weight is a critical issue for college students. Decline in physical activity is often a major contributor to college weight gain.

- Overweight and obesity are serious and common health problems, not just in the United States but around the world.

- BMI, waist circumference, and waist-to-hip ratio can give indicators of whether your weight will increase your risk for certain health conditions and diseases.

- To truly understand your weight and its effects on your health, you need to know your body composition, not just how much you weigh.

- Reaching a healthful weight requires consistent, long-term work on both eating habits and increasing physical activity. Short-term diets are often of limited help. Diet aids can be expensive, may not work, and may even be harmful.

- Medical options, including prescription drugs and bariatric surgery, may be beneficial for people who are extremely obese.

- To gain weight, boost your calories in healthful ways by eating nutritious foods like nuts, juices, peanut butter, and meal replacement bars to gain weight. Also, eat more often and get exercise to stimulate appetite.

- Maintaining a healthful weight is most effective when you establish and consistently follow eating and exercise habits you enjoy, and use them to keep your weight within a healthful range.

- Societal contradictions that encourage weight gain while glorifying thinness lead many of us to have negative views of our own bodies. These body image issues contribute to disordered eating and eating disorders.

- Eating disorders are complicated psychiatric conditions that are affected by family, social dynamics, and feelings of self-worth. Disordered eating behaviors are also unhealthful but don't qualify as psychiatric conditions.

Test Your Knowledge

1. A person who has a large waistline, high blood pressure, and high blood glucose most likely has what obesity-related health condition?
   a. osteoarthritis
   b. coronary heart disease
   c. metabolic syndrome
   d. gallbladder disease

2. Which of the following conditions is NOT related to being overweight?
   a. polycystic ovary syndrome
   b. high blood pressure
   c. fatty liver disease
   d. low LDL levels

3. What percentage of 21-year-olds engage in regular, vigorous physical activity?
   a. 75%
   b. 50%
   c. 35%
   d. 10%

4. When most students start college, how many pounds do they gain?
   a. 1 to 4
   b. 7 to 8
   c. 9 to 12
   d. 13 to 16

5. What is the healthful weight range for someone who is 5 feet 11 inches tall?
   a. 133 to 172 pounds
   b. 140 to 171 pounds
   c. 149 to 183 pounds
   d. 164 to 196 pounds

6. What is BMI?
   a. a ratio between your height and your weight, used to help assess health risks
   b. a measurement of how much fat you have
   c. a measurement of how much muscle you have
   d. a 100% reliable indicator of how healthy you are

7. What is the best approach to weight loss?
   a. Eat more protein and drink more water.
   b. Take in less calories and exercise more.
   c. Avoid foods containing carbohydrates.
   d. Take in more energy and eat less fat.

8. What term best describes our response to the sight, smell, thought, or taste of food?
   a. satiety
   b. craving
   c. hunger
   d. appetite

9. In order to maintain weight loss, you should
 a. eat as little as possible.
 b. stop working out; it makes you hungry.
 c. never allow yourself to have a high-calorie day.
 d. focus on eating fruits and vegetables.

10. Which of the following statements about body image is FALSE?
 a. A desire for thinness often begins in childhood.
 b. Men are not self-critical of their body size and shape.
 c. College is a prime time for self-judgment.
 d. Women become more self-accepting of their bodies with age.

Get Connected

🌐 **Health Online** Visit the following websites for further information about the topics in this chapter:

- American College of Sports Medicine Exercise Guidelines
 www.acsm.org
- American Dietetic Association
 www.eatright.org
- Centers for Disease Control and Prevention: Overweight and Obesity
 www.cdc.gov/obesity/index.html
- National Institute of Mental Health: Eating Disorders
 www.nimh.nih.gov/health/publications/eating-disorders/complete-index .shtml
- USDA Nutritional Database
 www.nal.usda.gov/fnic/foodcomp/search

- World Health Organization: Obesity
 www.who.int/topics/obesity/en
- Top 100 Weight Loss Blogs
 www.uspharmd.com/blog/2008/top-100-weight-loss-blogs
- Buddy Slim (find a weight-loss partner)
 www.buddyslim.com
- FitDay (free online weight-loss journal)
 www.fitday.com
- Inside Out Weight Loss audio podcasts
 http://personallifemedia.com/podcasts/216-inside-out-weight-loss

Website links are subject to change. To access updated Web links, please visit **www.pearsonhighered.com/choosinghealth.**

References

i. Centers for Disease Control/National Center for Health Statistics. (2009). FastStats: Overweight prevalence. Retrieved from http://www.cdc.gov/nchs/fastats/overwt .htm.

ii. American Obesity Association. (2005). AOA Fact Sheets. Retrieved from http:// obesity1.tempdomainname.com/subs/ fastfacts/Obesity_Consumer_Protect.shtml.

iii. Flegal, K. M., Graubard, B.I., Williamson, D.F., & Gail, M.H. (2005). Excess deaths associated with underweight, overweight, and obesity. *Journal of the American Medical Association.* 293:1861–1867.

iv. Economos, C. D., Hildebrandt, M. L., & Hyatt, R. R. (2008). College freshman stress and weight change: Differences by gender. *American Journal of Health Behavior, 32*(1), 16–25.

1. Centers for Disease Control/National Center for Health Statistics. (2009). FastStats: Overweight prevalence. Retrieved from http://www.cdc.gov/nchs/fastats/overwt .htm.

2. World Health Organization. (2009) Obesity and overweight. Fact sheet number 311. Retrieved from http://www.who.int/ mediacentre/factsheets/fs311/en/index.html.

3. Mayo Clinic. (2009). Obesity. Retrieved from http://www.mayoclinic.com/health/ obesity/DS00314.

4. National Institute of Diabetes and Digestive and Kidney Diseases/National Institutes of Health. (2007). Do you know the health risks of being overweight? NIH Publication No. 07–4098. Retrieved from http://win.niddk.nih.gov/publications/ health_risks.htm.

5. Nguyen, N. T., Magno, C. P., Lane, K. T., Hinojosa, M. W., & Lane, J. S. (2008, December). Association of hypertension, diabetes, dyslipidemia, and metabolic syndrome with obesity: Findings from the National Health and Nutrition Examination Survey, 1999–2004. *Journal of the American College of Surgeons, 207*(6), 928–934.

6. Grundy, S. M., Cleeman, J. I., Daniels, S. R., et al. (2005, October). Diagnosis and management of the metabolic syndrome: An American Heart Association/National Heart, Lung, and Blood Institute scientific statement. *Circulation, 1129*(17), 2735–2752.

7. Mayo Clinic. (2009). Metabolic syndrome. Retrieved from http://www.mayoclinic.com/ health/metabolic%20syndrome/DS00522.

8. Ford, E. D., Giles, W. H., & Modkad, A. H. (2004). Increasing prevalence of the metabolic syndrome among US adults. *Diabetes Care, 24*(10), 244–249.

9. Olshansky, S. J., Passaro, D. J., Hershow, M. D., et al. (2005). A potential decline in life expectancy in the United States in the 21st

century. *New England Journal of Medicine, 352*, 1103–1110.

10. National Institutes of Health. (2007). Statistics related to overweight and obesity, *National Institutes of Health.* (Electronic version). Retrieved from http://win.niddk.nih.gov/ statistics/index.htm#preval.

11. Farah, H., & Buzby, J. (2005, November). U.S. food consumption up 16 percent since 1970. *U.S. Department of Agriculture: Amber Waves.* Retrieved from http://www.ers.usda .gov/AmberWaves/November05/Findings/ USFoodConsumption.htm.

12. Newman C. (2004, August). Why are we so fat? *National Geographic, 206*(2), 46–61.

13. Centers for Disease Control and Prevention. (2010). State indicator report on physical activity 2010 national action guide. Retrieved from http://www.cdc.gov/ physicalactivity/downloads/PA_State_ Indicator_Report_2010_Action_Guide.pdf.

14. U.S. Department of Health & Human Services. (2000). Physical activity and fitness. In *HealthyPeople2010* [Online]. Retrieved from http://www.health.gov/ healthypeople/document/htm1/volume2/ 22physical.htm.

15. Matthews, C. E., Chen, K. Y., Freedson, P. S., Buchowski, M. S., Bettina, M., Beech, B. M., Pate, R. R., & Troiano, R. P. (2008). Amount of time spent in sedentary behaviors

in the United States, 2003–2004. *American Journal of Epidemiology, 167*(7), 875–881.

16. The Nielsen Company. (2009). *A2/M2 Three Screen Report, 1st quarter 2009.* Retrieved from http://it.nielsen.com/site/ documents/A2M2_3Screens_1Q09_ FINAL.pdf.

17. U.S. Census Bureau. (2005). Americans spend more than 100 hours each year commuting to work, Census Bureau Reports. American Community Survey, 2005. Retrieved from http://www.census.gov/ Press-Release/www/releases/archives/ american_community_survey_acs/004489 .html.

18. Duyff, R. L. (2006). *American Dietetic Association complete food and nutrition guide* (p. 26). New York: John Wiley and Sons.

19. Frayling, T. et al. (2007). A common variant in the FTO gene is associated with body mass index and predisposes to childhood and adult obesity. (Electronic version). *Science 12.* Retrieved from http://www .sciencemag.org/cgi/content/abstract/ 1141634v1.

20. Levi, A., Chan, K., & Pence, D. (2006). Real men do not read food labels: The effects of masculinity and involvement on college students' food decisions. *Journal of American College Health, 55*(2), 91–98.

21. Moczulski, V., McMahan, S., Weiss, J., Beam, W., & Chandler, L. (2007). Commuting behaviors, obesity risk, and the built environment. *American Journal of Health Behaviors, 22*(1), 26–32.

22. O'Connor, D., Jones, F., Conner, M., & McMillan, B. (2008). Effects of daily hassles and eating styles on eating behavior. *Health Psychology, 27*(1), 20–31.

23. McDonald's. McDonald's USA Nutrition facts for popular menu items. (Electronic version). Retrieved from http://www.mcdonalds.com/app_controller.nutrition.ind.ex1.html.

24. Economos, C. D., Hildebrandt, M. L., & Hyatt, R. R. (2008). College freshman stress and weight change: Differences by gender. *American Journal of Health Behavior, 32*(1), 16–25.

25. Nelson, T., Gortmaker, S., Subramanian, S., Cheung, S., & Wechsler, H. (2007). Disparities in overweight and obesity among US college students. *American Journal of Health Behaviors, 31*(4), 363–373.

26. Wharton, C., Adams, T., & Hampl, J. (2008). Weight loss practices and body weight perceptions among US college students. *Journal of American College Health, 56*(5), 579–584.

27. Jung, M., Bray, S., & Ginis, K. (2008). Behavior change and the "Freshman 15": Tracking physical activity and dietary patterns in 1st-year university women. *Journal of American College Health, (56)*5, 523–530.

28. Kasparek, D., Corwin, S., Valois, R., Sargent, R., & Morris, R. (2008). Selected health behaviors that influence freshman weight change. *Journal of American College Health, 56*(4), 437–444.

29. Ogden, C.L., Carroll, M.D., Curtin, L.R., McDowell, M.M., Tabak, C.J., & Flegal, F. (2006). Prevalence of overweight and obesity in the United States, 1999–2004. *Journal of the American Medical Association, 295*(13), 1549–1555.

30. Freedman, D., et al. (2005). The relation of childhood BMI to adult adiposity: The Bogalusa heart study. *Pediatrics, 115*(1), 22–27.

31. Centers for Disease Control and Prevention (CDC). (2009). *Behavioral risk factor surveillance system survey data.* Atlanta, GA: U.S. Department of Health and Human Services, Centers for Disease Control and Prevention.

32. Wang, Y. & Beydoun, M. (2007). The obesity epidemic in the United States—gender, age, socioeconomic, racial/ethnic, and geographic characteristics: A systematic review and meta-regression analysis. *Epidemiological Reviews, 29*, 6–28.

33. World Health Organization. (2004, April 19). *Diet, physical activity, and health: A report by the Secretariat.* (Electronic version). Retrieved from http://www.who.int.

34. Nappo-Dattoma, L. (2007, July). Part I: Obesity and its threat to your patients' health. *Access,* 36–40.

35. Brooks, Y. et al. (2007). Body mass index and percentage of body fat as health indicators for young adults. *American Journal of Health Behaviors, 31*(6), 687–700.

36. Bray, G. (2006). Obesity: The disease. *Journal of Medicinal Chemistry, 49*(14), 4001–4007.

37. Vartanian, L. R. et al. (2007, April). Effects of soft drink consumption on nutrition and health: A systematic review and meta-anaylsis. *American Journal of Public Health, 97*(4), 667–675.

38. Butchko, Harriett H. et al. (2002). Aspartame: Review of safety. *Regulatory Toxicology and Pharmacology, 35*, S1–S93, 200.

39. Elder, S., & Roberts, S. (2007). The effects of exercise on food intake and body fatness: A summary of published studies. *Nutrition Reviews, 65*(1), 1–19.

40. Dansinger, M., Gleason, J., Griffith, J., Selker, H., & Schaefer, E. (2005.) Comparison of the Atkins, Ornish, Weight Watchers, and Zone Diets for weight loss and heart disease risk reduction. *Journal of the American Medical Association, 293*(1), 43–53.

41. U.S. Food and Drug Administration. (2005, September/October). Revealing trans fats. *FDA Consumer Magazine.* Pub No. FDA05-1329C. Available online at http://www.fda.gov/FDAC/features/2003/503_fats.html.

42. Gardner, C. et al. (2007). Comparison of the Atkins, Zone, Ornish, and LEARN diets for change in weight and related risk factors among overweight premenopausal women. *Journal of the American Medical Association, 297*(9), 969–977.

43. Yancy, W. et al. (2004). A low-carbohydrate, ketogenic diet versus a low-fat diet to treat obesity and hyperlipidemia. *Annals of Internal Medicine, 140*, 769–777.

44. Marketdata Enterprises, Inc. (2007). *U.S. weight loss market to reach $58 billion in 2007.* (Electronic version). Available online at http://www.prwebdirect.com/releases/2007/4/prweb520127.php.

45. Celio, C. et al. (2006). Use of diet pills and other dieting aids in a college population with high weight and shape concerns. *International Journal of Eating Disorders, 39*(6), 492–497.

46. Jordan, M., & Haywood, T. (2007). Evaluation of Internet websites marketing herbal weight-loss supplements to consumers. *Journal of Alternative and Complementary Medicine, 13*(9), 1035–1043.

47. FDA warns consumers to stop using Hydroxycut products. (2009, May 1). FDA News. Available online at http://www.fda.gov/bbs/topics/NEWS/2009/NEW02006.html.

48. U.S. Food and Drug Administration. (2005). *FDA news release: FDA acts to seize ephedra-containing dietary supplements.* P05-94. Retrieved from http://www.fda.gov/NewsEvents/Newsroom/PressAnnouncements/2005/ucm108524.htm.

49. Gastric bypass sparks debate. (2008, December 14). *Biomedicine.* Available online at http://www.bio-medicine.org/medicine-news-1/Gastric-Bypass-Success-Sparks-Debate-32124-1/.

50. Kasparek, D., Corwin, S., Valois, R., Sargent, R., & Morris, R. (2008.) Selected health behaviors that influence college freshman weight change. *Journal of the American College Health Association, 56*(4), 437–444.

51. Carney, T., & Louw, J. (2006). Eating disorderd behaviors and media exposure. *Social Psychiatry and Psychiatry Epidemiology, 41*, 957–966.

52. Lowes, J., & Tiggemann, M. (2003). Body dissatisfaction, dieting awareness and the impact of parental influence in young children. *British Journal of Health Psychology, 8*, 135–147.

53. Keel, P., Baxter, M., Heatheron, T., & Joiner, T. (2007). A 20-year longitudinal study of body weight, dieting, and eating disorder symptoms. *Journal of Abnormal Psychology, 116*(2), 422–432.

54. Forrest, K., & Stuhldreher, W. (2007). Patterns and correlates of body image dissatisfaction and distortion among college students. *American Journal of Health Studies, 22*(1), 18–25.

55. American Psychiatric Association Work Group on Eating Disorders. (2000). Practice guideline for the treatment of patients with eating disorders (revision). *American Journal of Psychiatry, 157*(1 Suppl.), 1–39.

56. Eating Disorders Review. (2006, November/December). *In a recent poll, nearly 20 percent of students admit to disordered eating,* p. 8.

Drug Use and Abuse 7

An estimated **20.1 million** people in the U.S. currently use **illicit drugs.**[i]

Marijuana is the **most common** illicitly used drug.[i]

College students tend to **vastly overestimate** how many of their **peers** use drugs illicitly.[ii]

Do you use drugs?

LEARNING OBJECTIVES

DESCRIBE the prevalence of drug use among college students.

DEFINE *drug misuse, drug abuse, addiction,* and *dependence.*

DESCRIBE three common methods of drug administration.

IDENTIFY commonly abused drugs and describe their mechanisms, effects, and health risks.

DISCUSS the prevention and treatment of drug abuse.

Health Online icons are found throughout the chapter, directing you to web links, videos, podcasts, and other useful online resources.

Many of us might quickly say no, only to realize that the answer to that question is not so simple. A **drug** is any chemical that is taken in order to alter the body physically or mentally for a non-nutritional purpose. Drugs that alter feelings, mood, perception, or psychological functioning are considered **psychoactive.** Although you may not realize it, you likely use one or more psychoactive drugs on a daily basis. If you drink caffeinated beverages like coffee or cola, take aspirin or other pain relievers, or take allergy medicine, you are using a drug. Of course, there is a big difference between having a daily cup of coffee and being addicted to, say, cocaine or methamphetamine. There is a wide spectrum of drug types, and some drugs are much more harmful than others.

This chapter covers the use and abuse of legal as well as illegal drugs. We will also discuss addiction, dependence, and the prevention and treatment of drug abuse. We will reserve detailed discussion of the two most widely used drugs—alcohol and tobacco—for Chapter 8.

Drug Use on Campus

People use drugs for a variety of reasons. Some use drugs to seek pleasure, escape from problems, or relieve pain. Others turn to drugs to try to improve their performance at school, work, or on the field. Popular culture often glamorizes drugs—think of how many "stoner" characters you see featured in movies, and how often you see actors, actresses, and rock stars smoking or drinking. The social pressure to experiment with drugs can be intense—especially for college students living away from home, perhaps for the first time, and who have friends who use them.

A national study conducted by Columbia University found that nearly half of full-time college students binge drink or abuse prescription or illegal drugs.[1] Nearly one in four meets the medical criteria for drug addiction or dependence. Among the study's findings:

- The percentage of students who binge drink frequently (that is, three or more times in a 2-week period) has increased 16% since 1993. (Binge drinking is covered in depth in Chapter 8.)
- The proportion of students abusing stimulants such as Ritalin and Adderall has jumped 93% since 1993.
- The number of students who use marijuana every day now exceeds 300,000 (more than double the number in 1993).
- The proportion of students who use cocaine, heroin, and other illegal drugs (other than marijuana) increased 52% between 1993 and 2005.

The most recent National Survey on Drug Use and Health reports that patterns of illicit drug use varies by educational status.[2] In 2008, rates of current illicit drug use were lower for college graduates (5.7%) than for those without high school degrees (8.6%). However, college graduates were more likely to have experimented with illicit drugs during their lifetime compared to adults without high school degrees.

Interestingly, students tend to vastly overestimate the percentage of their peers who use drugs. For example, in a national survey conducted in the fall of 2008, students reported believing that 77% of their peers had used marijuana, when in reality only 14.5% of students reported actually using the drug.[3] It is important to realize that *not everyone is using drugs*—far from it. The number of students who abuse drugs, however, is in-

drug A chemical substance that alters the body physically or mentally for a non-nutritional purpose.

psychoactive A drug that alters feelings, mood, perceptions, or psychological functioning.

View a video of students telling personal stories about their drug addictions at http://pact360.org/youth360.

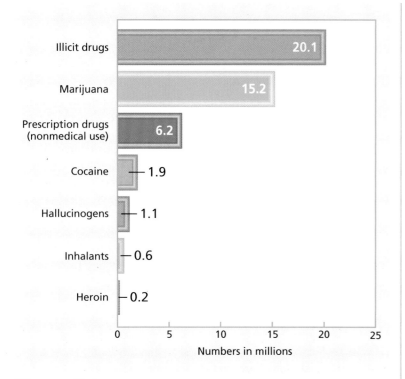

Figure 7.1 Illicit drug use in the United States.
Marijuana and the nonmedical use of prescription drugs top the list of illicit drugs used in the U.S.

Source: Data from *Results from the 2008 National Survey on Drug Use and Health: National Findings* by the Substance Abuse and Mental Health Services Administration, Office of Applied Studies, 2009, retrieved from http://oas.samhsa.gov/nsduh/ 2k8nsduh/2k8Results. Data represents past-month use of illicit drugs among persons aged 12 or older in 2008.

creasing, and the health risks to both themselves and to society are serious.

Figure 7.1 summarizes the most commonly used illicit drugs in the U.S. **Diversity & Health: Drug Use Through the Lenses of Sex, Race, Age, and Geography** on page 145 examines the differences in how patterns of drug use vary among different demographic groups.

Misuse, Abuse, Addiction and Dependence

Drug misuse is the inappropriate use of a legal drug, either for a reason for which it was not medically intended, or by a person without a prescription. Using your roommate's amoxicillin because you think you have a sinus infection is an example of drug misuse. **Drug abuse** is the use (most often the excessive use) of any legal or illegal drug in a way that is detrimental to your health. If, for example, you take prescription painkillers to get high or use street amphetamines to lose weight, you are abusing drugs. All drug use involves some level of health risks; however, the risks are significantly increased if you misuse or abuse drugs.

Drug **addiction** is a complex, relapsing condition that is characterized by uncontrollable drug craving and use—despite actual or potential harmful consequences. In the past, people believed that drug addiction was due to moral failure, laziness, or lack of will-power. We now know that addiction is much more complicated than that, and that it has both psychological and physical roots.

Drugs chemically tap into and interfere with the brain's communication system, altering how nerve cells send, receive, and process information. The most addictive substances trigger a rush of the neurotransmitter *dopamine*. Dopamine is the brain's "feel good" chemical and causes feelings of pleasure and satisfaction. When the brain is overstimulated chemically, users experience a sense of **euphoria** that primes their bodies to repeat the stimulation. Eventually the brain adapts to the drug by producing less of its own chemicals to regulate cognition and feelings of pleasure, other emotions, or motivation. As a result, when the drug is no longer externally supplied, users may feel "flat" or depressed, uninterested in things that used to bring them pleasure.

Prolonged or repeated use of chemical substances can actually alter the brain's structure and how it works. The body can eventually develop **tolerance,** meaning that the brain has grown so accustomed to the drug that more of the drug is required to achieve the effect that a smaller amount used to have. Tolerance may also cause users to need to keep using a drug just to feel "normal."

This cycle of drug use and tolerance feeds drug addiction. Although people do have control over the choice of whether to initiate drug use, once they start, the pleasurable effects often make them want or need to keep using. **Psychological dependence** ("psychological addiction") means a mental attachment to a drug—the belief that a drug is needed to relieve stress, anxiety, or other feelings of mental discomfort. With **physical dependence,** the body requires the regular use of a substance in order to function. A physically dependent person also develops tolerance; therefore, larger and larger doses are needed to achieve a high, or even feel normal. Both psychological dependence and physical dependence are characterized by an intense craving for a drug.

Withdrawal refers to the process and experience of ceasing to take a drug that has created a physical dependence. Withdrawal can make some common drugs extremely difficult to quit. Effects can include headaches, nausea, and vomiting, depending on the drug and degree of dependence.

The American Psychiatric Association defines substance dependence as a pattern of substance use that leads to "significant impairment or distress" and that is characterized by at least three or more of the following within a 1-year period:

- The development of tolerance to the substance

- The experience of withdrawal symptoms

drug misuse The inappropriate use of a legal drug, either for a reason for which it was not medically intended, or by a person without a prescription.

drug abuse The use (most often the excessive use) of any legal or illegal drug in a way that is detrimental to your health.

addiction A complex, relapsing condition characterized by uncontrollable craving for a substance or behavior despite the harmful consequences.

euphoria A feeling of intense pleasure.

tolerance Reduced sensitivity to a drug so that increased amounts are needed to achieve the usual effect.

psychological dependence A mental attachment to a drug.

physical dependence The physical need for a drug.

withdrawal Physical symptoms that develop when a person stops using a drug.

Drug Use Through the Lenses of
Sex, Race, Age, and Geography

A recent national survey of drug use in the United States revealed the following information.

Overall

- About 8% of the United States population (an estimated 20.1 million individuals

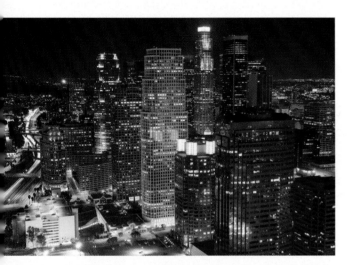

Rates of drug use are higher in metropolitan areas than in rural areas.

aged 12 or older) currently use illicit drugs. The most commonly used illicit drug is marijuana, followed by prescription drugs (used nonmedically), cocaine, hallucinogens, inhalants, and heroin.

Sex

- 9.9% of males are illicit drug users, compared to 6.4% of females. Males are more likely to be marijuana users than females (7.9% of males, compared to 4.4% of females). Females between the ages of 12 and 17 are more likely to use prescription drugs for nonmedical purposes than males in the same age group (3.3% of females, compared to 2.5% of males).

Age

- The age group with the highest percentage of illicit drug users is young adults aged 18–20 (21.5%). Adults aged 21–25 show the second highest percentage (18.4%), followed by teens aged 16–17 (15.2%).

Race

- Mixed race individuals reported the highest rates of illicit drug use (14.7%), followed by African-Americans (10.1%), Native Americans (9.5%), Caucasians (8.2%), Pacific Islanders (7.3%), Hispanics (6.2%), and Asian Americans (3.6%).

Geography

- Rates of illicit drug use are highest in the West (9.8%), followed by the Northeast (8.2%), Midwest (7.6%), and the South (7.1%). Illicit drug use is higher in metropolitan areas than nonmetropolitan areas. For instance, 8.5% of the population in large metropolitan counties are illicit drug users, compared to 6.1% in completely rural counties.

Source: Data from *Results from the 2008 National Survey on Drug Use and Health: National Findings* by the Substance Abuse and Mental Health Services Administration, Office of Applied Studies, 2009, retrieved from http://oas.samhsa.gov/nsduh/2k8nsduh/2k8Results.cfm.

View the complete results of the 2008 national survey on drug use and health at **http://oas.samhsa.gov/nsduh/2k8nsduh/2k8Results.cfm.**

- Using the substance in larger quantities or over a longer period than intended
- Inability to cut down or control one's use of the substance
- Spending an inordinate amount of time on activities aimed at obtaining the substance, using the substance, or recovering from the substance's effects
- Sacrificing important social, occupational, or recreational activities due to the substance use
- Continuing use of the substance despite knowledge that the substance has either caused or is exacerbating a physical or psychological problem.

How the Body Processes Drugs

By definition, psychoactive drugs all **intoxicate** the brain causing physical, psychological, and behavioral changes. How quickly and to what extent intoxication occurs depends on characteristics of the user such as sex, body size, physiological makeup, and use history. Intoxication is also related to the drug's action, the dosage, and how it enters and leaves the body.

Methods of Administration

There are five basic ways that people self-administer drugs **(Table 7.1):**

- **Ingestion** is the process of swallowing and absorbing a drug through the digestive system. For example, pills and alcoholic beverages are both ingested. Ingestion is the slowest way for a chemical to reach the brain.
- **Injection** is the process of using a syringe to inject a drug into the skin (*subcutaneous injection*), muscle (*intramuscular injection*), or bloodstream (*intravenous injection*). Injecting a drug can expose a user to diseases, including HIV, hepatitis B and C, and other types of infection that can enter the body on a shared or otherwise dirty needle. Injecting a drug into a vein also sends it more quickly to the brain. As a result, the drug can deliver a quicker rush, but the high can also fade faster, often prompting the user to use again. This pattern can increase the addictive power of a drug.
- **Inhalation** is the process of breathing a drug into the lung through the mouth or nostril,

intoxicate To cause physical and psychological changes as a result of the consumption of psychoactive substances.

Table 7.1: **Common Methods of Drug Administration**

Method	Description	Typical Drugs
Ingestion	Swallowing a drug and absorbing it through the digestive system	Alcoholic beverages, pills, LSD
Injection	Using a syringe to inject a drug directly into the skin, muscle, or bloodstream	Cocaine, methamphetamine, heroin
Inhalation	Breathing a drug into the lungs through the mouth or nostrils, that is, snorting or smoking	Marijuana, tobacco, cocaine (crack), inhalants such as paint thinner or glue
Mucosal absorption	Absorbing a drug through the mucous membranes	Chewing tobacco (absorbed through the membranes in the mouth); snorted cocaine (absorbed through the membranes in the nose)
Topical administration	Applying a drug directly on to a body surface, like the skin	Nicotine patch

that is, by sniffing ("snorting") or smoking it. Like injection, inhalation increases a drug's addictive potential because it speeds drugs into the bloodstream.

- **Mucosal absorption** is the absorption of a drug through the mucous membranes. Chewing tobacco is absorbed through the mucous membranes of the mouth. Cocaine that has been snorted is absorbed through the mucous membranes of the nose.
- **Topical administration** is typified by applying a drug directly on to a body surface like the skin. A nicotine patch, which is applied directly to the skin's surface, is an example of topical administration.

How Drugs Leave the Body

The organs involved in metabolizing (breaking down and eliminating, or "clearing") drugs are the same organs that break down and eliminate nutritional waste. The liver metabolizes drug chemicals into substances that can be excreted by the bowels in stool and by the kidneys in urine. Some substances, like alcohol, are also excreted through the skin or expelled by the lungs. Elimination can also occur through exhaled breath, sweat, saliva, or in the breast milk of nursing mothers.

Physiological Impact of Drugs

How long a drug remains active in the body depends on several factors. The *distribution half-life* is the amount of time it takes a drug to move from general circulation to body tissues such as muscle and fat. This information is important for treating overdose patients and is used to estimate the amount of a chemical in a patient's circulation at a given time.[4]

Physiological responses to drugs vary widely from individual to individual. Someone who is heavyset may require a greater amount of a drug than someone who is thin to achieve a similar psychoactive effect. Sex can also be a factor—women have a greater fat-to-muscle ratio and a lower amount of water in their bodies compared to men, both of which can influence how a drug affects their bodies. Ethnicity, too, can play a role. For instance, Caucasians generally transform antipsychotic and anti-anxiety medications in the body more quickly than Asians, and show lower concentrations of these drugs in their bloodstream. As a result, they may need relatively higher doses of these drugs than Asians do.[5] Additionally, an individual's history of drug use is an important factor, as long-term use can result in a tolerance to the drug that isn't seen in first-time users.

A drug's physiological effect on the body can also be affected when two or more drugs are combined. In *additive interactions,* the

toxicity The dosage level at which a drug becomes poisonous to the body.

effect of one drug is combined with the effect of another. In *antagonistic interactions,* the effect of one drug is diminished when combined with another drug. The dosage level where the drug becomes poisonous to the body and can cause temporary or permanent damage is referred to as **toxicity.**

Commonly Abused Drugs

Many people don't think of themselves as "drug users" because they have never experimented with illegal drugs like methamphetamine or cocaine. But not all drugs are illegal, and even drugs that seem a routine part of daily life can be harmful if they are used improperly. The following section surveys a spectrum of commonly abused drugs.

Prescription and Over-the-Counter Medications

The use of prescription and over-the-counter (OTC) medications is increasing. A record 3.4 billion prescriptions were handed out in 2005—an increase of nearly 60% since 1995.[6] An estimated 81% of adults in the U.S. now take at least one prescription or OTC medication every week, and 27% take at least five.[7] Taken as directed, medications can restore and improve health and boost quality of life, but all carry risks. "Off-the-label" abuse is growing, and unwanted side effects are not uncommon.

Prescription Medications

Many people do not take prescription medicines properly. An estimated half of all prescriptions dispensed each year in the United States are not taken according to directions, and fully 96% of patients fail to ask questions about how to use their medicine.[8] The four most common types of misuse are:

- Taking the incorrect dose
- Taking the medicine at the wrong time
- Forgetting to take a dose
- Failing to take all the medicine

For financial reasons, low-income populations (such as college students) sometimes put themselves at risk for disease complications by not purchasing and using as much of a medicine as they have been advised to take. Some people start to feel better and mistakenly assume they do not need to finish their prescription. That practice has contributed to the problem of new emerging antibiotic-resistant bacteria, so-called "super germs" that can no longer be treated by current medications.

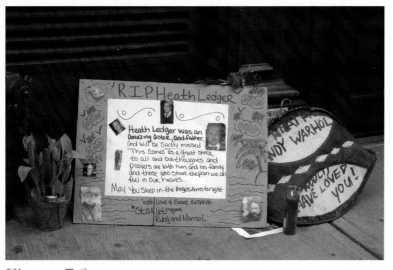

Figure 7.2 Misusing prescription drugs is dangerous. A lethal combination of prescription drugs caused the death of actor Heath Ledger.

Another serious issue is "off-the-label," nonmedical use of prescription drugs. An increasing number of non-sick college students are taking prescription drugs for psychoactive effects.[9] Some take prescription medication because it seems less harmful than taking an illicit drug. However, the nonmedical use of pain relievers was implicated in about 324,000 emergency room visits in 2006.[10] In addition, a national survey conducted by the American College Health Association found that 13.5% of college students reported using prescription drugs that were not prescribed to them.[3] The most commonly misused prescription drugs were painkillers, followed by stimulants, sedatives, antidepressants, and erectile dysfunction drugs. Misuse of prescription drugs—especially combinations of drugs—can be fatal **(Figure 7.2).**

> **View an ABC News segment on the increasing misuse and abuse of prescription drugs at www.abcnews.go.com/video/video?id=7663015.**

Over-the-Counter (OTC) Drugs

"Over-the-counter" drugs are medications available for purchase without a prescription. OTC drugs include aspirin, allergy pills, and cough or cold medications. There are now more than 700 OTC products available that contain ingredients that were available only by prescription three decades ago—some at greater dosage strength.[11]

OTC drugs pose many of the same challenges as prescription drugs. They need to be taken as directed and may interact with other medicines, herbal supplements, foods, or alcohol. Some OTC drugs are hazardous for people with certain medical conditions, such as asthma. Pregnant women should always check with a doctor before taking any OTC drug.

The U.S. Food and Drug Administration (FDA) cautions against the misuse of several common OTC medications. For example, too much acetaminophen (a common pain-relief drug, sold as Tylenol among other brand names) can lead to serious liver damage. If in-

gested with alcohol or after a long night of drinking, the risk of liver problems increases. In a review of the key studies on acetaminophen and alcohol, government researchers found that as few as four or five "extra-strength" acetaminophen pills taken over the course of a day could damage the liver if alcohol was also consumed.[12]

Cough and cold formulations can also be dangerous. In January 2008, the FDA advised against giving cough or cold medications to children under age two because "serious and potentially life-threatening side effects could occur." Side effects have included rapid heart rates, convulsions, and even death.

People tend to wrongly assume that if a little medicine is good, a lot must be better. Yet OTC medications are not meant to be taken in higher doses or for longer periods than is indicated on the label. If symptoms do not go away after a few days of using an OTC drug, it is time to see a doctor or nurse practitioner.

Marijuana

Marijuana is the most commonly used illegal drug in the United States.[2] According to the most recent National Survey on Drug Use and Health, 15.2 million Americans reported using marijuana in the past 30 days, representing about 6.1% of the population over the age of 12.[2]

marijuana The most commonly used illegal drug in the U.S.; derived from the plant *cannabis sativa*.

Marijuana (made from the plant *cannabis sativa*) grows wild and is farmed in many parts of the world. "Pot"—a dry, shredded mix of flowers, stems, seeds and leaves of the plant—is usually rolled and smoked as a cigarette (called a "joint"),

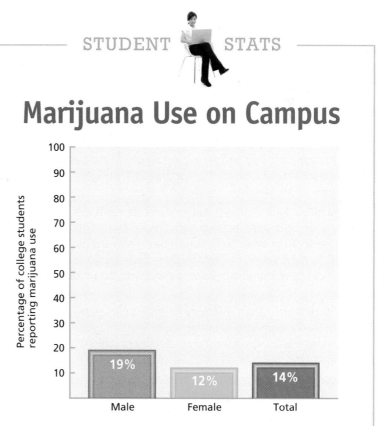

STUDENT STATS

Marijuana Use on Campus

Percentage of college students reporting marijuana use

Male: 19%
Female: 12%
Total: 14%

Source: Data from *American College Health Association National College Health Assessment (ACHA-NCHA II) Reference Group Executive Summary, Fall 2009* by the American College Health Association, 2009, retrieved from http://www.acha-ncha.org/reports_ACHA-NCHAII.html.

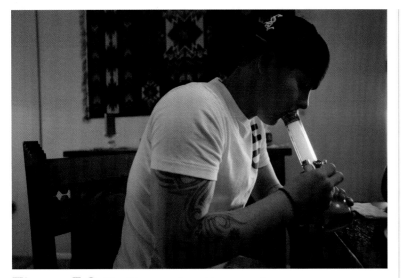

Figure 7.3 Marijuana. Smoking marijuana can cause lung damage and increase the risk of cancer.

or by using a water pipe (called a "bong") that passes the smoke through water to cool it **(Figure 7.3).** It is also sometimes mixed in food such as brownies, or brewed as a tea.

Over the years, marijuana growers have bred the plant so that pot has a much higher percentage of its psychoactive ingredient, THC (tetrahydrocannabinol) than it used to. At the same time, the strength of THC in marijuana today can vary widely, so most users cannot be sure of its strength in advance.

Effects on the Body
When you inhale THC in marijuana smoke, it takes just a few minutes to move from your lungs to your bloodstream to your brain. Ingesting marijuana from food is slower. In the brain, THC kicks off a series of cellular reactions that cause the high, essentially changing the physical and chemical balance in the brain. Ultimately, brain cells release the chemical dopamine, boosting sensations of pleasure. The heart beats faster (in some users, double the normal rate); the bronchi (large air passages in the lungs) become enlarged; and blood vessels in the eyes expand, reddening the whites of the eye. Other manifestations include dry mouth ("cotton mouth"), hunger, and sleepiness.

Users often like the drug because it makes them feel euphoric and because colors and sounds seem more intense. It can also make time seem to slow. Some report being relaxed by THC intoxication. Other short-term mental effects include confusion, lapses of memory, difficulty learning or solving problems, and reduced reaction time.

Attention, learning, and memory have all been shown to be impaired in heavy, chronic marijuana users. Students who chronically use the drug make more errors and have more difficulty processing information than those who use it just once a month.[13]

Because marijuana is usually smoked, users can end up with many of the long-term problems that tobacco smokers do. Problems may be heightened because pot smokers inhale deeply and hold the smoke in their lungs. Long-term health risks include daily cough and phlegm production, bronchitis and other respiratory problems, lung damage, impaired immune system functioning, impaired cognitive

functioning, and possibly increased risk of cancer of the respiratory tract and lungs.

Increasingly, research is finding that marijuana can be a hard habit to kick, and admissions to drug treatment centers for marijuana use have more than doubled since the early 1990s. Withdrawal symptoms can be similar to those experienced by people who stop smoking tobacco. Irritability, anger, and trouble sleeping are among the most common signs of marijuana withdrawal.

Note that there is no safe way to purchase drugs "on the street"— including marijuana. Drugs purchased through illegal dealers can be laced or "cut" with other drugs and contain impurities. They may even be sold as one drug but actually contain a different drug. Those who purchase drugs illegally for recreational use are undertaking a very serious risk to their health.

stimulants A class of drugs that stimulate the central nervous system causing acceleration of mental and physical processes in the body.

> For more information on the health effects of marijuana, visit **www.drugabuse.gov/Infofacts/marijuana.html**.

Stimulants

Stimulants are a class of drugs that stimulate the function of the central nervous system resulting in increased heart rate, higher blood pressure, and an elevated rate of mental function. Stimulants

Tainted Drugs

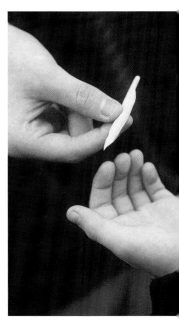

"Hi, I'm Andrea.* One Halloween, me and my friends were at a party and we got a call saying we had to pick up my friend's boyfriend. So we picked him up, and he had marijuana on him, which he offered to us. We smoked it, thinking it's her boyfriend, so it must be okay. Well, it ended up being laced with PCP and it was one of the worst things I've ever gone through. The day after that, when I woke up, I could not stop jittering. My chest felt like it was going to explode. It was a really bad experience and ultimately made me give up marijuana for good."

1: Was there any way Andrea could have known that the marijuana was laced with another drug?

2: If a friend offered you marijuana, how would you respond?

*Name changed at student's request

> **Do you have a story similar to Andrea's? Share it at www. pearsonhighered.com/choosinghealth.**

also elevate mood and increase feelings of happiness and well-being and are consequently called "uppers." Legal stimulants include nicotine, caffeine, and the prescription drug methylphenidate (marketed as Ritalin). Illegal stimulants include cocaine, amphetamines, and methamphetamine.

Caffeine

Caffeine is a central nervous system stimulant found in coffee, tea, soft drinks, chocolate, and some medications. In its pure form, caffeine is a white crystalline powder that tastes very bitter. It is the most popular mind-altering drug in the world. In the U.S., 87% of adults consume some type of caffeine regularly, many for the grand dose of energy that comes with a "grande"-sized cappuccino.[14] **Table 7.2** lists the caffeine content in some commonly consumed foods and beverages.

Effects on the Body. The effects of caffeine start in less than an hour after consumption. As the drug stimulates the body's central nervous system, users feel more alert and energetic. Caffeine can also put users in a better mood, improve their concentration, and even boost their athletic prowess and endurance.[15] However, while most people can safely drink two to four cups of coffee a day, excessive caffeine consumption can cause restlessness, anxiety, dehydration, and irritability. Caffeine can also trigger headaches and insomnia and lead to abnormal heart rhythms. Even relatively small amounts, such as a single cup of coffee, can significantly raise your blood pressure. Studies suggest that people who consume five or more cups of coffee per day may be at increased risk of coronary heart disease.[16] Pregnant women who drink a cup and a half of coffee a day may double their risk of having a miscarriage.[17]

Caffeine is physically addictive. As with other types of drugs, regular users can suffer withdrawal symptoms if they suddenly go "cold

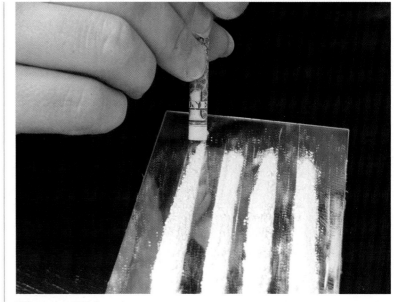

Figure 7.4 Cocaine. Cocaine use can result in heart damage, stroke, and sudden death.

caffeine A widely used stimulant found in coffee, tea, soft drinks, chocolate, and some medicines.

cocaine A potent and addictive stimulant derived from leaves of the coca shrub.

turkey." Withdrawal usually lasts for 2 to 9 days and may include headaches, anxiety, fatigue, drowsiness, and depression.

Cocaine

Cocaine is derived from South American coca leaves, which people have ingested for thousands of years. "Coke" refers to cocaine in its fine white powder form **(Figure 7.4)**. It is inhaled (snorted) or dissolved in water and injected intravenously. *Freebase cocaine* is a rock-like crystal that is heated so that its vapors can be smoked (inhaled). It is also known as "crack," which refers to the crackling sound that freebase makes when heated. Crack became extremely popular and a major drug of abuse in inner cities during the 1980s because it gives the user a high in less than 10 seconds and because it costs much less than powder cocaine.

Effects on the Body. Cocaine is a strong central nervous system stimulant that, like THC, triggers the release of the neurotransmitter dopamine, which is associated in the brain with pleasure. Almost immediately, cocaine use causes a rush of euphoria. These effects typically disappear within a few minutes or a few hours. To continue the euphoria, users must continue taking the drug.

Taken in small amounts, cocaine usually makes the user feel energetic and mentally alert. It can also temporarily reduce the need for food and sleep. While some people find it helps them perform simple physical and mental tasks more quickly, others notice the opposite effect. Paranoia is also common. Continued use of cocaine often leads to tolerance, so that higher doses and more frequent binges are needed to derive the same level of pleasure.

Some of cocaine's more common side effects include loss of appetite, increased heart rate, increased blood pressure, and increased respiration. They also include chest pain, blurred vision, fever, muscle spasms, and convulsions. Cocaine use, especially long-term use, may cause abnormal heart rhythms, seizures, heart damage, strokes, abdominal pain and nausea, coma, and death.

Table 7.2: **Caffeine Content of Selected Foods and Beverages**

Food/Beverage/Pill	Caffeine (milligrams)
Generic brewed coffee, 8 oz.	95–200
NoDoz, maximum strength, 1 tablet	200
Excedrin, extra strength, 2 tablets	130
Rockstar, 8 oz.	80
Red Bull, 8.3 oz.	76
Starbucks single espresso, 1 oz.	58–75
Mountain Dew, 12 oz.	54
Black tea, 8 oz.	40–120
Coca Cola Classic, 12 oz.	35
Nestea iced tea, 12 oz.	26
Generic decaffeinated brewed coffee, 8 oz.	2–12
Hershey's milk chocolate bar, 1.55 oz.	9

Source: Data from *Caffeine Content for Coffee, Tea, Soda and More,* by the Mayo Clinic, 2009, retrieved from http://www.mayoclinic.com/health/caffeine/AN01211.

Repeated snorting of cocaine can lead to nosebleeds, a hindered sense of smell, and a chronically runny nose. Ingesting cocaine can reduce blood flow, which can cause severe bowel gangrene. Injection can trigger allergic reactions and put users at risk for blood-borne diseases such as HIV and hepatitis. Injections also leave puncture marks called "tracks" on the forearms or other sites of injection. Another hazard of the powder is that dealers often dilute it with cornstarch, talcum powder, or sugar, or with other stimulants such as amphetamines.

Mixing cocaine and alcohol is especially dangerous. Taken together, the two drugs are converted by the body into cocaethylene, which is more toxic than either drug alone, and can cause death.

> Listen to a podcast about how a mechanism in the brain contributes to cocaine cravings in users: www.drugabuse.gov/newsroom/Podcasts/ 20080703.html.

Amphetamines

Amphetamines have a chemical structure similar to adrenaline and noradrenalin, stimulants produced by the human body. They stimulate the central nervous system, increasing a person's sense of alertness, decreasing appetite and the need for sleep, and enhancing physical performance. They also induce feelings of well-being and euphoria.

Adderall as a Study Aid?

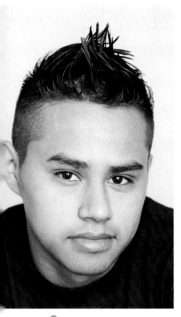

"Hi, I'm Wilmer. I'm a junior, majoring in business. I have a lot of family stuff going on—my mom lost her job, so I've started bagging groceries to help out with bills. I'm also taking 6 classes this semester because I had to go on medical leave for a broken leg last fall and want to catch up for my major. I usually start studying around 9 at night and I get sleepy by midnight, even though I always have more to do. My roommate takes Adderall and says it helps you stay up. I have other friends who take it and I'm tempted to try it. It seems like it's really common, and there don't seem to be any side effects. What's the harm?"

1: Is Wilmer right that there are no side effects or risks associated with Adderall?

2: Wilmer's stressed out and overworked. What could he do to improve his situation *without* resorting to taking drugs?

> **Do you have a story similar to Wilmer's? Share your story at www. pearsonhighered.com/choosinghealth.**

CONSUMER CORNER

Can Drugs Make You Smarter?

In recent years, there has been an increase in college students' use of prescription medications such as Adderall, Ritalin, Concerta, and Provigil (drugs intended for the treatment of attention-deficit disorders) as enhancement drugs to aid in concentration and study. Users believe these drugs help keep them alert and focused for extended periods of time, allowing them to study for much longer than without the drugs. Dr. Anjan Chatterjee, a University of Pennsylvania neurologist, coined the term "cosmetic neurology" to describe the practice of taking medications intended for specific medical conditions as cognitive enhancers.

How do these drugs work? They are amphetamine-based and act on the brain's reward system by increasing levels of dopamine. Although they can measurably increase concentration and motivation, there is a dark side to their use: They can cause nervousness, headaches, sleeplessness, decreased appetite, and increased heart rate, among other side effects. These drugs are also highly addictive. An FDA warning on Adderall's label states that "amphetamines have a high potential for abuse" and can lead to dependence.

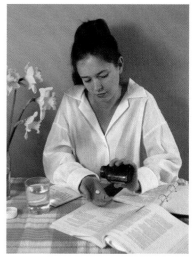

"Off-the-label" use of amphetamines like Ritalin and Adderall are an increasing problem on campus (see **Consumer Corner: Can Drugs Make You Smarter?**). Between 1993 and 2004, the percentage of college students abusing prescription stimulants nearly doubled (the increase was 93%).[1] More than 225,000 students were taking them for nonmedical reasons.[1]

Effects on the Body. The acute effects of amphetamines resemble those of cocaine. For 8–24 hours after the drug enters the body, breathing rate, heart rate, body temperature, and blood pressure increase. Users who are more experienced develop feelings of euphoria, decreased appetite, and a boost in alertness and energy. Adverse and potentially lethal changes can occur and may cause convulsions, chest pains, or stroke. Even healthy young athletes have suffered heart attacks after using amphetamines. Because amphetamines increases blood pressure and heart rate, long-term use can increase the risk of heart-related illness.

Amphetamines are addictive. Many users need to take amphetamines again and again to avoid the "down" they begin to

amphetamines Central nervous system stimulants that are chemically similar to the natural stimulants adrenaline and noradrenalin.

feel when the drug wears off. Eventually, users must take a larger amount to get the same effect. People who abruptly stop taking amphetamines experience a variety of physical effects, including fatigue, irritability, and depression.

Methamphetamine

The highly addictive **methamphetamine** is a chemical similar to amphetamines, but it is much more potent, longer lasting, and more harmful to the central nervous system. Methamphetamine can be prescribed medically for ADHD, extreme obesity, and narcolepsy. However, because of its high potential for abuse, it is legal only by a one-time, nonrefillable prescription. Most methamphetamine that sells on the street is made by small illegal labs from household materials. It can be ingested, injected, smoked, or snorted. "Crystal meth" refers to methamphetamine in its clear, chunky crystal form. Methamphetamine use has declined in recent years. Between 2006 and 2008, the number of methamphetamine users in the U.S. decreased by over half.[2] That said, more than 300,000 people in the U.S. still use methamphetamine.[2]

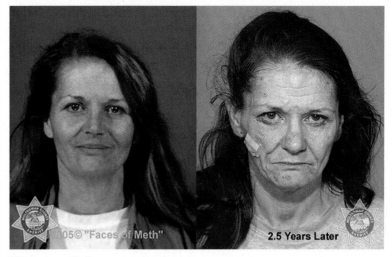

Figure 7.5 Methamphetamine. Methamphetamine use can take a dramatic physical toll.

Effects on the Body. Like many other psychoactive drugs, methamphetamine enhances mood and body movement by causing the brain to flood with dopamine. Smoking the drug causes an intense rush. Snorting it produces a longer high, which can last for more than a day. Users feel pleasantly aroused.

Even small amounts of methamphetamine can have big effects on the body. Methamphetamine can cause a rapid or irregular heartbeat, boost blood pressure, and reduce appetite. Other side effects include irritability, anxiety, insomnia, confusion, and tremors. High doses can elevate body temperature to dangerous or lethal levels, as well as cause convulsions. Cardiovascular collapse and death are not uncommon. Chronic abusers may experience aggressiveness, anorexia, memory loss, hallucinations, and a paranoia that sometimes causes homicidal or suicidal thoughts. Some users hallucinate that bugs are crawling all over them and therefore scratch themselves repeatedly.

Chronic methamphetamine use significantly changes how the brain functions. Long-term use can reduce motor speed and impair verbal learning.[23] Research also suggests that methamphetamine may alter areas of the brain associated with emotion and memory, which could account for many of the emotional and cognitive problems that have been observed in abusers.[23] Users develop tolerance, needing more of the drug to get the same high.

Over time, some methamphetamine users begin to develop what is known as "meth mouth"—severely stained teeth that appear to be rotting away or falling out. Methamphetamine can also damage tissues and blood vessels, promote acne, and slow down the healing of sores. Open sores, in fact, are a hallmark of methamphetamine use.

Despite such serious side effects, users often find themselves hooked **(Figure 7.5).** The addiction is very difficult to treat, and for

methamphetamine A highly addictive and dangerous stimulant that is chemically similar to amphetamine, but more potent and harmful.

hallucinogens Drugs that alter perception and are capable of causing auditory and visual hallucinations.

LSD (lysergic acid diethylamide) A powerful hallucinogen manufactured from lysergic acid, a substance found in a fungus that grows on rye and other grains.

View "before" and "after" images of people who became addicted to methamphetamine at www.facesofmeth.us.

chronic users withdrawal includes physical symptoms such as depression, anxiety, fatigue, aggression, and paranoia, as well as intense craving for the drug.

Injecting methamphetamine increases risk of contracting HIV, hepatitis, and other infectious diseases commonly spread through dirty needles. In individuals who already have HIV, health and cognition can decline more rapidly from use of methamphetamine, compared with HIV-positive patients who do not use the drug.

Methamphetamine labs affect the environment, too. For every pound of the drug produced clandestinely, an estimated five to six pounds of hazardous waste is created.[18] The waste can leave farmland or forests unsafe and useless until thoroughly cleaned up by hazmat teams. Several states now require that prospective home buyers and tenants be informed about residences that once housed a "meth lab."

Hallucinogens

Hallucinogens are so named because they cause hallucinations in addition to altering perceptions, thoughts, and mood. People who use hallucinogenic drugs often report seeing "real" things and hearing "real" sounds that others know do not exist. Some hallucinogens come from plants, like the button-shaped top of the mescal cactus that produces mescaline, and certain types of mushrooms. But other, manufactured hallucinogens can be more potent.

LSD

LSD (lysergic acid diethylamide) is one of the strongest moodaltering chemicals. Commonly known as "acid," it is derived from lysergic acid, which is found in a fungus called *ergot,* which grows on rye and other grains. Its hallucinogenic effects were discovered in 1943 when the scientist who first synthesized it accidentally swallowed some. LSD was heavily promoted in the 1960s by counterculture icon Timothy Leary who famously said, "Turn on, tune in, drop out." Liquid LSD is commonly dried into blotter paper and ingested by holding the paper in the mouth. LSD "trips" saw a resurgence among teens in the 1990s.

Effects on the Body. The effects of LSD are unpredictable in that they depend on the amount taken, the user's personality, and the surroundings in which the drug is used. First effects are often felt within 30 to 90 minutes, as the user moves from one emotion to another or feels several emotions simultaneously. A heavy dose can cause delusions and visual hallucinations. Physical changes include dilated pupils; increased body temperature, heart rate, and blood pressure; sweating; sleeplessness; and tremors.

Sometimes LSD users have "flashbacks," meaning they relive parts of a previous LSD experience even long after the drug has worn off. Flashbacks may occur a few days or even a few years after actual use.

LSD is not addictive, but some users grow tolerant, needing progressively larger doses to reach a previous level of high.

PCP

The street names for **PCP** (phencyclidine) include "angel dust," "killer weed," "embalming fluid," and "rocket fuel." As these names suggest, the drug can have volatile, bizarre, and fatal effects. Originally developed in the 1950s as an anesthetic, it was discontinued because of many side effects. Today, street PCP comes from illegal labs, its color ranging from tan to brown and its consistency from powdery to gummy. Users usually apply it to a smokable, leafy material such as parsley, mint, or marijuana. Many people take in PCP unknowingly when someone else adds it to marijuana, LSD, or methamphetamine.

Effects on the Body. PCP is a **dissociative drug,** meaning it produces feelings of detachment or dissociation from a person's surroundings. Dissociative drugs act by changing the distribution of a glutamate (like dopamine) in the brain. Glutamate is responsible, in part, for a person's memory and perception of pain. While some users say PCP makes them feel stronger—or at least gives them the perception of strength, power, and invulnerability—others have very bad reactions, including confusion, agitation, and delirium. To date, no one knows why reactions vary so much. Other effects can include shallow breathing, flushing, sweating, numbness of the extremities, and poor muscular coordination. In adolescents, use may interfere with hormones related to growth.

At high doses, the health risks become severe. Effects can range from nausea and vomiting to blurred vision and drooling. Seizures, coma, and death also occur. PCP is known for triggering violent behavior in people, and has been associated with many trips to hospital emergency rooms. Suicides associated with PCP have also been reported. Symptoms such as memory loss, difficulties with speech, and depression can last for up to a year after taking PCP.

Psilocybin (Magic Mushrooms)

Psilocybin, also known as "magic mushrooms" or "shrooms," is popular at raves, clubs, and in-

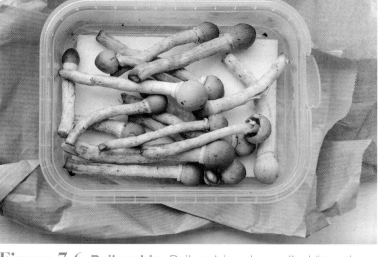

Figure 7.6 Psilocybin. Psilocybin, also called "magic mushrooms," induces hallucinations and can cause psychosis in some users.

creasingly on college campuses **(Figure 7.6).** This hallucinogen is found in certain mushrooms, available fresh or dried, and grown in South America, Mexico, and parts of the United States. The mushrooms are often brewed as a tea or eaten with foods that mask their bitter flavor.

Effects on the Body. Within 20 minutes of ingestion, users begin to notice changes, usually hallucinations and an inability to separate fantasy from reality. Panic attacks can also occur. The effects usually fade away after six hours. Psilocybin is not known to be addictive, and there seem to be no withdrawal effects. But serious risks include the onset of psychosis in susceptible users, and poisoning if another, deadlier mushroom (of which there are many) has been confused with the psilocybin mushroom.

"Club Drugs"

The National Institute on Drug Abuse uses the term **club drugs** to refer to LSD and four other psychoactive substances: MDMA (ecstasy), GHB, Rohypnol, and ketamine. These four drugs were first popularized by young adults at raves. They have begun to fall out of favor, but still attract some partygoers by their relatively low prices. More than 17,000 emergency room visits each year are a result of using club drugs.[19]

MDMA (Ecstasy)

Methylenedioxymethamphetamine (**MDMA**), commonly known as ecstasy, is a synthetic drug chemically similar to methamphetamine **(Figure 7.7).** Ecstasy is less popular now than it was during the heyday of raves, but it is still the drug of choice for some partygoers looking for mood enhancement and an energy boost. Ecstasy comes in tablets, often colorful round pills

PCP (phencyclidine) A dangerous synthetic hallucinogen that reduces and distorts sensory input and can unpredictably cause both euphoria and dysphoria.

dissociative drug A medication that distorts perceptions of sight and sound and produces feelings of detachment from the environment and self.

psilocybin A hallucinogenic substance obtained from certain types of mushrooms that are indigenous to tropical regions of South America.

club drugs Illicit substances, including MDMA (ecstasy), GHB, and ketamine that are most commonly encountered at nightclubs and raves.

MDMA (methylenedioxymethamphetamine) A synthetic drug, commonly called "ecstasy," that works as both a stimulant and hallucinogen.

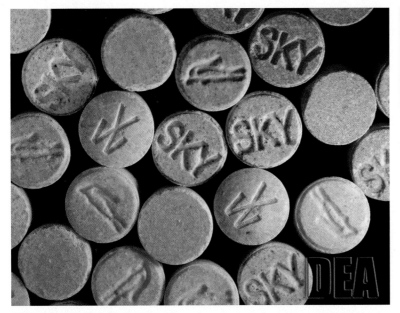

Figure 7.7 MDMA (Ecstasy). Ecstasy use can cause anxiety, confusion, and paranoia. Coupled with dehydration, it can also result in fatal organ failure.

imprinted with smiley faces, peace signs, and hearts. It is also known as "E", "X," and "XTC."

Effects on the Body. Typically, an ingested tablet takes about 15 minutes to enter the bloodstream and reach the brain. Ecstasy produces feelings of self-confidence, peacefulness, empathy, and increased energy. About 45 minutes later, the user feels the peak of the high. Some users then "bump" (take another tablet). The effects of a single tablet can last for 3 to 6 hours.

Ecstasy's negative effects are similar to those of amphetamines and cocaine. Psychological effects include confusion, sleep problems, anxiety, drug craving, and paranoia. More distinctly physical effects can include nausea, blurred vision, chills, sweating, muscle tension, rapid eye movement, involuntary teeth clenching, faintness, and increases in heart rate and blood pressure. Because the stimulant effects enable users to dance for long periods of time, many have suffered dehydration and heatstroke. Heatstroke can lead to kidney, liver, or cardiovascular failure, and can be fatal. In addition, regular and repeated use can cause depression, anxiety, and memory problems that last for up to a week. Studies have shown that some regular users of MDMA have significant memory loss and that chronic users perform more poorly on cognitive tasks than non-users.[24]

> **View the documentary "Ecstasy Rising: The History of MDMA" at http://current.com/news/90765380_ecstasy-rising-the-history-of-mdma-by-peter-jennings-abc-news.htm.**

GHB

For years, a central nervous system depressant nicknamed **GHB** (gamma-hydroxybutyric acid) was sold over-the-counter in health food stores throughout the U.S. Bodybuilders used GHB to help reduce fat and build muscle. Today, however, GHB is a controlled substance and is often referred to as a "date rape drug" because of its use as a substance commonly slipped into drinks in order to make victims unconscious and vulnerable. People also ingest GHB for its euphoric effects and for the perception of increased libido and sociability. Ingested usually as a liquid (often with alcohol), GHB is generally colorless, tasteless, and odorless.

Effects on the Body. Low doses of GHB can cause drowsiness, dizziness, nausea, and vision problems; higher doses are associated with seizures, respiratory distress, and comas. GHB is addictive, and users who try to kick the habit often experience insomnia, anxiety, tremors, and sweating.

Rohypnol (Roofies)

Rohypnol is a drug that induces sedative effects similar to those of Valium. Used legally in Latin America and Europe as a short-term treatment for insomnia, at high doses it can cause unconsciousness. Rohypnol has never been approved for medical use in the United States. Doctors cannot prescribe it, and pharmacists cannot sell it.

Effects on the Body. Rohypnol can cause decreased blood pressure, drowsiness, visual disturbances, dizziness, and confusion. It can also cause partial amnesia, rendering users unable to remember certain events that they experienced while under the influence of the drug. It is often called a "date rape drug" because it can be used to incapacitate unsuspecting victims. As a result, sexual assault victims may not be able to clearly recall the assault, the assailant, or the events surrounding the assault.

Because of increasing reports about the misuse of GHB and Rohypnol, Congress passed the Drug-Induced Rape Prevention and Punishment Act of 1996. This legislation increased the federal penalties for using any controlled substance to aid in a sexual assault.

Ketamine

Ketamine, commonly known as "special K," is a rapid-acting anesthetic most commonly used on animals. It is also snorted or swallowed by humans for an "out-of-body" or "near-death" experience known as a "K-Hole." Ketamine is odorless and tasteless, and so can be undetectable when added to beverages.

Effects on the Body. Ketamine is chemically similar to PCP. Like PCP, ketamine can cause a dream-like state and hallucinations, but is less associated with confusion, irrationality, and violent behavior. But the risk isn't light. Low doses of ketamine often result in impaired attention, learning ability, and memory. In high doses, it can cause delirium, amnesia, high blood pressure, depression, and severe respiratory problems.

Inhalants

Psychoactive **inhalants** include more than 1,000 common household items, such as paint, glue, and felt-tip markers, which people sniff in order to get high. They are cheap, legal, and easy to buy. Examples of inhalants include:

- **Solvents** (liquids in which chemicals are dissolved). Paint thinners or removers, gasoline, glue, dry-cleaning

GHB (gamma-hydroxybutyric acid) A central nervous system depressant known as a "date rape drug" because of its use to impair potential victims of sexual assault.

Rohypnol (roofies) A powerful sedative known as a "date rape drug" because of its use to impair potential victims of sexual assault.

ketamine An anesthetic that can cause hallucinations and a dream-like state; commonly known as "special K."

inhalants Chemical vapors that, when inhaled, produce mind-altering effects.

fluids, correction fluids, the ink in felt-tipped pens, electronic contact cleaners.

- **Aerosols** (particles of a liquid or solid that are suspended in a gas). Spray paints, hair or deodorant sprays, vegetable oil sprays, aerosol computer cleaning products, fabric protector sprays.
- **Gases.** Butane lighters, propane tanks, whipped cream dispensers, refrigerant gases, ether, chloroform, halothane, nitrous oxide ("laughing gas").
- **Nitrites** (a type of chemical compound that includes the element nitrogen). Various products often bottled and labeled as "video head cleaner," "room odorizer," "leather cleaner," or "liquid aroma."

Effects on the Body

Most psychoactive inhalants work somewhat like anesthetics, slowing down the body's functions. Inhalants can cause intoxication, usually for just a few minutes. By repeated sniffing, users extend the high for several hours. At first, inhalants make people feel slightly stimulated. After repeated inhalations, they can feel less inhibited but also less in control.

Health risks vary by type of inhalant. Some inhalants can lead to unconsciousness. Butane, propane, and the chemicals in aerosols have all been linked to what is known as "sudden sniffing death"—fatal heart failure within minutes of repeated inhalations. Some young users also cover their heads with a paper or plastic bag to inhale a higher concentration of chemical. This can backfire, as the practice can cause suffocation.

Chronic abuse of solvents can also cause severe damage to the brain, liver, and kidneys. Other side effects include hearing loss, limb spasms, bone marrow damage, and blood oxygen depletion.

Inhalant abuse often starts at an early age. According to a recent national survey, 28% of eighth graders reported experimenting with inhalants.[20] Some adolescents turn to inhalants because they are easier to obtain than alcohol. But inhalants are much more dangerous: Long-term users risk neurological and cognitive dysfunction, and may experience both psychological and social problems.

Depressants

Depressants (also known as "downers") include alcohol, barbiturates, and benzodiazepines. All are substances that depress the central nervous system and slow the brain's activity. The effect is a drowsy or calm feeling that can benefit people suffering from anxiety, sleep disorders, or pain. When improperly used, however, depressants can result in addiction, health problems, and even death.

Barbiturates and Benzodiazepines

Barbiturates are a type of central nervous system depressant often prescribed to induce sleep. They were extremely popular in the early 20th century, and have been used as sedatives, hypnotics, anesthetics, and anticonvulsants. Barbiturate sedation can range from mild and short-term to severe and long-term (inducing coma.) Because of their side effects, potential for abuse, and safety

concerns, fewer than 10% of all depressant prescriptions in the United States are for barbiturates.

Benzodiazepines are medications commonly prescribed to treat anxiety and panic attacks. They were first marketed in the 1960s and have become the depressant of choice in many medical practices. Considered safer and less addictive than barbiturates, they now account for about one in every five prescriptions for controlled substances.[25] They are most commonly used to sedate, induce sleep, relieve anxiety and muscle spasms, and help prevent seizures. More than a dozen benzodiazepines are approved for use in the United States, including lorazepam (Ativan), alprazolam (Xanax), diazepam (Valium), midazolam (Versed), and chlordiazepoxide (Librium).

Effects on the Body. People who take benzodiazepines to get high experience reduced inhibition and impaired judgment. Small doses can induce calmness and muscle relaxation; larger doses can slur speech, impair judgment, and hinder motor coordination. Benzodiazepines are not usually prescribed for long-term use. Symptoms of chronic use include memory loss, irritability, and changes in alertness. Long-term use can cause amnesia, hostility, irritability, and disturbing dreams. Very high doses of benzodiazepines can lead to respiratory distress, coma, and death.

Long-term users can develop tolerance and physical dependence. Withdrawal can be dangerous. Because depressants work by slowing the brain's activity, abruptly ending long-term use can cause the brain to race out of control. Insomnia and anxiety—the same symptoms that may have prompted a person to use these drugs in the first place—are common. Long-term users may also experience tremors and weakness upon withdrawal. More severe withdrawal can include seizures and delirium. Hospitalization may be required to ease and get through withdrawal. Anyone who is dependent on barbiturates or benzodiazepines should seek medical treatment before giving them up, to reduce the risk of seizures and death.

Another type of depressant is alcohol, which we will discuss in detail in Chapter 8.

depressants Substances that depress the activity of the central nervous system including barbiturates, benzodiazepines, and alcohol.

barbiturates A type of central nervous system depressant often prescribed to induce sleep.

benzodiazepines Medications commonly prescribed to treat anxiety and panic attacks.

opioids (narcotics) Drugs derived from opium or synthetic drugs that have similar sleep-inducing, pain-reducing effects.

heroin The most widely abused of opioids; typically sold as a white or brown powder or as a sticky black substance known as "black tar heroin."

Opioids

The opium poppy *Papaver somniferum* has a long history as the raw material of the type of drugs known as **opioids,** sometimes called *narcotics*. A milky fluid found in the unripe seedpods of its flower is drained and dried to produce the pain reliever known as *opium*. Literally tons of opioids are legally imported into the United States every year and medically prescribed, mainly for reducing pain. Prescription opioids include morphine, codeine, hydrocodone (Vicodin), and oxycodone (marketed under the brand name OxyContin, Percodan, and Percocet).

Heroin

The fastest-acting and most abused opiate is **heroin,** an illegal, highly addictive drug **(Figure 7.8).** Heroin is typically sold as a white or brown powder, or as a sticky black substance known as "black tar heroin." Heroin is known on the street as "smack," "H," and "junk," and is usually injected directly into a vein, though it can also be smoked. About

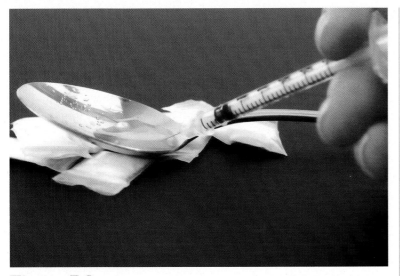

Figure 7.8 Heroin. Heroin users can develop collapsed veins, infections, and liver disease.

114,000 people in the U.S. try heroin for the first time each year. Relative to users of other drugs, heroin users tend to be older when they start, at a mean age of 23.[2]

Prescription Opioids

Also of growing concern is the nonmedical use of prescription opioids. An estimated 5.2 million people in the U.S. over the age of 12 reported misusing a prescription pain reliever over the previous year, with people aged 18 to 25 most likely to do so.[21] Between 1993 and 2005, there was a 343% increase in the percentage of students reporting they had abused legal opioids like Percocet, Vicodin, and OxyContin in the past month.[1]

Effects on the Body. Opioids attach to proteins in the brain, spinal cord, and gastrointestinal tract and block the perception of pain. They can also induce euphoria by affecting the brain region responsible for our perception of pleasure. Morphine is often given to patients before or after surgery to alleviate severe pain, whereas codeine is used for milder analgesia (pain relief) or serious coughs.

When taken as directed, prescription opioids can manage pain effectively. Side effects can include drowsiness, nausea, and constipation. If taken in a large enough dose, however, prescription opioids can result in respiratory depression or even death. The medications are not meant to be used with other substances that depress the central nervous system such as alcohol, antihistamines, barbiturates or benzodiazepines, as the combinations increase the risk of life-threatening respiratory distress.

Long-term use or misuse can lead to physical dependence and withdrawal symptoms if use is suddenly stopped. Withdrawal symptoms include restlessness, insomnia, diarrhea, vomiting, and involuntary leg movements.

Table 7.3 provides a summary of commonly abused drugs, their intoxication effects, and the health risks of using them.

Prevention and Treatment

Only 16% of the 7.5 million people in the U.S. who need drug abuse treatment receive it.[2] According to a national survey, lack of health-care insurance and not being ready to stop using were the top two reasons given for not receiving treatment.[2]

Preventing Drug Abuse

In 1920, a constitutional amendment prohibited alcohol for consumption on U.S. soil. What was then called a "noble experiment"

Table 7.3: **Commonly Abused Drugs**

Category	Representative Drugs	Method of Administration	Intoxication Effects & Health Risks
Cannabis	Marijuana (street names: pot, dope, weed, grass, joint, reefer)	Inhaled or ingested	Effects: Psychoactive agent THC causes a sense of euphoria. Heart rate increases, bronchi enlarge, blood vessels expand. Risks: Addiction, impaired cognition, lung damage, increased cancer risk
Stimulants	Cocaine (street names: crack, rock, blow, C, coke, snow)	Inhaled or injected	Effects: Derived from coca leaves, this drug first produces feelings of increased energy and euphoria. Heart rate and blood pressure increase, appetite drops. Risks: Addiction, irritability, anxiety, paranoid or violent behavior, damage to heart, brain, and other vital organs
	Amphetamines (street names: speed, uppers, crank)	Inhaled, ingested, injected	Effects: This large, varied group of synthetic drugs improve mood and alertness. Heart rate and blood pressure increase. Risks: Addiction, restlessness, appetite suppression, hallucinations, erratic or violent behavior
	Methamphetamines (street names: meth, crystal, ice, glass, tina) *Shown at left*	Inhaled, ingested, injected	Effects: A common form of amphetamine, this highly addictive drug quickly produces a sense of euphoria followed by a dramatic drop in emotion and energy as the drug wears off. Risks: Addiction, appetite suppression, dental damage, brain damage, psychosis, paranoia, aggression

(continued)

Table 7.3: **Commonly Abused Drugs** (continued)

Category	Representative Drugs	Method of Administration	Intoxication Effects & Health Risks
Hallucinogens	LSD (street names: acid, blotter) *Shown at left*	Ingested	Effects: Effective even at very low doses, this drug is known for producing powerful hallucinations. Other effects include nausea, increased heart rate, tremors, and headaches. Risks: Shortened attention span, miscarriage and pre-term labor in pregnant women, paranoia, disordered thinking
	PCP (street name: angel dust)	Inhaled, ingested, injected	Effects: This synthetic drug can lead to both euphoria and extreme unhappiness, and can also produce hallucinations. Risks: Slurred speech, poor coordination, vomiting, loss of sensitivity to pain, nausea, vomiting, coma, violent behavior, coma, and even death
	Psilocybin (street names: shrooms, magic mushrooms)	Ingested	Effects: This group of mushrooms, if ingested, has effects similar to that of LSD. Effects last for up to six hours. Risks: Paranoia, disordered thinking, nausea, erratic behavior
Club Drugs	MDMA (street names: ecstasy, E, X, XTC)	Ingested	Effects: This synthetic drug creates feelings of warmth and friendliness, and also increases heart rate and blood pressure. Risks: Hallucinations, brain damage, disordered thinking, disturbed sleep. Extremely dangerous if mixed with alcohol.
	GHB (street name: G)	Ingested	Effects: A central nervous system depressant that disrupts memory and can lead to unconsciousness. Risks: Temporary amnesia, nausea, vomiting, seizures, memory loss, hallucinations, coma
	Rohypnol (street name: roofies)	Ingested	Effects: This drug is a powerful tranquilizer that slows physical and mental responses, and is the best known of the so-called "date rape" drugs. Risks: Temporary amnesia, slowed physical and mental reactions, semi-consciousness, unconsciousness
	Ketamine (street names: K, special K) *Shown at left*	Inhaled or injected	Effects: Used legally as an anesthetic for animals, this drug produces hallucinations. Risks: Sensory distortion, disordered thinking , sensory detachment, impaired attention, delirium
Inhalants	Solvents (e.g., paint thinner), aerosols (e.g. spray paint), gases (e.g. nitrous oxide), nitrites (e.g. leather cleaner)	Inhaled	Effects: Found in ordinary household products, these substances can produce a feeling of being "high" or drunk. Risks: Dizziness, impaired speech, impaired physical coordination, vomiting, hallucinations, loss of consciousness, death
Depressants	Barbiturates (street name: barbs, downers)	Ingested or injected	Effects: This group of drugs slows the functions of the central nervous system and is legally prescribed for anxiety and insomnia. Risks: Slowed pulse and breathing, slurred speech, impaired memory, addiction, sleep problems, impaired
	Benzodiazepines (street names: downers, benzos) *Shown at left*	Ingested or injected	Effects: This subset of barbiturates function as tranquilizers, and includes common medications such as Valium. Risks: Same as for other barbiturates
Opioids	Heroin (street names: smack, H, brown sugar, junk, horse) *Shown at left*	Injected or inhaled	Effects: This depressant produces a feeling of drowsiness, dreaminess, and euphoria, and can also lead to dramatic mood swings. Risks: Addiction, cardiovascular damage, respiratory illnesses, internal infections, death
	Prescription opioids (street names: Oxy, Captain Cody)	Ingested	Effects: This group of drugs produces feelings of sleepiness, dreaminess, and a reduced sensitivity to pain. Risks: Addiction, dangerous interactions with other drugs, nausea, vomiting, lack of physical coordination

ended in failure in 1933; alcohol consumption did fall at the beginning of Prohibition, but subsequently rose again. Since that time, government prevention efforts have tended to focus on reducing the supply of illicit drugs on U.S. streets, but unfortunately, these efforts have done little to curb the global drug trade. The government has also spent millions of dollars on public awareness campaigns meant to discourage drug use, but the effectiveness of these campaigns is inconclusive.

In an effort to discourage people from using drugs—and to catch those who do—some schools, hospitals, and other workplaces conduct *random drug testing*. This process usually involves taking a urine sample and testing for such common drugs as marijuana, cocaine, amphetamines, and opiates. Despite being controversial, random drug testing has become increasingly popular in the United States and is conducted on many middle and high school campuses.

None of this contradicts the obvious—that at an individual level, the best strategy for avoiding drug abuse is to not use drugs in the first place. Like everyone else, students need to be their own personal advocates. Just as you surely have been advised to "think before you drink," health experts encourage you to consider all of the ramifications before you light up or shoot up. Do you understand the short- and long-term health risks involved in drug use? Is a temporary high worth the risk of addiction, health problems, and even death? It's important to recognize that the risk of drug abuse increases greatly during times of transition, such as changing schools or moving.[22] If you find yourself tempted to use drugs—or are already using them—seek help. Also, remember that there are many healthful ways to achieve "natural highs," including exercise, spending time with people you love, and pursuing non-drug related activities that you find exciting and pleasurable.

relapse The return to an addictive substance or behavior after a period of conscious abstinence.

residential programs Live-in drug treatment centers.

12-step programs Addiction recovery self-help programs based on the principles of Alcoholics Anonymous.

intervention A technique used by family and friends of an addict to encourage the addict to seek help for a drug problem.

Treatment for Drug Dependence

Historically, drug abuse in the United States was seen as more of a moral problem than as a public health problem. The legacy of that stance is that arrest and punishment took precedence over placing drug users into treatment programs. However, courts now often try to strike a balance between punishment and the goal of recovery. Many people now enter drug treatment without ever coming into contact with the legal system.

The long-term goal of drug treatment programs, of course, is to get people off harmful drugs for good. But programs also aim to bring about positive short-term effects, including improving a person's ability to function and minimizing the health and social risks of addiction. Programs move through stages of *detoxification*, *treatment* per se, and steps to minimize chances of **relapse** (returning to abuse after a period of conscious abstinence). A program may require substitute medication such as methadone or buprenorphine, behavioral therapy, or a combination of these.

Addiction is considered a chronic, recurring illness, and abusers often repeat stints of treatment before they reach abstinence. Some people have better luck with **residential programs,** residing at a treatment center and away from old habits and social circles for weeks or months at a time. Others have embraced **12-step programs,** such as Alcoholics Anonymous or Narcotics Anonymous. The concept behind these organizations is simple: Men and women come together to share their problems with drugs or alcohol and give strength and hope to each other. The 12 steps take addicts through a process of self-growth, such as asking them to admit they have no control over their addiction and to make amends to all the people they have harmed.

Often, addicts do not realize they have a problem or that it is interfering with their lives. In such cases, friends and family may stage what is called an **intervention,** an organized attempt by an individ-

☺ *Practical Strategies for Health*

What Are the Signs of Drug Addiction?

How can you tell if you or someone you care about has an addiction? Look for the following signs:

- **Compulsion.** Does the person have an obsession with doing drugs and getting high?

- **Loss of control.** Does the person have a pattern of behaving recklessly, such as missing class because of drug use?

- **Negative consequences.** Does the person have a pattern of continuing a destructive behavior despite negative effects such as academic failure, financial ruin, injury or illness, arrest, or poor relationships with others?

- **Denial.** Does the person fail to recognize or acknowledge that the addiction is causing problems?

An excellent resource for helping a loved one with a drug addiction is the Partnership for a Drug-Free America website at www.drugfree.org, where you will find articles, information about treatment programs, fact sheets, personal stories, and more.

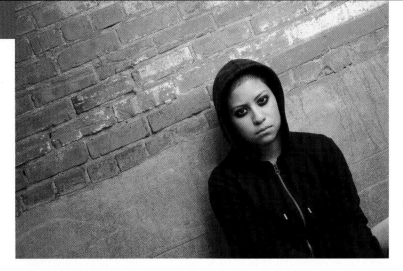

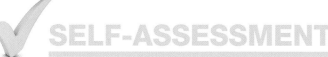

✓ SELF-ASSESSMENT

To complete this self-assessment online, visit **www.pearsonhighered.com/choosinghealth**.

Should You Seek Drug Treatment?

Answer Yes or No to the following 20 questions.

1. Have you used drugs other than those required for medical reasons?
2. Have you abused prescription drugs?
3. Do you abuse more than one drug at a time?
4. Do you use drugs more than once a week?
5. Have you tried to stop using drugs and were not able to do so?
6. Have you had blackouts or flashbacks as a result of drug use?
7. Do you ever feel bad or guilty about your drug use?
8. Does your spouse or parents ever complain about your involvement with drugs?
9. Has drug abuse created problems between you and your spouse or your parents?
10. Have you lost friends because of your use of drugs?
11. Have you neglected your family because of your use of drugs?
12. Have you been in trouble at work because of your use of drugs?
13. Have you lost a job because of drug abuse?
14. Have you gotten into fights when under the influence of drugs?
15. Have you engaged in illegal activities in order to obtain drugs?
16. Have you been arrested for possession of illegal drugs?
17. Have you ever experienced withdrawal symptoms (felt sick) when you stopped taking drugs?
18. Have you had medical problems as a result of your drug use, such as memory loss, hepatitis, convulsions, bleeding, etc.?
19. Have you gone to anyone for help for a drug problem?
20. Have you been involved in a treatment program especially related to drug use?

HOW TO INTERPRET YOUR SCORE

The more "yes" answers you gave, the more likely it is that you should seek treatment for your drug use.

Source: DAST-20 Drug Abuse Screening Test reproduced by permission of Dr. Harvey A. Skinner. © Copyright 1982 by Harvey A. Skinner, PhD and the Centre for Addiction and Mental Health, Toronto, Canada.

---

ual, family, or other group to encourage a sufferer to get professional help. Interventions usually involve direct, face-to-face demonstrations of love, support, and encouragement to enter treatment.

Recovery from addiction is often more complicated for a **polyabuser**—a user of multiple drugs. Many drug abusers are polyabusers. Abusers under the age of 20 are most likely to be polyabusers.[26] Polyabuse has been linked to many deaths. It is dangerous in part because it can increase the collective toxicity of the drugs in the body. Of the nearly 2 million people who enter drug treatment programs every year in the United States, more than half abuse multiple drugs.[26] Alcohol, marijuana, and cocaine are the most common elements in polyabuse.

> View personal stories of hope and recovery from drug addiction at **http://lifeafter.drugfree.org.**

Codependency and Enabling

Addiction is a disease that affects others besides just the user. Loving family and close friends usually suffer as well. Often the relationship between a drug user and his or her loved ones involves **codependency**—a situation in which family members or friends are part of a pattern that may perpetuate behaviors that sustain addiction. In a codependent situation, family or friends may be controlled or manipulated by the addict. They may tend to put the addict's needs before their own and devote themselves to trying to help a person who may not want their help.

Many codependents are also **enablers,** a rather positive-sounding word that actually has negative consequences. Enablers make it possible for a loved one to continue with self-destructive behavior by making excuses for them—or even protecting them from the negative consequences of their behavior. Paying an addict's rent or legal bills because he or she has squandered money on drugs is one example

> **polyabuser** A person who abuses more than one drug.
>
> **codependency** When a friend or family member is part of a pattern that may perpetuate behaviors that sustain addiction.
>
> **enablers** People who protect addicts from the negative consequences of their behavior.

of enabling. Drug abusers do not feel the true financial pinch of their abuse as long as someone else bails them out. Although enabling may sound admirable, it is most often counterproductive.

Preventing Relapse

As mentioned, *relapse* is a return to the addictive substance or behavior after a period of abstinence. Unfortunately, it is a common and unfortunate fact of drug treatment. Experts stress that "falling off the wagon" does not mean treatment does not work or that a user will never be free of the disease. Relapse can, however, be extremely demoralizing. It is better to look at relapse not as a failure, but as practice. As with every challenge in life, you may need to try several times before finally getting something right.

Research points to three factors that can trigger intense renewed drug craving and cause a relapse:[27]

- **Priming.** One small exposure to a formerly abused substance can cause an addict to use again, sometimes more heavily than before. For a recovering addict, "just one joint" is rarely that.

- **Environmental cues.** Seeing people, places, or things that were heavily associated with past drug use can sometimes prompt a recovering addict to use again.

- **Stress.** Acute and chronic stress can contribute to the resumption of drug abuse.

It can take years to kick a habit, but through proper treatment and perseverance, people with drug addictions can recover and lead productive lives. Few health-related behaviors are harder to change than those tied to addictive drugs. All of us trying to make healthy changes can draw inspiration from those who have successfully overcome a drug habit. A common misperception is that a person has to hit "rock bottom" before he or she can recover from a drug addiction. This is not true; early treatment or intervention is often successful and effective.

Beyond Drugs:
Other Addictive Behaviors

Beyond drug use, "addiction" can refer to other behaviors that become obsessive and potentially harmful. Two—gambling and compulsive spending—are worth considering here because they may arise in part from psychological challenges similar to those that lead to drug abuse.

Gambling

About 85% of adults in the U.S. have gambled at least once in their life.[1] For the vast majority of us, slot machines or the occasional game of poker do not pose a problem. However, for an estimated 2 million people in the United States, roughly 1% of adults, gambling is an addiction.[1] Although gambling is illegal for anyone under age 21 in many states, most addicted gamblers get their start before finishing high school, and young adults are especially vulnerable.

The American Psychiatric Association considers a gambling habit to be *pathological* (harmful) when players experience destructive traits such as being preoccupied with gambling, spending excessive amounts of money, and being unable to cut back or stop gambling. Other telltale signs include lying to friends and family to hide the extent of the problem and borrowing from others or stealing to finance the habit.

Compulsive Spending

Compulsive spending is an addictive behavior for more than one in 20 U.S. adults.[2] Most "shopaholics" are young and have incomes under $50,000. Most are also four times less likely than the average person to pay off their credit card balances in full.[2]

In a random sample national telephone survey, researchers found that people addicted to spending "took greater pleasure in shopping and buying, more often make senseless and impulsive purchases, more often feel depressed after shopping, and more often experience uncontrollable buying binges."[2] Other preliminary studies suggest compulsive buyers may suffer from abnormally high levels of depression and anxiety, as well as substance abuse and eating disorders.[3]

Scientists believe that the effects on the brain experienced by those with "behavior addictions" (such as gambling, spending, and pornography) are very similar to those experienced by people with drug addictions. For example, when a compulsive spender buys something, the act triggers the release of certain chemicals in the brain that cause a rush of euphoria. The compulsive spender or gambler is actually addicted to that pleasurable feeling, not the shopping or gambling per se.

Source: 1. National Council on Problem Gambling. (n.d.). FAQs: Problem gamblers, retrieved from http://www.ncpgambling.org/i4a/pages/Index.cfm?pageID=3315. 2. Koran, L. M. et. al. (2006). Estimated prevalence of compulsive buying behavior in the United States. *American Journal of Psychiatry, 163*(10), 1806-1812. 3. Christensonk, G. A. et.al. (1994). Compulsive buying: descriptive characteristics and psychiatric comorbidity. *Journal of Clinical Psychiatry,* 55:5–11.

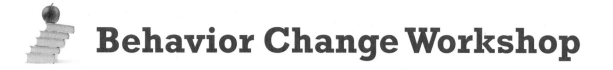

Behavior Change Workshop

To complete this workshop online, visit www.pearsonhighered.com/choosinghealth.

You may not realize how many drugs you already take on a daily basis. When you think of "drugs," you may only think of illegal drugs such as marijuana or cocaine or perhaps prescription medications. However, common substances such as alcohol, caffeine, and nicotine are also drugs. Try monitoring your drug use for one day.

Part I. Keep a Drug Diary
List the drugs you consumed daily over the course of a week. Did you drink coffee? List the number of cups. How about energy drinks or soda pop? Tea? Did you smoke cigarettes? How many? Did you take meds? Drink alcohol?

Example:

Substance	Amount	Drug	What Did It Do for You?
Coffee	3 cups	Caffeine	Helped me wake up

Your turn:

	Substance	Amount	Drug	What Did It Do for You?
Day 1				
Day 2				
Day 3				
Day 4				
Day 5				
Day 6				

	Substance	Amount	Drug	What Did It Do for You?
Day 7				

Part II. Reduce or Eliminate Drugs from Your Daily Life

Review your 1-week drug diary. Are you consuming more drugs than you realized? Are you using drugs as a coping mechanism? Looking at your list, are there any substances you would like to reduce or eliminate?

1. Focus on one specific drug you use and write it down here:

_____

2. What need is the drug meeting for you?

_____

_____

3. How committed are you to reducing or eliminating this drug from your daily routine? What stage of behavior change are you in?

_____

_____

4. Assuming you are committed to behavior change, write down a healthier way you can meet the need for which you currently use the drug.

_____

_____

5. What resources do you have that will help you achieve your goal?

_____

_____

Don't forget to utilize campus and community resources, as well as the support of family and friends.

Chapter Summary

- Many college students overestimate how many of their peers are actually using illicit drugs. However, nearly half of all students admit to binge drinking or abusing drugs at some point during their college years.
- *Drug misuse* is the inappropriate use of a legal drug. *Drug abuse* is the use of any drug that results in harm to your health.
- *Addiction* is a relapsing condition characterized by uncontrollable drug craving and use, despite the consequences.

- *Psychological dependence* is a mental attachment to a drug. *Physical dependence* is when the body requires the regular use of a drug in order to function.
- Five common ways that people self-administer drugs are ingestion, injection, inhalation, mucosal absorption, and topical administration.
- Physiological responses to drugs vary widely from individual to individual. Factors may include the individual's physical build, sex, ethnicity, and history of drug use.

- Commonly abused drugs include prescription and over-the-counter medications, marijuana, stimulants (e.g., caffeine, cocaine, amphetamines, and methamphetamine), hallucinogens (e.g., LSD, PCP, and psilocybin), "club drugs" (e.g., MDMA, GHB, Rohypnol, and ketamine), inhalants, and depressants (e.g., opioids, barbiturates, and benzodiazepines).

- Most people who need drug treatment do not receive it.
- *Relapse* is the return to drug abuse after a period of conscious abstinence.
- Types of drug treatment include on-site residential programs and off-site 12-step programs.

Test Your Knowledge

1. What are *drugs*?
   a. chemical substances prescribed by a doctor only
   b. only prescription medications and over-the-counter medications
   c. illegal substances only
   d. any chemical taken in order to alter the body physically or mentally for a non-nutritional purpose

2. Using a prescription drug that is not prescribed to you is an example of
   a. drug misuse.
   b. drug abuse.
   c. drug addiction.
   d. tolerance.

3. Uncontrollable craving for a drug, despite harmful or potentially harmful consequences, is characteristic of
   a. drug misuse.
   b. drug abuse.
   c. euphoria.
   d. addiction.

4. Using a syringe to direct a drug into the bloodstream is an example of
   a. ingestion.
   b. absorption.
   c. injection.
   d. inhalation.

5. Which of the following can affect an individual's physiological response to a drug?
   a. physical build
   b. sex
   c. past drug history
   d. all of the above

6. What is the most commonly abused illicit drug in the country?
   a. heroin
   b. cocaine
   c. marijuana
   d. prescription drugs for nonmedical use

7. What is the second most commonly abused illicit drug in the country?
   a. heroin
   b. cocaine
   c. marijuana
   d. prescription drugs for nonmedical use

8. Caffeine is an example of a(n)
   a. depressant.
   b. opioid.
   c. hallucinogen.
   d. stimulant.

9. What is psilocybin more commonly known as?
   a. ecstasy
   b. roofies
   c. hashish
   d. magic mushrooms

10. The return to drug abuse after a period of conscious drug abstinence is called
    a. intervention.
    b. remediation.
    c. relapse.
    d. codependency.

Get Critical

What happened:

In June 2009, the "King of Pop," Michael Jackson, died at his home in Los Angeles. The misuse of the powerful anesthetic propofol was the cause of death. Authorities also reported that Jackson had been having trouble sleeping and had been taking up to seven prescription drugs in the months before his death, including the anti-anxiety drugs Xanax and Zoloft and the painkiller Demerol.

What do you think?

- What kind of factors do you think led Jackson to seek help in the form of prescription drugs?
- What is it about prescription drugs that may mislead users into thinking they are safer than they really are?

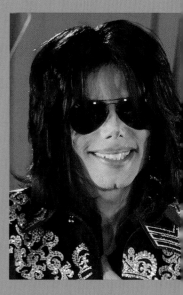

Get Connected

Health Online Visit the following websites for further information about the topics in this chapter:

- The Science of Addiction
  www.nida.nih.gov/scienceofaddiction
- Drugs of Abuse Information
  www.drugabuse.gov/drugpages.html
- Partnership for a Drug-Free America
  www.drugfree.org
- Narcotics Anonymous
  www.na.org

- National Center on Addiction and Substance Abuse at Columbia University
  www.casacolumbia.org
- Clubdrugs gov: A Service of the National Institute on Drug Abuse
  www.clubdrugs.gov

Website links are subject to change. To access updated Web links, please visit **www.pearsonhighered.com/choosinghealth**.

References

i. Substance Abuse and Mental Health Services Administration, Office of Applied Studies. (2009). *Results from the 2008 national survey on drug use and health: National findings*. Retrieved from http://oas.samhsa.gov/nsduh/2k8nsduh/2k8Results.cfm.

ii. American College Health Association. (2009). *American College Health Association national college health assessment (ACHA-NCHA II): Reference group executive summary, fall 2009.* Retrieved from http://www.acha-ncha.org/reports_ACHA-NCHAII.html

1. The National Center on Addiction and Substance Abuse at Columbia University. (2007). *Wasting the best and the brightest: Substance abuse at America's colleges and universities.* Retrieved from http://www.casacolumbia.org

2. Substance Abuse and Mental Health Services Administration, Office of Applied Studies. (2009). *Results from the 2008 national survey on drug use and health: National findings.* Retrieved from http://oas.samhsa.gov/nsduh/2k8nsduh/2k8Results

3. American College Health Association. (2009). *American College Health Association national college health assessment (ACHA-NCHA II): Reference group executive summary, fall 2009.* Retrieved from http://www.acha-ncha.org/reports_ACHA-NCHAII.html

4. Gelenberg, A. J., & Bassuk, E. (eds.). (1997). *The practitioner's guide to psychoactive drugs* (4th ed.). New York, NY: Plenum.

5. Levinthal, C. F. (2002). *Drugs, behavior, and modern society* (3rd ed.). Boston, MA: Allyn & Bacon.

6. Miller, L. (Ed.). (2006). *Chain pharmacy industry profile* (9th ed.). Alexandria VA: NACDS Foundation.

7. Kaufman, D. W., Kelly, J. P., Rosenberg, L., Anderson, T. E., & Mitchell, A. A. (2002). Recent patterns of medication use in the ambulatory adult population of the United States: The Slone survey. *Journal of the American Medical Association, 287*(3), 337–344.

8. Robert Wood Johnson Foundation. (2004). *California pilot program creates Rx fact sheets, ads to inform consumers.* Retrieved from http://www.rwjf.org/reports/grr/041745.htm

9. McCabe, S. E., Schulenberg, J. E., Johnston, L., O'Malley, P. M., Bachman, J., & Kloska, D. D. (2005). Selection and socialization effects of fraternities and sororities on US college student substance use: A multicohort national longitudinal study. *Addiction, 100*, 512–524.

10. Substance Abuse and Mental Health Services Administration, Office of Applied Studies. (2008). *Drug abuse warning network, 2006: National estimates of drug-related emergency department visits.* Retrieved from http://dawninfo.samhsa.gov/files/ED2006/DAWN2K6ED.pdf

11. U.S. Food and Drug Administration and the Consumer Healthcare Products Association. (2010). *Over-the-counter medicines: What's right for you?* Retrieved from http://www.fda.gov/Drugs/ResourcesForYou/Consumers/BuyingUsingMedicineSafely/UnderstandingOver-the-CounterMedicines/Choosingtherightover-the-counter medicineOTCs/ucm150299.htm

12. National Institute on Alcohol Abuse and Alcoholism. (1997). Alcohol metabolism. *Alcohol Alert*, No. 35; PH 371.

13. Block, R. I., & Ghoneim, M. M. (1993). Effects of chronic marijuana use on human cognition. *Psychopharmacology, 100*(1–2), 219–228.

14. Frary, C., Johnson, R., & Wang, M. (2005). Food sources and intakes of caffeine in the diets of persons in the United States. *Journal of the American Dietetic Association, 105*(1), 110–113.

15. Graham, T. E. (2001). Caffeine and exercise: Metabolism, endurance and performance. *Sports Medicine, 31*(11), 785–807.

16. Higdon, J., & Frei, B. (2006). Coffee and health: A review of recent human research. *Critical Reviews in Food Science & Nutrition, 46*(2), 101–123.

17. Weng, X., Odouli, R., & Li, D. (2008). Maternal caffeine consumption during pregnancy and the risk of miscarriage: A prospective cohort study. *American Journal of Obstetrics & Gynecology, 198*(3), 279e1–279e8.

18. Scott, M. (2002). *Clandestine drug labs* (2nd ed.). Rockville, MD: National Criminal Justice Reference Service.

19. Substance Abuse and Mental Health Services Administration, Office of Applied Studies. (2008). Drug abuse warning network, 2006: National estimates of drug-related emergency department visits. Retrieved from http://dawninfo.samhsa.gov/files/ED2006/DAWN2K6ED.pdf

20. Johnston, L. D., O'Malley, P. M., Bachman, J. G., & Schulenberg, J. E. (2009). *Monitoring the future: National survey results on drug use, 1975–2008, volume I: Secondary school students* (NIH Publication No. 09-7402). Bethesda, MD: National Institute on Drug Abuse. Retrieved from http://monitoringthefuture.org

21. Substance Abuse and Mental Health Services Administration, Office of Applied Studies. (2009, February 5). *The NSDUH Report: Trends in nonmedical use of prescription pain relievers: 2002 to 2007.* Rockville, MD: Substance Abuse and Mental Health Services Administration.

22. Krohn, M. D., Lizotte, A. J., & Perez, C. M. (1997). The interrelationship between substance use and precocious transitions to adult statuses. *Journal of Health and Social Behavior, 38*(1), 87–103.

23. National Institute on Drug Abuse. (2010). NIDA InfoFacts: Methamphetamine. Retrieved from http://www.drugabuse.gov/infofacts/methamphetamine.html.

24. National Institute on Drug Abuse. (2010). NIDA InfoFacts: MDMA (Ecstasy). Retrieved from http://www.drugabuse.gov/Infofacts/ecstasy.html.

25. U.S. Drug Enforcement Administration. (n.d.). Depressants. Retrieved from http://www.justice.gov/dea/concern/depressants.html.

26. Drug and Alcohol Services Information System. (2005). Polydrug admissions: 2002. *The DASIS Report.* Retrieved from http://www.oas.samhsa.gov/2k5/polydrugTX/polydrugTX.htm.

27. Hanson, G. (2002). New insights into relapse. *NIDA Notes, 17*(3). Retrieved from http://www.drugabuse.gov/NIDA_Notes/NNVol17N3/DirRepVol17N3.html

Alcohol and Tobacco Use and Abuse

8

● **Alcohol** is a factor in about 60% of fatal burn **injuries**, drownings, and homicides; 50% of severe trauma injuries and sexual assaults; and 40% of fatal motor vehicle **crashes**, suicides, and fatal falls.[i]

● 26.9% of U.S. **college** students **do not drink** at all.[ii]

● 1 out of every 5 **deaths** in the U.S. is caused by a **smoking-related** illness.[iii]

● **Secondhand smoke** contains more than 250 chemicals known to be **toxic** or cancer-causing, including **arsenic**, ammonia, formaldehyde, and benzene.[iv]

LEARNING OBJECTIVES

DISCUSS the prevalence of alcohol and tobacco use in the United States.

DESCRIBE how the body absorbs and metabolizes alcohol.

DESCRIBE the short-term and long-term health effects of alcohol use.

LIST strategies for preventing alcohol abuse and for treating alcoholism.

EXPLAIN the effects of nicotine on the body.

IDENTIFY the short-term and long-term health effects of nicotine use.

LIST strategies for quitting smoking.

 Health Online icons are found throughout the chapter, directing you to web links, videos, podcasts, and other useful online resources.

There will be many times in college when you are exposed to two of the most popular drugs

in the U.S.: alcohol and tobacco. Both are easily accessible on college campuses, and students often feel pressure to try them. Although experimenting with these drugs may seem like a harmless rite of passage, their use can carry serious consequences. Just one drunken night can result in a fatal vehicle accident, or make you vulnerable to sexual assault. Alcohol and tobacco are also both highly addictive. Many alcoholics trace the roots of their alcoholism to their college years, and smoking is notoriously hard to quit. The long-term health consequences of heavy drinking and smoking can be devastating, and include diseases like cirrhosis (scarring of the liver), cancer, and heart disease.

Students tend to underestimate how easy it is to develop a drinking or smoking problem, and how difficult it is to overcome one. By setting limits—or by abstaining from alcohol and tobacco altogether—you can reduce the likelihood that these addictive drugs might one day control you.

Alcohol Use in the U.S.

According to national surveys, slightly more than half the adults in the U.S. drink alcohol—about 129 million people.[1] Among men, 57% report being current drinkers, compared to 45% of women. However, among those aged 12–17, the percentages of male and female drinkers are very similar (both about 14–15%). Among Caucasian adults of either sex, 56% drink alcohol—a higher percentage than reported by any other racial or ethnic group.[1] See the **Diversity & Health** box on page 166 for a more detailed snapshot of drinking in the U.S.

The 1984 Federal Uniform Drinking Age Act (FUDAA) financially penalizes any state that fails to prohibit the purchase or public possession of any alcoholic beverage by a person under 21. Because all states ultimately complied, the act effectively raised the national minimum legal drinking age to 21. Research shows that the FUDAA has had positive effects on health and safety, primarily in decreasing traffic crashes and fatalities, suicide, and decreased consumption by those under age 21.[2–5]

Alcohol Use and Binge Drinking on Campus

An estimated 85% of college students nationwide have tried alcohol, and 40% report **binge drinking.**[6] Binge drinking, or *heavy episodic drinking*, is defined by the National Institute of Alcohol Abuse and Alcoholism as a pattern of drinking alcohol that results in a blood alcohol concentration (BAC) of 0.08% or above (we will discuss BAC in more detail shortly.)[7] For a typical adult, this corresponds to consuming five or more drinks (for men), or four or more drinks

binge drinking A pattern of drinking alcohol that results in a blood alcohol concentration of 0.08 or above (about five or more alcoholic drinks within 2 hours for men, or four or more alcoholic drinks within 2 hours for women).

Alcohol Use Through the Lenses of
Sex, Race/Ethnicity, Age, Education, and Geography

Although alcohol use and abuse cuts across all demographic groups, some groups show heavier patterns of drinking than others. A recent national survey conducted by the Substance Abuse and Mental Health Services Administration revealed the following patterns.

Overall

- Among people aged 12 or older, 51.6% reported being current drinkers: about 129 million people.

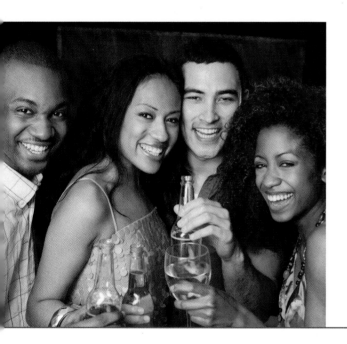

- Among people aged 12 or older, 6.9% reported heavy drinking (having five or more drinks on one occasion, on at least 5 days over the course of the previous month).

Sex

- Of males aged 12 or older, 57.7% reported being current drinkers, compared to 45.9% of females in the same age group.
- Among those aged 12 to 17, there was less of a difference between male and female drinkers: 14.2% of males in this age group were current drinkers, compared to 15% of females.

Race/Ethnicity

- Among Caucasians, 56.2% report being current drinkers, the highest rate of any racial/ethnic group.
- Among mixed race individuals, 47.5% report being current drinkers.
- Among Native Americans, 43.3% report being current drinkers.
- Among Hispanics, 43.2% report being current drinkers.
- Among African Americans, 41.9% report being current drinkers.
- Among Asian Americans, 37% report being current drinkers.
- Rates of binge drinking (defined in this survey as having five or more drinks on at least one occasion over the previous month) were highest among Hispanics (25.6%), followed by Native Americans (24.4%), Caucasians (24%), those of mixed-race (22%), African Americans (20.4%), and Asian Americans (11.9%).

Age

- Among individuals aged 21–25, 69.5% reported being current drinkers, the highest rate of any age group.

Education

- Among individuals aged 26 and older, the rates of binge drinking or heavy drinking were lower among college graduates than among those without a college degree. For binge drinking, 19.5% of college graduates reported engaging in that behavior, compared to 23.2% of non-college graduates. For heavy drinking, 4.6% of college graduates reported doing so, compared to 7% of non-college graduates.

Geography

- The rates of alcohol use are lower in the South (47.3%) than in the Northeast (56.8%), Midwest (54.2%) or the West (51.8%).

Data from: *Results from the 2008 National Survey on Drug Use and Health: National Findings,* by the Substance Abuse and Mental Health Services Administration, 2009, retrieved from http://www.oas.samhsa.gov/nsduh/2k8nsduh/2k8Results.cfm.

(for women), in about 2 hours. Note that some organizations define binge drinking even more narrowly, i.e., as equivalent to consuming four or more drinks (for men) and three or more drinks (for women) within 2 hours.

The incidence of binge drinking is highest among young adults aged 18–24, whether they are in college, the military, or the workforce. In fact, the highest prevalence of alcohol dependence occurs in this age group.[6] Studies indicate 12th graders heading to college are consistently less likely than their non–college-bound counterparts to report binge drinking.[8] However, once at college, these same students report more binge drinking than their peers who entered the workforce.

Binge drinking is arguably the most significant health risk behavior among college students today. If you consider the consequences—and just how widespread binge drinking is—it is easy to see why. Alcohol is a factor in about 60% of fatal burn injuries, drownings, and homicides; 50% of severe trauma injuries and sexual assaults; and 40% of fatal motor vehicle crashes, suicides, and fatal falls.[9] Additionally, binge drinking can lead to drunk driving, violence, vandalism, risky sex, forced sex, and poor academic performance.[10] Binge drinkers not only place themselves in harm's way, but also raise risks for those around them. Those who live with or near heavy drinkers are exposed to more property damage, fights, and noise disturbances than those who do not.[11] Nationwide, 43% of

Alcohol Use on Campus

A recent national survey of college students revealed that:

26.9% —— Students who had never tried alcohol

13.9% —— Students who had tried alcohol, but did not have any in the last 30 days

59.2% —— Students who had consumed alcohol at least once in the last 30 days

Data from: *American College Health Association National College Health Assessment (ACHA-NCHA II) Reference Group Executive Summary Fall 2009* by the American College Health Association, 2009.

some interesting use patterns. Alcohol consumption among freshmen varies considerably from week to week within a single academic year. Consumption increases significantly during time periods that corresponded to Thanksgiving, Christmas, New Year's, and Spring Break. An increase in drinking also occurred during the third week of school (immediately after students arrived on campus), though this increase was not as dramatic as those during holidays.[15,16]

> Listen to a Centers for Disease Control podcast on the dangers of binge drinking at www2c.cdc.gov/podcasts/player.asp?f=11157.

Why Students Drink

Students cite many different reasons for reaching for a drink. Researchers have classified the motivations into four different categories: coping (to avoid problems), conformity (to gain peer acceptance), enhancement (to induce a positive mood), and social (to make parties and outings more enjoyable).[17]

Peer pressure is often a major factor. When students are frequently offered alcoholic beverages at parties or goaded into consuming multiple drinks at a time by their friends, they may come to think that heavy drinking is normal behavior and therefore acceptable. Aware of the impact of social norms on students' drinking behaviors, alcohol abuse prevention experts try to counter student perceptions of their peers' drinking behaviors with the fact that the overwhelming majority of students drink responsibly. In fact, in a recent national survey, 13.9% of U.S. college students who had tried alcohol reported that they had not had a single alcoholic beverage within the past 30 days, and 17.2% reported they had only indulged 1 to 2 days out of the past 30. In addition, 26.9% of college students in this survey reported that they had never tried alcohol at all.[18]

Parents are also a major influence on the drinking patterns of college students. Parents who allow their children to drink alcohol in high school are not protecting their children from abusing alcohol when they leave the home for college. On the contrary, students whose parents allowed alcohol consumption in high school were significantly more at risk for alcohol misuse and its consequences in college.[19] Meanwhile, parental disapproval of drinking in high school does seem to have a protective effect against alcohol misuse in college.[19]

> Is your drinking pattern risky? Assess yourself at http://rethinkingdrinking.niaaa.nih.gov/IsYourDrinkingPatternRisky/WhatsYourPattern.asp.

The Makeup of Alcohol

Alcohol is a chemical substance that is toxic to the body. The key ingredient in every can of beer, glass of wine, and shot of tequila is **ethyl alcohol,** or **ethanol.** This intoxicating substance is produced through a process called *fermentation,* in which natural sugars are converted into alcohol and carbon dioxide with the help of yeast. To produce beer and wine, manufacturers add other ingredients, such as water, that dilute the drinks. To create hard liquor, they put the ethyl alcohol through another process, known as *distillation.* Distillation involves heating and then cooling the fermented liquid so that it ends up with a higher alcoholic concentra-

college students reported difficulties sleeping or studying because of someone else's drinking, and 44% reported having to "babysit" another student who had had too much to drink.[12] Of even more concern is the fact that each year, more than 696,000 students between the ages of 18 and 24 are assaulted by another student who has been drinking, and more than 97,000 students between the ages of 18 and 24 are victims of alcohol-related sexual assault or date rape.[13]

Although college students of all types may binge drink, it is most common in athletes, sports fans, fraternity and sorority members, and extremely social students. Women and minorities, and religious, married and older students tend to drink less.[14] The **Student Stats** feature provides a snapshot of overall drinking patterns on campus, based on a recent nationwide survey of college students.

Another recent study focused on students' weekly alcohol consumption and discovered

ethyl alcohol (ethanol) The intoxicating ingredient in beer, wine, and distilled liquor.

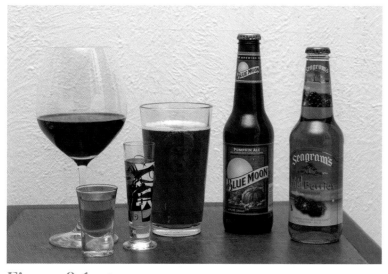

Figure 8.1 "Standard" serving sizes. A 5-ounce glass of wine, a 1.5-ounce shot of liquor, and a 12-ounce can of beer are all "standard" servings containing about the same amount of alcohol: 14 grams (1/2 ounce).

tion than before. These stronger beverages are often referred to by their **proof value,** a measure of their ethyl alcohol content. A proof is double the actual alcohol percentage—for example, 100 proof bourbon contains 50% alcohol by volume. Many red wines have an alcohol percentage of around 13%, or a proof value of 26.

Because different beverages have such varying levels of alcohol, a "standard" serving size also varies by drink type. A **standard drink** contains about 14 grams (or 1/2 ounce) of pure alcohol. That is the equivalent of a 12-ounce can of beer, or 8 to 9 ounces of malt liquor. A 5-ounce glass of table wine is considered standard, as is 1.5 ounces of 80-proof liquor—roughly one shot glass **(Figure 8.1)**. Although these amounts may seem intuitive enough, researchers at the University of California at Berkeley found that when people were asked to serve themselves a standard drink at home, they poured considerably more alcohol than they should have.[20]

How the Body Absorbs and Metabolizes Alcohol

When you consume an alcoholic beverage, the alcohol passes from your stomach and small intestine into your bloodstream, a process known as **absorption.** The alcohol then travels to your liver, where it is broken down by enzymes in a process known as **metabolism (Figure 8.2)**. (A small amount of alcohol is metabolized in the stomach as well, but 80% of alcohol metabolism takes place in the liver.) One enzyme in particular, *alcohol dehydrogenase* (ADH), converts alcohol into a by-product called *acetaldehyde.* The acetaldehyde is then quickly transformed into acetate by other enzymes and is eventually metabolized to carbon dioxide and water. Some alcohol, however, is not metabolized by the body, and is excreted in urine, sweat, and breath. It can be detected in breath and urine tests that gauge blood alcohol levels.

For more information on what constitutes a "standard drink," visit http://pubs.niaaa.nih.gov/publications/Practitioner/pocketguide/pocket_guide2.htm.

The liver can metabolize only a small amount of alcohol at a time, roughly one standard drink per hour, although metabolism varies among individuals. Alcohol that is not immediately metabolized by the liver continues to circulate in the bloodstream to other parts of the body, including the brain. If a person consumes alcohol at a faster rate than the liver can break it down, alcohol poisoning, also called **acute intoxication,** can occur.

Blood Alcohol Concentration

The amount of alcohol contained in a person's blood is known as **blood alcohol concentration (BAC).** BAC is measured in grams of alcohol per deciliter of blood, and is usually expressed in percentage terms. Having a BAC of 0.08% means that a person has 8 parts alcohol per 10,000 parts blood in the body. Also referred to as *blood alcohol level,* BAC can be affected by several factors, including:

- **How much and how quickly you drink.** Binge drinking causes a large amount of alcohol to enter your body in a very short period of time. Because your body cannot process alcohol at a fast pace, this results in a higher BAC.

- **What you drink.** All drinks are not created equal. The water in beer and wine acts as a buffer for alcohol so that people feel the effects of these beverages a little less than if they had downed a straight shot of hard liquor. Champagne, on the other hand, contains carbon dioxide, which increases the rate of alcohol absorption and causes a more rapid intoxication. Mixers can also make a big difference. Water and fruit juices mixed with alcohol may slow the absorption and intoxication process, whereas soda and other carbonated beverages speed it up. The temperature of the alcohol also affects absorption, with a hot toddy moving into the bloodstream more quickly than a frosty margarita.

- **Your sex.** Women are more vulnerable to alcohol than men and will have a higher BAC after drinking the same amount of alcohol. This occurs for several reasons. First, women typically are smaller, and consequently have less blood volume than men. They also have a higher percentage of body fat. Because alcohol is not easily stored in fat, it will enter the bloodstream more quickly in women. Men have significantly more muscle and consequently have a higher percentage of water in their bodies. The added water helps dilute the alcohol men consume. Women absorb about 30% more alcohol into the bloodstream than men do.

proof value A measurement of alcoholic strength, corresponding to twice the alcohol percentage (13% alcohol equals 26 proof).

standard drink A drink containing about 14 grams pure alcohol (one 12-oz. can of beer, one 5-oz. glass of wine, or 1.5 oz. of 80-proof liquor).

absorption The process by which alcohol passes from the stomach or small intestine into the bloodstream.

metabolism The breakdown of food and beverages in the body to transform them into energy.

acute intoxication (alcohol poisoning) Potentially fatal concentration of alcohol in the blood.

blood alcohol concentration (BAC) The amount of alcohol present in blood, measured in grams of alcohol per deciliter of blood.

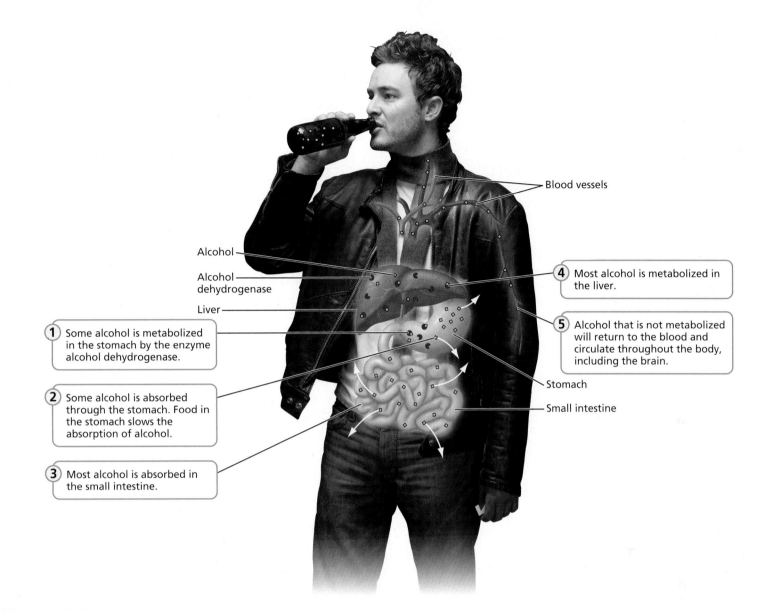

Blood vessels

Alcohol

Alcohol dehydrogenase

Liver

(1) Some alcohol is metabolized in the stomach by the enzyme alcohol dehydrogenase.

(2) Some alcohol is absorbed through the stomach. Food in the stomach slows the absorption of alcohol.

(3) Most alcohol is absorbed in the small intestine.

(4) Most alcohol is metabolized in the liver.

(5) Alcohol that is not metabolized will return to the blood and circulate throughout the body, including the brain.

Stomach

Small intestine

Figure 8.2 **Alcohol absorption and metabolism.** Alcohol is absorbed into the bloodstream through the stomach and small intestine. Metabolism takes place in the stomach and in the liver.

This is primarily because women produce less alcohol dehydrogenase, the enzyme responsible for the breakdown of alcohol in the stomach. **Figure 8.3** shows how BAC levels differ between men and women of similar weights.

- **Your age.** Research indicates that as people age, they become more sensitive to alcohol's effects.[21] The same amount of alcohol can have a greater effect on an older person than on a younger one.
- **Your weight.** The less you weigh, the less blood and water you have in your body to dilute alcohol. As a result, a lighter person will have a higher BAC than a heavier person who drinks the same amount.
- **Your physical condition.** People who are fatigued or stressed out tend to be more affected by moderate amounts of alcohol.

- **Your food intake.** Eating a meal before drinking, especially one high in protein and fat, helps slow the absorption of alcohol into the bloodstream. Conversely, drinking on an empty stomach speeds absorption. BAC rises more rapidly when you have not eaten because there is no food in your stomach in which to dilute the alcohol.
- **Medications.** Aspirin and other medications, including many sold over the counter, prevent the enzyme ADH from breaking down alcohol. This causes alcohol to accumulate in the blood faster (resulting in a higher BAC) and have longer lasting effects. Women on birth control pills process alcohol more slowly than other women, and remain drunk longer.

Use this calculator to estimate your blood alcohol concentration under a variety of circumstances: **http://health.discovery.com/tools/calculators/alcohol/alcohol.html**.

For Women

Drinks per hour	Body Weight in pounds					
	100	120	140	160	180	200
1	0.05	0.04	0.03	0.03	0.03	0.02
2	0.09	0.08	0.07	0.06	0.05	0.05
3	0.14	0.11	0.10	0.09	0.08	0.07
4	0.18	0.15	0.13	0.11	0.10	0.09
5	0.23	0.19	0.16	0.14	0.13	0.11
6	0.27	0.23	0.19	0.17	0.15	0.14
7	0.32	0.27	0.23	0.20	0.18	0.16
8	0.36	0.30	0.26	0.23	0.20	0.18
9	0.41	0.34	0.29	0.26	0.23	0.20
10	0.45	0.38	0.32	0.28	0.25	0.23

For Men

Drinks per hour	Body Weight in pounds					
	100	120	140	160	180	200
1	0.04	0.03	0.03	0.02	0.02	0.02
2	0.08	0.06	0.05	0.05	0.04	0.04
3	0.11	0.09	0.08	0.07	0.06	0.06
4	0.15	0.12	0.11	0.09	0.08	0.08
5	0.19	0.16	0.13	0.12	0.11	0.09
6	0.23	0.19	0.16	0.14	0.13	0.11
7	0.26	0.22	0.19	0.16	0.15	0.13
8	0.30	0.25	0.21	0.19	0.17	0.15
9	0.34	0.28	0.24	0.21	0.19	0.17
10	0.38	0.31	0.27	0.23	0.21	0.19

Figure 8.3 Blood alcohol concentration (BAC) tables. The orange areas indicate legal intoxication.

Source: Adapted by permission of the Pennsylvania Liquor Control Board's Bureau of Alcohol Education, from "Alcohol Impairment Charts," published by the Pennsylvania Liquor Control Board, with data gathered from The National Clearinghouse for Alcohol and Drug Information, Substance Abuse, and Mental Health Services Administration.

Intoxication

In the most basic sense, **alcohol intoxication** is just another term for being drunk. In a legal sense, it means having a BAC of 0.08% or greater. Intoxication levels vary, but generally a person weighing 150 pounds can expect the following symptoms:[22]

- At a BAC of 0.03% (after about one drink), you feel relaxed and slightly exhilarated.
- At a BAC of 0.06% (after two drinks), you feel warm and relaxed, as well as experience decreased fine motor skills.
- At a BAC of 0.09% (after three drinks), you notice a slowed reaction time, poor muscle control, slurred speech, and wobbly legs.

- At a BAC of 0.12% (after four drinks), you have clouded judgment, a loss of self-restraint, and an impaired ability to reason and make logical decisions.
- At a BAC of 0.15% (after five drinks), you have blurred

---

alcohol intoxication The state of physical and/or mental impairment brought on by excessive alcohol consumption (in legal terms, a BAC of 0.08% or greater).

---

vision, unclear speech, an unsteady gait, and impaired coordination.
- At a BAC of 0.18% (after six drinks), you find it difficult to stay awake.
- At a BAC of 0.30% (after ten to twelve drinks), you are in a stupor or deep sleep.
- At a BAC of 0.50% you are in a deep coma and in danger of death.

The Effects of Alcohol on the Body

Excess alcohol consumption negatively affects the health of the drinker on many different levels **(Figure 8.4)**. Not only do heavy drinkers put themselves at a higher risk of accidental injury and violence, they also increase their risks of developing lasting neurological problems and serious diseases, such as cancer, heart disease, and liver disease.

Immediate Effects of Alcohol on the Body

Within moments of ingestion, alcohol begins to cause changes in the body. As mentioned, as BAC increases, the drinker will experience symptoms such as lightheadedness, relaxation, loss of inhibition, compromised motor coordination, slowed reaction times, slurred speech, dulled senses (i.e., less acute vision, hearing, smelling, and taste), and clouded judgment. Other short-term effects of alcohol use include:

- **Dehydration.** Alcohol is a diuretic, triggering more frequent urination. This can lead to dehydration and an electrolyte imbalance. Symptoms of mild to moderate dehydration include thirst,

---

STUDENT STORY

Differences in Intoxication

"Hi, I'm Rita. My college has an annual event called "Slope Day" which celebrates the end of the school year and where pretty much everyone drinks until they fall down. I don't usually drink much, but this year my friend gave me a thermos full of soda mixed with vodka. It didn't taste very alcoholic, and I drank almost the whole thing. I got SO SICK later that evening. Meanwhile, my friend seemed to drink twice as much as me and didn't get sick at all. What gives?"

1: What factors probably contributed to Rita's intoxication?

2: What questions would you have about Rita and her friend in order to explain the differences in how their bodies responded to the same alcoholic beverage?

Do you have a story similar to Rita's? Share your story at **www.pearsonhighered.com/choosinghealth.**

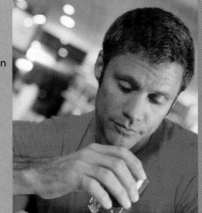

Short-term effects:
- Lightheadedness
- Relaxation
- Loss of inhibition
- Compromised motor coordination
- Slowed reaction times
- Slurred speech
- Dulled senses (i.e., less acute vision, hearing, smelling, taste)
- Clouded judgment
- Dehydration
- Digestive problems
- Sleep disturbance
- Low blood sugar levels due to alterations in metabolism
- Hangover

Long-term effects:
- Increased risk of cancer
- Increased risk of cardiovascular disease
- Increased risk of liver disease (fatty liver disease, hepatitis, cirrhosis)
- Neurological problems
- Fetal alcohol syndrome in infants (if alcohol is consumed during pregnancy)

Figure 8.4 Short- and long-term health effects of alcohol use.

weakness, dryness of mucous membranes, dizziness, and lightheadedness.

- **Gastrointestinal problems.** Alcohol irritates the stomach and intestines, causing inflammation and indigestion. This is especially true when a person drinks a beverage with an alcohol concentration greater than 15%.[23]

- **Sleep disturbances.** Although alcohol has sedative effects that can make people feel sleepy, it actually tends to *disrupt* sleep and throw off the biological rhythms of the body. As a result, alcohol-induced sleep is often shorter in duration and poorer in quality. In addition, alcohol relaxes the throat muscles, facilitating snoring.

- **Alterations in the metabolic state of the liver and other organs.** These changes result in low blood sugar levels.

The effect many drinkers fear most, however, is a **hangover,** which begins within several hours after drinking has stopped and can last for up to 24 hours. A hangover is the constellation of unpleasant physical and mental symptoms that accompany a bout of heavy drinking. They include fatigue, headache, increased sensitivity to light and sound, redness of the eyes, dry mouth, muscle aches, thirst, vomiting, diarrhea, dizziness, vertigo, depression, and irritability.

Researchers believe that key contributors to hangovers are compounds found in alcoholic beverages known as *congeners*.[24] Congeners contribute to the taste, smell, and appearance of alcoholic drinks, but the body metabolizes them very slowly, and they are more toxic than ethanol. Research has shown that beverages containing a large number of congeners, such as whiskey, brandy, and red wine, cause greater hangover effects than beverages composed of more pure ethanol, such as gin and vodka.[25] In general, the more alcohol people drink, the more likely they are to develop a hangover.

Alcohol Poisoning

Every year, dozens of students from universities and colleges across the country die from **alcohol poisoning** as a result of a dangerously high level of alcohol consumption and the toxic byproducts that result when alcohol is metabolized by the body. When the body absorbs too much alcohol, it can depress the central nervous system, slowing breathing, heart rate, and the gag reflex that is needed to prevent choking. Inebriated students can lose consciousness, choke on their own vomit, and die from asphyxiation. In addition, victims can experience *hypothermia* (low body temperature) and *hypoglycemia* (too little blood sugar), which can lead to seizures. Vomiting can also cause seizures, resulting in permanent brain damage.

Signs of alcohol poisoning include mental confusion, vomiting, seizures, slow or irregular breathing, low body temperature, and skin that is pale or bluish in color. If a person cannot be roused, that is another indication that emergency medical care is needed.

Alcohol poisoning should be taken as seriously as any other kind of poisoning. Giving a grossly intoxicated person a cup of coffee or a cold shower will not help. Neither will having him or her sleep or "walk it off." A person's blood alcohol concentration can continue to rise even while he or she is passed out. It is dangerous to assume the person will be fine if left alone to sleep. If you encounter someone who you suspect may have alcohol poisoning, call 911 immediately if the person:

- Is unconscious and you can't rouse him or her even by shaking.
- Has consumed other drugs.
- Is experiencing seizures.
- Is injured.
- Has a respiration rate of fewer than 8 breaths per minute.
- Is experiencing shallow or irregular breathing (10 seconds or more between breaths).

Long-Term Effects of Alcohol on the Body

It is difficult to find a part of the body that alcohol does not damage if it is abused for long periods of time. Chronic, heavy use of alcohol has been linked to cancer, heart disease, liver problems, neurological ailments, and stomach disorders.

hangover Alcohol withdrawal symptoms, including headache and nausea, caused by an earlier bout of heavy drinking.

alcohol poisoning Dangerously high level of alcohol consumption, resulting in depression of the central nervous system, slowed breathing and heart rate, and compromised gag reflex.

Cancer

Study after study has linked cancer and excessive alcohol use.[26] Cancers of the liver, breast, esophagus, mouth, larynx, and throat have all been associated with chronic drinking patterns.[26] Oral cancers are six times more common in alcohol users than in non-drinkers.[26] Drinkers who also smoke are at an even higher risk.[26]

Certain populations may be more at risk for certain alcohol-related cancers. Scientists have known that approximately 36% of East Asians (Japanese, Chinese, and Koreans) experience a facial flushing response to alcohol.[27] This flush occurs because of an inherited deficiency in an enzyme that helps metabolize alcohol, aldehyde dehydrogenase 2 (ALDH2). There is accumulating evidence that ALDH2-deficient people are at much higher risk of esophageal cancer from alcohol consumption than those with fully active ALDH2.

Cardiovascular Disease

Although there is some evidence that *moderate* alcohol use may lower the risk of some types of heart disease (see **Spotlight: Can Alcohol Have Health Benefits?**), excessive chronic alcohol use can raise the blood levels of triglycerides, a type of fat. It can also lead to high blood pressure, heart failure, and, in some chronic drinkers, stroke. Excessive use of alcohol can also have a direct toxic effect on the heart muscle cells, causing *cardiomyopathy*. Cardiomyopathy is a serious disease in which the heart muscle becomes inflamed and weakened. As a result, it cannot pump blood efficiently. The lack of blood flow affects all parts of the body, resulting in damage to multiple tissues and organ systems.

Liver Disease

Alcohol can cause three kinds of liver disease:

- **Fatty liver.** A buildup of fat cells in the liver that can cause abdominal discomfort.
- **Alcoholic hepatitis.** Also called inflammation of the liver. About a third of heavy drinkers will develop alcoholic hepatitis, which causes progressive liver damage and is marked by nausea, vomiting, fever, and jaundice.
- **Alcoholic cirrhosis.** The most serious type of alcohol-related liver disease. An estimated 40% of the 26,000 people who die from cirrhosis each year have a history of alcohol abuse, according to the American Liver Foundation.[28] With cirrhosis, normal liver tissue is replaced with scar tissue, causing life-threatening damage.

Neurological Effects

Alcohol can cause severe and possibly lasting brain damage in people under age 21, according to the American Medical Association. The brain grows and changes during adolescence and into the college years and alcohol can negatively affect two brain areas involved in learning and behavior. Moderate drinking impairs learning

MYTH OR FACT?

Can Coffee Cure a Hangover?

A hangover is the body's reaction to being poisoned . . . poisoned with too much alcohol. Excessive drinking traumatizes the central nervous system, resulting in headaches, dizziness, nausea, dehydration, and even a weakened immune system.

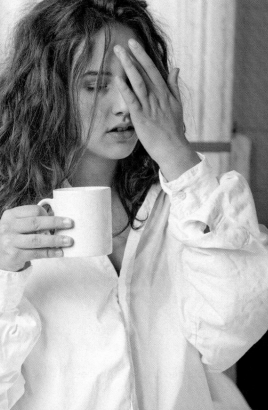

Alcohol is a diuretic and consequently increases urination, which leads to dehydration. Coffee is not an effective hangover cure because the caffeine in it causes even more dehydration. In fact, coffee could actually make your hangover worse! The morning after, you should avoid caffeinated beverages and stick to water for rehydration. Sports drinks might also be a good choice because they will both counter dehydration and replace lost electrolytes.

While we're at it, let's examine a few additional supposed hangover "cures":

- Can a Bloody Mary (vodka and spiced tomato juice) cure a hangover? No. Drinking additional alcohol the morning after may *postpone* the symptoms of a hangover, but cannot prevent them.
- Will eating before you go to bed help alleviate your hangover symptoms the next day? No. In order for food to have any impact, it needs to be in your stomach *while* you are drinking, when it can slow the absorption of alcohol and reduce your level of intoxication. Eating after the fact isn't going to help.
- What about taking over-the-counter painkillers before going

to bed? No. These painkillers peak in about four hours, so unfortunately, the effect of a bedtime dose will be gone by morning. Also, note that taking acetaminophen (e.g., Tylenol) immediately after drinking can be downright dangerous. Alcohol disrupts how the liver processes acetaminophen, which can lead to liver inflammation and permanent damage.

The only surefire way to avoid the effects of a hangover is to not drink to excess in the first place.

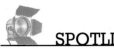
Can Alcohol Have Health Benefits?

There is some evidence that people who regularly consume *small* amounts of alcohol may have a decreased risk of coronary heart disease, type II diabetes, high blood pressure, and stroke compared with people who do not drink at all.[1] Other studies have shown that moderate drinkers (defined as people who regularly have 1–2 drinks per day) have the lowest mortality rate, while heavy drinkers have the highest, and teetotalers (those who don't drink) and light drinkers have rates that fall somewhere in the middle.[2]

That said, researchers caution that many people find it difficult to limit themselves to one or two drinks a day, and would be better off not to drink at all. Women should also be aware that alcohol use, even moderate use, has been linked to an increased risk of breast cancer.[3] Among young people in particular, alcohol use is associated with *increased* risk of premature death from accidents or injuries. College students should not take up drinking or drink more frequently with the goal of improving their health.

References: **1.** "Alcohol Consumption in the New Millennium: Weighing Up the Risks and Benefits for Our Health" by R. K. Foster and H. E. Marriott, 2006, *Nutrition Bulletin, 31*(6), pp. 286–331. **2.** "The Health Benefits of Moderate Drinking Revisited: Alcohol Use and Self-Reported Health Status" by M. T. French and S. K. Zavala, 2007, *American Journal of Health Promotion, 21*(6), pp. 484–491. **3.** "Moderate Alcohol Intake and Cancer Incidence in Women" by N. E. Allen, V. Beral, D. Casabonne, S. W. Kan, G. K. Reeves, A. Brown, and J. J. Green, 2009, *Journal of the National Cancer Institute, 101*(5), pp. 296–305.

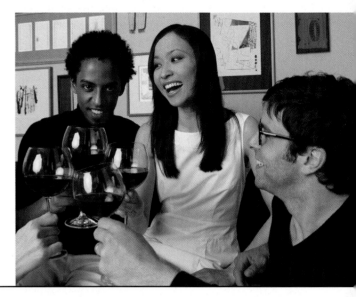

and memory far more in youth than adults, with adolescents only needing to drink half as much to suffer the same negative brain effects.[29]

Alcohol and Pregnancy

A pregnant woman is not only "eating for two," she is also "drinking for two." The ingestion of high levels of alcohol during the first trimester of a pregnancy can cause a miscarriage. Alcohol that is ingested at other points in the pregnancy can lead to health problems and even brain damage in the fetus. Scientists coined the term **fetal alcohol syndrome** more than three decades ago to describe a pattern of birth defects that appeared in the children of mothers who drank while pregnant. The telltale signs of the condition include facial abnormalities, retarded growth, and permanent intellectual and behavioral problems.

Today, drinking while pregnant is recognized as the leading cause of birth defects, developmental disabilities, and mental retardation. The prevalence of fetal alcohol syndrome is estimated to be between 0.5 and 2 for every 1000 births, and approximately 40,000 newborns are affected by an alcohol-related disorder each year.[30] Despite the known risks, an estimated 10.6% of pregnant women reported consuming alcohol while pregnant in a recent national survey.[31]

The highest risk is to babies whose mothers are heavy drinkers, but scientists are unsure whether there is any safe level of alcohol use during pregnancy. In 2005, the U.S. surgeon general issued an advisory to pregnant women urging them to abstain from alcohol altogether. Stating that it is "in the child's best interest for a pregnant woman to simply not drink alcohol," Dr. Richard Carmona said studies also indicate babies can be affected by alcohol just after conception, before a woman even knows she is pregnant. For that reason, the federal government has begun recommending that women who may possibly be pregnant avoid alcohol.

> **fetal alcohol syndrome** A pattern of mental and physical birth defects found in some children of mothers who drank excessively during pregnancy.

> The Mothers Against Drunk Driving (MADD) website includes statistics on drunk driving, victim services, and opportunities to help eliminate drunk driving: **www.madd.org.**

The Effects of Alcohol on Behavior

Alcohol does not just have physical effects on the body—it is also associated with poor decision making and risky behavior. Among the most serious risks associated with alcohol use are drunk driving and alcohol-related sexual activity.

Drinking and Driving

Every year, more than 160 million incidents of *driving while intoxicated*, also known as DWI, occur in the United States. They result in more than 36 deaths every day on our roadways—jumping to 45 per day during winter vacation and 54 per day over the New Year's holiday.[32]

College students are disproportionately affected by drunk driving. In 2005 alone, more than 1,825 students aged 18–24 died from alcohol-related car crashes and unintentional injuries.[33] More than one-fourth of college students in the United States drove under the influence of alcohol.[33]

Having a BAC of 0.08% or greater will qualify you for a DWI arrest in all 50 states if you are 21 years of age or older. It is illegal to have *any* alcohol in your system if you are underage. Teenagers who are caught operating a motor vehicle after having just a little to drink could have their license suspended. They may also be charged with a DWI even if they have a BAC of less than 0.08%.

Alcohol and Sexual Activity

Engaging in sexual intercourse while inebriated can be just as dangerous as riding in two tons of steel after the driver has had a few too many drinks. In one study, 21.3% of college students reported participating in unplanned sexual activities after having too much to drink.[34] More than one in ten said they did not use protection while having sex under the influence, possibly exposing themselves to sexually transmitted diseases such as AIDS or hepatitis B, as well as unplanned pregnancy.[34]

For women, the risks can be even greater. Heavy drinking increases the odds that a woman will become a victim of violence or rape. Conservative estimates of sexual assault indicate that one in four women in the U.S. have experienced sexual assault, with alcohol being involved in approximately half the cases.[35]

Alcohol and Other Problems

Students who engage in heavy drinking also increase their risks of other problems. About 11% of college drinkers report that they have damaged property while under the influence of alcohol. And 25% say they have missed class, fallen behind, flunked exams, or received lower grades as a result of their drinking.[36] Alcohol use is also closely associated with depression, and can increase the risk that a depressed person will attempt suicide.

A common refrain on vintage T-shirts states, "I don't have a drinking problem. I drink, I get drunk. I fall down. No problem!" Health experts, however, are not laughing. More than 500,000 college students are hurt or injured each year because of their drinking.[36]

Alcohol Abuse

Excessive drinking is a pervasive problem in American society. In the U.S., 17.6 million adults meet the criteria for either alcohol abuse or alcohol dependence.[37] **Alcohol abuse** refers to drinking that gets in the way of work, school or home life, and causes interpersonal, social, or legal problems. **Alcoholism,** technically known as **alcohol dependence,** is problem drinking taken a step further—alcoholics do not just enjoy drinks, they crave them and experience withdrawal symptoms whenever they stop drinking.

Alcoholism

Approximately one-third of college students meet the diagnostic criteria for alcohol abuse, and 1 in 17 meet the criteria for alcoholism.[38] Alcoholism is defined as exhibiting at least three of the following symptoms during a one-year period:

alcohol abuse Drinking alcohol to excess, either regularly or on individual occasions, resulting in disruption of work, school, or home life and causing interpersonal, social, or legal problems.

alcoholism (alcohol dependence) A physical dependence on alcohol to the extent that stopping drinking brings on withdrawal symptoms.

- **Tolerance.** Needing to drink more and more alcohol to get drunk.
- **Withdrawal symptoms.** Having a physical dependence on alcohol to the extent that nausea, sweating, shakiness, tremors, seizures, and anxiety are experienced after stopping drinking.
- **Loss of control.** Drinking more or longer than intended.

How to Protect Yourself from Risky Alcohol-Related Behavior

Accidents or injuries resulting from alcohol-related behavior are all too common on college campuses. The following guidelines can help keep you safe.

- **Don't drink to get drunk.** Alcohol-related risks increase dramatically with intoxication, so if you drink, drink moderately. Eat before you start consuming any alcohol, and keep eating while you drink. During the evening, take breaks between drinks by alternating alcoholic beverages with non-alcoholic ones. Avoid drinking games that can cause you to drink alcohol more quickly than your body can handle.

- **Pair-up with a friend.** If you are drinking away from home, don't do it alone. Always pair-up with a friend and make a pact to stick together.

- **Make arrangements for getting home safely.** If you are heading to a drinking event, arrange for a sober driver or contact a cab company ahead of time. Most colleges have "safe ride" systems that pro-vide safe late night transportation services from popular night spots.

- **Don't accept drinks from strangers.** While at a party, club, or bar, don't give anyone the opportunity to slip drugs like Rohypnol or GHB into your drink. Never put your drink down. If your drink is out of sight, even for a few minutes, don't finish it. Get yourself a new one. Don't accept an open drink from anyone. If you order a drink in a bar, make sure you watch the bartender open the bottle or mix your drink.

- **Know the signs of alcohol poisoning.** Be prepared so that you can help a friend if the situation arises. If the person is unconscious, cannot be roused, has consumed other drugs, is experiencing seizures, is injured, and/or is exhibiting shallow or irregular breathing, call 911 immediately. Remember that other signs of alcohol poisoning include mental confusion, vomiting, low body temperature, and skin that is pale or bluish in color.

- **Desire or an inability to quit.** Having a persistent desire to cut down on drinking or attempting unsuccessfully to do so.
- **Overwhelming time commitment.** Spending an excessive amount of time buying alcohol, drinking it, and recovering from its effects.
- **Interference with life.** Experiencing a reduction in social, recreational, or work activities due to alcohol use.
- **Continued use.** Drinking despite the knowledge that it is causing physical or psychological problems.

Risk Factors for Alcoholism

Genetic, physiological, psychological, and social factors all play a role in determining a person's susceptibility to alcoholism. To what extent each factor influences a person's susceptibility depends on the individual. The risk of alcoholism is higher for people who have a parent who abused alcohol, for instance, but not all children of alcoholics become alcoholics themselves. Other factors that increase a person's risk for abusing alcohol include low self-esteem, impulsiveness, a need for approval, peer pressure, poverty, and being a victim of physical or sexual abuse. Individuals who are under a great deal of chronic stress are also vulnerable. They may turn to alcohol to cope with their problems and try to make themselves feel better, a potentially destructive behavior that is called **self-medicating.**

The age at which a person begins drinking can also raise his or her risk for alcohol abuse. People who begin drinking as teenagers are more likely to develop problems with alcohol. Gender is another risk factor; statistics show that men are much more likely to become dependent on alcohol than women are.[1]

No matter what the cause, once people begin abusing alcohol, the problem often perpetuates itself. Heavy drinking can deplete or increase the levels of some chemicals in the body, causing it to crave or need alcohol to feel good again. Some people keep drinking simply to avoid the uncomfortable withdrawal symptoms.

Common Profiles of Alcoholics

Alcoholism knows no demographic boundaries. It can affect men and women of any race, class, age, and social group. That said, researchers have identified five types of alcoholics that are the most prevalent in our society.

- **The young adult subtype.** Usually alcoholics by their 21st birthday, these young adult drinkers typically do not abuse other drugs and are free of mental disorders. They usually lack a family history of alcoholism, and rarely seek help for their drinking problem. They may drink less often than other alcoholics, but tend to binge drink when they do. They account for 31.5% of alcoholics in the U.S.

- **The young antisocial subtype.** These drinkers start at an earlier age than the young adult subtype, and tend to come from families suffering from alcoholism. About half could be considered antisocial, and many have major depression, bipolar disorder, or anxiety problems. They are more likely to smoke cigarettes and marijuana, as well as use cocaine. They account for 21% of all alcoholics.

- **The functional subtype.** Typically middle-aged, well-educated, and smokers, these drinkers have stable jobs, good incomes, and families. About one-third have a family history of alcoholism, and about one-fourth have had a major bout of depression. They make up 19.5% of the alcoholic population.

- **The intermediate familial subtype.** These middle-aged drinkers tend to have alcoholic parents. About half have been depressed. Most smoke cigarettes, and nearly one in five have had problems with cocaine and marijuana use. They account for 19% of alcoholics.

- **The chronic severe subtype.** Chronic severe drinkers typically start drinking early in life—and develop alcohol problems at a young age, too. They tend to be middle-aged, antisocial, and prone to psychiatric disorders, including depression. They exhibit high rates of smoking, marijuana use, and cocaine dependence. Although they account for only 9% of U.S. alcoholics, about two-thirds of chronic severe drinkers seek help for their drinking problems, making them the most prevalent type of alcoholic in treatment.[39]

self-medicating Using alcohol or drugs to cope with sadness, grief, pain, or mental health problems.

Although 22 is the average age when alcohol dependence begins, the onset varies from the mid-teens to middle age.[40]

Are you at risk for developing alcoholism or alcohol abuse? Take the **Self-Assessment** on page 176.

Getting Help for a Drinking Problem

Few people who abuse alcohol acknowledge that they have a drinking problem. Fewer still seek treatment or counseling for it. It can take a major health problem, accident, or hitting "rock bottom" to motivate a problem drinker to change his or her behavior. Even when drinkers decide that they want to quit, they may not know how to do so on their own. An estimated 19 million people in the U.S. need treatment for an alcohol use problem (about 7.6% of the population aged 12 or older), but only 1.6 million receive treatment at a specialized facility.[1] Among youths between the ages of 12 and 17, an estimated 1.2 million need treatment for an alcohol use problem, but only 77,000 receive treatment.[1]

Treatment Options

Advances in alcoholism treatment in recent years have provided more choices than ever for patients and health professionals. They include:

- **Medications.** Newer medications (naltrexone, topiramate, and acamprosate) can make it easier to quit drinking by offsetting changes in the brain caused by alcoholism and reducing the craving for alcohol. They don't make you sick if you drink, unlike an older medication (disulfiram). None of these medications are addictive. They can also be combined with support groups or alcohol counseling.

- **Alcohol counseling or "talk therapy."** There are several counseling approaches that are about equally effective—12 step, cognitive-behavioral, motivational enhancement, or a combination of these. Getting help in itself appears to be more important than the particular approach used, as long as it offers empathy, avoids heavy confrontation, strengthens motivation, and provides concrete ways to change drinking behavior. These programs usually focus on abstinence from alcohol. They may offer individual or group therapy, connect patients with alcoholism support groups, provide informational lectures, or lead activity therapy sessions. Specialized counseling may focus on the individual or family, and may involve months of sessions or just occasional appearances. Short, one-on-one counseling sessions known as "brief interventions" have been increasing in popularity in recent years. Unlike traditional alcoholism treatments that emphasize complete abstinence from alcohol, interventions encourage sensible drinking at healthy levels. They require minimal follow-up and can be very effective.[41]

- **Self-help groups.** Mutual help organizations include the 12-step program Alcoholics Anonymous. People in these groups attend general meetings and support each other by sharing advice and their personal experiences with alcohol abuse and recovery.

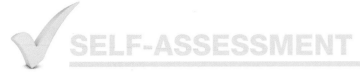
SELF-ASSESSMENT

To complete this self-assessment online, visit **www.pearsonhighered.com/choosinghealth**.

Do You Have Symptoms of an Alcohol Use Disorder?

Generally known as alcoholism and alcohol abuse, alcohol use disorders are medical conditions that doctors can diagnose when a patient's drinking causes distress or harm. See if you recognize any of these symptoms in yourself. In the past year, have you:

- ☐ had times when you ended up drinking **more, or longer,** than you intended?
- ☐ more than once wanted to **cut down or stop** drinking, or tried to, but couldn't?
- ☐ more than once gotten into situations while or after drinking that **increased your chances of getting hurt** (such as driving, swimming, using machinery, walking in a dangerous area, or having unsafe sex)?
- ☐ had to drink **much more** than you once did to **get the effect** you want? Or found that your **usual number** of drinks had **much less effect** than before?

- ☐ continued to drink even though it was making you feel **depressed or anxious** or adding to **another health problem**? Or after having had a **memory blackout**?
- ☐ spent a **lot of time** drinking? Or being sick or getting over other aftereffects?
- ☐ continued to drink even though it was causing **trouble** with your **family** or **friends**?
- ☐ found that drinking—or being sick from drinking—often **interfered with taking care** of your **home** or **family**? Or caused **job** troubles? Or **school** problems?

- ☐ **given up** or **cut back** on **activities** that were important or interesting to you, or gave you pleasure, in order to drink?
- ☐ more than once gotten **arrested,** been held at a police station, or had other **legal problems** because of your drinking?
- ☐ found that when the effects of alcohol were wearing off, you had **withdrawal symptoms,** such as trouble sleeping, shakiness, restlessness, nausea, sweating, a racing heart, or a seizure? Or sensed things that were not there?

HOW TO INTERPRET YOUR SCORE

Depending on the symptoms and their severity, even one symptom can indicate alcohol abuse, and as few as three can indicate alcohol dependence, or alcoholism. The more symptoms you have, the more urgent the need for change.

    You can do something to reduce your risks.

- **Cut back or quit.** Some people with a few, mild symptoms can cut back effectively, but for others, it's safest to quit.

- **Change on your own or with help.** Many people change on their own, whereas others may opt for support.
- **Ask a health professional for advice.** Advances in alcohol research have provided new treatment options. A health care professional can look at the number, pattern, and severity of your symptoms to help you decide the best course of action.

Source: National Institutes of Health. (2010). What are symptoms of an alcohol-use disorder? Retrieved from the Rethinking Drinking website at http://rethinkingdrinking.niaaa.nih.gov/WhatsTheHarm/WhatAreSymptomsOfAnAlcoholUseDisorder.asp.

- **Intensive treatment programs.** These include 14- to 28-day residential programs which typically employ a 12-step approach combined with individual and group therapy in a strictly scheduled abstinence environment. They also include longer-term (3–4 month) programs and halfway houses that offer life skill and job training as well as treatment for substance dependence and mental health problems.

    Looking for an alcohol treatment center? Visit **http://findtreatment.samhsa.gov**, which allows you to search for a treatment program near you.

    This site provides self-help strategies for cutting back on or quitting drinking: **http://rethinkingdrinking.niaaa.nih.gov/Support/ChooseYourApproach.asp**.

Dealing with Relapse

Once an alcoholic has decided to curb or stop drinking altogether, he or she must confront the possibility of *relapse*. **Relapse**—resuming the behavior of drinking to excess, or "falling off the wagon"— is experienced by up to 90% of drinkers when they first try to quit.[42] With hard work and commitment, however, it can be overcome. Research from the National Institute on Alcohol Abuse and Alcoholism reveals that 20 years after the onset of alcohol dependence, about three-fourths of individuals were fully recovered.[40] Even more surprising, more than half of these individuals were able to drink at low levels without showing symptoms of alcohol dependence.[40] That said, many alcoholics find that abstinence is ultimately the only way to keep alcohol use from disrupting their lives.

    Beating any addiction requires both patience and prac-

---

relapse Returning to drinking after a period of sobriety.

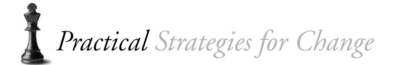

Practical Strategies for Change

Beating Relapse

If you relapse while trying to quit drinking, don't give up. Follow these tips:

- **Get right back on track.** Stop drinking—the sooner the better.
- **Remember, each day is a new day to start over.** Although it can be unsettling to slip, you don't have to continue drinking. You are responsible for your choices.
- **Understand that setbacks are common when people undertake a major change.** It's your progress in the long run that counts.
- **Don't run yourself down.** It doesn't help. Don't let feelings of discouragement, anger, or guilt stop you from asking for help and getting back on track.
- **Get some help.** Contact your counselor or a sober and supportive friend right away to talk about what happened, or go to an AA or other mutual-help meeting.
- **Think it through.** With a little distance, work on your own or with support to better understand why the episode happened at that particular time and place.
- **Learn from what happened.** Decide what you need to do so that it won't happen again, and write it down. Use the experience to strengthen your commitment.
- **Avoid triggers to drink.** Get rid of any alcohol at home. If possible, avoid revisiting the situation in which you drank.
- **Find alternatives.** Keep busy with things that are not associated with drinking.

tice. The body has to be weaned off a substance it has been dependent upon, and the mind has to give up a long-time emotional crutch. Recovering alcoholics often have to change their social patterns and entire lifestyle. The box **Practical Strategies for Change: Beating Relapse** provides some tips for recovering from a relapse.

Smoking in the U.S.

Each year, 443,000 people in the United States die prematurely because of smoking-related illnesses.[43,44] That translates to 1 of every 5 deaths in the U.S. Tobacco use causes more deaths each year than HIV, illegal drug use, alcohol use, car accidents, suicides, and murders combined.[43,45] Although smoking rates have dropped in recent years, approximately 46 million U.S. adults remain smokers.[46]

The **Diversity & Health** box on page 178 provides a closer look at the prevalence of smoking among different demographic groups.

Smoking on Campus

Among college students, 15% have tried smoking at least once, according to a recent national survey; 4.6% reported smoking cigarettes daily.[18] The **Student Stats** box examines actual versus perceived use of tobacco and marijuana products among college students.

Of all tobacco users, 41.4% are between the ages of 18 and 25.[1] One-fifth of high school students are current smokers by the time they graduate.[47] The younger people are when they start smoking, the more likely they are to become adult smokers. Research findings conclude that approximately 90% of adults who are regular smokers began at or before the age 19.[48]

Why Students Smoke

It would be difficult to find a student who has *not* heard that smoking can kill you. Why, then, do students start smoking? There are as many different factors and reasons as there are individuals, but the following are among the most common:

- **Rebellion and experimentation.** For a young person, smoking a cigarette can be a symbolic act. The fact that smoking is something "bad" can actually make it more appealing. It may be a teenager's way of challenging authority. The desire to experiment with recreational drugs is another reason young people take up smoking.
- **Peer pressure.** If their friends smoke, teens may begin smoking so that they can maintain acceptance from their peer group.
- **Family exposure.** Research shows that if children have one or more parents who smoke, they are twice as likely to become smokers themselves by the time they finish high school.[49]
- **Aggressive advertising and marketing.** The major cigarette manufacturers spend more than $35 million every day to promote their products, and many of their efforts directly reach young adults.[50] One study found that adolescents who owned a tobacco promotional item and could name a brand whose advertisements attracted their attention were more than twice as likely to become established smokers than adolescents who did neither.[51]
- **Desire to lose weight.** Though it is true that nicotine can be an appetite suppressant, taking up smoking to lose weight is one of the worst decisions a young person can make. The damage to

health caused by smoking far outweighs any short-term benefits in weight management.
- **Stress.** Schoolwork, stressful family environments, and complicated social relationships with classmates have all been cited as reasons why students smoke. In one study of adolescent girls, almost half of those who smoked said they started because they had a lot of stress in their lives.[52]

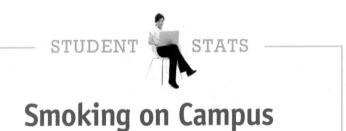 **View video clips about the addictiveness of nicotine, the effects of tobacco advertising, and more at www.tobaccofree.org/clips.htm.**

What's in a Cigarette?

Smoking cigarettes is by far the most common form of tobacco use. A typical cigarette in the U.S. contains 50% shredded tobacco leaf, 30% reconstituted tobacco (made from other parts of the tobacco plant, such as the stem), and 20% expanded tobacco (tobacco that has been "puffed up" like popcorn and functions as "filler").[53] It also contains nearly 600 additives with a wide range of functions. Cocoa, licorice, and vanilla, for example, are among the additives that help hide the harsh taste of tobacco. Meanwhile, ammonia—a chemical commonly used for household cleaning—boosts the delivery of

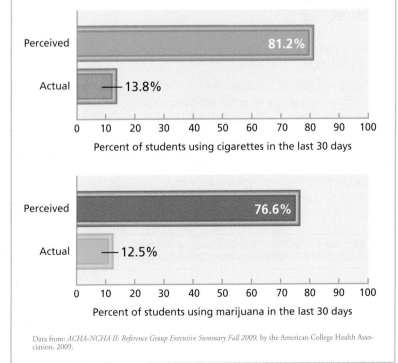

STUDENT STATS

Smoking on Campus

A recent national survey revealed that students tend to greatly overestimate how many of their peers regularly smoke cigarettes or marijuana.

Perceived — 81.2%
Actual — 13.8%

Percent of students using cigarettes in the last 30 days

Perceived — 76.6%
Actual — 12.5%

Percent of students using marijuana in the last 30 days

Data from: *ACHA-NCHA II: Reference Group Executive Summary Fall 2009*, by the American College Health Association, 2009.

Tobacco Use Through the Lenses
of Sex, Race/Ethnicity, Age, Education, and Geography

A recent national survey conducted by the Substance Abuse and Mental Health Services Administration revealed the following:

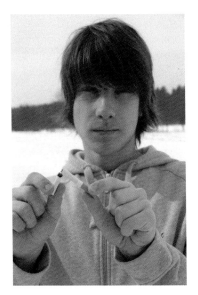

Smoking rates are highest among those aged 18–25.

Overall

- An estimated 28.4% of those aged 12 or older (about 70.9 million people) use a tobacco product; 23.9% smoke cigarettes, 5.3% smoke cigars, and 3.5% use smokeless tobacco.

Sex

- Men are more likely to use a tobacco product than women. Of males aged 12 or older, 34.5% use a tobacco product, compared to 22.5% of females.
- However, among those aged 12 to 17, there is not much difference in the rate of smoking in males (9%) versus females (9.2%).

Race/Ethnicity

- Among Native Americans, 48.7% report current tobacco use, the highest of any racial/ethnic group.
- Among people of mixed race background, 37.3% use tobacco.
- Among Caucasians, 30.4% use tobacco.

- Among African Americans, 28.6% use tobacco.
- Among Hispanics, 21.3% use tobacco.
- Among Asian Americans, 13.9% use tobacco.

Age

- People aged 18–25 report a higher rate of current tobacco use (41.4%) than any other age group.

Education

- Adults with college degrees are less likely to use tobacco than those with less education.

Geography

- Rates of smoking are higher in the South (25.5%) and Midwest (25.9%) than in the West (21%) and Northeast (22.2%).

Data from Results from the 2008 National Survey on Drug Use and Health: National Findings *by the Substance Abuse and Mental Health Services Administration, 2009, retrieved from http://www.oas.samhsa.gov/nsduh/2k8nsduh/2k8Results.cfm.*

---

nicotine (the key psychoactive ingredient in tobacco) into the lungs and bloodstream.

When a cigarette is lit and smoked, it releases approximately 4,000 chemicals, more than 60 of which are **carcinogenic,** meaning they cause cancer. These carcinogens include arsenic (a poison), formaldehyde (used in embalming fluid), polonium-210 (a radioactive substance), and **tar.** Tar is a sticky, thick brown residue that forms when tobacco is burned and its chemical particles condense. Other harmful chemicals in cigarette smoke include hydrogen cyanide, benzene (found in gasoline), and **carbon monoxide,** an especially dangerous gas that inhibits the delivery of oxygen to the body's vital organs.

> **Learn more about the chemicals found in cigarette smoke at http://tobaccofreekids.org/microsites/whatareyousmoking.**

Effects of Smoking on Health

Smoking harms nearly every organ of the body, including the lungs, kidneys, bladder, heart, pancreas, stomach, and esophagus. It weakens the immune system and shortens life expectancy. Adults

who smoke die an average of 13 to 14 years earlier than those who don't smoke.[54] About half of long-term smokers will die because of their habit, according to the American Cancer Society.[55]

Short-Term Health Effects

From the moment a person takes the first puff of a cigarette, physiological changes take place in the body. Within 8 seconds of entering the body, nicotine is absorbed by the lungs and quickly moved into the bloodstream, where it is circulated throughout the brain. There, it triggers the release of large amounts of **dopamine,** a neurotransmitter that stimulates feelings of pleasure. Once smokers develop a tolerance to nicotine, they need

nicotine An alkaloid derived from the tobacco plant that is responsible for smoking's psychoactive and addictive effects.

carcinogenic Cancer-causing.

tar A sticky, thick brown residue that forms when tobacco is burned and its chemical particles condense.

carbon monoxide A gas that inhibits the delivery of oxygen to the body's vital organs.

dopamine A neurotransmitter that stimulates feelings of pleasure.

Quitting Cold Turkey

"Hi, I'm Addison. When I first started smoking I was 16 years old. I've tried to quit numerous times—always cold turkey. I'd last maybe a week if I was lucky. Recently I tried to quit again. This time I went cold turkey *and* I started working out too. I tried to replace a bad habit with a healthier habit. I go to the gym every day, I haven't smoked in two weeks, and I hope to keep it that way."

1: What stage of behavior change is Addison in? (Review Chapter 1 if you can't remember the stages of behavior change.)

2: What do you think of Addison's plan to "replace" smoking with working out?

3: How can Addison improve his chances of quitting smoking for good?

Do you have a story similar to Addison's? Share your story at **www.pearsonhighered.com/choosinghealth.**

more and more of it to achieve the same effects they experienced when they first began smoking. Eventually, smokers need to keep smoking just to feel "normal," as the body becomes addicted to nicotine. Stopping smoking can cause withdrawal symptoms such as cravings, irritability, insomnia, headache, inability to concentrate, and dry mouth.

Other short-term health effects of smoking include:

- **Increased heart rate and blood pressure.** Nicotine causes the heart to beat faster. It also raises blood pressure.
- **Shortness of breath and reduction in stamina.** The carbon monoxide in cigarette smoke binds to a protein in red blood cells, disrupting these cells' ability to effectively deliver oxygen to the rest of the body.
- **Coughing.** Cigarette smoke damages the respiratory passageways, increasing the production of mucus and triggering the need to cough.
- **Heightened alertness.**
- **Decreased skin temperature.** Nicotine constricts blood vessels, resulting in less blood flow to the skin (reducing its temperature) and to the legs and feet.
- **Increased blood sugar.**
- **Dulled sense of smell and taste.**
- **Bad breath.**
- **Smelling like smoke.**

chronic obstructive pulmonary disease (COPD) A category of diseases that includes emphysema, chronic bronchitis, and asthma.

emphysema A chronic disease in which the air sacs in the lung become damaged, making breathing difficult.

- Decreased urine production.
- Risks to a developing fetus.

Long-Term Health Effects

Cigarette smoking is so harmful that the surgeon general has called it "the leading preventable cause of disease and deaths in the United States." It raises the risk of cancer and cardiovascular disease, and contributes to a host of other negative health effects.

Cancer

In the United States, smoking is responsible for 90% of lung cancer deaths in men and nearly 80% in women.[54] Smoking is also associated with cancers of the kidney, bladder, pancreas, stomach, esophagus, mouth, throat, larynx, cervix, and blood. A smoker's risk of developing these cancers increases with the number of cigarettes and the number of years they smoke. The risk, however, does begin to drop over time in those who are able to quit for good.

The risk of developing cancer is not insignificant. The odds of getting lung cancer are more than 23 times higher among men who smoke cigarettes than men who do not.[54] Women who smoke are 13 times more likely to develop the disease than women who do not.[56]

Cardiovascular Disease

Smoking is a key risk factor for three major types of cardiovascular disease:

- **Coronary heart disease.** The leading cause of death in the United States, coronary heart disease often stems from the development of *atherosclerosis*, a progressive hardening of the coronary arteries. Smoking contributes to the development of atherosclerosis, which can result in a heart attack. Indeed, you are four times more likely to die of coronary heart disease if you smoke.[54]
- **Stroke.** A stroke occurs when a blood vessel carrying oxygen and nutrients to the brain either bursts or is blocked by a clot. When that happens, part of the brain cannot get the blood and oxygen it needs and starts to die. It can cause speech problems, vision problems, memory loss, and paralysis on one side of the body. It can also be fatal. Cigarette smoking doubles a person's odds of having a stroke. The risk, however, steadily decreases after quitting smoking, with former smokers having roughly the same stroke risk as nonsmokers do 5 to 15 years after quitting.[54]
- **Abdominal aortic aneurysm.** An aortic aneurysm is a dangerously weakened and bulging area in the aorta, the major blood vessel that supplies blood to the body. A ruptured aortic aneurysm can cause life-threatening bleeding. Smoking is clearly associated with the condition. Several studies show that the risk of death from abdominal aortic aneurysm more than quadruples in smokers and doubles in former smokers.[54]

Respiratory Disease

Smoking damages the airways and alveoli of the lungs and can lead to **chronic obstructive pulmonary disease** (COPD), a category of diseases that includes emphysema, chronic bronchitis, and asthma.

In **emphysema,** the walls of the lungs' air sacs lose their elasticity and are destroyed. It becomes difficult for the lungs to transfer oxygen to the bloodstream, causing shortness of breath. Em-

Are "Light" Cigarettes Safe to Use?

You have probably seen advertisements for cigarettes that are "low-tar," "mild," "light," or "lite." Some even purport to be "ultra-light." But are such cigarettes really any less dangerous than regular cigarettes?

Although it's true that some of these cigarettes deliver less tar or nicotine than regular cigarettes in machine-based tests, health experts say there is no convincing evidence that they are less harmful to a person's health. On the contrary, studies have shown that when smokers switch to low-tar cigarettes, they change the way they smoke, smoking more cigarettes, taking bigger puffs, and holding smoke in their lungs longer.[1]

- The U.S. surgeon general has concluded that "smoking cigarettes with lower machine-measured yields of tar and nicotine provides no clear benefit to health."[2]
- The National Cancer Institute has determined that people who switch to light cigarettes are likely to inhale the same amount of hazardous chemicals as those smoking regular

or "full-flavored" cigarettes. They also remain at high risk for developing smoking-related cancers and other diseases.[3]

- There is no evidence that switching to light cigarettes actually helps smokers kick their habit.

The bottom line: "Light" cigarettes are still harmful to a person's health.

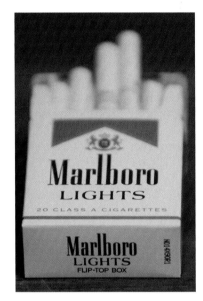

References: **1.** *The Health Consequences of Smoking: The Changing Cigarette, a Report of the Surgeon General* by the U.S. Department of Health and Human Services, 1981. **2.** *The Health Consequences of Smoking, a Report of the Surgeon General* by the U.S. Department of Health and Human Services, 2004. **3.** *Risks Associated with Smoking Cigarettes with Low Machine-Measured Yields of Tar and Nicotine* (Monograph 13) by the National Cancer Institute, October 2001, retrieved from http://cancercontrol.cancer.gov/tcrb/monographs/.

In 2005, COPD was one of the leading causes of death in the United States, killing more than 126,000 people.[57] More than 90% of those deaths were attributed to smoking, according to the surgeon general.[57]

Other Health Effects

Aside from the increased risks for cancer, cardiovascular disease, and respiratory disease, smoking can have additional health consequences:

- Erectile dysfunction in men.
- Loss of bone density in women following menopause.
- Periodontitis, a gum infection that can lead to tooth loss.
- Increased risk of developing cataracts, a leading cause of blindness.
- Decreased fertility in women.
- Premature aging and wrinkling of skin.
- Stained teeth.

Figure 8.5 summarizes the short- and long-term health effects of smoking.

Smoking and Pregnancy

When a pregnant woman smokes, so does her unborn baby. The nicotine, carbon monoxide, benzene, and other cancer-causing chemicals that enter her bloodstream are passed on to her fetus. Nicotine also reduces the amount of oxygen that reaches the fetus, negatively affecting its growth.

Smoking while pregnant is like gambling—with the baby's life. Babies born to women who smoke are two to three times more likely to die of *sudden infant death syndrome* than babies born to women who did not smoke.[58] They also have 30% higher odds of being born prematurely, and are more likely to weigh less than 5.5 pounds when they are born, increasing their risk for illness or death.[58] Smoking during pregnancy has also been linked to miscarriages and stillbirths. Up to 5% of infant deaths would be prevented if women did not smoke during their pregnancy.[59]

Secondhand Smoke

Secondhand smoke is a mixture of **sidestream smoke**—the smoke emanating from the burning end of a cigarette or pipe—and **mainstream smoke,** which is exhaled from the lungs of smokers. Also called *environmental tobacco smoke,* it contains more than 250 chemicals known to be toxic or capable of causing cancer, including arsenic, ammonia, formaldehyde and benzene.[60]

The smoke that nonsmokers are exposed to actually has higher concentrations of some harmful chemicals than the smoke inhaled by the smoker, according to the American Lung Association. This is because

chronic bronchitis Inflammation of the main airways in the lungs that continues for at least three months.

asthma A chronic pulmonary disease in which the air passages become inflamed, making breathing difficult.

secondhand smoke (environmental tobacco smoke) The smoke nonsmokers are exposed to when someone has been smoking nearby; a combination of sidestream smoke and mainstream smoke.

sidestream smoke Smoke emanating from the burning end of a cigarette or pipe.

mainstream smoke Smoke exhaled from the lungs of smokers.

physema sufferers often have trouble performing simple physical activities such as shopping or climbing the stairs. As the disease progresses, many emphysema patients must rely on an oxygen tank to help them breathe.

Chronic bronchitis is an inflammation of the main airways in the lungs that continues for at least three months. Symptoms include a chronic cough that produces mucus, shortness of breath, wheezing, and frequent respiratory infections.

Asthma is a chronic pulmonary disease in which the air passages become inflamed. The inflammation causes a narrowing of the airways, making breathing very difficult. Asthma symptoms include wheezing, coughing, shortness of breath, and chest tightness.

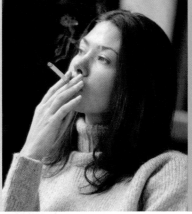

Short-term effects:	Long-term effects:
• Feeling of euphoria • Increased heart rate • Increased blood pressure • Shortness of breath • Reduction in stamina • Coughing • Heightened alertness • Decreased skin temperature • Increased blood sugar • Dulled sense of smell and taste • Bad breath • Smelling like smoke • Decreased urine production • Health risks to developing fetus	• Greatly increased risk of cancer • Increased risk of heart disease • Increased risk of emphysema, bronchitis, asthma • Erectile dysfunction • Loss of bone density in women following menopause • Periodontitis • Increased risk of cataracts • Decreased fertility in women • Premature aging and wrinkling of skin • Stained teeth

Figure 8.5 Short- and long-term health effects of smoking.

sidestream smoke is not filtered through a cigarette filter or a smoker's lungs. As a result, secondhand smoke has at least twice the amount of nicotine and tar as mainstream smoke. It also has five times the amount of carbon monoxide, and has higher levels of ammonia and cadmium (chemicals found in glass cleaner and batteries, respectively).

Millions of people in the United States are essentially *passive smokers:* people who breathe in secondhand smoke from their environment. In national surveys, 43% of passive smokers have been found to have detectable levels of *cotinine*—the major breakdown product of nicotine—in their blood.[60]

The health risks to passive smokers are no less serious than if they were the ones lighting up a cigarette or puffing on a cigar. The U.S. surgeon general concluded in 2006 that "the scientific evidence indicates that there is no risk-free level of exposure to secondhand smoke." In fact, secondhand smoke can kill.

Health Effects of Secondhand Smoke

Secondhand smoke, which can linger in the air for hours after cigarettes have been extinguished, can exacerbate—or cause—a number of health conditions, including cancer, respiratory infections, and asthma. On a basic level, it can irritate the eyes, nose, throat, and lungs. It can also cause chest pain, coughing, and production of excessive phlegm. In a report spanning more than 700 pages, the U.S. surgeon general concluded that secondhand smoke can also:

- Cause premature death and disease in children and adults who do not smoke.
- Increase a nonsmoker's risk of heart disease by 25 to 30%.
- Cause lung cancer in people who have never smoked.
- Cause respiratory illnesses, including asthma, in children.
- Cause ear infections in children.
- Cause sudden infant death syndrome in some babies.[60]

"The health effects of secondhand smoke exposure are more pervasive than we previously thought," the report summarized. "The scientific evidence is now indisputable: secondhand smoke is not a mere annoyance. It is a serious health hazard that can lead to disease and premature death in children and nonsmoking adults."[60]

Check out this article on the dangers of secondhand smoke from *Time* magazine: www.time.com/time/health/article/0,8599,1638535,00.html.

Health experts estimate that secondhand smoke causes 3,400 lung cancer deaths and between 22,700 and 69,600 heart disease deaths in adult nonsmokers in the United States each year.[61] It causes more than 750,000 middle ear infections in children and increases the number and severity of asthma attacks in more than 200,000 asthmatic children.[61]

Other Forms of Tobacco

Cigars, clove cigarettes, bidis, pipes, and smokeless "spit" tobacco are other commonly used tobacco products **(Figure 8.6)**. Like cigarettes, they are also associated with numerous health problems.

Cigars

Cigars contain many of the same addictive, toxic, cancer-causing substances that cigarettes do. The smoke from cigars also contains many of the toxins found in cigarette smoke, including ammonia,

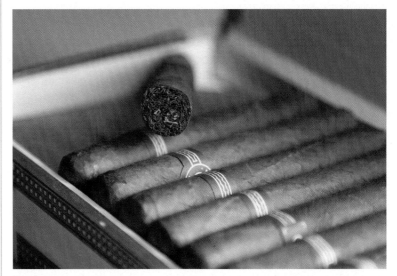

Figure 8.6 All tobacco products pose health risks. Cigars (above), clove cigarettes, bidis, and smokeless tobacco all increase the risk of cancer and heart disease.

carbon monoxide, and benzene, but in much higher concentrations. A single cigar can contain as much tobacco as an entire pack of cigarettes.[62]

Because most cigar smokers do not inhale, their risk of developing lung cancer is lower than it is for cigarette smokers. However, cigar smokers still have higher rates of lung cancer, heart disease, and chronic obstructive pulmonary disease than nonsmokers do.[63]

Clove Cigarettes

Clove cigarettes, which have a distinctly sweet, pungent odor, are shaped like traditional cigarettes and are imported from Indonesia or other Southeast Asian countries. Also called *kreteks*, they usually contain tobacco, cloves, and other additives. Although they may smell and taste different from conventional cigarettes, there is no evidence that they are any safer. Some analyses, in fact, have demonstrated that they deliver more nicotine, carbon monoxide, and tar than traditional cigarettes.[64] Clove cigarette smokers have higher rates of asthma and up to 20 times the risk for abnormal lung function, compared with nonsmokers.[65]

New federal laws ban the sale of flavored cigarettes, including clove cigarettes. It is not illegal to smoke them, but it is illegal to sell them.

Bidis

Bidis (pronounced bee-dees) are thin, hand-rolled cigarettes that come in a variety of flavors, including cherry, chocolate, grape, and mango. Imported from India and other Southeast Asian countries, they are packed with tobacco and wrapped in leaf, sometimes tied at the ends by a colorful string.

Contrary to a popular misconception, bidis are *not* safer than cigarettes. Bidi smoke contains 3 to 5 times more nicotine than found in a regular cigarette.[65] Bidi smokers are at increased risk for several types of cancer, including oral, lung, stomach, and esophageal cancer, as well as coronary heart disease, emphysema, and chronic bronchitis.[65]

Smokeless ("Spit") Tobacco

Baseball fans are used to seeing their heroes use smokeless tobacco, also known as "spit" or "chew." Indeed, one in three major league baseball players uses smokeless tobacco.[66] Viewers watching one game of the 2004 World Series were exposed to a full 9 minutes and 11 seconds of players' perceptible use of smokeless tobacco.[67] No wonder, then, that many boys and young men have followed in the footsteps of their role models, using smokeless tobacco at alarming rates.

About 1 in every 10 male college students is a current user of smokeless tobacco, compared with just 1 in every 250 female college students.[68] Caucasian students are most likely to use it.[68] Smokeless tobacco is especially popular among students enrolled in colleges in rural areas or small towns. Highlighting the influence baseball players have had on their young fans, smokeless tobacco use is also common among intercollegiate athletes.[68]

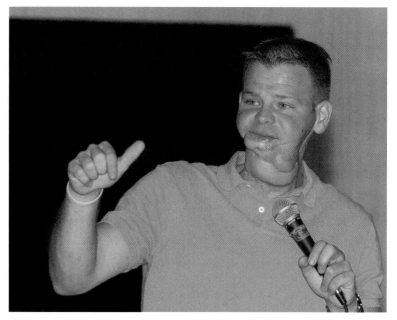

Gruen Von Behrens was hooked on chewing tobacco at age 14 and diagnosed with oral cancer at age 17. He has lost his jaw, lower teeth, and part of his tongue in his fight to beat the disease.

leukoplakia White spots on the mucous membranes in the mouth that may become cancerous.

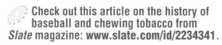

Check out this article on the history of baseball and chewing tobacco from *Slate* magazine: www.slate.com/id/2234341.

Smokeless tobacco comes in two forms. *Snuff* is a fine-grain tobacco that is often sold in teabag-like pouches that users "pinch" or "dip" between their lower lip and gum. *Chewing tobacco* comes in wads of shredded or "bricked" tobacco leaves that people put between their cheek and gum. No matter the type, smokeless tobacco is meant to stew in the mouth for minutes at a time. Users suck on the tobacco juices and then spit to get rid of the saliva that builds up, hence the nickname "spit."

Chewing tobacco is made from tobacco leaves that have had their stems removed. Snuff is made from both the leaf and stem. Both are typically loaded with sweeteners and flavorings to make them taste more pleasant. Although they don't emit harmful plumes of smoke like cigarettes and cigars do, smokeless tobacco contains plenty of addictive nicotine. It is absorbed into the bloodstream through the mucous membranes that line the mouth, and users can become physically hooked without ever swallowing the tobacco soup that builds up in their mouths. The average dose of smokeless tobacco, in fact, contains up to four times the amount of nicotine found in the average cigarette. One can of snuff is equivalent, nicotine-wise, to about four packs of cigarettes.

The health effects of using smokeless tobacco are varied. Regular use increases a person's risk for cancers of the lip, tongue, cheeks, gums, and mouth. The products stain and wear down the teeth, cause gums to recede, and can cause a condition called **leukoplakia,** characterized by whitish lesions in the mouth. These lesions may become cancerous, and are frequently found in snuff and chew users in their 20s.

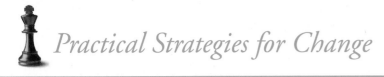
Quitting Smoking

The National Institutes for Health promote the START method as an effective smoking cessation strategy.

S = Set a quit date.
Choose a date within the next two weeks as your official quit date. Smoking cessation experts suggest that you pick a special date as your quit date. Consider your birthday, a special anniversary, New Year's Day, 4th of July, "World No-Tobacco Day" (May 31st), or the "Great American Smoke-out" (the third Thursday of November).

T = Tell family, friends, and coworkers that you plan to quit.
If you are going to be successful in your attempt to quit, you will need the help and support of others. So inform the important people in your life and let them know exactly how they can help you in your efforts.

A = Anticipate and plan for the challenges you'll face while quitting.
Studies show that most people who return to smoking do so within the first three months. Make plans ahead of time for dealing with cravings and withdrawal symptoms when they hit.

R = Remove cigarettes and other tobacco products from your home, car, and work.
Get rid of everything you can that reminds you of smoking. Change your routine, so that certain events and places don't prompt a cigarette craving. Throw away all cigarettes and smoking paraphernalia such as lighters, matches, and ashtrays.

T = Talk to your doctor about getting help to quit.
Your health-care provider can prescribe medication that can help you quit. There are also effective over-the-counter products that are helpful in dealing with nicotine withdrawal. These products include:

- Nicotine gum
- Nicotine inhaler
- Nicotine lozenge
- Nicotine nasal spray
- Nicotine patch
- Bupropion SR pills (prescription only)
- Varenicline pills (prescription only)

For more help: Call 1-877-44U-QUIT (1-877-448-7848) to talk to a smoking cessation counselor from the National Cancer Institute. For help within your own state, call 1-800-QUITNOW (1-800-784-8669 / TTY 1-800-332-8615) or visit www.smokefree.gov.

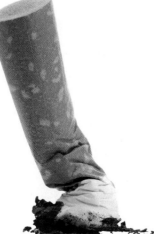

Getting Help to Quit Smoking

If you smoke, the odds are that you have thought about quitting. Perhaps you have already tried to quit. An estimated 38–50% of smokers under the age of 65 try to break their addiction each year—often without the help of medications or counseling.[69] Usually they are unsuccessful.

Stopping smoking is not a simple matter. Nicotine activates the pleasure and reward centers of the brain and raises levels of the "feel good" neurotransmitter, dopamine. Consequently, nicotine can be as addictive as heroin or cocaine. Those attempting to quit often must deal with withdrawal symptoms such as restlessness, depression, hunger, insomnia, and headaches. A smoker's brain develops an abundance of nicotine-binding receptors to accommodate the large doses of nicotine. Recent research findings conclude that for up to 6 weeks after people stop smoking, these receptors still exist.[69] Unfortunately, these nicotine-receptor brain cells contribute to the cravings and other discomforts of smoking withdrawal and probably explain why the first months of smoking cessation are very difficult for many people. The good news is that after 6–12 weeks of abstinence, the former smoker's nicotine receptor levels match those of a nonsmoker and consequently relapse is less likely.

Despite the challenges, making the decision to quit—and getting assistance to do so—can pay off for those who are determined enough. Indeed, the number of smokers able to quit has so outpaced the rate of young adults taking up smoking that today there are more former smokers than current ones.[70] The box **Practical Strategies for Change: Quitting Smoking** offers advice on taking the first steps toward quitting.

The health benefits of quitting smoking begin almost immediately. **Figure 8.7** illustrates the short- and long-term benefits of quitting.

Treatment Options

Several products are available to aid smokers who wish to quit. Most of them, including nicotine gum, inhalers, lozenges, nasal sprays, and patches, are *nicotine replacement therapies* designed to help smokers gradually reduce their dependence on nicotine and reduce the severity of nicotine withdrawal symptoms. Others, such as bupropion (Zyban) and varenicline (Chantix), do not contain nicotine at all, but reduce the smoker's craving for tobacco and ease withdrawal symptoms (note that serious safety concerns have recently arisen about both of these drugs). You should talk with your doctor or a pharmacist before taking any smoking cessation products, especially if you have any allergies, health problems, are taking any medications, or are pregnant or planning to become pregnant.

Note that nicotine replacement therapies are only available to those aged 18 and older. You should not continue smoking while taking a smoking cessation product. You should also avoid taking more than one smoking cessation product at the same time without consulting a doctor, as improper use can result in nicotine overdose.

In addition to nicotine replacement therapies, smoking-cessation programs are effective for approximately 20–40% of smokers.[60] There are several types of treatment options, including residential, individual or group therapy, and education and support groups.

QUIT SMOKING

First 48 hours:

20 minutes	8 hours	24 hours	48 hours
• Blood pressure drops to normal. • Pulse rate drops to normal. • Body temperature of hands and feet increases to normal.	• Carbon monoxide level in blood drops to normal. • Oxygen level in blood increases to normal.	• Chance of heart attack decreases.	• Nerve endings start regrowing. • Ability to smell and taste is enhanced.

First year:

2 weeks to 3 months	1 to 9 months	1 year
• Circulation improves. • Walking becomes easier. • Lung function increases up to 30%.	• Coughing, sinus congestion, fatigue, and shortness of breath decrease. • Cilia regrow in lungs, increasing ability to handle mucus, clean the lungs, and reduce infection. • Overall energy level increases.	• Excess risk of coronary heart disease is half that of a smoker.

Future years:

5 years	10 years	15 years
• Lung cancer death rate for average former smoker (one pack a day) decreases by almost half.	• Lung cancer death rate similar to that of nonsmokers. • Precancerous cells are replaced • Risk of cancer of the mouth, throat, esophagus, bladder, kidney, and pancreas decreases.	• Risk of cornary heart disease is that of a nonsmoker.

Figure 8.7 **Benefits of quitting smoking.** The health benefits of quitting smoking begin the moment you stop.

Ready to quit smoking today? Visit www.smokefree.gov. The American Cancer Society also offers helpful tips for quitting smoking at www.cancer.org/Healthy/StayAwayfromTobacco/GuidetoQuittingSmoking/index.

Dealing with Relapse

Smokers commonly experience withdrawal symptoms when they first quit smoking, including difficulty concentrating, a negative mood, and the urge to smoke. These symptoms usually peak within one or two weeks. Not surprisingly, smokers are most likely to relapse early in the quitting process, although sometimes relapse can occur months or even years after quitting. Any smoking—even taking one single puff—increases the likelihood of a full relapse.

Watch videos of real students discussing their experiences with alcohol and tobacco at www.pearsonhighered.com/choosinghealth.

> " *The number of smokers able to quit has so outpaced the rate of young adults taking up smoking that today there are more former smokers than current ones.* "

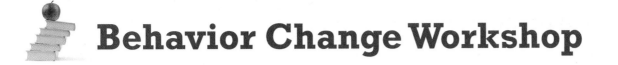

Behavior Change Workshop

To complete this workshop online, visit **www.pearsonhighered.com/choosinghealth**.

Alcohol and tobacco are highly addictive drugs that can be very difficult to curb or eliminate from your daily life. If these drugs are seriously disrupting your life, seek help. The following websites are two great places to start: http://findtreatment.samhsa.gov and www.smokefree.gov. Also, keep in mind that most college campuses have student health centers staffed with counselors who can help support you in breaking an alcohol or smoking habit.

In the meantime, consider the situations that cause you to want to drink or smoke, and then ask yourself what you might do instead of reaching for a beer or for a cigarette.

Part I. Identify Emotional or Situational "Triggers"

1. What are your top five "triggers"? What situations or emotions make you most want to drink or smoke? Common triggers include stress, boredom, sadness, loneliness, taking a work break, and socializing with friends. List these if any apply to you, or list others.

_____

_____

_____

2. Target one of the above triggers. Ask yourself honestly: How ready are you to commit to a behavior change that will help you deal with that trigger without turning to drinking or smoking? What stage of behavior change are you in? (See Chapter 1 for a review of the stages of behavior change.)

Target trigger: _____

_____

Current stage of behavior change: _____

_____

Part II. Take Action
1. Assuming you are truly committed to changing your behavior, describe what you might do to deal with your target trigger *instead* of smoking or drinking.

Example: *Instead of having a drink the next time I am stressed, I will take a walk outside to clear my head.*

Next step: _____

_____

_____

2. Describe how you will fight the temptation to drink or smoke.

Example: *I will try a nicotine replacement therapy like nicotine gum in order to gradually reduce my dependence on nicotine.*

_____

_____

Chapter Summary

- Alcohol and tobacco are the most commonly used drugs in the United States and on college campuses.
- Alcohol is absorbed into the bloodstream from the stomach and small intestine. It is metabolized by the liver. If a person consumes alcohol at a faster rate than the liver can break it down, intoxication occurs.
- Blood alcohol concentration (BAC) is affected by numerous factors, including how much and how quickly alcohol is consumed, type of alcohol, sex, age, weight, physical condition, food intake, and medications.
- The short-term effects of alcohol use include lightheadedness, loss of inhibition, compromised motor coordination, slowed reaction times, slurred speech, dulled senses, clouded judgment, dehydration, and hangover. Long-term effects include increased risk of cancer, cardiovascular disease, liver disease, and neurological problems.
- Residential treatment programs, medications, internet resources, and counseling can help problem drinkers quit drinking and avoid relapse.
- Smoking is the leading cause of preventable death in the United States.

- The short-term effects of smoking include increased heart rate and blood pressure, shortness of breath, coughing, alertness, decreased skin temperature, increased blood sugar, dulled senses, bad breath, smelling like smoke, and decreased urine production.
- The long-term effects of smoking include increased risk of cancer, cardiovascular disease, respiratory disease, and erectile dysfunction as well as loss of bone density, gum disease, decreased fertility, and premature aging of skin.
- Secondhand smoke contains higher concentrations of some harmful chemicals than the smoke inhaled by smokers. People who inhale secondhand smoke can suffer from the same health problems as smokers.
- Nicotine replacement therapies (such as nicotine gums, inhalers, and patches) are designed to help smokers gradually reduce their dependence on nicotine and reduce the severity of withdrawal symptoms.
- Quitting smoking has numerous immediate and long-term health benefits.

Test Your Knowledge

1. Blood alcohol concentration can be affected by all of the following except
   a. how expensive the alcohol is.
   b. how much a person drinks.
   c. how fast a person drinks.
   d. how much a person has eaten prior to drinking.

2. A standard drink is
   a. equivalent to 1.5 ounces of 80-proof liquor.
   b. equivalent to 5 ounces of table wine.
   c. equivalent to 12 ounces of beer.
   d. all of the above.

3. *Binge drinking* is defined as
   a. consuming five or more drinks within 2 hours for men, or four or more drinks within 2 hours for women.
   b. drinking once a day every day.
   c. consuming five or more drinks over the course of a week.
   d. drinking hard liquor.

4. Alcoholism is best characterized as
   a. simply another term for alcohol abuse.
   b. problem drinking that is accompanied by symptoms like tolerance, withdrawal symptoms when alcohol is not consumed, loss of control, and an inability to quit drinking.
   c. only a problem for older people.
   d. binge drinking.

Get Critical

What happened:

Images of movie stars smoking on-screen can play an influential role in determining whether or not young people start smoking. Research findings indicate that up to 75% of all Hollywood films feature characters smoking, and that these images influence at least 200,000 American youth to start smoking each year.[1,2] Photos depicting the real-life smoking habits of actors and actresses can also influence teens and young adults to copy the behavior.

What do you think?

- Does showing attractive actors and actresses smoking on-screen glamorize smoking?
- Does a movie that features a lead character smoking make you want to have a cigarette?
- Do movie studios and movie stars have any responsibility to consider the social impact of featuring on-screen smoking?

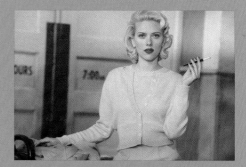

References: **1.** "Early Exposure to Movie Smoking Predicts Established Smoking by Older Teens and Young Adults," by M. Dalton, 2009, *Pediatrics, 12*(4), pp. e551–e558. **2.** *Smoking Presentation Trends in U.S. Movies 1991–2008* by K. Titus, 2009, University of California-San Francisco Center for Tobacco Control Research and Education.

5. The long-term effects of alcohol on the body include
   a. increased risk of cancer.
   b. increased risk of cardiovascular disease.
   c. increased risk of liver disease.
   d. all of the above.

6. What is the key psychoactive ingredient in cigarettes?
   a. ammonia
   b. licorice
   c. nicotine
   d. formaldehyde

7. The immediate physical effects of smoking include all of the following except
   a. increased heart rate and blood pressure.
   b. increased skin temperature.
   c. increased level of blood sugar.
   d. shortness of breath.

8. Babies born to mothers who smoked while pregnant
   a. are more likely to die of sudden infant death syndrome.
   b. are less likely to be born prematurely.
   c. are more likely to weigh more than 6 pounds at birth.
   d. are immune to the health effects associated with tobacco.

9. Secondhand smoke is
   a. not as dangerous as mainstream smoke.
   b. always filtered through a smoker's lungs.
   c. a mixture of sidestream smoke and mainstream smoke.
   d. smoke that contains smaller levels of carbon monoxide.

10. All of the following are forms of tobacco except
   a. cigars.
   b. bidis.
   c. cocaine.
   d. snuff.

Get Connected

Health Online Visit the following websites for more information about the topics in this chapter:

- Rethinking Drinking: Alcohol and Your Health
  http://rethinkingdrinking.niaaa.nih.gov
- Alcoholics Anonymous
  www.aa.org
- Alanon-Alateen
  www.al-anon.alateen.org
- Facts on Tap
  www.factsontap.org

- American Lung Association's Freedom from Smoking Online
  www.ffsonline.org
- Centers for Disease Control and Prevention
  www.cdc.gov/tobacco
- National Cancer Institute
  www.smokefree.gov

Website links are subject to change. To access updated web links, please visit **www.pearsonhighered.com/choosinghealth.**

References

i. National Institute on Alcohol Abuse and Alcoholism. (2010). *Rethinking drinking: Alcohol and your health.* Retrieved from http://rethinkingdrinking.niaaa.nih.gov/WhatsTheHarm/WhatAreTheRisks.asp

ii. American College Health Association. (2009). *American College Health Association National College Health Assessment (ACHA-NCHA II) reference group data report, Fall 2009.* Retrieved from http://www.acha-ncha.org/docs/ACHA-NCHA_Reference_Group_Report_Fall2009.pdf

iii. Centers for Disease Control and Prevention. (2008, November 14). Smoking-attributable mortality, years of potential life lost, and productivity losses: United States, 2000–2004. *Morbidity and Mortality Weekly Report, 57*(45), 1226–1228. Retrieved from http://www.cdc.gov/mmwr/preview/mmwrhtml/mm5745a3.htm

iv. U.S. Department of Health and Human Services. (2006). *The health consequences of involuntary exposure to tobacco smoke: A report of the surgeon general.*

1. Substance Abuse and Mental Health Services Administration. (2009). *Results from the 2008 national survey on drug use and health: National findings.* Retrieved from http://www.oas.samhsa.gov/nsduh/2k8nsduh/2k8Results.cfm

2. National Institutes of Health. (2010). *Fact Sheet: Alcohol-related traffic deaths.* Retrieved from http://www.nih.gov/about/researchresultsforthepublic/AlcoholRelatedTrafficDeaths.pdf

3. Wagenaar, A. C., & Toomey, T. L. (2002). Effects of minimum drinking age laws: Review and analyses of the literature from 1960 to 2000. *Journal of Studies on Alcohol and Drugs, Supplement 14*, 206–225. Retrieved from http://www.jsad.com/jsad/article/Effects_of_Minimum_Drinking_Age_Laws_Review_and_Analyses_of_the_Literature/1478.html

4. Voas, R. B., Tippetts, A. S., & Fell, J. C. (2003). Assessing the effectiveness of minimum legal drinking age and zero tolerance laws in the United States. *Accident Analysis & Prevention, 35*(4), 579–587.

5. Fell, J. C., (2008). The relationship of underage drinking laws to reductions in drinking drivers in fatal crashes in the United States. *Accident Analysis and Prevention, 40*(4), 1430–1440.

6. Johnston, L. D., O'Malley, P. M., Bachman, J. G., & Schulenberg, J. E. (2009). *Monitoring the future: National survey results on drug use, 1975–2008. Volume II: College students and adults ages 19–50* (NIH Publication No. 09-7403). Bethesda, MD:

National Institute on Drug Abuse. Retrieved from http://monitoringthefuture.org/new.html

7. National Institute on Alcohol Abuse and Alcoholism. (2004). Binge drinking defined. *NIAAA Newsletter,* Winter 2004, No. 3. Retrieved from http://pubs.niaaa.nih.gov/publications/Newsletter/winter2004/Newsletter_Number3.pdf

8. Timberlake, D. S., Hopfer, C. J., Rhee, S. H., Friedman, N. P., Haberstick, B. D., Lessem, J. M., & Hewitt, J. K. (2007). College attendance and its effect on drinking behaviors in a longitudinal study of adolescents. *Alcoholism: Clinical and Experimental Research, 31*(6), 1020–1030.

9. National Institute on Alcohol Abuse and Alcoholism. (2010). *Rethinking drinking: Alcohol and your health.* Retrieved from http://rethinkingdrinking.niaaa.nih.gov/WhatsTheHarm/WhatAreTheRisks.asp

10. DeSimone, J. (2007). Fraternity membership and binge drinking. *Journal of Health Economics, 26,* 950–967.

11. Perkins, H. W. (2002). Surveying the damage: A review of research on consequences of alcohol misuse in college populations. *Journal of Studies on Alcohol Supplement 14,* 91–100.

12. Wechsler, H., Moeykens, B., Davenport, A., Castillo, S., & Hansen, J. (1995). The adverse impact of heavy episodic drinkers on other college students. *Journal of Studies on Alcohol, 56,* 628–634.

13. Hingson, R., Heeren, T., Winter, M., & Wechsler, H. (2005). Magnitude of alcohol-related mortality and morbidity among U.S. college students ages 18–24: Changes from 1998 to 2001. *Annual Review of Public Health, 26,* 259–279.

14. Wechsler, H., Dowdall, G. W., Davenport, A., Davenport, A. & Castillo, S. (1995). Correlates of college student binge drinking. *American Journal of Public Health, 85*(7), 921–926.

15. Greenbaum, P. E., Del Boca, F. K., Darkes, J., Darkes, J., Wang, C. P. & Goldman, M. S. (2005). Variation in the drinking trajectories of freshmen college students. *Journal of Consulting and Clinical Psychology, 73,* 229–238.

16. National Institute on Alcohol Abuse and Alcoholism. (2008). *What colleges need to know now: An update on college drinking research* (NIH Publication No. 07–5010). Rockville, MD: National Institute on Alcohol Abuse and Alcoholism.

17. Cooper, M. L. (1994). Motivations for alcohol use among adolescents: Development and validation of a four-factor model. *Psychological Assessment, 6,* 117–128.

18. American College Health Association. (2009). *American College Health Association National College Health Assessment (ACHA-NCHA II) reference group data report, Fall 2009.* Retrieved from http://www.acha-ncha.org/docs/ACHA-NCHA_Reference_Group_Report_Fall2009.pdf

19. Abar, C., Abar, B., & Turrisi, R. (2009). The impact of parental modeling and permissibility on alcohol use and experienced negative drinking consequences in college. *Addictive Behaviors, 34*(6–7), 542–547.

20. Kerr, W. C., Greenfield, T. K., Tujague, J., & Brown, S. E. (2005). A drink is a drink? Variation in the amount of alcohol contained in beer, wine and spirits drinks in a U.S. methodological sample. *Alcoholism: Clinical and Experimental Research, 29*(11), 2015–2021.

21. Meier, P., & Seitz, H. K. (2008). Age, alcohol metabolism, and liver disease. *Current Opinion in Clinical Nutrition and Metabolic Care, 11*(1), 21–26.

22. Milgram, G. (1990). *Facts on the effects of alcohol.* New Jersey Alcohol/Drug Resource Center and Clearinghouse, Center of Alcohol Studies, Rutgers University. Retrieved from http://www.eric.ed.gov/ERICDocs/data/ericdocs2sql/content_storage_01/0000019b/80/16/17/68.pdf

23. Lieber, C. S. (1995). Medical disorders of alcoholism. *New England Journal of Medicine, 333*(16), 1058–1065.

24. Wiese, J. G., Shlipak, M. G., & Browner, W. S. (2000). The alcohol hangover. *Annals of Internal Medicine, 132*(11), 897–902.

25. Swift, R., & Davidson, D. (1998). Alcohol hangover mechanisms and mediators. *Alcohol Health & Research World, 22*(1), 54–60.

26. National Cancer Institute. (2006). *Alcohol and cancer.* Retrieved from http://www.cancer.org/downloads/PRO/alcohol.pdf

27. Brooks, P. J., Enoch, M. A., Goldman, D., Li, T. K., & Yokoyama, A. (2009). The alcohol flushing response: An unrecognized risk factor for esophageal cancer from alcohol consumption. *PLoS Medicine, 6*(3), e1000050.

28. American Liver Foundation. (2007). *Cirrhosis.* Retrieved from http://www.liverfoundation.org/education/info/cirrhosis

29. American Medical Association. (2010). Harmful consequences of alcohol use on the brains of children, adolescents, and college students. Retrieved from http://www.ama-assn.org/ama/no-index/physician-resources/9416.shtml

30. SAMHSA Fetal Alcohol Spectrum Disorders Center for Excellence. (2007). *What You Need to Know: Fetal Alcohol Spectrum Disorders by the Numbers.* DHHS Pub. No. (SMA)-06-4236. Rockville, MD: Center for Substance Abuse Prevention Substance Abuse and Mental Health Services Adminstration.

31. Substance Abuse and Mental Health Services Administration. (2009). *Results from the 2008 national survey on drug use and health: National findings.* Retrieved from http://www.oas.samhsa.gov/nsduh/2k8nsduh/2k8Results.cfm

32. National Highway Traffic Safety Administration. (2007, December). Fatalities related to alcohol-impaired driving during the Christmas and New Year's Day holiday periods. *Traffic Safety Facts* (DOT HS 810 870). Retrieved from http://www-nrd.nhtsa.dot.gov/Pubs/810870.PDF

33. Hingson, R. W., Zha, W., & Weitzman, E. R. (2009). Magnitude of and trends in alcohol-related mortality and morbidity among U.S. college students ages 18–24, 1998–2005. *Journal of Studies on Alcohol and Drugs,* Supplement 14, 12–20.

34. Wechsler, H., Lee, J. E., Kuo, M., Seibring, M., Nelson, T. F., & Lee, H. (2002). Trends in college binge drinking during a period of increased prevention efforts: Findings from 4 Harvard School of Public Health college alcohol study surveys: 1993–2001. *Journal of American College Health, 50*(5), 203–217.

35. Abbey, A., Zawacki, T., Buck, P. O., Clinton, A. M., & McAuslan, P. (2001). Alcohol and sexual assault. *Alcohol Research & Health, 25*(1), 43–51.

36. Hingson, R. W., Heeren, T., Zakocs, R. C., Kopstein, A., & Wechsler, H. (2002). Magnitude of alcohol-related mortality and morbidity among U.S. college students ages 18–24. *Journal of Studies on Alcohol 63*(2), 136–144.

37. Grant, B., Dawson, D., Stinson, F., Chou, S., Dufour, M., & Pickering, R. (2004). The 12-month prevalence and trends in DSM–IV alcohol abuse and dependence in the United States, 1991–1992 and 2001–2002. *Drug and Alcohol Dependence, 74*(3), 223–234.

38. Knight, J. R., Wechsler, H., Kuo, M., Seibring, M., Weitzman, E., & Schuckit, M. (2002). Alcohol abuse and dependence among U.S. college students. *Journal of Studies on Alcohol, 63*(3), 263–270.

39. Moss, H. B., Chen, C. M., & Yi, H. Y. (2007). Subtypes of alcohol dependence in a nationally representative sample. *Drug and Alcohol Dependence, 91*(2–3), 149–158.

40. National Institute on Alcohol Abuse and Alcoholism. (2010, February). Alcoholism isn't what it used to be. *NIAAA Spectrum, 2*(1). Retrieved from http://www.spectrum.niaaa.nih.gov/features/Alcoholism.aspx

41. Ehrlich, P. F., Haque, A., Swisher-McClure, S., & Helmkamp, J. (2006). Screening and brief intervention for alcohol problems in a university student health clinic. *Journal of American College Health, 54*(5), 279–287.

42. National Institute on Alcohol Abuse and Alcoholism. (1989). Relapse and craving. *Alcohol Alert,* No. 6; PH 277. Retrieved from http://pubs.niaaa.nih.gov/publications/aa06.htm

43. Centers for Disease Control and Prevention. (2008, November 14). Smoking-attributable mortality, years of potential life lost, and productivity losses: United States, 2000–2004. *Morbidity and Mortality Weekly Report, 57*(45), 1226–1228. Retrieved from http://www.cdc.gov/mmwr/preview/mmwrhtml/mm5745a3.htm

44. National Center for Health Statistics. (2008). *Health, United States, 2008, with special feature on the health of young adults.* Retrieved from http://www.cdc.gov/nchs/data/hus/hus08.pdf

45. Mokdad, A., (2004). Actual causes of death in the United States, 2000. *Journal of the American Medical Association, 291*(10), 1238–1245.

46. Centers for Disease Control and Prevention. (2009). Cigarette smoking among adults and trends in smoking cessation: United States, 2008. *Morbidity and Mortality Weekly Report, 58*(44), 1227–1232.

47. Johnston, L. D., O'Malley, P. M., Bachman, J. G., & Schulenberg, J. E. (2004). *Overall teen drug use continues gradual decline; but use of inhalants rises.* Ann Arbor, MI: University of Michigan News and Information Services. Retrieved from http://www.monitoringthefuture.org/data/04data.html

48. Campaign for Tobacco-Free Kids. (2009). *The path to smoking addiction starts at very young ages.* Retrieved from http://www.tobaccofreekids.org/research/factsheets/pdf/0127.pdf

49. Jackson, C., & Dickinson, D. (2006). Enabling parents who smoke to prevent their children from initiating smoking. *Archives of Pediatric and Adolescent Medicine, 160*(1), 56–62.

50. U.S. Federal Trade Commission. (2007). *Cigarette report for 2004 and 2005.* Retrieved from http://www.ftc.gov/reports/tobacco/2007cigarette2004-2005.pdf

51. Biener, L., and Siege, M. (2000). Tobacco marketing and adolescent smoking: More support for a causal inference. *American Journal of Public Health, 90*(3), 407–411.

52. Lloyd, D. A., & Taylor, J. R. (2004). *Stress as a distal predictor of heavy smoking initiation in young people.* Paper presented at the Annual Meeting of the American Sociological Association, San Francisco, CA. Retrieved from http://www.allacademic.com/meta/p108960_index.html

53. Sean Dash & Bruce Nash. (2006). Tobacco [Television series episode]. In *Modern Marvels.* New York, NY: History, A&E Television Networks.

54. U.S. Department of Health and Human Services. (2004). *The health consequences of smoking: A report of the surgeon general.* Retrieved from http://www.cdc.gov/tobacco/data_statistics/sgr/2004/complete_report/index.htm

55. American Cancer Society. (2009). *Cigarette smoking.* Retrieved from http://www.cancer.org/docroot/PED/content/PED_10_2x_Cigarette_Smoking.asp

56. Miniño, A., Heron, M., Murphy, S., & Kochanek, K. (2007). Deaths: Final data for 2004. *National Vital Statistics Reports, 55*(19). Retrieved from http://www.cdc.gov/nchs/data/nvsr/nvsr55/nvsr55_19.pdf

57. Centers for Disease Control and Prevention. (2008). Deaths from chronic obstructive pulmonary disease, United States, 2000–2005. *Morbidity and Mortality Weekly Report, 57*(45), 1229–1232.

58. Centers for Disease Control and Prevention. (2009). *Tobacco use and pregnancy.* Retrieved from http://www.cdc.gov/reproductivehealth/tobaccoUsePregnancy/index.htm

59. Salihu, H. M., Aliyu, M. H., Pierre-Louis, B. J., & Alexander, G. R. (2003). Levels of excess infant deaths attributable to maternal smoking during pregnancy in the United States. *Maternal and Child Health Journal, 7*(4), 219–227.

60. U.S. Department of Health and Human Services. (2006). *The health consequences of involuntary exposure to tobacco smoke: A report of the surgeon general.* Retrieved from http://www.surgeongeneral.gov/library/secondhandsmoke/report/index.html

61. California Environmental Protection Agency. (2005). *Identification of environmental tobacco smoke as a toxic air contaminant: Executive Summary.*

62. American Cancer Society. (2009). *Cigar smoking.* Retrieved from http://www.cancer.org/docroot/PED/content/PED_10_2X_Cigar_Smoking.asp

63. National Cancer Institute. (2009). *Cigar smoking and cancer* (Fact Sheet). Retrieved from http://www.cancer.gov/cancertopics/factsheet/Tobacco/cigars

64. Malson, J. L., Lee, E. M., Murty, R., Moolchan, E. T., & Pickworth, W. B. (2003). Clove cigarette smoking: Biochemical, physiological, and subjective effects. *Pharmacology Biochemistry and Behavior, 74,* 739–745.

65. Centers for Disease Control and Prevention. (2009). *Bidis and kreteks.* Retrieved from http://www.cdc.gov/tobacco/data_statistics/fact_sheets/tobacco_industry/bidis_kreteks

66. Severson, H. H., Klein, K., & Lichtenstein, E. (2005). Smokeless tobacco use among professional baseball players: Survey results, 1998 to 2003. *Tobacco Control, 14,* 31–36.

67. Smith, S. (2006, April 11). Team of destiny had a dirty habit: Study finds heavy use of chew by '04 Sox. *The Boston Globe,* Retrieved from http://www.boston.com/sports/baseball/redsox/articles/2006/04/11/team_of_destiny_had_a_dirty_habit/

68. Rigotti, N. A., Lee, J. E., & Wechsler, H. (2000). U.S. college students' use of tobacco products: Results of a national survey. *Journal of the American Medical Association, 284*(6), 699–705.

69. Cosgrove, K. P. (2009). B_2-nicotinic acetylcholine receptor availability during acute and prolonged abstinence from tobacco smoking. *Archives of General Psychiatry, 66*(6), 666–667.

70. Centers for Disease Control and Prevention. (2006). Cigarette smoking among adults: United States. *Morbidity and Mortality Weekly Report, 56,* 1157–1161.

9

Relationships and Communication

- 86–88% of college students have experienced "hooking up." [i]

- The average Facebook user has 130 "friends" on the site. [ii]

- An estimated 50–60% of couples in the U.S. now live together before getting married. [iii]

- Between 85% and 90% of the U.S. population will eventually marry during their lifetime. [iv]

IDENTIFY the characteristics of effective communication.

UNDERSTAND how self-perception, early relationships, and gender roles influence relationships.

DESCRIBE Sternberg's Triangular Theory of Love.

IDENTIFY the characteristics of healthy versus dysfunctional intimate relationships.

DESCRIBE at least three different types of committed relationships.

EXPLAIN the factors that should be considered before starting a family.

Health Online icons are found throughout the chapter, directing you to web links, videos, podcasts, and other useful online resources.

We are social beings, craving connections with others and the support, love, and sense

of contentment they give us. Our families teach us and guide us through the highs and lows of life. Our friends listen to us, laugh with us, and share in our successes and failures. Our lovers provide us with intimacy, companionship, and comfort. Our relationships with others fulfill us, define us, nurture us, and make us feel safe. Good relationships can relieve stress and, indeed, help keep us healthy.

Relationships, however, take effort to maintain. Being able to speak up, listen well, and resolve conflicts are critical skills to develop for all personal relationships. In this chapter, we will discuss the characteristics of effective communication, examine what constitutes a healthy relationship, identify signs of dysfunctional relationships, and explore various categories of committed relationships. Along the way, we will introduce methods of building relationship skills that strengthen healthy ties to friends, colleagues, family, and partners. We will emphasize that although there is no such thing as a perfect relationship or a perfect family, strong unions are based on mutual affection, respect, commitment, companionship, and honesty.

Communication in Relationships

The cornerstone of every successful relationship is effective communication. That idea seems straightforward enough, but in real life, true communication can be challenging. All of us, at times, will experience difficulty in making our thoughts, feelings, and needs known. In addition, understanding the intentions and concerns of others isn't always easy. Effective communication is a skill that can be developed and continually improved. Without it, many relationships fail.

Communicating Feelings

True communication entails much more than just making small talk. It involves sharing honest feelings and other personal information about ourselves—our hopes, our dreams, our secrets, our fears. This kind of sharing, called **self-disclosure,** was first described by psychologist Sidney M. Jourard in his 1971 work, *The Transparent Self.* "If we want to be loved, we must disclose ourselves. If we want to love someone, he must permit us to know him," he wrote. "This would seem to be obvious. Yet most of us spend a great part of our lives thinking up ways to avoid becoming known."[1]

It is not always comfortable to share one's feelings. To do so can leave a person feeling vulnerable and exposed. If you think back through your own life, odds are you have known someone who had difficulty saying "I love you" or telling you what he or she was feeling or thinking. In order to be truly close to another person, however, we need to occasionally let our guard down and speak freely and honestly about what is on our minds.

---

self-disclosure The sharing of honest feelings and personal information about yourself with another person.

Communication Skills

Especially when dealing with conflict or other uncomfortable situations, certain communication strategies are helpful:

- **Stay focused.** Focus on the current issue, your feelings about it, and finding a solution.

- **Take responsibility.** Own what is yours and admit when you've made mistakes.

- **Use "I" messages.** Begin the discussion with an "I feel" statement. Making the discussion about the other person may make him or her feel attacked and trigger defensiveness.

- **Listen effectively.** A big part of being a good communicator is being an effective listener.

- **Be solution-focused.** Try to look for a win-win compromise. Effective communication requires that you find a resolution that both parties can be happy with.

- **Step away if necessary.** Sometimes the timing isn't right for resolving a relationship conflict. If tempers flare and the conversation is headed toward an unproductive verbal fight, take a break. But don't just forget about it. Problems don't disappear because you don't talk about them. So return to the issue when it can be approached with a more constructive attitude.

- **Avoid jumping to conclusions or making quick judgments.** Let the other person complete his or her thought before judging. If you have a question about what another person means, ask for a clarification.

- **Resist antagonizing the other person.** For example, resist correcting grammatical errors or nitpicking at other details that do not matter to the real issue at hand.

- **Seek help if you need it.** If you or your partner continues to have difficulty communicating about relationship issues in a constructive way, it may be time to seek help from a counselor or other professional who can help.

Nonverbal Communication

Sometimes you can get a message across without saying a single word. Imagine a teenager who has been out way past her curfew. When she arrives home, she unlocks the front door and tiptoes inside, hoping to make it to her bedroom unnoticed. But in the living room, she sees her father, still awake in his easy chair, tapping his feet, arms crossed, face scowling. Message received.

Savvy communicators know that it isn't just what you say but *how* you say it that matters. Nonverbal cues such as posture, gestures, eye contact, and even touch help us broadcast our thoughts, whether we realize it or not. This is known as **nonverbal communication,** sometimes called *body language*. If a friend has a glazed-over look in her eyes or is yawning while you are talking, that body language can communicate that she is bored. A person with upright posture and good eye contact conveys confidence, whereas someone who is hunched over and whose eyes dart back and forth communicates nervousness and discomfort. Crossed arms can convey defensiveness—or simply that someone is cold. The ability to ensure that your body language is in tune with what you intend to say is a key characteristic of an effective communicator.

nonverbal communication
Communication that is conveyed by body language.

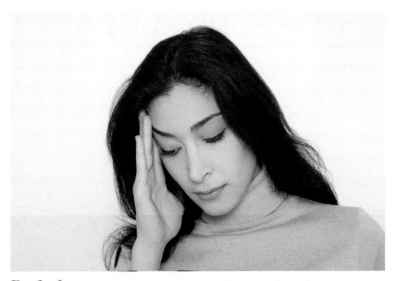

Body language can communicate a lot of information. Do you think this person is relaxed, or anxious?

Being a Good Listener

Listening is an integral part of successful communication. Though it might seem like a simple skill, good listening actually requires concentration, focus, and attentiveness. Some strategies for effective listening include:

- **Be silent while another person is sharing his or her feelings or concerns.** Speak up only when you have a question or want to summarize what you have heard.

- **Empathize with what the other person is saying.** If you put yourself in the other person's shoes, you will gain a better perspective of his or her viewpoint.

- **Overcome the urge to interrupt.** Let others complete their thoughts before you speak.

- **Try to set aside any anger or resentment you may be feeling.** These emotions can interfere with your ability to truly listen.

- **Make other people feel comfortable speaking to you.** This can be done by maintaining eye contact, keeping a relaxed posture, and nodding and smiling so that others know you are listening. Avoid smirking, frowning, or crossing your arms.

- **Give the speaker your undivided attention.** Get rid of any distractions. Close the door and turn off your cell phone.

Resolving Conflicts

Put any relationship under a microscope and you will see conflicts arise. Conflict is a normal part of relationships because people have different needs, viewpoints, interests, and backgrounds. However, not everyone handles conflicts in the same way. Some people actively avoid discussing their concerns or annoyances, believing it is better to keep the peace than start what could become an ongoing feud. This communication style is commonly

He Said, She Said:
Gender Roles and Communication

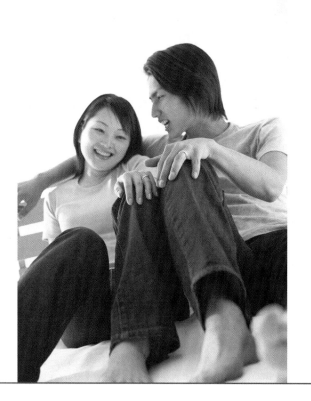

Although both men and women share a common need to communicate information, thoughts, and feelings, research reveals that there are differences in how they go about it. One of the most fundamental differences is the motivation, or driving force, behind a man and woman's communication.[1] Men communicate in order to achieve social status and to avoid failure, whereas women communicate to build personal connections and avoid social isolation. So a man wants to *report* and a woman wants *rapport*. Though individuals may vary, in general:

- Women seek to connect to others in conversation, whereas men want to be independent information givers.

- Women want to build consensus before making a decision, whereas men want to make decisions expediently on their own.

- Women avoid competitive conversation and attempt to minimize differences, whereas men are more comfortable giving orders and pointing out areas of superiority.[1]

There are also gender differences in overall communication style. In general, these include the following:

- Men speak significantly fewer words each day than women, probably because men like to get to the bottom line and women like to notice and share details.

- Women process their problems out loud. They will use conversation to think through a problem and work toward a solution. In contrast, men think through a problem silently, and then verbalize their solution.

- Men are more likely to speak bluntly and state requests directly. Women are more likely to be tactful, use indirect speech, listen, and to offer feedback or make requests. Similarly, women are more likely to give feedback with sensitivity to another person's feelings. Men give feedback more directly, making the assumption that the other person won't take it personally.

- Women are more likely to use "circular" speech and often change the topic in the middle of a conversation, returning to it later. Men are more likely to be linear communicators and thinkers; they want to finish one topic before going on to another.[2]

Neither communication style is better or worse, just different. And understanding the differences can improve male-female communication and relationships.

References: **1**. *You Just Don't Understand: Women and Men in Conversation*, by D. Tannen, 1991, New York: Ballantine Books. **2**. *Men Are from Mars, Women Are from Venus*, by J. Gray, 1992, New York: HarperCollins.

---

referred to as **conflict avoidance.** Others prefer to be more direct and confrontational, and have no problems making it clear when they are unhappy with a situation.

conflict avoidance The active avoidance of discussing concerns, annoyances, and conflict with another person.

conflict resolution Resolving a conflict in a manner that both people can accept and that minimizes future occurrences of the conflict.

conflict escalation Increasing conflict to a more confrontational, painful, or otherwise less comfortable level.

The most effective way to resolve conflict is for two people to voice their concerns maturely and engage in constructive criticism, rather than resort to name calling and finger pointing. Settling disagreements, of course, is not always easy. **Conflict resolution** is an acquired skill. To avoid **conflict escalation,** the opposing parties should agree to fight fair, be respectful, and stay away from personal attacks and put-downs.

Strategies for effective conflict resolution include:

- Strive to resolve conflict, rather than to "win."

- Voice your frustrations as soon as possible, rather than allowing them to build up.

- Approach the conflict as you would any other problem that needs to be solved: Define the problem, express the facts (and your feelings) regarding the problem, and listen to possible solutions. You should evaluate each possible solution, agree upon one, and make specific plans on how and when to implement it. After a solution is adopted, evaluate it. Is everyone satisfied with the outcome, or would another solution work better?

- Communicate your concerns and opinions clearly, honestly, and directly, instead of expecting the other person to read your mind.

- Listen to the other person's feedback and summarize what you think he or she has said.

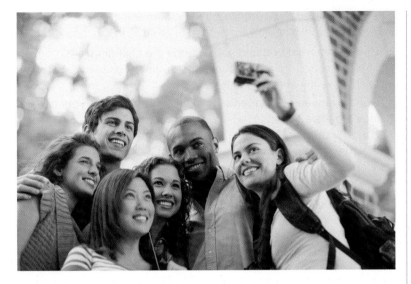

Friendships with others can boost emotional and physical health.

- Do not ridicule the other person's feelings.
- Stay on the subject, arguing only one point at a time.
- Make sure you are fighting about what is truly bothering you.
- Do not fight while drunk or drinking.
- Postpone a discussion to an agreed upon time if one person is tired or not ready to work on the problem.
- Admit when you are wrong.
- Compromise when at all possible.
- Forgive, forget, and start over.[2]

Developing Relationships

Most of us are social creatures from the time we are born, craving closeness and connections to others. And whether we are at home, school, or work, we spend much of our time in the presence of other people. Several personal factors influence how we develop relationships with others, including our self-perception, our early relationships, and cultural gender roles.

Self-Perception

How we relate to others depends, in part, on how good we feel about ourselves, our self-concept. As discussed in Chapter 2, self-esteem is a sense of positive self-regard that results in elevated levels of self-respect, self-worth, self-confidence, and self-satisfaction. People with low self-esteem are more likely to feel lonely and socially isolated. They tend to be pre-occupied with the thought of rejection and often behave agreeably toward others because they want to be liked.[3] One psychology professor found that college students with low self-esteem often blame themselves for a boyfriend's or girlfriend's unhappiness, even when other factors are clearly responsible.[3] The study stated that overly insecure people may "read nonexistent meaning into their partners' ambiguous cues," and wind up sabotaging their relationships, "thus leading their relation-

ships to the outcome they wish to avoid." The finding is true not only of young lovers but of couples in long-term relationships. Researchers have found that even after a decade of marriage, people with low self-esteem misread subtle cues and believe their partners love them far less than they actually do.[4]

Early Relationships

The first relationship we ever experience is the family relationship. Early experiences with our families are important because they help form the template for all subsequent relationships we experience in our lives. Some experts theorize that our relationships with others are patterned after the attachment we had with parents and other caregivers when we were children, a concept known as **attachment theory.**[5] These early interactions may shape our expectations of adult relationships and be responsible for the individual differences in relationship behaviors and needs.[6]

Exactly what constitutes a "family" changes over time, but it is generally defined as a domestic group of people with some degree of kinship, be it through marriage, blood, or adoption. Families today take many different forms, including households headed by single parents, blended families with stepparents and stepsiblings, extended family households with relatives or family friends all living under the same roof, foster families, and gay and lesbian partnerships, to name just a few. There is no perfect or "right" kind of family, but in a healthful family environment, children are respected and nurtured, and learn how to have strong relationships of their own.

Gender Roles

Gender roles are the behaviors and tasks considered appropriate by society based upon whether we are a man or a woman. Just as many girls are trained at an early age to play with dolls and stuffed animals, boys are encouraged to appreciate cars and trains and to emulate seemingly all-powerful "super heroes." As we grow up, some experts think that beginning in adolescence, girls' tendencies to place greater value on interpersonal connections than boys do can even leave them more vulnerable to depression and lower self-esteem.[7]

Gender roles often extend into adulthood. However, we live in a time of changing gender roles. A generation ago, men were traditionally expected to work and support the family while women were encouraged to stay home to raise the children. Today, many women opt to juggle both family and career, while some men make the decision to be stay-at-home fathers. Yet attitudes and stereotypes about gender roles remain. In addition, some research has shown that traditional gender roles become more pronounced in married couples after the birth of a child.[8]

attachment theory The theory that the patterns of attachment in our earliest relationships with others form the template for attachment in later relationships.

gender roles Behaviors and tasks considered appropriate by society based on whether someone is a man or a woman.

Friendships

Do you have a "BFF" (Best Friend Forever)? If so, you benefit in more ways than one. Besides providing someone to hang out with and confide in, friendships are important for good health. In one landmark study, researchers tracked thousands of residents in a Northern California county for nine years and found that people who lacked social and community ties were two to three times more likely to die during that time than those with

Good Friends

"Hi, I'm Brittany and this is my friend Sandy. We're both freshmen and we've been friends for about a semester now, ever since we became neighbors in our dorm. We started eating dinner together occasionally and then began hanging out more and more often. We like the same music, we study together, go to the gym, and just hang out and have fun. Recently both of my parents were laid off, and Sandy has been really great in helping me deal with it; she listens to me talk and I feel like she's really there for me. In a few weeks, a group of us are going to Florida for spring break, and next year, we're even going to get an apartment together. I thought it was going to be difficult making friends in college but I'm so glad I've found such a good one already!"

1: What are the benefits of Brittany and Sandy's friendship? What personal and environmental factors helped make them friends?

2: Why do you think Brittany confided in Sandy about her parents being laid off? How did Sandy help?

3: What can Brittany and Sandy do to make sure that they have a good living situation when they move in together next year?

Do you have a story similar to Brittany and Sandy's? Share your story at **www.pearsonhighered.com/choosinghealth.**

a solid social network.[9] A separate study found that people who are isolated are at increased risk of dying from a number of causes, and that social support is especially related to survival after a heart attack.[10] The quality of that social support matters: it must provide both a sense of belonging and intimacy and must help people to be more competent and feel more capable.

Unfortunately, friendships are less numerous today than they have been in the past. A recent study found that between 1985 and 2004, the number of Americans who felt they have someone to discuss important matters with dropped by almost a third. The study also found that the percentage of people who spoke about important matters only with family members jumped from 57% to 80%.[11] Declining rates of friendship don't make it any less important, however; loneliness can harm your health. One study showed that college freshmen who have a small social circle and consider themselves lonely had a weaker immune response to a flu vaccine than non-lonely students.[12] Loneliness is also associated with stress, depression, and poor life satisfaction.[13] See Chapter 2 for more on loneliness.

Maintaining Old Friendships

Friendships can be some of the longest, most-fulfilling relationships in your life, outlasting romantic relationships and even marriages. But the demands of being a student can make it hard to keep up with

older friendships. If you are struggling with maintaining your tried-and-true relationships now that you're in college, follow these tips:

- **Understand that you and your friends are changing.** Don't be afraid to show how you're changing, and don't expect your friends to stay exactly the same either.
- **Don't overwhelm old friends with information about your college life.** It's exciting to fill in your friends with what you are doing now, but be sure to listen to their stories as well. Avoid dominating the conversation with too much talk about your new friends or school.
- **Keep in touch.** Phone, email, voice over Internet services like Skype, instant messaging, and social networking applications like Facebook and Twitter, are all great ways to update your friends about what you're doing and hear from them. However, be warned, the strongest friendships can't exist on your Facebook status updates alone. If you really want to maintain a friendship with someone, take the time to send him or her a personal message or pick up the phone.
- **Don't be afraid to reconnect.** If you've lost touch with an old friend, research indicates that you can still rekindle the friendship even after years without contact.[14]

Listen to this National Public Radio story on college friendships: **www.npr.org/templates/story/story.php?storyId=112330125.**

These videos explore the effects of social networking: **www.pbs.org/wgbh/pages/frontline/digitalnation/relationships/socializing.**

Intimate Relationships

Intimacy is the emotionally open and caring way of relating to another person. An intimate relationship is usually one that is deep and has evolved over time, in which two people feel safe and comfortable sharing their innermost thoughts and secrets.

intimacy A sense of closeness with another person formed by being emotionally open and caring.

Sternberg's Triangular Theory of Love

Psychologist Robert Sternberg theorized that there are three primary components of healthy, loving relationships:

- **Intimacy.** The emotional component. Intimacy is the feeling of closeness and connectedness experienced in loving relationships.
- **Passion.** The motivational component. Passion is the intensity that fuels romance, physical attraction, and sex.
- **Commitment.** The cognitive component. Commitment is the short-term decision to love another person and the long-term decision to stay committed to maintaining that love.[15]

Sternberg used the shape of a triangle to illustrate his theory, which he called the Triangular Theory of Love **(Figure 9.1)**. Sternberg postulates that the type and intensity of love a couple experiences depends upon the strength of each of the three components in their relationship. The factors can be combined to characterize seven different types of love:

- **Liking.** Liking is intimacy alone. A closeness to another person, without passionate feelings or a long-term commitment.

the Facebook
REVOLUTION

On February 4, 2004, Harvard computer science student Mark Zuckerberg launched "Thefacebook" and forever changed the world of social connections and friendships.[1] Originally used only by Harvard students, the network quickly spread to colleges across the U.S. and Canada. In 2005, Facebook launched a high school version and by late 2006, anyone with a valid email address could join. Facebook is the leading social networking site with more than 400 million active members throughout the world.[2] Half of its members visit the site every day.[2]

Despite the popularity of Facebook, it is not without its critics. Privacy proponents worry that members' information is too easily accessed by those with both personal and business motives. Facebook has also received criticism for hosting controversial group pages, including ones that support anorexia and holocaust denial. Other critics point out that Facebook has been used to facilitate cyberbullying and stalking. University professors complain that students are wasting a tremendous amount of time on Facebook that could be spent studying and that students are distracted in class because they are using Facebook. Professors at some U.S. colleges have even banned laptops from classrooms because of Facebook.[3]

Critics also contend that Facebook and other social network sites are redefining the very meaning of "relationship" or "friend," and not for the better. They worry that people's increasing reliance on online communication is reducing their ability to communicate meaningfully and build relationships in person.[4]

Regardless of their critics, social networking sites like Facebook are probably here to stay. You can learn to use them safely and effectively by following a few tips:

- **Limit your number of friends.** Do you really care about all of those thousands of Facebook "friends" you've been collecting since high school? Limit your friends list to those you really care about and don't let it become a way of keeping score of your popularity or a substitute for social interaction with your real friends.

- **Don't accept friend requests from people you don't know.**

- **Don't tag friends in unflattering photos.**

- **Manage your profile settings.** You may not want your boss or professor seeing your photos from last weekend. So, if you have both personal and professional "friends," make sure you know how to use the custom settings to edit what specific people can see.

- **Think before you post.** Don't post anything you wouldn't say in real life or don't want the entire Internet to read.

- **Use personal messaging instead of wall posts.** Be careful about posting something on your or a friend's wall that might get one or both of you in trouble. Instead, use Facebook's personal message feature to say anything you don't want thousands of people to read about.

- **Don't list personal info.** Never post your address, phone number, class schedule, or any other personal information that you don't want thousands of people to know.

- **Activate privacy settings.** Facebook has several privacy settings that you can use to control the amount of information other people see.[5]

- **Limit the amount of time you spend on Facebook.** Because information (even if it is trivial information) is updated constantly on Facebook, it can become addicting. Why not ignore your virtual friends for a while and spend some face-to-face time with your real live friends?[6]

References: **1.** "Hundreds Register for New Facebook Website," by Alan Tabak, February 9, 2004, *Harvard Crimson*, retrieved from http://www.thecrimson.com/article.aspx?ref=357292.

2. *Statistics,* Facebook Press Room, retrieved March 15, 2010, from http://www.facebook.com/press/info.php?statistics.

3. "Facing the Facebook," by M. Bugeja, January 3, 2006, *The Chronicle of Higher Education*, retrieved from http://chronicle.com/article/Facing-the-Facebook/46904.

4. "Archbishop Vincent Nichols Voices Fears over Social Networking Sites," August 2, 2009, *The Guardian*, retrieved from http://www.guardian.co.uk/media/2009/aug/02/vincent-nichols-social-networking-bebo.

5. "10 Privacy Settings Every Facebook User Should Know," by N. O'Neill, February 2, 2009, *All Facebook*, retrieved from http://www.allfacebook.com/2009/02/facebook-privacy.

6. "Are Social Networks Messing with Your Head?" by D. DiSalvo, Jan/Feb 2010, *Scientific American Mind*, pp. 48–55.

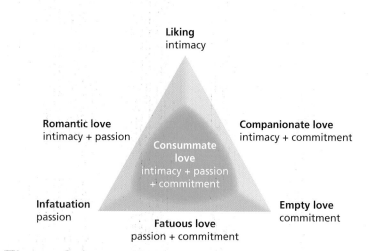

Source: "A Triangular Theory of Love," by R. J. Sternberg, 1986, *Psychological Review, 93*, pp. 119–135. © 1986. Reprinted by permission of Robert J. Sternberg.

Figure 9.1 Sternberg's triangular theory of love.

- **Infatuation.** Infatuation is passion alone. Also known as "love at first sight."
- **Empty love.** Empty love is commitment alone. The passion is not there and neither is the intimacy. This can be found in some stagnant relationships or just before a couple breaks up.
- **Romantic love.** Romantic love is passion and intimacy without commitment. Physical attraction with an emotional bond.
- **Companionate love.** Companionate love is commitment and intimacy without passion. It is essentially a committed friendship in which the passion has died down, as sometimes occurs in people who have been married a long time.
- **Fatuous love.** Fatuous love is commitment and passion without intimacy. A whirlwind romance that often does not last very long.
- **Consummate love.** Consummate love is the whole package: intimacy, passion, and commitment. The kind of love many of us strive for.[15]

Sternberg also identified an eighth category—nonlove—which is the absence of intimacy, passion, and commitment. This type of casual interaction makes up the majority of our relationships with other people.

What Causes Attraction?

You have probably heard the saying "opposites attract," but scientists have found the opposite to be true. Studying the factors that bring two people together for a romantic relationship reveals that we tend to pick partners who are a lot like us—who are of similar economic class, educational level, religion, and racial or ethnic group and who share the same interests or values. Emerging research indicates that we even seek out partners who have similar body shapes to our own.[16] This tendency to be attracted to people who share some of our characteristics is known as **assortative mating.** Some studies have also found that we look for people who share a similar level of physical attractiveness to us, with more attractive people being more particular about the physical attractiveness of their potential partners.[17]

Beauty, of course, is more than skin deep. Who we are and how we behave also influence whether others are attracted to us. One study found that men and women who were honest or helpful were perceived as better looking. Those who were rude or unfair or displayed other negative traits were generally considered to be less attractive.[18]

Although similarities in physique may bring us together, it is similarity in personality that appears to be most indicative of whether the relationship will be a happy one.[19] Why? "Once individuals are in a committed relationship, it is difficult to ignore personality differences," the study concluded. And personality differences, the researchers noted, "may result in more friction and conflict in daily life."[20] In the couples they studied, there were very few signs that opposites attract—or last—as a couple.

Dating

Dating—that is, spending time with another person one-on-one to determine whether there is an attraction or a desire to see more of one another—has evolved over the years. In earlier generations, men would typically ask women out on a formal date, and steady dating would be considered a "courtship" intended to lead to marriage. In a 2002 report by Rutgers University's National Marriage Project, many men reported that they rarely asked women out on dates anymore, preferring to meet people through groups of friends

assortative mating The tendency to be attracted to people who are similar to us.

How to Be a Healthy Couple

"Hi, we're Jonathan and Yeani, and we've been a couple for six months. There are a lot of obstacles that we face in our relationship, especially when it comes to juggling our schoolwork in addition to all the other aspects of our lives. At times, things seem hard. We each get stressed out by school and we can get on each others' nerves, but it's nice to have someone to lean on, and to know that you don't have to go through all your problems alone. For us, communication and trust have really helped make our relationship successful. Our best advice to new couples trying to make things work in college is to be open with one another, and don't be afraid to express your concerns, doubts, fears, or any other emotions with your partner."

1: Do you think juggling a relationship with school is a common source of stress for college couples? What can you do to help balance school and relationship time?

2: Why do you think Jonathan and Yeani chose to be in a relationship rather than just hooking up?

3: Do you agree with their advice for new couples in college? What else do you think college couples should do to keep their relationship healthy?

Do you have a story similar to Jonathan and Yeani's? Share your story at **www.pearsonhighered.com/choosinghealth.**

and spending time together more casually. A formal date is "the old way," said one man. "I'll meet them and we'll just hang out," added another.[21]

Hooking Up

On campus, the concept of dating has largely been replaced with **hooking up**—casual, noncommittal, physical encounters that may range from kissing and "making out" to oral sex and intercourse. "Dating has been replaced by hooking up as the dominant script for heterosexual interaction on campus," argues Kathleen Bogle, author of *Hooking Up: Sex, Dating, and Relationships on Campus*.[22] As the **Student Stats** box reveals, hooking up is common on college campuses, although many students have had negative "hook-up" experiences. Because hooking up is often fueled by alcohol, your judgment during the encounter can be impaired. Some of the negative effects from hooking up include negative impact on psychological well-being and social status; regrets; decreased relationship skills; and sexual risk taking, including an increased likelihood of STIs and unplanned pregnancy.[23, 24]

Since formal dating is becoming less common, the old courtship rules and rituals no longer apply. Unfortunately, according to National Marriage Project research, no new rules and rituals have been developed to replace the old discarded ones and singles are "mystified, frustrated, and confused."[21] Some experts are concerned that today's singles are not learning the skills to build intimacy and test out whether someone would be a good marriage partner.

hooking up Casual, noncommittal, physical encounters that may range from kissing and "making out" to oral sex and intercourse.

homosexual A person sexually attracted to someone of the same sex.

heterosexual A person sexually attraction to someone of the opposite sex.

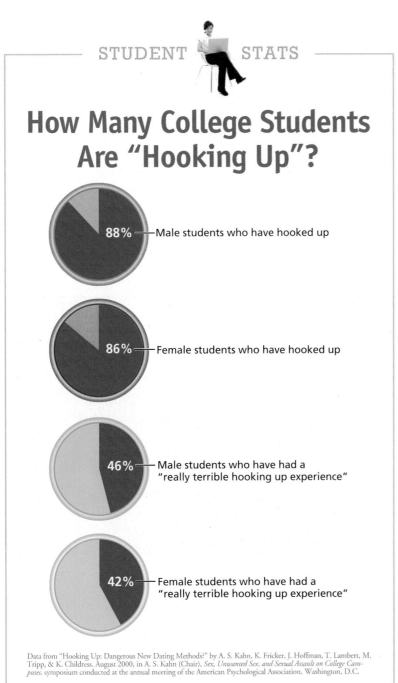

STUDENT STATS

How Many College Students Are "Hooking Up"?

88%—Male students who have hooked up

86%—Female students who have hooked up

46%—Male students who have had a "really terrible hooking up experience"

42%—Female students who have had a "really terrible hooking up experience"

Data from "Hooking Up: Dangerous New Dating Methods?" by A. S. Kahn, K. Fricker, J. Hoffman, T. Lambert, M. Tripp, & K. Childress. August 2000, in A. S. Kahn (Chair), *Sex, Unwanted Sex, and Sexual Assault on College Campuses*, symposium conducted at the annual meeting of the American Psychological Association, Washington, D.C.

Online Dating

Online dating has gained in popularity over recent years. Dating services are a booming business. Popular sites such as eHarmony.com, Match.com, and Yahoo! Personals report millions of users each month. These services assist members in finding suitable partners by providing a place where they can both advertise themselves online with a personal profile and view the profiles of others looking for partners. Members search profiles using criteria such as sex, age, location, and interests. Online dating easily and effectively increases the pool of potential partners, a real selling point for the busy, technologically savvy 21st century dater. Also, because face-to-face meetings are not immediate, potential partners have the opportunity to build their relationships via phone calls, texting, email, and other technology before that first face-to-face encounter.

It's important to remember that online dates are basically strangers. So in order to stay safe while using an online dating service, keep these precautions in mind:

- Never give out your full name, address, or other personal information until you have met the person and are sure he or she is trustworthy.
- Make sure to meet your date in a public place, like a restaurant or café. Avoid going to isolated places with a new date. Always tell a friend beforehand what you are doing and where you are going.
- Do not have a new date pick you up at your home. Wait to reveal where you live until you trust the person.
- If something doesn't feel right when you meet the person, don't be afraid to cut your date short.

Same-Sex Relationships

Around 8.8 million people in the U.S. identify as lesbian, gay, or bisexual (LGB).[25] In many ways committed **homosexual** couples are similar to committed **heterosexual,** or straight, couples.[25] Studies conclude that long-term same-sex couples are just as committed and satisfied in their relationships as heterosexual married couples.[26, 27] In at least one study, same-sex couples reported more positive feelings toward their partners and less conflict than married straight couples.[27] Indeed, same-sex couples often have more egalitarian or equal relationships because they do not subscribe to traditional gender roles. If there is a major difference, it is seen in lesbian couples—whom scientists have found are "especially effective at working together harmoniously."[26]

Yet one striking difference for LGB couples is the disapproval and discrimination same-sex couples often face from society or even from family. Many states do not allow homosexual couples to marry or adopt children, and some religions frown upon homosexuality. This can make homosexual couples feel stigmatized, isolated, and powerless. **Homophobia,** the fear and hatred of homosexuality, can also discourage intimacy between same-sex friends if it makes them fear being labeled as gay or lesbian.[28]

Healthy Relationships

Successful relationships are built on trust, respect, and communication. They enable each individual to retain his or her own identity and foster personal growth rather than smothering it.

Some people have an idealized view of healthy relationships, believing that they are free of conflict and require little effort to maintain. However, no deep, intimate relationship is without challenges. Well-adjusted couples learn how to steer clear of avoidable problems and to be respectful, supportive, and sensitive to each others' feelings when they encounter challenges they must overcome. With cooperation and compromise, as well as a commitment to work together, couples can help each other through some of the most trying times

---

homophobia Fear and hatred of homosexuality.

Online support for students struggling with their sexual identities can be found at http://nsrc.sfsu.edu, www.hrc.org/issues/coming_out.asp, www.glsen.org, and www.thegyc.com.

---

of life—the loss of a job, the death of a parent or child, the onset of a chronic, debilitating disease. **Practical Strategies for Health** provides tips for maintaining a strong and healthy relationship.

How do you know if your intimate relationship is a healthy one? Are there aspects of your relationship that concern you or that could be improved? Are you at a point in your relationship where the negatives are outweighing the positives? Taking a step back and assessing the strength of your relationship with a boyfriend, girlfriend, or partner can be illuminating. The **Self-Assessment** on the next page is one place to start.

Dysfunctional Relationships

Whereas some relationships are uplifting, others are toxic, becoming more of a burden than a joy. Dysfunctional relationships can come in many forms, with one or both partners being manipulative, controlling, mean, disrespectful, or even verbally or physically abusive.

This kind of negative behavior is often learned early in the home. Children observe how their parents relate to each other, and often think the hostile or unhealthy ways they interact are normal. Research has shown that adolescents who witnessed their parents' marital violence were more likely to be physically aggressive toward romantic partners themselves.[29] Similarly, adolescents exposed to marital discord tended to have conflict in their own marriages many years later.[30]

☺ *Practical Strategies for Health*

Tips for Maintaining a Strong Relationship

Although there is no simple recipe for success, the following strategies can help you maintain a strong, healthy relationship with your boyfriend, girlfriend, spouse, or partner:

- **Be honest with the other person.** Strive to maintain a warm, comfortable relationship in which you can confide in each other about virtually anything.

- **Trust each other.**

- **Respect each other.** Be able to disagree without using put-downs or threats. Try to understand the other person's feelings, even if you don't share his or her ideas.

- **Communicate effectively.** Ask how your loved one thinks and feels, rather than expecting him or her to be a mind reader. Offer

empathy when needed. Take the time to make sure you understand what the other person is attempting to say.

- **Give your loved one freedom and encouragement.** Recognize that each person has the right to his or her own opinions, feelings, friends, and dreams. Encourage each other's enjoyment and success in life.

- **Encourage common interests and shared activities.** Engage in activities and hobbies you both like. Be able to enjoy each other's company.

- **Be kind to one another.** Help each other out and show care through consistent respect rather than abuse followed by apologies.

- **Have mutual affection for one another.** Be appreciative and re-

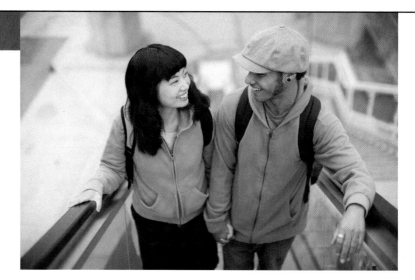

mind yourself of all the good things that you like about your loved one.

- **Share decision making.** Make decisions together, rather than tell each other what to do.[1]

Reference: **1.** Adapted from "Characteristics of a Healthy and Enjoyable Friendship or Dating Relationship," *Employee Assistance,* retrieved from http://www.eap.partners.org/WorkLife/Relationships/Healthy_Relationships/Characteristics_of_a_Healthy_and_Enjoyable_Friendship_or_Dating_Relationship.asp. Originally from Liz Claiborne, Inc.

Are We a Happy Couple?

Circle "yes" or "no" in response to each of the following questions.

1. I am very satisfied with how we talk to each other.   yes no
2. We are creative in how we handle our differences.   yes no
3. We feel very close to each other.   yes no
4. My partner is seldom too controlling.   yes no
5. When discussing problems, my partner understands my opinions and ideas.   yes no
6. I am completely satisfied with the amount of affection from my partner.   yes no
7. We have a good balance of leisure time spent together and separately.   yes no
8. My partner's friends or family rarely interfere with our relationship.   yes no
9. We agree on how to spend money.   yes no
10. I am satisfied with how we express spiritual values and beliefs.   yes no

HOW TO INTERPRET YOUR SCORE

The more you replied "yes" to these statements, the more likely you are to be part of a happy couple.

Source: Adapted from Olson, D. H. & Olson, A. K. (2000). *Empowering Couples: Building on Your Strengths.* Minneapolis, MN: Life Innovations, Inc. Reproduced by permission.

To complete this self-assessment online, visit www.pearsonhighered.com/choosinghealth.

Often, the signs that a relationship is dysfunctional or somehow amiss are subtle:[31]

- You focus on the other person at the expense of yourself.
- You feel pressured to change to meet your partner's ideals.
- Your partner expects you to justify what you do and whom you see, or you expect your partner to.
- You don't have any personal space.
- One of you makes all the decisions without listening to the other's input.
- You are afraid to disagree, and your ideas are criticized.
- You lie to each other.
- You feel stifled and trapped, unable to escape the pressures of the relationship.
- You or your partner is addicted to drugs or alcohol and it impacts your relationship.

If you have noticed any of these signs in your relationship, it may be time to think about whether it is indeed a good match for you.

Another problem that can damage relationships is **jealousy.** In relationships, jealousy is defined as the response to a threat to a relationship from an actual or imagined rival for a partner's attention.[32] Although it is natural to feel jealous once in a while, jealousy becomes serious when it is a precursor to domestic violence or interferes with the relationship in other ways. Jealousy is associated with low self-esteem, irrational thinking, depression, divorce, and physical violence. It is not a marker of true love, but rather insecurity, immaturity, and a need to be in control. An underlying cause of extreme jealousy is a fear of abandonment. Ironically, the behavior of extremely jealous partners often makes these fears come true. Not only can it destroy a relationship, it can be destructive to everyone in it.

Experts suggest that couples deal with jealousy directly and attempt to talk about the feelings underlying it. Often, talking about what sparks the jealousy may be enough to reduce it. If you are suffering from jealousy yourself, work on building your self-esteem, since low self-esteem is one of the sources of jealousy. If your partner is jealous, be available and respond to his or her concerns, offer reassurance, and keep in mind that changes do not happen immediately and sometimes counseling may even be needed to help you and your partner move forward.[33]

There is one situation that demands that you immediately leave a relationship: physical abuse. If a partner is threatening you physically or being physically abusive to you or your children, remove yourself and your children from the relationship as soon as possible. Chapter 14 discusses physical abuse and domestic violence in more detail.

When Relationships End

Despite our best efforts, many relationships eventually end. Those that lead to marriage are still vulnerable to the problems that can eventually result in a split: infidelity, jealousy, competitiveness, illness, money problems, and growing apart. Raising children can also put a strain on a relationship.

Breaking up, however, can be difficult, especially if you were not the initiator. Recovering from a failed relationship takes time and effort. Strategies that can facilitate the recovery process include:

- **Talk about it.** Share your feelings with a good friend or family member.
- **Focus on what is good about you.** Resist the urge to blame yourself and exaggerate your faults while mending a broken heart.
- **Take care of yourself.** Exercise, eat well, and get plenty of sleep.
- **Let your emotions out.** Do not be afraid to cry.
- **Do things you normally enjoy.** Have some fun.
- **Keep yourself busy.** Get your mind off your pain for awhile.
- **Give yourself time to recover.** Recognize that your hurt will not go away overnight.[34]

Committed Relationships

Most adults value having a committed relationship with another person. Nationwide surveys reveal that about two-thirds of unmarried adults say a long-term committed relationship is integral to having a fulfilling life.[35] Committed relationships come in various forms, including cohabitation, marriage, and domestic partnerships.

Cohabitation

One of the greatest transformations in family life in the U.S. during the last century has been the significant increase in **cohabitation**—unmarried couples living together under the same roof. Whereas

jealousy The response to a threat to a relationship from an actual or imagined rival for a partner's attention.

cohabitation The state of living together in the same household; usually refers to unmarried couples.

traditional courtship progressed from dating to engagement to marriage, many couples today opt to live together before getting engaged or married. Some continue in long-term, committed relationships without ever tying the knot. Cohabitation is now so common and accepted in our society that an estimated 50–60% of couples in the U.S. now live together before getting married.[36] For some, cohabitation represents a chance to get to know each other better before taking marriage vows. Others choose to cohabitate to benefit from the companionship, intimacy, and shared living costs cohabitation allows.

There is a down side to cohabitation. Most cohabitating couples are denied the legal and financial benefits afforded to married couples. These include family leave, Social Security benefits after the death of a partner, and access to a lover's pension, health insurance coverage, and un-taxed retirement savings.[37] In addition, cohabitating couples in the U.S. report the lowest levels of wealth among household types. Research indicates that nearly half the couples that live together remain unmarried five years later, and that most of them are no longer in a relationship with each other.[38] Those who do get married are actually more likely to get divorced. Couples who cohabitate or who cohabitated before marriage report higher rates of depression and marital conflict, lower marital satisfaction, higher relational dependency, more infidelity, less life satisfaction, lower self-esteem, and lower levels of marital interaction compared with couples who did not live together before marriage. One theory for these differences is that marriage fosters certain behavior changes by the couple and those around them that cohabitation just doesn't encourage.[39] The newest research is hopeful, however, indicating that these trends may be changing as cohabitation becomes more common and accepted in society. It also shows that cohabitating couples who are engaged before they move in together may be more successful than couples who live together but have no plans to marry.[40]

Marriage

Between 85% and 90% of Americans will marry during their lifetime.[41] An overwhelming majority of high school seniors say that having a happy marriage is "extremely important" to them.[42] Same-sex couples, meanwhile, have been waging an intense legal and political battle to have their unions recognized and legalized around the country.

Aside from its romantic associations, marriage has practical implications, benefits, and obligations. It is a legally binding contract, giving a sense of legitimacy to the relationship in the eyes of society and the law.[43] It signals to others that each spouse has entered into a long-term commitment that carries with it expectations of fidelity, mutual support, and lifetime partnership.

Benefits of Marriage

Study after study has shown that marriages in general—and good marriages in particular—provide a wealth of physical, psychological, and financial benefits. The longer a person stays married, in fact, the more the benefits accrue.[43] The benefits include:

- **Better mental health.** Married people tend to be happier and more satisfied with their lives, on average, than unmarried people, according to an analysis of 22 studies.[44]

- **Better physical health and longer life expectancies.** Being married is linked to fewer sick days, less use of hospital facilities and less likelihood of having chronic health conditions.[45] Married men

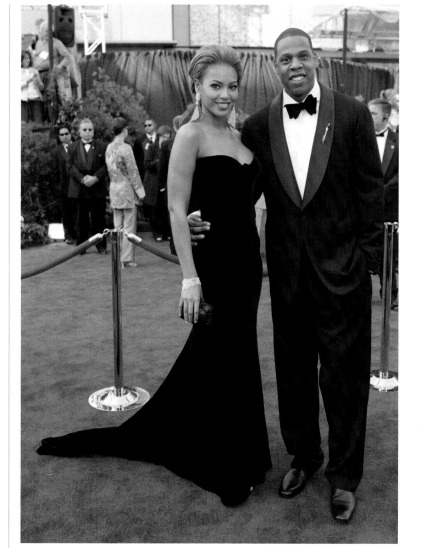

Beyoncé and Jay-Z married in 2008.

can expect to live, on average, at least seven years longer than never-married men, while married women tend to live at least three years longer than their never-married counterparts.[46]

- **Better financial health.** Married couples tend to have higher household incomes than unmarried people.[42]

Are married people healthier because they are married? Or is it that healthier people are somehow more likely to get married? Although researchers suspect that both could be at play, there is evidence that marriage fosters healthful and helpful behaviors. For example, married couples generally drink less, exercise more, get more sleep, and visit the doctor more often than people who are not married.[47]

Separation and Divorce

"Till death do us part" is a phrase that is often included in marriage vows. For about half the couples getting married for the first time, however, the marriage will end not when one person passes away, but when one decides to file for divorce.[48] Divorce has become an increasingly common and accepted practice in the United States, as the moral and social stigmas surrounding it have greatly diminished. Divorce rates actually peaked in the early 1980s, and the rate of divorces and annulments has gone down slightly since then; over the past seven years they have stabilized at around 50%.[49]

Researchers attribute the divorce rate to a number of factors, including society's increasingly high expectations for marriage. During the 1950s and early 1960s, surveys of college students demonstrated that marriage was sought after because of the opportunities it afforded couples—namely, the chance to own a home, live a stable lifestyle, and have children. Nowadays, college students say they value marriage because they believe it will provide them with emotional fulfillment.[50] As people's expectations for marriage go up, marital satisfaction goes down. About half of divorces today occur in couples that seem to have a relatively stable marriage. They do not bicker all the time, are moderately happy with their marriages, and have many positive interactions. Yet they do not believe marriage needs to be a lifelong commitment, see few barriers obstructing their leaving, and anticipate that being single or being with someone else will be better than being married to their current partner.[50] Other risk factors for divorce include a pattern of negative interactions between spouses, having parents who are divorced, marrying under the age of 21, and reacting strongly or defensively to problems and disappointments.[51] For those in really bad marriages, divorce can represent a relief, an end to seemingly never-ending marital woes.[52] For most people, though, divorce results in a crisis that causes severe emotional pain and distress to the entire family. Whereas adults often experience temporary stress and sadness, their children may develop long-term emotional problems that can get worse as they grow older.[53] Children of divorced parents are 50% more likely to get a divorce themselves one day.[54]

There are factors that decrease your risk of divorce. Divorce rates are lowest for people with at least some college, who have annual incomes over $50,000, who are religious, who have parents who are married, and who wait until the age of 25 to marry and have children.[42]

Domestic Partnerships

Although same-sex marriages are still not permitted in many states, **domestic partnerships** often are. In a domestic partnership, a couple lives together, stays in a long-term committed relationship, and legally registers as domestic partners. In return, they often have access to their partner's employer-sponsored benefits such as health insurance and bereavement leave. Domestic partnerships are also recognized by some states, counties, and cities, and give couples access to other privileges, including the ability to visit a partner in the hospital. Yet the benefits vary widely by location, and fall far short of those provided through marriage. Domestic partners, for example are often not allowed to make any medical decisions on behalf of an incapacitated partner. Domestic partnerships are open to committed couples—homosexual or heterosexual—who have lived together usually for more than one year.

Staying Single

In 1980, the median age at marriage was 22 years for women and 24.7 years for men. Fast-forward a quarter century and the age rose to 25.9 years for women and 28.1 years for men—the oldest in U.S. history.[55] In 2008, 22% of men ages 35–44 had never been married, and 17%

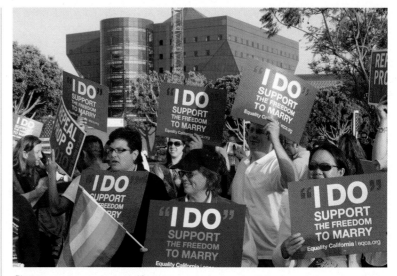

Same-sex marriage continues to be a controversial issue in the U.S.

of women that age had also never married.[56] The trend to stay single is occurring in all racial groups in the U.S. but is most pronounced in African Americans.[56]

Why are Americans waiting longer to marry, or avoiding marriage entirely? Some opt to focus on their education and career. Rising cohabitation rates have also meant that many adults enjoy intimacy and companionship while remaining legally single. Women today are also much more financially independent and less pressured to marry in order to attain economic stability. Attitudes about marriage and childrearing have also changed, with far fewer couples believing marriage is necessary to raise children.[57]

Singles can, and do, lead very fulfilled lives, enjoying successful careers, close personal friendships, and strong family ties. Some date frequently, others rarely. Some choose to live with a partner long-term. Singles are often stereotyped as being alone and lonely, but, in reality, they are likely to have networks of important people and friendships that have lasted years beyond many marriages.[58]

Starting a Family

Most people in the United States anticipate that they will be parents one day. For some, raising children is one of the life achievements they most look forward to. The American family, however, has undergone a dramatic transformation in recent decades. Women are waiting longer to have children, spacing births further apart, and ending their fertility at earlier ages than ever before. In addition, almost 9% of women now say they do not want to have any children.[59] Consequently, the U.S. birth rate is at an all-time low.

Nontraditional families are also on the rise, with single-parent households increasing more than six-fold since 1950, and unmarried-couple households more than quadrupling.[60] Only 67% of children in 2009 lived with two married, biological parents.[61] These changes in the traditional organization of the American family don't

domestic partnership A legal arrangement in which a couple lives together in a long-term committed relationship and receives some, but not all, of the rights of married couples.

This interactive map can help you learn about same-sex marriage and domestic partnership legislation for each state: www.npr.org/templates/story/story.php?storyId=112448663.

necessarily signal the decline of our social structure. They do, however, point to how flexible and complex American family arrangements have become and remind us that there is no such thing as a "typical" family.

Choosing Children

Having a baby can be one of the most rewarding experiences in life. It can also be one of the most difficult, trying a new parent's patience and testing a couple's relationship. Parenthood is often associated with less intimacy in marriage, as well as a reduction in marital satisfaction and individual well-being, as a new baby places many demands on a parent's time and competes with a partner for attention.[62] If a child is born out of wedlock, the demands of parenthood can be even more challenging.

If you are considering parenthood, ask yourself whether you are ready for the following dramatic changes:

- **Relationship changes.** Caring nonstop for a newborn baby can leave little time for couples to focus on their own relationship. Especially during the child's first year, parents are likely to fight more and be intimate less. Married couples often experience a decrease in their overall satisfaction with their marriage.[62]

- **Changes in your relationships with family and friends.** Your parents may have ideas about what your priorities should be, and they may differ from yours. They may have strong feelings about how you should care for your children, and the religious beliefs you should pass on to them. Your friendships could also change, as your confidants find that new babies mean new schedules and new priorities, and leave much less time for socializing with friends.[63]

- **Less time for yourself.** Having little time to sleep or take good care of yourself is a complaint of many new parents. The amount of work it takes to care for a newborn can be overwhelming.[63]

In addition, assess the following:

- **Your health.** If you are a prospective mother, you should evaluate how healthy you are and what you should do to prepare your body for a pregnancy. If you smoke or drink, quit. Reduce your caffeine consumption. Eat nutritious foods, get regular exercise, and begin taking prenatal vitamins right away. If you are a prospective father, you should also work at adopting a more healthful lifestyle including avoiding tobacco, alcohol, and recreational drugs, because using these substances before conception could affect male fertility or perhaps even contribute to poor fetal health.[64]

- **Your finances.** Consider your monthly budget and the added expenses that come with a baby, including food, diapers, clothing, and furniture. Assess the decrease in income you will see if one of you takes time off work. Come up with a plan on how to cover the medical bills and the cost of daycare, if you will need it.

- **Your home environment.** Babies have special needs—and often require a lot of gear. Will a new baby fit into your current living arrangement? Do you need a larger place to live? Are there alterations you will have to make to your home to make it acceptable for a baby, ensuring it has a functioning heater or air-conditioner, for example?

- **Your childcare arrangements.** Agree on who will care for your child. You? Your partner? A family member? A daycare center? Are any of these options affordable?

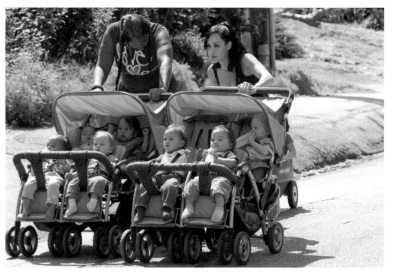

The childcare challenges of "Octomom" Nadya Suleman, who gave birth to octuplets in 2009, are an extreme example of the challenges faced by all parents.

- **How you will divide the labor.** Relationship satisfaction has been linked to how satisfied couples are with the way housework is divided. Some couples become more traditional in their division of labor after a baby arrives, and this can cause tension in some relationships. Talk about your expectations of who will do what.

- **Parenting styles.** What values do you want to emphasize? Do you have similar beliefs on discipline? Do you know what religious beliefs you would like to share with your child?

Balancing Work and Family Life

Decades ago, there was one fairly common family construct: Men went to work and earned money for their families, while women stayed home and tended to the children. These days, however, many families find they need both parents to hold down full-time jobs outside the home in order to pay the bills. You're likely to see families headed by a "Supermom," a woman who balances a full-time career with household chores and parenting duties. In the U.S., 57% of women who have a child less than a year old are in the labor force.[65] And more men are opting to be "Mr. Mom"—taking years off from work to be stay-at-home dads.

Parents are seeing an increasing demand on their time from all directions. The number of double-income families has continued to rise, as has the number of single-parent families and parents caring for their children and their aging parents at the same time. There has also been a cultural shift toward more intensive parenting, with parents wanting to spend more time interacting with their children.[66] All this can leave many parents feeling as though they are engaged in a nonstop juggling act.

Surveys of working parents show that parenting can leave little time for pursuing individual interests. In one survey, researchers found that women with children spend more than 100 hours a week on housework, caregiving, and professional responsibilities, whereas men spend about 85 hours a week on those tasks.[67] The men and women spent nearly equal amounts of time on the job and toiling away in the house. The time discrepancy stems from the amount of time actually spent with the children, with women being much more involved.

Stepfamilies

One out of every three Americans is now either a stepchild, a stepsibling, a stepparent, or another member of a stepfamily.[68] These "blended families" have become commonplace in modern society, as more parents have opted to divorce and later remarry. Indeed, about three-fourths of divorced adults do go on to remarry, many of them within the first few years of their original marriage's end.[69] In about 65% of these remarriages, one or both partners have children from a previous relationship, according to the National Stepfamily Resource Center.[70]

When a stepfamily is first coming together, life can be unpredictable and chaotic. It can take several years for members of previously distinct families to integrate, and they do not always succeed.[71] Members of a stepfamily need to form new roles and norms within their new family, rather than trying to re-create the original family. Setting realistic expectations and encouraging open communication can be extremely useful in fostering strong stepfamily relationships.

Single Parenthood

Even if you were not raised by a single parent, odds are you know someone who was. Of the 74.2 million children living in the United States in 2009, 26% lived with only one parent.[72] The statistics reflect not only the high divorce rate and the small proportion of partners who are widowed, but the growing number of parents who have never been married. One-third of children today are born to unmarried mothers and end up being raised in a single-parent home—or spending part of their childhood living with other relatives or stepparents.[73] Most often, single parents are female.

One of the greatest hurdles single mothers face is economic hardship. An estimated 30% of women who have a child born out of wedlock live in poverty, compared with just 8% of women who were married at the time of their child's birth.[74] Single mothers, on average, also have lower levels of education than other women, which can hurt their job prospects and lower their earnings potential.

Just how children fare growing up in a single-parent household varies, and has been the source of some controversy. Experts know it is not always the family's structure that is important, but how it functions. Yet research suggests that this type of living arrangement is detrimental to many kids. "Children who grow up in a household with only one biological parent are worse off, on average, than children who grow up in a household with both of their biological parents, regardless of the parents' race or educational background," state the authors of *Growing Up with a Single Parent: What Hurts, What Helps*.[75] Children from single-parent families have a risk of negative life outcomes that is two to three times higher than children from married, two-parent families.[42] Children born out of wedlock are more likely to experience a wide range of behavioral and emotional problems, reaching adulthood with less education and earning less income. They are more likely to be "idle"—out of school and out of work—in their late teens and early 20s. They experience more symptoms of depression, and have more troubled marriages and higher rates of divorce. They are also more likely to have a child out of wedlock themselves.[76]

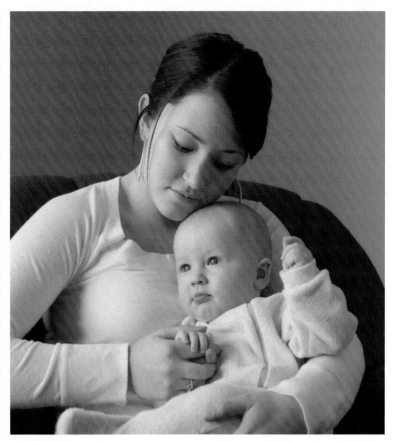

Single mothers often face economic hardship.

Characteristics of Happy Families

Researchers have devoted a great deal of time to looking at strong families, measuring their affection and communication, trying to decipher their secrets for success. What they found is that a happy family is not one without trouble or weaknesses. Some have experienced financial difficulties, health problems, or other setbacks. But strong families learn how to adapt and endure, taking a constructive approach to dealing with crises.[77]

Members of strong families share and value these traits:

- **Commitment.** They are dedicated to the family and promoting each other's happiness. They are honest, faithful, and dependable.
- **Appreciation and affection.** They care for each other and are not afraid to express it. They give compliments and show their affection freely.
- **Positive communication.** They are good talkers and good listeners. They do argue, but avoid blaming each other and are able to compromise.
- **Time together.** They spend quality time together as often as they can, and arrange their schedules to ensure that this happens.
- **Spiritual well-being.** They have hope, faith, and compassion, as well as shared ethical values.
- **The ability to manage stress and crises.** They see crises as both challenges and opportunities for growth. They pull together during tough times and give support to each other.[78]

Watch videos of real students discussing communication and relationships at www.pearsonhighered.com/choosinghealth.

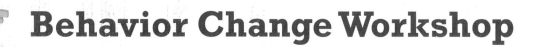

Behavior Change Workshop

To complete this workshop online, visit www.pearsonhighered.com/choosinghealth.

Part I. Assessing Your Communication Skills

1. Think about the communication skills that are listed on page 191. List the skills that you feel you have mastered in your own life. Then, list one area in particular that you would like to improve.

Mastered: _____

_____

Needs improvement: _____

_____

2. Reflect on a recent conversation that would have benefited from changes to the communication skill that you felt needed improvement. Now that you are more informed about successful communication, what could you have done differently?

_____

_____

_____

3. Describe what you might do or think about as a "next step" for improving your communication skills. Also list your timeline for making this next step.

Next step: _____

_____

Timeline: _____

_____

4. Listening is a major component of communication. Consider the good listening skills that were discussed on page 191. Which techniques can you try to become a better listener? Provide examples of how you will apply these skills in your life.

Techniques: _____

_____

Examples: _____

_____

Part II. Building Stronger Relationships

1. Think about a relationship that you would like to improve. What could be done to make the relationship stronger?

_____

_____

_____

2. One way to improve a relationship is to try to see things through the other person's eyes. Take a moment to think about your friend or partner and write down key factors in that person's life and situation. Answer the following questions: Who are the important people in his or her life and why? What other people is he or she having problems with and why? What are his or her current stressors? What is he or she looking forward to or worried about?

_____

_____

_____

_____

3. Imagine that you are writing a note to the person with whom you want to improve relations. What would you say? Write it down.

_____

_____

_____

_____

● Chapter Summary

- Good communication includes being able to articulate your honest thoughts and feelings, being a good listener, and being aware of how body language can affect how others interpret what you are saying.
- Effective conflict resolution requires that both parties voice their concerns maturely and engage in constructive criticism, rather than resorting to personal attacks and put-downs.
- Self-perception, early relationships, and gender roles affect how we develop relationships throughout life.
- Strong friendships and social ties contribute to greater overall health.
- Sternberg's Triangular Theory of Love identifies intimacy, passion, and commitment as the three primary components of healthy, loving relationships.

- Healthy relationships are based on trust, respect, and communication. Dysfunctional relationships are characterized by physical or verbal abuse, manipulation, disrespect, or cruelty.
- Cohabitation, marriage, and domestic partnerships are examples of different kinds of committed relationships.
- Raising children can be rewarding as well as stressful. Couples should ask themselves how having a baby would change their lives, and whether they are truly ready for those changes.
- Strong families are characterized by commitment, appreciation, affection, positive communication, time together, spiritual well-being, and the ability to adapt to changes.

Test Your Knowledge

1. Sharing your feelings and other personal information with another person is called
   a. self-assuredness.
   b. self-love.
   c. self-appreciation.
   d. self-disclosure.

2. All of the following are examples of non-verbal communication except
   a. eye contact.
   b. email.
   c. arm movements.
   d. facial expressions.

3. In Sternberg's Triangular Theory of Love, the primary components of healthy relationships include all of the following except
   a. passion.
   b. contentment.
   c. commitment.
   d. intimacy.

4. Assortative mating refers to the tendency of people to
   a. be attracted to people who have opposite interests to their own.
   b. fall in love at first sight.
   c. "hook up" instead of date.
   d. select romantic partners who are similar to themselves.

5. Healthy relationships are characterized by all of the following except
   a. honesty.
   b. respect.
   c. good communication.
   d. constant contact.

6. How many people in the U.S. identify themselves as LGB?
   a. 880,000
   b. 8.8 million
   c. 18.8 million
   d. 80 million

7. What is the best way to deal with jealousy in an intimate relationship?
   a. Ignore it.
   b. Limit what you do until your partner is no longer jealous.
   c. Talk openly about it.
   d. Reduce the jealous person's self-esteem.

8. In general, married people
   a. enjoy better mental and physical health than unmarried people.
   b. live longer than unmarried people.
   c. are financially better off than unmarried people.
   d. all of the above

9. What is the divorce rate in the United States?
   a. around 50%
   b. around 75%
   c. around 33%
   d. increasing

10. What proportion of people in the U.S. are part of a stepfamily?
    a. one in two
    b. one in three
    c. one in four
    d. one in five

Get Critical

What happened:

Is there such a thing as love at first sight? Researchers at Ohio State University decided to find out, recruiting 164 first-year students and pairing them off on the first day of class. Students were instructed to introduce themselves and spend just a few minutes talking. They were then given a questionnaire and asked to predict how close they would become to each other over the course of the next few months. Nine weeks later, were they on target? Researchers found that most students did indeed guess correctly during that first brief meeting the kind of relationship that would develop.

In a separate study, Florida State University psychologists found that it takes just half a second to decide whether someone is attractive and a potential mate. They also noticed that people gazed at attractive faces for a little bit longer than the faces that were not appealing to them.

What do you think?

- Do you find these studies compelling proof that "love at first sight" exists?

- How do you define "love"? Do you agree with Sternberg's Triangular Theory of Love? Why or why not?

1. At First Sight: Persistent Relational Effects of Get Acquainted Conversations, by M. Sunnafrank and A. Ramirez, 2004, *Journal of Social and Personal Relationships, 21*, pp. 361–379. 2. Can't Take My Eyes Off You: Attentional Adhesion to Mates and Rivals, by J. K. Maner, M. T. Gailliot, D. A. Rouby, and S. L. Miller, 2007, *Journal of Personality and Social Psychology, 93*, pp. 389–401.

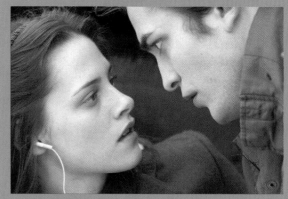

In the movie *Twilight,* Edward and Bella experienced love at first sight.

Get Connected

Health Online Visit the following websites for further information about the topics in this chapter:

- Conflict Management Information Source
  www.crinfo.org
- American Psychological Association
  www.apa.org
- Human Rights Campaign
  www.hrc.org
- National Teen Dating Abuse Helpline
  www.loveisrespect.org

- The National Marriage Project
  www.virginia.edu/marriageproject
- American Association for Marriage and Family Therapy
  www.aamft.org
- Go Ask Alice
  www.goaskalice.columbia.edu

Website links are subject to change. To access updated web links, please visit **www.pearsonhighered.com/choosinghealth.**

References

i. Kahn, A. S., Fricker, K., Hoffman, J., Lambert, T., Tripp, M., & Childress, K. (2000, August). Hooking up: Dangerous new dating methods? In A. S. Kahn (Chair), *Sex, unwanted sex, and sexual assault on college campuses.* Symposium conducted at the annual meeting of the American Psychological Association, Washington, D.C.

ii. Facebook Press Room. (2010). Statistics. Retrieved from http://www.facebook.com/press/info.php?statistics

iii. Stanley, S. M., Rhoades, G. K., & Markman, H. J. (2006). Sliding versus deciding: Inertia and the premarital cohabitation effect. *Family Relations, 55,* 499–509.

iv. Karasu, S. R. (2007). The institution of marriage: Terminable or interminable? *American Journal of Psychotherapy, 61*(1), 1–16.

1. Jourard, S. M. (1971). *The Transparent Self.* New York: D. Van Nostrand Company.

2. University of Pennsylvania Faculty/Staff Assistance Program. (n.d.). *Conflict resolution: How to fight fair so that everyone wins.* Retrieved from http://www.upenn.edu/fsap/conflict.htm

3. Schuetz, A. (1998). Autobiographical narratives of good and bad deeds: Defensive and favorable self-description moderated by trait self-esteem. *Journal of Social and Clinical Psychology, 17,* 466–475.

4. Bellavia, G., & Murray, S. (2003). Did I do that? Self-esteem–related differences in reactions to romantic partners' moods. *Personal Relationships, 10*(1), 77–95.

5. Bowlby, J. (1982). *Attachment and loss: Vol. 1., Attachment* (2nd ed.). New York: Basic Books.

6. Kilmann, P. R., Urbaniak, G. C., & Parnell, M. M. (2006). Effects of attachment-focused versus relationship skills-focused group interventions for college students with insecure attachment patterns. *Attachment & Human Development, 8*(1), 47–62.

7. Gurian, A. (n.d.). *Depression in adolescence: Does gender matter?* NYC Child Study Center. Retrieved from http://www.aboutourkids.org/articles/depression_in_adolescence_does_gender_matter

8. Katz-Wise, S. L., Priess, H. A., & Hyde, J. S. (2010). Gender-role attitudes and behavior across the transition to parenthood. *Developmental Psychology, 46*(1), 18–28.

9. Berkman, L. F., & Syme, S. L. (1979). Social networks, host resistance, and mortality: A nine-year follow-up study of Alameda County residents. *American Journal of Epidemiology, 109*(2), 186–204.

10. Berkman, L. F. (1995). The role of social relations in health promotion. *Psychosomatic Medicine, 57*(3), 245–254.

11. McPherson, M., Smith-Lovin, L., & Brashears, M. E. (2006). Social isolation in America: Changes in core discussion networks over two decades. *American Sociological Review, 71*(3), 353–375.

12. Pressman, S. D., Cohen, S., Miller, G. E., Barkin, A., Rabin, B. S., & Treanor, J. J. (2005). Loneliness, social network size, and immune response to influenza vaccination in college freshmen. *Health Psychology, 24*(3), 297–306.

13. Swami, V., Chamorro-Premuzic, T., Sinniah, D., Maniam, T., Kannan, K., & Stanistreet, D. (2007). General health mediates the relationship between loneliness, life satisfaction and depression. *Social Psychiatry and Psychiatric Epidemiology, 42,* 161–166.

14. Ledbetter, A. M., Griffin, E. M., & Sparks, G. G. (2007). Forecasting "friends forever": A longitudinal investigation of sustained closeness between best friends. *Personal Relationships, 14*(2), 343–350.

15. Sternberg, R. J. (1986). A triangular theory of love. *Psychological Review, 93,* 119–135.

16. Rowett Research Institute (2007, August 13). Love at first sight of your body fat. *ScienceDaily.* Retrieved from http://www.sciencedaily.com/releases/2007/08/070812095324.htm

17. Association for Psychological Science. (2008, February 14). Beauty bias: Can people love the one they are compatible with?. *ScienceDaily.* Retrieved from http://www.sciencedaily.com/releases/2008/02/080211094943.htm

18. Blackwell Publishing, Ltd. (2007, November 30). Personality traits influence perceived attractiveness. *ScienceDaily.* Retrieved from http://www.sciencedaily.com/releases/2007/11/071129145852.htm

19. Luo, S., & Klohnen, E. C. (2005). Assortative mating and marital quality in newlyweds: A couple-centered approach. *Journal of Personality and Social Psychology, 88*(2), 304–326.

20. Luo, S., & Klohnen, E. C. (2005). Assortative mating and marital quality in newlyweds: A couple-centered approach. *Journal of Personality and Social Psychology, 88*(2), page 323.

21. Whitehead, B. D., & Popenoe, D. (2002). *The state of our unions: The social health of marriage in America.* Piscataway, NJ: National Marriage Project, Rutgers University. Retrieved from http://www.virginia.edu/marriageproject/pdfs/SOOU2002.pdf

22. Bogle, K. A. (2007). The shift from dating to hooking up in college: What scholars have missed. *Social Psychology & Family, 1*(2), 775–788.

23. Daniel, C., & Fogarty, K. (2007). *"Hooking up" and hanging out: Casual sexual behaviaor among adolescents and young adults today* (Publication FCS2279). Department of Family, Youth and Community Sciences, Florida Cooperative Extension Service, Institute of Food and Agricultural Sciences, University of Florida. Retrieved from http://edis.ifas.ufl.edu/fy1002

24. Kruse, A. (2009, December 2). Liquid courage: The dangers of drinking and hooking up. *California University Cal Times.* Retrieved from http://sai.cup.edu/caltimes/index.php/2009/12/02/liquid-courage-the-dangers-of-drinking-and-hooking-up

25. Romero, A. P., Baumle, A. K., Lee Badgett, M. V., & Gates, G. J. (2007, December). *Census snapshot: The United States.* The Williams Institute, UCLA School of Law. Retrieved from http://www.law.ucla.edu/williamsinstitute/publications/USCensusSnapshot.pdf

26. Roisman, G. I., Clausell, E., Holland, A., Fortuna, K., & Elieff, C. (2008). Adult romantic relationships as contexts of human development: A multimethod comparison of same-sex couples with opposite-sex dating, engaged, and married dyads. *Developmental Psychology, 44*(1), 91–101.

27. Balsam, K. F., Beauchaine, T. P., Rothblum, E. D., & Solomon, S. E. (2008). Three-year follow-up of same-sex couples who had civil unions in Vermont, same-sex couples not in civil unions, and heterosexual married couples. *Developmental Psychology, 44*(1), 102–116.

28. Madureira, A. F. A. (2007). The psychological basis of homophobia: Cultural construction of a barrier. *Integrative Psychological & Behavioral Science, 41,* 225–247.

29. O'Leary, K. D., & Cascardi, M. (1998). Physical aggression in marriage: A development analysis. In T. N. Bradbury (Ed.), *The developmental course of marital dysfunction* (pp. 343–374). New York: Cambridge University Press.

30. Amato, P. R., & Booth, A. (2001). The legacy of parents' marital discord: Consequences for children's marital quality. *Journal of Personality and Social Psychology, 81,* 627–638.

31. Lyness, D. (2008). Am I in a healthy relationship? *TeensHealth from Nemours.* Retrieved from http://kidshealth.org/teen/your_mind/relationships/healthy_relationship.html

32. Barelds, D. P. H., & Dijkstra, P. (2006). Reactive, anxious and possessive forms of jealousy and their relation to relationship quality among heterosexuals and homosexuals. *Journal of Homosexuality, 51*(3), 183–198.

33. HealthyPlace.com. (2009, January 13). How to deal with a jealous partner. *HealthyPlace: America's Mental Health Channel.* Retrieved from http://www.healthyplace.com/relationships/jealousy/how-to-deal-with-a-jealous-partner/menu-id-1624

34. Cheyne, K. L., & Pendley, J. S. (2007). Getting over a breakup. *TeensHealth from Nemours.* Retrieved from http://kidshealth.org/teen/your_mind/relationships/broken_heart.html

35. Harris Interactive. Retrieved from http://iac.mediaroom.com/index.php?s=43&item=869

36. Stanley, S. M., Rhoades, G. K., & Markman, H. J. (2006). Sliding versus deciding: Inertia and the premarital cohabitation effect. *Family Relations, 55,* 499–509.

37. Human Rights Campaign. (n.d.) *FAQs: Questions about same-sex marriage.* Retrieved from http://www.hrc.org/issues/5517.htm

38. Bumpass, L. L., & Sweet, J. A. (1989). National estimates of cohabitation. *Demography, 26,* 615–625.

39. Harms, W. (2000, March 2). Research looks at cohabitation's negative effects. *The University of Chicago Chronicle, 19*(11). Retrieved from http://chronicle.uchicago.edu/000302/cohabit.shtml

40. Goodwin P. Y., Mosher W. D., & Chandra, A. (2010). Marriage and cohabitation in the United States: A statistical portrait based on cycle 6 (2002) of the National Survey of Family Growth. In *Vital and Health Statistics* (Series 23, Number 28). National Center for Health Statistics, Centers for Disease Control and Prevention.

41. Karasu, S. R. (2007). The institution of marriage: Terminable or interminable? *American Journal of Psychotherapy, 61*(1), 1–16.

42. Popenoe, D., & Whitehead, B. D. (2007). *The state of our unions, 2007: The social health of marriage in America.* Piscataway, NJ: The National Marriage Project, Rutgers University. Retrieved from http://www.virginia.edu/marriageproject/pdfs/SOOU2007.pdf

43. Wilcox, W. B., Doherty, W., Glenn N., & Waite, L. (2005). *Why marriage Matters: Twenty-six conclusions from the social sciences* (2nd ed.). New York: Institute for American Values.

44. Wood, W., Rhodes, N., & Whelan, M. (1989). Sex differences in positive well-being: A consideration of emotional style and marital status. *Psychological Bulletin, 106,* 249–264.

45. Verbrugge, L. M. (1979). Marital status and health. *Journal of Marriage and the Family, 41,* 267–285.

46. Waite, L., & Gallagher, M. (2000). *The case for marriage: Why married people are happier, healthier, and better off financially.* New York: Doubleday.

47. Garrison, M. (2007). The decline of formal marriage: Inevitable or reversible? *Family Law Quarterly, 41*(3), 491–520.

48. Falke, S. I., & Larson, J. H. (2007). Premarital predictors of remarital quality: Implications for clinicians. *Contemporary Family Therapy, 29,* 9–23.

49. National Center for Health Statistics, Centers for Disease Control and Prevention. *National marriage and divorce rate trends: 2000–2007.* Retrieved from http://www.cdc.gov/nchs/nvss/marriage_divorce_tables.htm

50. Amato, P. R., & Hohmann-Marriott, B. (2007). A comparison of high- and low-distress marriages that end in divorce. *Journal of Marriage and Family, 69,* 621–638.

51. American Psychological Association. (2004). *Marital education programs help keep couples together.* Retrieved from http://www.apa.org/research/action/marital.aspx

52. Kalmijn, M., & Monden, C. W. S. (2006). Are the negative effects of divorce on well-being dependent on marital quality? *Journal of Marriage and Family, 68,* 1197–1213.

53. Popenoe, D., & Whitehead, B. D. (2001). *Information brief: The top ten myths of divorce.* Piscataway, NJ: The National Marriage Project, Rutgers University. Retrieved from http://www.virginia.edu/marriageproject/pdfs/MythsDivorce.pdf

54. Riggio, H. R., & Fite, J. E. (2006). Attitudes toward divorce: Embeddedness and outcomes in personal relationships. *Journal of Applied Social Psychology, 36*(12), 2935–2962.

55. U.S. Census Bureau. (2006). Table MS-2: Estimated median age at first marriage, by sex: 1890 to the present. In *Current Population Survey, March and Annual Social and Economic Supplements, 2005 and earlier.* Retrieved from http://www.census.gov/population/socdemo/hh-fam/ms2.pdf

56. U.S. Census Bureau. (2008). *Marital status, 2006–2008 American community survey 3-year estimates* (S1201). Retrieved from http://factfinder.census.gov/servlet/STTable?_bm=y&-geo_id=01000US&-qr_name=ACS_2008_3YR_G00_S1201&-ds_name=ACS_2008_3YR_G00_

57. Sharp, E. A., & Ganong, L. (2007). Living in the gray: Women's experiences of missing the marital transition. *Journal of Marriage and Family, 69,* 831–844.

58. DePaulo, B. (2008, February 8). *Single and happy.* National Sexuality Research Center. Retrieved from http://nsrc.sfsu.edu/article/single_and_happy

59. National Center for Health Statistics, Centers for Disease Control and Prevention. (2009). Birth expectations. In *Key statistics from the National Survey of Family Growth.* Retrieved from http://www.cdc.gov/nchs/nsfg/abc_list_b.htm#birthexpectations

60. Jiang, L., & O'Neill, B. C. (2007). Impacts of demographic trends on household size and structure. *Population and Development Review, 33*(3), 567–591.

61. U.S. Census Bureau. (2010). Table C3: Living arrangements of children under 18 years/1 and marital status of parents, by age, sex, race, and Hispanic origin/2 and selected characteristics of the child for all children: 2009. In *Current Population Survey, 2009, Annual Social and Economic Supplement.* Retrieved from http://www.census.gov/population/socdemo/hh-fam/cps2009/tabC3-all.xls

62. Ahlborg, T., & Strandmark, M. (2006). Factors influencing the quality of intimate relationships six months after delivery – First-time parents' own views and coping strategies. *Journal of Psychosomatic Obstetrics & Gynecology, 27*(3), 163–172.

63. Holzworth, A. N., & Radunovich, H. L. (2007). *Questions to ask as you consider parenthood: A couples' guide* (Publication FCS2271). Department of Family, Youth and Community Sciences, Florida Cooperative Extension Service, IFAS, University of Florida, Gainesville. Retrieved from http://edis.ifas.ufl.edu/fy928

64. Ansari, A. S., Sharma, A., & Lohiya, N. K. (2007). Does paternal occupation and lifestyle affect embryo quality? *Journal of Endocrinology & Reproduction, 11*(1), 15–22.

65. Dye, J. L. (2008). *Fertility of American women: 2006* (Publication P20-558). U.S. Census Bureau. Retrieved from http://www.census.gov/prod/2008pubs/p20-558.pdf

66. Valcour, M. (2007). Work-based resources as moderators of the relationship between work hours and satisfaction with work-family balance. *Journal of Applied Psychology, 92*(6), 1512–1523.

67. Mason, M. A., & Goulden, M. (2004). Do babies matter? Part II Closing the baby gap. *Academe, 90*(6), 10–15.

68. Larson, J. (1992). Understanding stepfamilies. *American Demographics, 14,* 360.

69. Michaels, M. (2007, March). Remarital issues in couple therapy. *Journal of Couple & Relationship Therapy, 6*(1/2), 125–139.

70. National Stepfamily Resource Center. (2010). *Stepfamily fact sheet.* Retrieved from http://www.stepfamilies.info/stepfamily-fact-sheet.php

71. Speer, R. B., & Trees, A. R. (2007). The push and pull of stepfamily life: The contribution of stepchildren's autonomy and connection-seeking behaviors to role development in stepfamilies. *Communication Studies, 58*(4), 377–394.

72. U.S. Census Bureau. (2010). Table C2: Living arrangements of children under 18 years/1 and marital status of parents, by age, sex, race, and Hispanic origin/2 and selected characteristics of the child for all children: 2009. In *Current Population Survey, 2009, Annual Social and Economic Supplement.* Retrieved from http://www.census.gov/population/socdemo/hh-fam

73. Kreider, R. M. (2008). *Living Arrangements of Children: 2004* (Publication P70-114). U.S. Census Bureau. Retrieved from http://www.census.gov/prod/2008pubs/p70-114.pdf

74. Williams, K., Sassler, S., & Nicholson, L. M. (2008). For better or for worse? The consequences of marriage and cohabitation for single mothers. *Social Forces, 86*(4), 1481–1511.

75. McLanahan, S., & Sandefur, G. (1997). *Growing up with a single parent: What hurts, what helps.* Cambridge: Harvard University Press.

76. Amato, P. R. (2005). The impact of family formation change on the cognitive, social, and emotional well-being of the next generation. *The Future of Children, 15*(2), 75 96.

77. Krysan, M., Moore, K. A., & Zill, N. (1990). *Research on successful families.* U.S. Department of Health and Human Services. Retrieved from http://aspe.hhs.gov/daltcp/Reports/ressucfa.htm

78. DeFrain, J., & Asay, S. M. (2007). Strong families around the world: An introduction to the family strengths perspective. *Marriage & Family Review, 41*(1/2), 1–10.

- About 34% of college students report that they have never engaged in vaginal intercourse.[i]

- In a recent study, 20% of teens and 33% of young adults reported sending or posting nude or semi-nude photos or videos of themselves over their cell phones.[ii]

- In the United States, half of all pregnancies are unplanned —about 3 million each year.[iii]

Sexuality, Contraception, and Reproductive Choices

DESCRIBE the primary structures in male and female sexual anatomy.

DESCRIBE the key events in the female menstrual cycle.

IDENTIFY the phases of the sexual response cycle and discuss common sexual dysfunctions.

DEFINE *abstinence, non-intercourse sexual activity*, and *sexual intercourse*.

DISCUSS three basic sexual orientations.

COMPARE and contrast different methods of contraception.

DISCUSS surgical and medical abortion.

DESCRIBE the key stages of pregnancy, from conception to birth.

 Health Online icons are found throughout the chapter, directing you to web links, videos, podcasts, and other useful online resources.

Sex is something people rarely think about intellectually.

Sure, you may fantasize about it, but pondering the physiological and wellness aspects of sex is usually not high on a college student's list of priorities. Yet sex is worth deeper thought than we often give it. Sex influences how we see ourselves and how we relate to others. It affects our health, our sense of pleasure, our romantic relationships, and our decisions about whether and when to have a family. Understanding your **sexuality,** knowing your reproductive options, and making choices that best fit your values and goals are important elements of your overall health and well-being.

Sexual Anatomy and Health

Whether we engage in sexual activity or not, our bodies are continually preparing for reproduction. A woman's ovaries release an egg each month, while a man's testes are constantly manufacturing new sperm. Given these biological realities, the sexual decisions we make in a split second can alter the course of our lives dramatically, by leading to an unplanned pregnancy or a sexually transmitted infection (see Chapter 11) that permanently affects fertility.

Female Sexual Anatomy

A woman's sexual anatomy includes both external and internal sex organs **(Figure 10.1).** The term **vulva** refers to all of the female external organs collectively—also known as *genitals*. These include the following structures:

- **Mons pubis.** The fatty, rounded area of tissue in front of the pubic bone; covered in pubic hair after puberty.
- **Labia majora.** The fleshy, larger outer lips (*labia* means lips) surrounding the labia minora.
- **Labia minora.** The thin, inner folds of skin, which rest protectively over the *clitoris,* the *vaginal opening,* and the *urethral opening*, through which urine is released from the body.
- **Clitoris.** An organ composed of spongy tissue with an abundance of nerve endings that make it very sensitive to sexual stimulation. During sexual arousal, the clitoris fills with blood and plays a key role in producing the female orgasm. In fact, the clitoris is the only organ in either sex with the sole purpose of sexual arousal and pleasure.

The internal organs include the following:

- **Vagina.** The tube that connects a woman's external sex organs with her *uterus*. It serves as the passageway through which menstrual flow leaves the body, as well as the passageway through which sperm enters the body during heterosexual intercourse. During childbirth, it functions as the birth canal.

sexuality The biological, physical, emotional, and psychosocial aspects of sexual attraction and expression.

vulva All of the female external organs, collectively. Also called *genitals*.

mons pubis The fatty, rounded areas of tissue in front of the pubic bone.

labia Two pairs (majora and minora) of fleshy lips surrounding and protecting the clitoris and the vaginal and urethral openings.

clitoris An organ composed of spongy tissue and nerve endings which is very sensitive to sexual stimulation.

vagina The tube that connects a woman's external sex organs with her uterus.

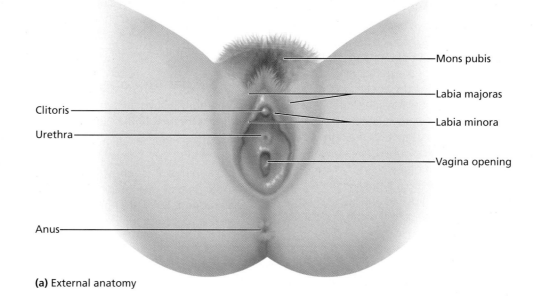

(a) External anatomy

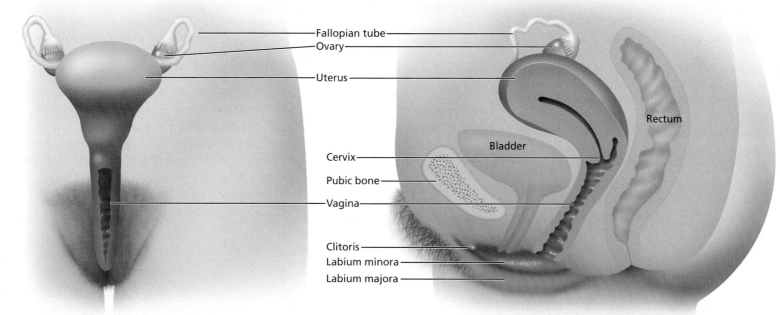

(b) Internal anatomy

Figure 10.1 Female sexual anatomy.

- **Uterus.** Also known as the *womb*. The uterus is a pear-shaped organ, normally about the size of a fist. It is here that a growing fetus is nurtured. The innermost lining of the uterus is called the *endometrium*. It is shed monthly in nonpregnant women of childbearing age. The narrowed end of the uterus that projects into the top of the vagina is called the *cervix*. Sperm deposited into the vagina swim through the opening of the cervix into the body of the uterus.

- **Ovaries.** The two chambers, one on either side of the pelvic cavity, where a woman's eggs, or

uterus (womb) The pear-shaped organ where a growing fetus is nurtured.

ovaries The two female reproductive organs where ova (eggs) reside.

menstrual cycle A monthly physiological cycle marked by *menstruation*.

fallopian tubes A pair of tubes that connect the ovaries to the uterus.

ova, are stored. Every month, at approximately midway through her **menstrual cycle,** a woman *ovulates*; that is, one of her ovaries releases an egg. The ovaries produce the hormone *estrogen*.

- **Fallopian tubes.** The tubes—one on either side of the uterus—that connect the uterus to the ovaries. After ovulation, the egg is swept into the nearby fallopian tube. It then travels through the tube to the uterus. If it encounters sperm within the tube, the egg may become fertilized. Either fertilized or not, the egg will continue to be swept into the uterus.

Common Sexual Health Problems in Females

Good sexual health includes good preventive care. According to the American Congress of Obstetricians and Gynecologists (ACOG), girls should have their first gynecologic visit between the ages of 13 and 15. Unless a girl is sexually active or is experiencing problems, these first visits will most likely not include a pelvic exam. New ACOG guidelines indicate that women should have their first pelvic exam and pap smear by age 21 and most women under 30 should receive cervical screening once every two years until the age of 30. Those age 30 and older, who have had three consecutive negative pap smears, can wait three years between pap smears. Unfortunately, about half of all college-age women do not get screened regularly.[1] Not only does this reduce the odds that any medical problems will be detected early, it also deprives women of the opportunity to discuss important sexual health issues and reproductive concerns with a trusted expert.

Among the most common sexual health problems in women are menstrual irregularities, discussed on page 215. Sexually transmitted infections (see Chapter 11) are another major health concern, not only for the harm they cause directly, but also because of their association with other serious disorders. For example, sexually transmitted infection can result in *pelvic inflammatory disease*, a common cause of infertility. And infection with the human papillomavirus (HPV), which is also sexually transmitted, is now known to be the most important risk factor for cervical cancer.[2]

Another infection affecting females is *vulvovaginal candidiasis* (VVC), an inflammation of the vagina that can produce itching, pain, and discharge. Although it is not sexually transmitted, the condition is common and often referred to as a "yeast infection." It is typically caused by an overgrowth of *Candida albicans,* a species of yeast (a type of fungus) that is normally present in the vagina in controlled amounts. VVC most commonly occurs when a woman takes a broad-spectrum antibiotic that kills off the normal vaginal bacteria that usually compete with *Candida* for nutrients.

Male Sexual Anatomy

A man's reproductive anatomy also includes both internal and external organs **(Figure 10.2)**. The external organs are the following:

- **Penis.** The male sexual and reproductive organ, which consists of the shaft (body), and a slitted tip called the glans (head). Made up of soft, spongy tissue, the penis fills with blood during sexual arousal and becomes firm and enlarged, a state known as an **erection.** Boys are born with a hood of skin, known as the *foreskin,* covering the head of the penis. In more than half of boys born in the United States, parents opt to have the skin surgically removed through a procedure called **circumcision** (see **Myth or Fact: Should Boys Be Circumcised for Health Reasons?**).

- **Scrotum.** The skin sac at the base of the penis that contains the *testes* (testicles). The scrotum is responsible for regulating the temperature of the testes, which need to be kept cool to facilitate production of *sperm*, the male reproductive cells.

The internal male organs are the following:

- **Testes (testicles).** The reproductive glands that manufacture sperm.

- **Epididymis.** The coiled tube—one above each testicle—where sperm are held until they mature.

- **Vas deferens.** The tube that ascends from the epididymis—one on each side of the scrotum—and transports sperm into the *ejaculatory duct.*

penis The male sexual and reproductive organ.

erection The process of the penis filling up with blood as a result of sexual stimulation.

circumcision The surgical removal of the foreskin.

scrotum The skin sac at the base of the penis that contains the testes.

testes (testicles) The two reproductive glands that manufacture sperm.

epididymis A coiled tube on top of each testicle where sperm are held until they mature.

vas deferens A tube ascending from the epididymis that transports sperm.

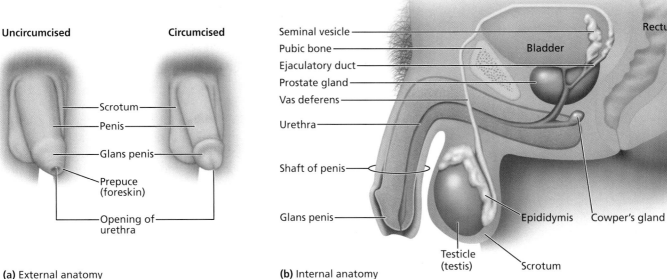

(a) External anatomy

Uncircumcised   Circumcised

Scrotum
Penis
Glans penis
Prepuce (foreskin)
Opening of urethra

(b) Internal anatomy

Seminal vesicle
Pubic bone
Ejaculatory duct
Prostate gland
Vas deferens
Urethra
Shaft of penis
Glans penis
Rectum
Bladder
Epididymis   Cowper's gland
Testicle (testis)   Scrotum

Figure 10.2 Male sexual anatomy.

- **Accessory glands.** A set of glands that lubricate the reproductive system and nourish the sperm. They include the *seminal vesicles,* small sacs that store *seminal fluid,* which provides sugars and other nutrients that feed and activate sperm. The seminal vesicles secrete seminal fluid into the ejaculatory duct, which also receives sperm from the vas deferens. This mixture of sperm and seminal fluid is called **semen.** Another accessory gland that contributes to semen is the *prostate gland,* a walnut-shaped structure below the bladder. It secretes into semen an alkaline fluid that helps protect sperm from the acidic environment of the vagina. Below the prostate are the *Cowper's glands,* pea-shaped glands on each side of the urethra that discharge a lubricating secretion into the urethra just before ejaculation.

accessory glands Glands (seminal vesicles, prostate gland and Cowper's gland) which lubricate the reproductive system and nourish sperm.

semen The male ejaculate consisting of sperm and other fluids from the accessory glands.

urethra A duct that travels from the bladder through the shaft of the penis, carrying fluids to the outside of the body.

- **Urethra.** Within the prostate, the ejaculatory duct joins the urethra, a much longer duct that travels from the bladder through the shaft of the penis, and carries fluids to the outside of the body. Both urine from the bladder and semen from the ejaculatory duct pass through the urethra, although not at the same time.

Common Sexual Health Problems in Males

Like women, men should take their sexual health seriously and get regular medical checkups. Sexually active men are also encouraged to perform self-exams of their genitals, looking in particular for any sores or warts. These may be signs of a sexually transmitted infection (see Chapter 11). If you notice these—or any other changes to your genitals—be sure to discuss them promptly with a doctor. A hard lump in a testicle may be a sign of testicular cancer, which is most often diagnosed in young men in their 20s and 30s.

MYTH OR FACT?

Should Boys Be Circumcised for Health Reasons?

Infant boys are born with a hood of skin, known as the *foreskin,* covering the head of the penis. In more than half of boys born in the United States, parents opt to have the foreskin surgically removed through a procedure called *circumcision.*

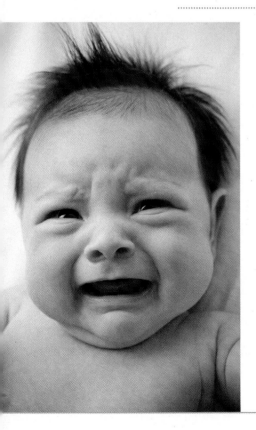

Circumcision rates vary greatly across the country and throughout the world, with the surgery being much more popular in the Midwest and Northeast than in the West, where slightly less than one-third of boys were circumcised in 2005.[1] Circumcision is also widely performed in the Middle East and Canada, but in Europe, Latin America, China, and India it is uncommon.

In some families, the decision to circumcise is primarily a religious one. In both the Jewish and Muslim faiths, circumcision is a common rite of passage. In others, it is more of a cultural determination—boys are circumcised because their fathers were. What remains most controversial is circumcising for health-related reasons.

Most medical experts agree on certain potential health benefits of circumcision. They point out that circumcision boosts personal hygiene,

making it somewhat easier to clean the penis. It also reduces the risk of urinary tract infections in infancy. Men who have been circumcised have lower rates of penile cancer, and several types of research studies have documented a reduced risk of both acquiring and transmitting some sexually transmitted infections, including HIV.[2] Safe sex practices, however, are much more important at stopping the spread of those diseases than circumcision is.

Opponents of circumcision point out that the procedure can be painful. It also comes with risks, including the potential for infection and excessive bleeding. Rarely, the penis may not heal properly or a second surgery may be needed. Some opponents argue that circumcision reduces penile sensation and sexual function; however, well-designed studies of these issues are few and inconclusive.[2]

The American Academy of Pediatrics has declared that "existing scientific evidence demonstrates potential medical benefits of newborn male circumcision; however, these data are not sufficient to recommend routine neonatal circumcision."[3] Whether to circumcise their son is a decision that parents should make after weighing both the benefits and the risks, the organization determined. When parents do go forward with a circumcision, the Academy advises that pain medication be given to the newborn.

References: **1.** [Raw Data] by the National Center for Health Statistics, 2007, retrieved from http://nchspressroom.files.wordpress.com/2007/07/circumcision-1979-2005.pdf. **2.** *Male Circumcision and Risk for HIV Transmission and Other Health Conditions: Implications for the United States* by the Centers for Disease Control, 2008, retrieved from http://www.cdc.gov/hiv/resources/factsheets/circumcision.htm. **3.** "Circumcision Policy Statement" by the American Academy of Pediatrics, 1999, *Pediatrics, 103*(3), pp. 686–693.

Talking Honestly About Sex

"Hi, I'm Abbey. I absolutely think that people have a responsibility to tell someone if they have a sexually transmitted disease before they have sex. That is definitely something that their partner should know ahead of time, and it's deceitful to hide that from them. If someone asked me if I had an STI right before sex, I would answer honestly. I wouldn't be put off. I would understand why they would want to know that, and respect that they want to be safe and responsible with their body. How would I ask someone if they had an STI? I would just straightforwardly ask them."

1: Why is it so important to discuss sexual histories and exposure to sexually transmitted infections with a new partner prior to sex?

2: Why is it risky for sexually active individuals to skip regular medical check-ups?

Do you have a story similar to Abbey's? Share your story at www. pearsonhighered.com/choosinghealth.

---

prostate gland A walnut-sized gland that produces part of the semen.

menarche The first onset of menstruation.

menstruation The cyclical discharge of blood and tissue from the vagina.

menopause The time when a woman stops having menstrual cycles.

menstrual phase Phase of the menstrual cycle characterized by menstrual flow, the release of follicle-stimulating hormone from the pituitary gland to the brain, and the release of estrogen into the bloodstream.

For more information on testicular cancer, see Chapter 12.

Several common sexual health problems in men involve the prostate:

- **Prostatitis.** An infection or inflammation of the **prostate gland.** Symptoms range from the frequent need to urinate to pain in the pelvic region and lower back.
- **Prostate gland enlargement.** An excessive growth of prostate tissue that presses on the urethra, impairing or blocking the flow of urine. This usually develops in men over age 60.
- **Prostate cancer.** A typically slow growth of cancerous tissue from which cancer cells can spread to other parts of the body (see Chapter 12). Prostate cancer most commonly affects men over age 65.[3]

The Menstrual Cycle

A rite of passage for girls as they transition into womanhood is **menarche** (pronounced *me-NAR-kee*), the onset of **menstruation,** the discharge of blood and endometrial tissue from the vagina. Also called a *period* or *menstrual period,* menstruation usually lasts from three to seven days. In the United States, the average age at menarche is 12, although it is considered normal to start as early as 8 or as late as 15.[4] **Menopause,** the time at which women stop menstruating, usually occurs in a woman's early 50s.

Menstruation is just one of several physiologic events in a woman's *menstrual cycle* **(Figure 10.3).** Because it is controlled by hormones, the menstrual cycle can be interrupted by anything that affects hormone production. This includes illness, excessive dieting with or without excessive exercise, and breast-feeding. Of course the menstrual cycle also ceases during pregnancy. Otherwise, in women of childbearing age, it repeats approximately every month, spanning from 21 to 35 days (the average is 28 days) each time.[4]

> **View an animation of the menstrual cycle at www.womenshealth.gov/faq/ menstruation.cfm#c. (Click Start in the lower right corner of the diagram.)**

Phases of the Menstrual Cycle

The menstrual cycle is characterized by a series of events involving both the uterus and the ovaries. As indicated in Figure 10.3, fluctuations in the levels of four female reproductive hormones control these events, which are typically grouped into three phases: the **menstrual phase,** the **proliferative phase,** and the **secretory phase.**

Menstrual Phase

The first day of a woman's menstrual flow is arbitrarily designated as day 1 of the menstrual cycle. Menstruation results from the break-

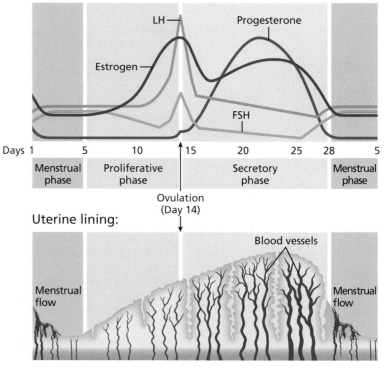

Figure 10.3 **Phases of the menstrual cycle.** The menstrual cycle consists of a menstrual phase, a proliferative phase, and a secretory phase.

proliferative phase Phase of the menstrual cycle characterized by a thickening of the lining of the uterus and discharge of cervical mucus. This phase ends when luteinizing hormone triggers the release of a mature egg.

secretory phase Phase of the menstrual cycle characterized by the degeneration of the follicle sac, rising levels of progesterone in the bloodstream, and further increase of the endometrial lining.

ovulate To release an egg from the ovary.

premenstrual syndrome (PMS) A collection of emotional and physical symptoms that occur just prior to menstruation.

down of the endometrium after the body "recognizes" that a pregnancy has not occurred. During this phase, a hormone called *FSH—follicle-stimulating hormone*—is released from the pituitary gland in the brain. A woman's ovary contains thousands of egg sacs called *follicles.* FSH stimulates the maturation of the immature egg within a few of these follicles. As they develop, the follicles begin releasing an ovarian hormone, *estrogen,* into the bloodstream. As estrogen reaches the uterus, it causes menstruation to end (around day 6).

Proliferative Phase
Estrogen is also responsible for causing the lining of the uterus to thicken (proliferate) in preparation for the entry into the uterus of a fertilized egg. Also during this phase, a woman may notice a copious, slippery discharge of mucus from her vagina. This characteristic *cervical mucus* helps facilitate the mobility of sperm and protect them from the otherwise acidic environment of the vagina. Its presence also indicates that a woman is about to **ovulate,** that is, release an egg. In fact, the proliferative phase ends when, around day 14 of a 28-day cycle, the pituitary gland releases another hormone, *LH,* or *luteinizing hormone,* which triggers just one of the several maturing follicles to release a mature egg (an ovum). In some women, ovulation is accompanied by a sharp pain on one side of the lower abdomen. This pain is caused by irritation from the stretching of the ovary wall and the release of fluid into the lower abdominal cavity. Although it may last for several minutes to several hours, this "mid-cycle pain" is entirely normal and can help a woman pinpoint more precisely the time when she is fertile.

Secretory Phase
Once the ovum has been ejected, the remaining follicle sac degenerates into a *corpus luteum,* a tiny gland that begins releasing a fourth reproductive hormone, progesterone. Rising levels of progesterone enter the bloodstream and travel to the uterus, further thickening the endometrial lining in preparation for the arrival of a fertilized egg.

As noted earlier, the released ovum is swept into the nearby fallopian tube and begins to travel toward the uterus. If sperm are present in sufficient numbers in the fallopian tube, fertilization is likely to occur. The fertilized egg will then produce the hormone *human chorionic gonadotropin* (hCG), which is needed to sustain a pregnancy. In fact, over-the-counter pregnancy test kits work by detecting the presence or absence of hCG in a woman's urine. Within 3 to 4 days, the fertilized ovum reaches the uterus.

A woman's ovum is viable only for about 12 to 24 hours. If fertilization does not occur within this time period, it will quickly deteriorate, and the levels of all four reproductive hormones will begin to dramat-

ically decrease. Thus, around day 25, the endometrium will start to degenerate. Within approximately 3–4 days, menstruation will begin and the cycle repeats itself again.

Disorders Associated with the Menstrual Cycle
Although normal menstruation is a sign of health and maturity, in some women it's accompanied by pain, excessive bleeding, or other problems that interfere with their ability to carry out their daily activities. We discuss the most common of these disorders here.

Premenstrual Syndrome
As many as 85% of women experience mildly disturbing emotional and physical symptoms just prior to menstruation.[5] These symptoms can include breast tenderness, fluid retention, headaches, backaches, uterine cramping, irritability, mood swings, appetite changes, depression, and anxiety. Approximately 15% of women experience a constellation of the symptoms at a "sufficient severity to interfere with some aspect of life" and consequently are considered to have **premenstrual syndrome,** or PMS.[6] The symptoms of PMS typically appear in the week or two before the period begins, and dissipate after menstrual bleeding starts.

Exactly what causes PMS isn't entirely clear. Some women may simply be more sensitive to the changes in female reproductive hormones that occur during the menstrual cycle. Chemical changes in the brain may also play a role. Stress and psychological problems do not cause the syndrome, although there is evidence that they can exacerbate it.[7]

Some lifestyle changes can reduce the symptoms of PMS. These include avoidance of smoking, alcohol, caffeine, salt, and sugary foods. A balanced diet rich in whole grains, fruits, and vegetables is important, along with regular exercise and adequate, restful sleep. In addition, some women find that a multivitamin and mineral supplement providing adequate levels of B vitamins, magnesium, and vitamin E is helpful, and women aged 19–50 should consume 1,000 milligrams of calcium daily. Over-the-counter remedies such as aspirin and ibuprofen can also relieve symptoms. In more severe cases of PMS in women who do not want to become pregnant, a woman's

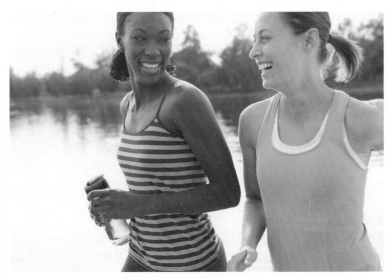

Exercise can help relieve the symptoms of **premenstrual syndrome**.

physician may prescribe birth control pills, which stop ovulation and reduce menstruation.[7]

Premenstrual Dysphoric Disorder (PMDD)

Some women experience the psychological symptoms of PMS in a more severe and debilitating way. This condition, known as **premenstrual dysphoric disorder** (PMDD), can interfere with daily functioning and social relationships. (*Dysphoria* refers to a generalized feeling of sadness, anxiety, or discontent.) Although any woman who has experienced a crying jag or a bout of irritability in the days before her period may assume her symptoms are severe, only 3–8% of women actually suffer from true PMDD.[8] A diagnosis of PMDD means that a woman experiences at least five of its symptoms, which include:

- anxiety
- panic attacks
- mood swings
- feelings of despair
- persistent irritability or anger
- sleep disturbances
- food cravings
- low energy
- difficulty focusing
- a loss of interest in daily activities and relationships

As with PMS, engaging in regular exercise, getting adequate rest, and following a balanced diet may help. Treatment may also include vitamins and over-the-counter pain relievers. In addition, the woman's physician may prescribe a type of antidepressant called a *selective serotonin reuptake inhibitor*, or SSRI, to modulate the brain's level of the neurotransmitter serotonin.

Dysmenorrhea

More than half of all menstruating women experience some pain for 1–2 days each month.[9] In most of these women, the pain is mild; however, sometimes the pain is severe enough to interfere with normal activities. This is called **dysmenorrhea,** or painful menstruation, and can include severe abdominal cramps, back or thigh pain, diarrhea, or even headaches in the days immediately preceding and during menstruation.[10] Dysmenorrhea is the leading cause of absenteeism from school in adolescent girls.[10]

The cramping pain of dysmenorrhea is due to *prostaglandins,* chemicals that regulate many body functions, including contraction of smooth muscle—like the muscle in a woman's uterus. Prostaglandins cause uterine muscle cells to contract, expelling the uterine lining. This is why over-the-counter prostaglandin inhibitors like ibuprofen and naproxen are usually effective in treating dysmenorrhea. The discomfort also usually wanes spontaneously with age and often disappears after pregnancy.

Endometriosis

Endometriosis is a condition in which endometrial tissue grows in areas outside of the uterus such as the fallopian tubes, ovaries, and other structures in the pelvic region.[11] This tissue responds to the same hormonal signals that affect the uterus, and so breaks down and bleeds monthly into the abdominopelvic cavity. The condition can cause severe pain in the pelvic region that may be associated with the menstrual cycle, as well as scarring that can result in infertility. Endometriosis occurs most commonly in women in their 30s and 40s, but can occur at any time during the reproductive years. Although a physician can evaluate a woman for endometriosis during a physical examination, it is confirmed by laparoscopic surgery, in which a thin, lighted tube is inserted into the abdominopelvic cavity. If endometrial tissue is found, it can often be removed during the same procedure.[11]

Amenorrhea

As much as some young women would love to stop menstruating, a lack of periods can be a sign that the body is in distress. Missed periods, also known as **amenorrhea,** can usually be traced to severe weight loss with or without excessive exercise, a hormonal imbalance, or significant stress. Some medications, including certain birth control pills, can also suppress menstruation.

Amenorrhea is clinically defined as having no periods for at least three consecutive months.[12] It occurs normally in women who are pregnant, and usually throughout the first few months of breast-feeding. However, it can also signal a serious underlying disorder of the reproductive organs. Amenorrhea is also a common consequence of disordered eating. For example, it is somewhat common among athletes—especially gymnasts and long-distance runners—who train vigorously while restricting their calorie intake to maintain a competitive weight.

Amenorrhea is not without long-term consequences. Symptoms can include headaches and vaginal dryness, but doctors are most concerned about its affect on bone health. Recall that the female reproductive hormone estrogen is produced by the ovaries during the normal menstrual cycle. Estrogen plays a key role in building new bone tissue, so amenorrhea puts women at significant risk for low bone density. This means that women who experience long-term amenorrhea can suffer from osteoporosis and bone fractures at a relatively early age.

Toxic Shock Syndrome

In 1980, scientists had an alarming announcement for women who used one brand of super absorbent tampons: They could kill you. The feminine hygiene products were linked to **toxic shock syndrome,** a rare disease characterized by a sudden high fever, vomiting, diarrhea, chills, muscle aches, a rash, and low blood pressure leading to dizziness or fainting. The bacterium *Staphylococcus aureus* is the primary culprit, and researchers determined that super absorbent tampons, especially when left in place for longer than 8 hours, could encourage the growth of the bacteria, which release a virulent toxin. Before the tampons were removed from store shelves, they sickened hundreds and killed dozens of women.[13]

Today, toxic shock syndrome is extremely rare, but can still occur in women—usually aged 15 to 24—who use tampons. To reduce the risk of developing the syndrome, experts recommend that women use the lowest absorbency tampons needed, and alternate between tampons and pads. Tampons should also be changed at least every 4 to 8 hours.

---

premenstrual dysphoric disorder (PMDD) Severe and debilitating psychological symptoms experienced just prior to menstruation.

dysmenorrhea Pain during menstruation that is severe enough to limit normal activities or require medication.

endometriosis A condition in which endometrial tissue grows in areas outside of the uterus.

amenorrhea Cessation of menstrual periods.

toxic shock syndrome (TSS) A rare bacterial infection linked to tampon use.

The Sexual Response Cycle

Famed sex researchers William H. Masters and Virginia E. Johnson were the first to scientifically study the body's physiological reaction to sexual stimulation and subsequent release through orgasm. They called this process the **human sexual response cycle.** According to Masters and Johnson's model, the cycle is made up of four distinct phases extending from the first moment of sexual desire until the calm after sexual fulfillment:

- **Excitement.** The first phase occurs as the result of any erotic mental or physical stimulation that leads to arousal. In both sexes it is characterized by increased heart and respiration rate and also increased blood pressure. Nipple erection, especially as the result of direct stimulation, occurs in almost all females and in approximately 60% of males. Both may also experience a "sex flush," which is the reddening of the skin due to vasocongestion (blood vessel engorgement). In males, the penis becomes mostly erect and the testicles draw upward. In females, the labia increases in size and the clitoris swells. Lubrication occurs as the result of vasocongestion of the vaginal walls.

- **Plateau.** This more intense excitement takes partners to the edge of orgasm, leaving hearts beating rapidly and genitals sensitive to touch. In males, the urethral sphincter, a valve at the base of the penis that prevents urination during ejaculation, closes. Muscles at the penis base also begin to contract rhythmically. Males also secrete a pre-ejaculatory fluid (that may contain small amounts of sperm) and the testicles rise closer to the body. In females, the outer third of the vagina swells and the pelvic muscle tightens, creating what Masters and Johnson refer to as the *orgasmic platform.*

- **Orgasm.** This event concludes the plateau phase and is the peak or climax of sexual response. It is accompanied by rhythmic muscle contractions of the genitals and surrounding areas. Most describe it as an intensely pleasurable feeling of release of sexual tension. In men, orgasm is accompanied by ejaculation.

- **Resolution.** In this phase the body returns to normal functioning. It often includes a sense of both well-being and fatigue.[14]

Men usually experience a *refractory period,* a period of time when they are not immediately able to respond to stimulation with an erection and may actually find continued stimulation unwelcome, or even painful. Most women do not experience a refractory period and may be able to immediately return to the plateau stage, allowing for the possibility of multiple orgasms.

Sexual Dysfunctions

Sexual dysfunctions are problems that can occur during any stage of the sexual response cycle—curbing desire, interrupting arousal, reducing pleasure, or preventing orgasm. An estimated 43% of women and 31% of men report having had at least one symptom of sexual dysfunction at some point in their life.[15]

Female Sexual Dysfunctions

A variety of problems can keep a woman from enjoying sex. These include painful intercourse, low level of sexual desire, and inability to achieve orgasm:[16]

- **Painful intercourse.** Up to 20% of women experience episodes of pain just before, during, or after intercourse.[17] Often the pain occurs only under certain circumstances, such as when the penis first enters the vagina or during vigorous thrusting. In other cases, the woman experiences a general burning or aching sensation. The causes vary with the type of pain reported, but some of the most common are insufficient vaginal lubrication, prior injury, infection or inflammation, an allergic reaction to a birth control product such as a spermicide or a latex condom, or an underlying disorder. Emotional factors such as stress, low self-esteem, or a history of sexual abuse occasionally play a role. Often, simply a change in position or the use of a commercial lubrication product can correct the problem. Underlying infection or other disorders should also be treated. In some cases, hormonal medications or therapy can help.

- **Low level of sexual desire.** About 5–15% of women experience a persistently low sex drive.[18] Common physical causes include fatigue, medication side effect, alcohol abuse, pregnancy, breast-feeding, and menopause. In addition, psychological problems and unresolved issues within the relationship can be factors. Lifestyle changes such as regular exercise and stress management can help, as can couples counseling. Hormonal therapy is also available. Finally, some women find that *Kegel exercises*—tightening the pelvic floor muscles as if stopping the flow of urine, holding for a few seconds, and releasing—can help put them back in touch with their sexual anatomy and their sex drive.

- **Inability to achieve orgasm.** About 1 in 5 women worldwide have difficulty experiencing orgasm.[19] The problem can occur as a side effect of prescription medications, including certain antidepressants. Medical problems, relationship problems, embarrassment, or a history of sexual abuse or rape can also prevent some women from reaching orgasm. However, one common factor is simply insufficient stimulation of the clitoris. Switching sexual positions can produce more clitoral stimulation during intercourse. Masturbation or use of a vibrator during sex can also help.[19]

Male Sexual Dysfunctions

Being unable to perform sexually can be damaging to a man's self-esteem and place stress on the relationship. Problems related to male sexual function include the following:

- **Erectile dysfunction (ED)** is the inability of a man to get or maintain an erection firm enough

---

human sexual response cycle Distinct phases extending from the first moment of sexual desire until the calm after orgasm.

excitement The first phase of the sexual response cycle, marked by erection in men, and lubrication and clitoral swelling in women.

plateau The second phase of the sexual response cycle, characterized by intense excitement, rapid heartbeat, genital sensitivity, the secretion of pre-ejaculatory fluid in men, and vaginal swelling in women.

orgasm The peak, or climax, of sexual response, characterized by rhythmic muscle contractions of the genitals and surrounding areas, and ejaculation in men.

resolution The stage of the response cycle in which the body returns to normal functioning.

sexual dysfunctions Problems occurring during any stage of the sexual response cycle.

erectile dysfunction (ED) The inability of a male to obtain or maintain an erection.

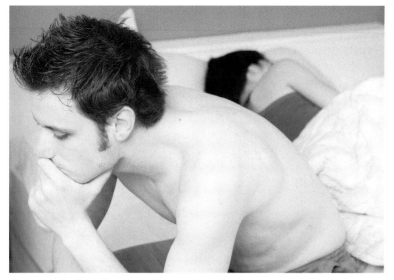

Sexual dysfunctions can occur in both men and women.

for sexual intercourse.[20] The problem is most prevalent among older men. Erectile dysfunction most commonly results from injury or underlying disease, but it can stem from fatigue, stress, depression, use of certain medications, or excessive alcohol or tobacco use. As treatment, a physician may prescribe lifestyle modifications such as weight loss or quitting smoking. Oral medications such as Viagra, Cialis, or Levitra can help by boosting the flow of blood to the penis, enabling an erection to occur; however, they can have serious side effects and are not intended for men with certain underlying health conditions. Surgery may be recommended in cases of underlying injury, and counseling or sex therapy is also an option.

- **Premature ejaculation (PE)** is a condition in which a man ejaculates earlier than he would like to, or than his partner would like him to. Although in the past, sex researchers and therapists attempted to define PE based on a quantitative time frame (i.e. how long it took to ejaculate), today most agree that a male has a problem when poor ejaculatory control interferes with the sexual satisfaction of one or both partners. PE can result from physical factors, but in most cases it is due to psychological factors such as anxiety. In college-aged men it frequently occurs because of lack of experience, intense arousal, and alcohol use.[21] However, hormonal imbalance, infection, nervous system disorders, and other physical causes should be ruled out if PE is chronic. Treatment of any underlying physical problem is important. In many cases, sexual counseling and incorporating into sexual activity a delaying tactic called the "squeeze technique" can resolve the problem.[22]

For more information on the "squeeze technique," visit the Mayo Clinic website at **www.mayoclinic.com/health/premature-ejaculation/DS00578/DSECTION=treatments-and-drugs.**

premature ejaculation (PE) A condition in which a male ejaculates earlier than he would like to.

abstinence The avoidance of sexual intercourse.

masturbation Manipulation of one's own genitals for sexual pleasure.

outercourse Sexual intimacy without penetration of the vagina or anus.

oral sex Stimulation of the genitals by the tongue or mouth.

fellatio Oral stimulation of the penis.

cunnilingus Oral stimulation of the vulva or clitoris.

Sexual Behavior

A wide range of human sexual behaviors and interests are considered "normal." Before biologist Alfred Kinsey's research in the late 1940s and early 1950s, Americans had no basis for determining what was the norm. Kinsey's research provided a basis for social comparison and helped answer a question many people wondered about: "Who's doing what with whom and how often are they doing it?" Since Kinsey, many researchers studying this question have concluded that the continuum of "normal" sexual behavior in our society is broad and varied.

Abstinence and Celibacy

Abstinence refers to the avoidance of sexual intercourse. Whether it is by active choice or as a matter of circumstance, many people find themselves abstaining from sexual activity for extended periods of time. This long-term abstinence is referred to as *celibacy*. Some choose celibacy for religious or moral reasons; others out of a desire to avoid becoming pregnant or developing a sexually transmitted infection.[23] The **Spotlight** box takes a closer look at abstinence and celibacy among young adults.

Non-Intercourse Sexual Activity

There are a number of ways people experience sexual pleasure without actually engaging in sexual intercourse. Among them are masturbation, sexual fantasies, kissing, "outercourse," and oral sex.

Fantasy and Masturbation

Sexual fantasies are sexual or romantic thoughts, daydreams, and imagined scenarios that can be very detailed and explicit, featuring fictional characters or actual people. They may reflect a person's unconscious desires, allowing the person to imagine sexual experiences that they may not feel comfortable acting out in real life.

Masturbation is the manipulation of one's own genitals for sexual pleasure. Masturbation is a healthy and common expression of sexuality. Research indicates that 92% of male college students and nearly half (48%) of female college students have masturbated.[24]

"Outercourse" and Oral Sex

Although the definition can vary, **outercourse** generally refers to sexual intimacy without penetration of the vagina or anus. Outercourse includes everything from kissing and "making out" to manual stimulation of the genitals and mutual masturbation. Because no semen enters the vagina during outercourse, there is no risk of pregnancy. The risk of sexually transmitted infections is also minimized, although infections like herpes and HPV can still spread through simple skin-to-skin contact of the genitals.

Oral sex is the stimulation of the genitals by the tongue or mouth. **Fellatio** is oral stimulation of the penis, and **cunnilingus** is oral stimulation of the vulva or clitoris. Some couples use oral sex as *foreplay*, stimulation that is erotic and is intended to increase arousal prior to sexual intercourse. Others engage in oral sex in place of sexual intercourse. Still others avoid the practice. Although oral sex does not

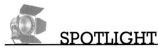

SPOTLIGHT

Celibacy: The New Sexual Revolution?

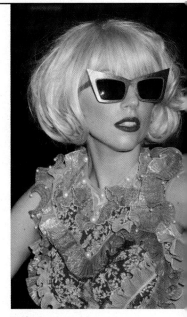

Fans worldwide were stunned in the spring of 2010, when pop star Lady Gaga announced in an interview that—despite her steamy MTV image—she's celibate. Moreover, she encouraged her fans to choose celibacy, too: "I can't believe I'm saying this—Don't have sex. It's not really cool anymore to have sex all the time. It's cooler to be strong and independent. It's okay not to have sex. It's okay to get to know people. I'm celibate. Celibacy's fine."[1]

Young adults do seem to be waiting longer before having sex. In a national survey conducted in 2009, about 34% of college students reported that they have never had vaginal intercourse—an increase of more than 5% from 2000.[2] An even bigger increase (8%) was reported in abstention from oral sex: in 2009, 32.8% had never had oral sex, whereas in 2000, 24.8% had never done it.[2] This modest increase in absti-

nence correlates with the statistics from surveys of high school students: in a 2005 survey, 53% identified themselves as virgins (someone who has never had intercourse), up 7% from 1991.[3]

At the same time, celibacy programs are increasingly visible on college campuses. The campus newspaper at the Lutheran Gustavus Adolphus College in Minnesota recently ran an article titled "Celibacy: The New Hipster Trend?" It proposed that, "On a campus where condoms are handed out like candy ... celibacy is becoming as hip as organic coffee." But Christian colleges are not alone in reporting the trend: a 2008 *New York Times Magazine* article reported on the emergence of "abstinence clubs" at Ivy League schools, including the Anscombe Societies at Princeton University and MIT, and True Love Revolution at Harvard. The clubs include among their mem-

bers not only students from conservative religions, but also so-called "new feminists" and philosophy students who use ethical arguments to ground their choice of celibacy.[4]

Not everyone agrees that celibacy is compatible with feminism—or a superior ethical choice for single adults. The movement has drawn a fair amount of controversy, with opponents claiming that the clubs perpetuate gender stereotypes that value women who are virgins and denounce those who are not. Some have accused the clubs of manipulating statistics about unplanned pregnancies and sexually transmitted infections to frighten students into celibacy.

Still, even opponents admit that the clubs provide a valuable service to students who want to abstain from sexual behavior during their college years, giving them a safe space—via meetings and a club website—where

they can debate social, scientific, philosophical, and religious positions on celibacy, and simply share information. Perhaps most importantly, they give members a circle of companions who know and respect their choices. And that can mean—as Lady Gaga herself might put it—that they won't get caught in a bad romance.

References: **1.** *Lady Gaga joins the list of celibate stars* by Kate Torgovnick, April 13, 2010, CNN Entertainment, retrieved from http://www.cnn.com/2010/SHOWBIZ/04/12/pro.abstinence.celebs.tf/index.html. **2.** *American College Health Association-National College Health Assessment (ACHA-NCHA II) Reference Group Executive Summary, Fall 2009* by the American College Health Association, 2009, retrieved from http://www.acha-ncha.org/docs/ACHA-NCHA_Reference_Group_ExecutiveSummary_Fall2009.pdf. **3.** "QuickStats: Never-Married Females and Males Aged 15–19 Years Who Have Ever Had Sexual Intercourse—National Survey of Family Growth, United States, 1988–2008," by the Centers for Disease Control, 2010, *Morbidity and Mortality Weekly Report, (59)* 26 p. 819, retrieved from http://www.cdc.gov/mmwr/preview/mmwrhtml/mm5926a8.htm?s_cid=mm5926a8_w **4.** "Students of Virginity" by Randall Patterson, March 30, 2008, *New York Times*, retrieved from http://www.nytimes.com/2008/03/30/magazine/30Chastity-t.html.

Lady Gaga

---

result in pregnancy, it is not necessarily "safe" sex. Unprotected oral sex can leave a partner vulnerable to the transmission of herpes, syphilis, hepatitis B, and gonorrhea. Using a condom or dental dam during oral sex can help prevent the spread of sexually transmitted infections. See Chapter 11 for more information on preventing sexually transmitted infections.

"Sexting"

Sexting is the use of cell phones or similar electronic devices to send sexually explicit text, photos, or videos. In a recent study, 20% of teens and 33% of young adults reported sending or posting nude or semi-nude photos or videos of themselves. In addition, 39% of teens and 59% of young adults reported they are sending or posting sexually suggestive messages. One-third of male teens and one-fourth of female teens report receiving nude or semi-nude images that were originally meant to be private.[25]

Sexting most frequently occurs in one of three circumstances:

- Exchanges of images only between two romantically involved partners.
- Exchanges between partners and shared outside the relationship.
- Exchanges involving people who are not in a relationship, but at least one of them hopes to be.[26]

Many states are enacting legislation to regulate sexting. Arizona passed a bill in March of 2010 making it a class-two misdemeanor for minors to possess or send sexually explicit text messages to another minor.[27] This law sets an important precedent because it is specific to the offense. Before its passage, prosecutors could only use child pornography laws, which were written long before the development of wireless technologies and were thus difficult to apply. It is likely that the new bill will prompt more prosecutions and more research examining sexting among college students.

sexting The use of cell phones or similar electronic devices to send sexually explicit text, photos, or videos.

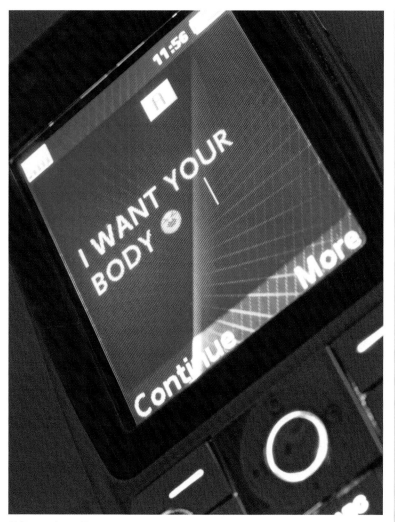

"Sexting" can leave you vulnerable to privacy breaches and embarrassment.

Use of Pornography

Pornography is explicit sexual material that is used for sexual excitement and erotic stimulation. It can be found in a wide host of media, including books, magazines, photos, sculpture, painting, animation, film, video, and video games. The pornography industry is big business, and in 2006 alone, the revenues were $96.06 billion. Topping the list in revenues are video sales and rentals, closely followed by Internet sales. Approximately 12% of all websites (4.2 million) are pornographic, and 25% of all search engine requests (68 million) are related to pornography.[28]

A study conducted by East Carolina University found that 92.4% of college students reported ever having looked at pornography and 43.1% reported doing so between one and two times a week. Almost 32% of college men reported viewing pornography three to five times per week, whereas less than 4% of women reported doing so. Men also expressed greater approval of pornography, and women reported feeling more threatened by it. The findings from this study also suggest that the Internet is the primary source of pornography for college students.[29]

---

vaginal intercourse Intercourse characterized by the insertion of the penis into the vagina.

anal intercourse Intercourse characterized by the insertion of the penis into a partner's anus and rectum.

sexual orientation Romantic and physical attraction toward others.

Along with commercial pornography websites, there has been an increase in noncommercial sites where visitors can post their own photos and videos. Some of these sites are devoted to college students and are referred to as "dorm porn." Some experts contend that both sexting and noncommercial pornographic websites reflect a larger trend toward digital self-exploitation.[30]

> Do you have questions about sex that you are afraid to ask? *Go Ask Alice* is a website sponsored by Columbia University that answers many frequently asked questions: www.goaskalice.columbia.edu.

Sexual Intercourse

Sexual intercourse, or *coitus,* is sexual union involving genital penetration. For many heterosexuals, the term is synonymous with **vaginal intercourse,** the insertion of the penis into the vagina. Unless they are trying to conceive, couples engaging in vaginal intercourse are encouraged to practice "safe sex." The use of condoms is advised to avoid unintended pregnancy while reducing the couple's risk for sexually transmitted infection.

Long considered a taboo in U.S. society, **anal intercourse** has increasingly become accepted, especially among younger generations. According to surveys from the Centers for Disease Control and Prevention (CDC), about 40% of men and 35% of women aged 25–44 have had anal sex with a partner of the opposite sex.[31] The CDC also reports that 6% of men aged 15–44 have had anal sex with another man at some point in their lives. The practice involves penile penetration of the anus and rectum. Since these tissues are much more fragile than those of the vagina, anal intercourse is one of the riskiest of sexual behaviors in terms of both injury and transmission of infectious disease. It represents one of the primary risk factors for acquiring HIV, the virus that causes AIDS, and is also associated with the spread of syphilis and gonorrhea. Condoms can be used, but they tend to break during anal sex. Sex educators advise couples engaging in anal sex to use a lubricant along with a condom.

Communicating About Sex

Each year, there are more than 15 million sexually transmitted infections among people in the United States, and well over 1 million terminations of unplanned pregnancies.[32] Given these statistics, it seems obvious that practicing safe sex is crucial. But before you can practice it, you have to talk about it. It's also important to communicate what you're comfortable with in terms of sexual behaviors, frequency, and other potentially sensitive issues. So how do you get up the nerve to talk candidly about sex? See **Practical Strategies for Health: Communicating Effectively About Sex.**

Sexual Orientation and Gender Identity

At a very early age, humans begin to develop their **sexual orientation,** their romantic and physical attraction toward others. Experts believe that our natural tendency to be attracted to men or women—or both—is shaped by a confluence of biological, environmental,

Communicating Effectively About Sex

If you are thinking about beginning a sexual relationship with someone, it's important to be able to communicate effectively about topics like sexual history, sexual health, contraceptive preferences, and how comfortable you each are with different types of sexual activity.

- **Do some preparation.** Jot down thoughts, concerns, and questions in advance. For instance, it's important to know your partner's sexual history. What can you do to feel more comfortable asking about it? Rehearsing the words in advance doesn't commit you to following a script, but it can help you frame your message in the moment with greater ease, clarity, and sensitivity.

- **Set a time to talk.** Once you're secure about the content of the conversation you want to have, reserve a time when you're both relaxed and not distracted, and a place that's comfortable and private. You might want to tell your

partner that there are some things you'd like to talk about, and suggest that the two of you go for a walk together.

- **Express your questions, concerns, and desires from a personal perspective.** Use "I" statements consistently, as in, "I'd like to know about your sexual history, and I will be honest in sharing mine." Pay attention to your partner's responses. Take in not only the words used, but your partner's body language as well.

- **Near the end of the conversation, recap any decisions you've mutually made.** Include steps that you'll take, such as, "Okay, so tomorrow we'll both schedule appointments at the campus health center to get screened for STIs."

Adapted from *Tips to Talk to Your Partner About Sex* by the Society of Obstetricians and Gynaecologists of Canada, 2006, retrieved from http://www.sexualityandu.ca/adults/tips-1.aspx#.

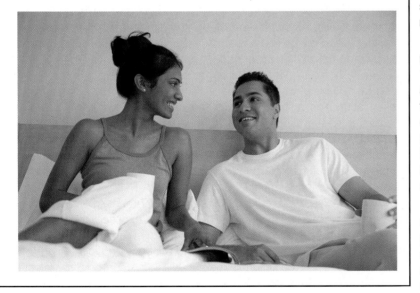

and cognitive factors, with sexual orientation being neither a conscious choice nor something that can be readily changed.

Sex researcher Alfred Kinsey theorized that sexual orientation could be delineated on one basic continuum, broken down into seven parts. At one end of the Kinsey Scale are **heterosexuals,** "straight" people who are solely attracted to the opposite gender. On the other end are **homosexuals,** *gays* or *lesbians* who are attracted

to people of the same gender. In the middle are **bisexuals,** individuals who are attracted to members of their own sex as well as the opposite sex. In between these points on the scale are varying levels of bisexuality.

Heterosexuality

Throughout the world, the majority of people describe themselves as heterosexual. In the United States, 95.9% of men and women aged 18–44 identify themselves as heterosexuals, and 4.1% of men and women identify themselves as homosexual or bisexual, according to a survey conducted by the Centers for Disease Control and Prevention (CDC).[31]

Heterosexuality is the only sexual orientation that receives full social and legal legitimacy in most countries, including the U.S. As a result of this and other cultural factors, homosexuals and bisexuals can be subjected to "heterosexism," a system of negative attitudes, bias, and discrimination in favor of heterosexual relationships. Those with a heterosexist view think that their orientation is the only "normal" one.

Homosexuality

Homosexuality is deep-rooted in many world cultures, having been an accepted practice in some parts of the ancient world. In other regions it has been and is still shunned. For example, psychiatrists in some countries, including China, India, and Brazil, still consider it a mental illness.

In the United States, the American Psychiatric Association removed homosexuality from its manual of psychiatric disorders in 1973, in response to a growing understanding of homosexuality as an entirely normal variant of sexual orientation. Correspondingly, there has been an increasing acceptance of homosexuality in U.S. culture. For example, in a 1973 survey, 70% of people in the U.S. reported believing that homosexual relations are always sinful; but in 2009, only 49% expressed this belief.[33] In 1992, only one Fortune 500 company offered health insurance benefits to domestic partners. By 2006, that number had grown to 253—more than half.[34]

Still, many homosexuals continue to face discrimination and harassment in the United States, a fact acknowledged by 64% of the population.[33] **Homophobia** is the irrational fear of, aversion to, or discrimination against homosexuals or homosexuality. The harassment often begins at an early age. In one survey of Massachusetts youths, researchers found that twice as many homosexual and bisexual students reported being threatened or injured with a weapon at their public high school that year than heterosexual students.[35] They were also twice as likely to have skipped school in the previous month out of a concern for their own safety. In another study, 92% of homosexual and bisexual students in middle and high school said they frequently were subjected to homophobic remarks and slurs, with some of the derogatory expressions even being uttered by faculty or staff.[36] Homophobia sometimes erupts into criminal violence: in

heterosexuals People who are sexually attracted to partners of the opposite sex.

homosexuals People who are sexually attracted to partners of the same sex.

bisexuals People who are attracted to partners of both the same and the opposite sex.

homophobia The irrational fear of, aversion to, or discrimination against homosexuals or homosexuality.

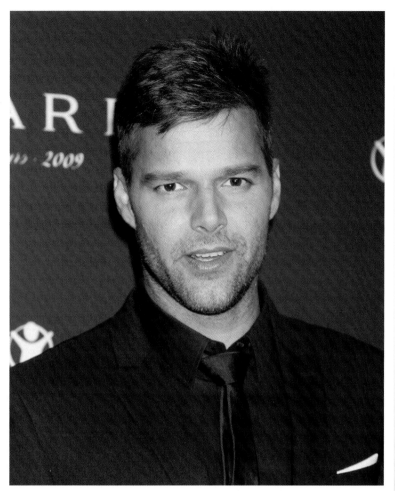

In 2010, singer Ricky Martin publicized his **homosexuality**.

2008, the FBI reported more than 1,200 incidents of hate crimes against homosexuals.[37]

Bisexuality

One rigid definition of bisexuality is having romantic or sexual relations with people of the same and opposite gender. Yet some bisexuals choose not to act on their innate impulses, while others have not had the opportunity to do so. A better gauge of bisexuality is having an attraction to both men and women. The intensity of the attraction can waver over time, but bisexuality should not be seen as a "phase" that a person is going through. In one long-term study of bisexual women, the subjects reported being attracted to both sexes throughout the 10-year study period.[38] Bisexuality, the experts wrote, is a "stable identity" rather than a "transitional stage."

Transgenderism and Transsexuality

Whereas the term *sex* refers to an individual's biological status as male or female, *gender* includes the ways people act, interact, and feel about themselves. **Transgenderism** is the condition where someone's *gender identity* (sense of his- or herself as male or female) or gender expression is different from his or her *assigned sex*. Sex assignment oc-

curs at birth—as long as a baby is born with typical male or female external genitalia. The term *transgenderism* is not used in cases when an infant is born with ambiguous genitalia. This condition is known as a *disorder of sexual development*, and in such cases, sex assignment is delayed until genetic and hormonal testing is conducted.

Once assigned, sex usually becomes a profound component of a growing child's gender identity. But for some people, the sex they have been assigned and the gender they identify with differ. The American Psychological Association states that "Anyone whose identity, appearance, or behavior falls outside of conventional gender norms can be described as transgender. However, not everyone whose appearance or behavior is gender-atypical will identify as a transgender person."[39]

Transsexuals are transgendered individuals who live, usually full-time, as the gender opposite to their assigned sex. Female-to-male (FTM) transsexuals are biological females who now live as males, while male-to-female (MTF) transsexuals are the opposite. Some choose to have hormonal treatments and surgical procedures to complete the physical transformation from one sex to the other. Others do not.

Conception and Contraception

About half of pregnancies in the United States are unintended. The U.S. abortion rate, although off its all-time high, continues to be among the highest in the industrialized world. In addition, failure to use protective birth control options such as condoms exposes millions of people in the U.S. each year to sexually transmitted infections that can cause life-threatening disease as well as infertility. So whether you are planning to have children or not, it is important to understand your fertility, how to protect it, and the methods for family planning.

Conception

At birth, a female's ovaries are filled with more than 1 million ovarian follicles, each containing an immature egg. After puberty, a woman's body prepares itself for pregnancy each month by ovulating—releasing one egg. Meanwhile, a man's testes are constantly creating sperm, millions of which are released into the woman's vagina during ejaculation. The vast majority of these sperm will never find their way to their target—millions will leak from the woman's vagina or be destroyed in its acidic environment. The few thousand sperm that do reach the egg—typically while it is still within the fallopian tube—next face the difficult task of penetrating the egg's tough outer layer. Thousands more of these remaining sperm are "used up" secreting enzymes that dissolve a region of the egg's membrane. As soon as a minute portion of the egg is exposed, the next sperm that approaches will be able to make contact with the egg, and will be pulled into the egg cell interior. The egg will then undergo a chemical change that will block any further sperm from penetrating its membrane. The "winning sperm" then travels to the egg's nucleus, and fertilization—or **conception,** the combination of the genetic material (DNA) of an egg and sperm cell—occurs.

Even then, pregnancy is not guaranteed. The fertilized egg, now called a **zygote,** must complete its journey through the fallopian tube and emerge into the uterus, where it can implant in

transgenderism The state in which someone's gender identity or gender expression is different from his or her assigned sex at birth.

transsexual A transgendered individual who lives as the gender opposite to their assigned sex.

conception The fertilization of a female egg with male sperm.

zygote A fertilized egg.

implantation The lodging of a fertilized egg in the endometrium of the uterus.

contraception Any method used to prevent pregnancy.

the endometrium (**implantation**). Any scar tissue within the tube can "snag" the zygote so that it attaches to the wall of the tube, where it cannot grow. In some cases the zygote will make it into the uterus but fail to implant, and the entire process from menstruation to ovulation will begin all over again.

Figure 10.4 summarizes the processes of conception through implantation.

Contraceptive Options

Contraception is any method used to prevent pregnancy. Contraceptive options differ in technique, price, effectiveness, and side effects, but they all have the same goal: to keep eggs and sperm apart. They do this in a number of ways:

- *Natural methods* involve no pills or devices and are therefore always available and cost-free.
- *Barrier methods* work to prevent sperm from reaching an egg.
- *Hormonal methods* deliver hormones to a woman that prevent ovulation. If no egg is released it can't be fertilized.
- *Surgical methods* are available for women and for men, and are the most permanent of options.

Table 10.1 summarizes different forms of contraception, organized into four general categories: cost-free methods, methods available

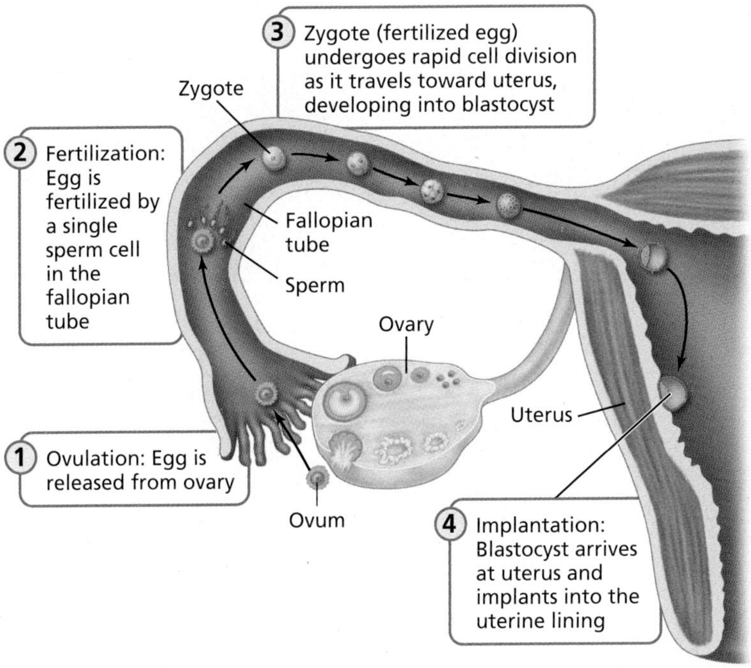

Figure 10.4 Events involved in conception. The process of conception includes ovulation, fertilization, and implantation.

Table 10.1: A Summary of Contraceptive Options

Method	Description	Advantages	Disadvantages	Typical Failure Rates (# of women out of 100 that may become pregnant during the first year of use)	Average Cost
Cost-Free Methods					
Intimacy without intercourse	Engaging in sexual or sensual behavior without vaginal penetration	Prevents pregnancy and STIs	Requires mutual commitment, trust, and self-control	No statistics available	No cost
Fertility awareness (rhythm or calendar method)	Understanding the monthly menstrual cycle and avoiding intercourse on fertile days	No cost	No protection against STIs; not as effective if cycle is irregular; high possibility of failure	1–25	No cost
Withdrawal	Withdrawing the penis before ejaculation	No cost	No protection against STIs; high risk of pregnancy; requires physical and psychological control and awareness	19	No cost
Over-the-Counter Methods					
Male condom	Very thin sheath that fits over an erect penis to prevent semen from entering vagina; made of latex, polyurethane, or lambskin	No need for a prescription, medical procedure, or examination; side effects are uncommon; latex and polyurethane condoms protect against many STIs	Only about 80–94% effective at preventing pregnancy; if not used correctly, unintended pregnancies can occur; requires planning	2–15	$0.50–$3.00 each use
Female condom	A soft polyurethane pouch with a soft outer ring and a pliable inner ring; the condom covers the inside of the entire vagina	Protects against STIs	Some users may have difficulty inserting the condom correctly	5–21	$0.50–$3.00 each use

(continued)

Table 10.1: **A Summary of Contraceptive Options** (continued)

Method	Description	Advantages	Disadvantages	Typical Failure Rates (# of women out of 100 that may become pregnant during the first year of use)	Average Cost
Contraceptive sponge	A round, soft foam sponge containing spermicide with a nylon loop for removal	Easy to obtain, no medical exam required; easy to carry; can be left in place for up to 30 hours	No protection against STIs and increases risk of STIs and other infections; may cause irritation in some women	9–16	$9–$15 for a packet of three sponges
Spermicides	Chemical compounds that kill or immobilize sperm	Easy to obtain, no medical exam required; variety of forms for convenience	May leak; high failure rate if used alone; doesn't protect against STIs; increases risk of urinary tract infection	18–29 if used alone, but spermicides increase protection when used with other barrier methods	$0.50–$3.00 each use
Emergency contraception (EC)/ Plan B	Marketed as "Plan B," a pill containing levonorgestrel, a synthetic hormone which can prevent pregnancy from occurring. Also known as the "morning after pill"	Effective when used within 72 hours after unprotected intercourse to prevent pregnancy, although it is most effective within the first 24 hours following intercourse	Begins to lose effectiveness 24–72 hours after intercourse. Does not protect against STIs	No statistics available.	$35–$60

Methods Requiring Prescriptions

Method	Description	Advantages	Disadvantages		Average Cost
Diaphragm	A soft dome-shaped cup with a flexible rim that is filled with spermicide and fits inside the vagina, covering the cervix	Does not require the ingestion of hormones; may be left in place for up to 24 hours	No protection against STIs; can not be used during menstruation; some women find insertion difficult; may become dislodged; requires an exam and fitting by a health-care provider; may cause urinary tract infection or vaginal irritation in some users	6–16	$100–$200 for device, fitting, and spermicide
Cervical cap	A pliable cup filled with spermicide that fits inside the vagina covering the cervix	Does not require the ingestion of hormones; may be left in place for up to 48 hours	No protection against STIs; can not be used during menstruation; some women find insertion difficult; may become dislodged; requires an exam and fitting by a health-care provider; may cause urinary tract infection or vaginal irritation in some users	6–16	$100–$200 for device, fitting, and spermicide
Intrauterine device (IUD)					
ParaGard	A small T-shaped plastic device that releases copper	No action necessary before, during, or after sex; can be left in place for 10–12 years	No protection against STIs; in rare cases, may cause infections or the device may slip out	Less than 1	$200–$300
Mirena	A small T-shaped plastic device that releases progestin	No action necessary before, during, or after sex; may lessen periods or they may cease; can be left in place for up to 5 years	No protection against STIs; in rare cases, may cause infections or the device may slip out	Less than 1	$200–$300
Birth control pills *A variety of combination pills are available. Monophasic pills each contain the same dose of hormone, whereas multiphasic pills contain varying doses of hormone. Both are available in 28-day packs. Other types are used on longer schedules.*	Pills containing the hormones estrogen and progestin, which prevent pregnancy; one pill should be taken at the same time each day; active pills are taken for 3 weeks, the 4th week's pills do not contain the hormone	Convenient; helps protect against cancer of the ovaries and uterus; some women have lighter periods and milder cramps	No protection against STIs; requires taking a pill each day, which may be hard to remember; refills must be on hand; requires ingesting artificial hormones; several adverse effects possible; consultation with health-care provider is essential	1–8	$20–35 per month
Emergency contraception (EC)/ ella	A "morning-after pill" that can be taken up to 5 days after sexual intercourse to prevent pregnancy	Unlike over-the-counter EC, can be taken up to 5 days after sexual intercourse and still be effective in preventing pregnancy	Does not protect against STIs. Not available in the U.S. until fall 2010	No statistics available.	No information available at press time
"Mini-pill"	Pills containing the hormone progestin, which prevents pregnancy	Convenient; helps protect against cancer of the ovaries and uterus; some women have lighter periods and milder cramps; better choice for women who are at risk for developing blood clots	No protection against STIs; requires taking a pill each day, which may be hard to remember; refills must be on hand; requires ingesting artificial hormones; several adverse effects possible; consultation with health-care provider is essential	1–8	$20–35 per month

Table 10.1: A Summary of Contraceptive Options (continued)

Method	Description	Advantages	Disadvantages	Typical Failure Rates (# of women out of 100 that may become pregnant during the first year of use)	Average Cost
Transdermal patch	A thin plastic patch that is placed on the skin, which releases the hormones estrogen and progestin slowly into the body	Convenient—woman does not have to remember to take a pill every day; may reduce risk of endometrial cancer and other cancers, relieve PMS and menstrual cramping, and improve acne	No protection against STIs; may cause bleeding between periods, breast tenderness, or nausea and vomiting; may cause skin irritation at patch site; may alter a woman's sexual desire; may be less effective in women who weigh more than 198 pounds; several long-term adverse effects possible; consultation with health-care provider is essential	1–8	$25–$30 per month
Vaginal ring	A small flexible ring that releases the hormones estrogen and progestin slowly into the body	Convenient—woman does not have to remember to take a pill every day; may reduce risk of endometrial cancer and other cancers, relieve PMS and menstrual cramping, and improve acne	No protection against STIs; may cause bleeding between periods, breast tenderness, or nausea and vomiting; may increase vaginal discharge and lead to irritation or infection; may alter a woman's sexual desire; several long-term adverse effects possible; consultation with health-care provider is essential	1–8	Cost of initial health-care appointment plus $15–$50 per month
Monthly injections	An injection containing the hormones estrogen and progestin	Convenient, may help reduce risk of certain cancers and promote lighter, shorter periods	No protection against STIs; requires monthly visit to health-care provider; side effects may include bloating/weight gain, headaches, vaginal bleeding, and irregular periods; women over the age of 35 or who smoke or have certain health conditions are at risk for serious adverse effects	1–3	$30–$35 month
Quarterly injections	An injection containing the hormone progestin	Convenient; requires only one injection four times a year; helps protect against endometrial cancer; reduces monthly bleeding and anemia; in most cases, women stop having their periods	No protection against STIs; side effects may include amenorrhea, bloating, weight gain, headaches, depression, loss of interest in sex, and hair loss; side effects can continue for several months after last injection; fertility may be delayed for as long as 18 months after stopping injections; not advised for women who want less than a year of birth control	1–3	$60–$75 for 3 months
Implant	A thin plastic rod containing the hormone progestin	Convenient; lasts for 3 years; helps protect women from endometrial cancer	No protection against STIs; insertion and removal of implants requires a small cut in the skin, and scarring may occur; if implants fail, there is a greater chance of a fertilized egg implanting in the fallopian tubes; side effects may include acne, headaches, weight gain, and hair loss	1	$450–$750 for 5 years
Surgical Methods					
Tubal ligation	The fallopian tubes are surgically tied or otherwise sealed	Convenient; no hormonal effect; permanent solution to birth control	No protection against STIs; sterilization is permanent—woman should consider possible life changes such as divorce, remarriage, or death of children, in which case pregnancy may be desired; invasive surgical procedure may be undesirable	Less than 1	$1,500–$6,000
Hysterectomy	Surgical removal of a woman's uterus, sometimes along with her ovaries and fallopian tubes	May be necessary to treat health conditions such as excessive menstrual bleeding or tumors	Irreversible	No statistics available	No information available
Vasectomy	A minor surgical procedure performed at a hospital or clinic in which the vas deferens is tied off and cut on both sides of the scrotum	Convenient; procedure does not affect sexual desire or hormone levels; male may resume sex as soon as it is comfortable; permanent solution to birth control	No protection against STIs; after the procedure the male will still have viable sperm for a period of time; sterilization is permanent	Less than 1	$350–$1000 including sperm count

Data from *Comparing Effectiveness of Birth Control Methods* by Planned Parenthood (n.d.), retrieved from http://www.plannedparenthood.org/health-topics/birth-control/birth-control-effectiveness-chart-22710.htm.

Sex and the College Student

Number of sexual partners college students reported having over the past year

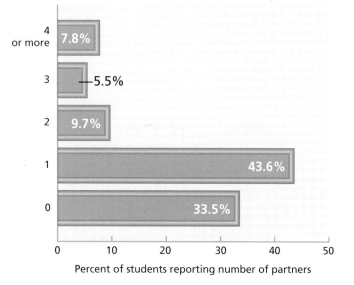

- 4 or more: 7.8%
- 3: 5.5%
- 2: 9.7%
- 1: 43.6%
- 0: 33.5%

Percent of students reporting number of partners

Top methods of contraception used by college students*

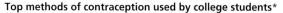

- Male condom: 61.8%
- Birth control pills: 58.7%
- Withdrawal: 26.1%
- Fertility awareness: 5.7%
- Spermicide (foam, jelly, cream): 5.4%
- Intrauterine device: 4.9%
- Vaginal ring: 4.6%

Percent of students reporting type of birth control

* Who engaged in vaginal intercourse and used contraception

Data from *American College Health Association-National College Health Assessment (ACHA-NCHA II) Reference Group Executive Summary, Fall 2009* by the American College Health Association, 2009, retrieved from http://www.acha-ncha.org/docs/ACHA-NCHA_Reference_Group_ExecutiveSummary_Fall2009.pdf.

over-the-counter, methods requiring a prescription, and surgical methods. As we take a closer look at these methods, take note of differences in availability, cost, effectiveness, ease of use, and whether or not the method provides protection against sexually transmitted infection. Meanwhile, the **Student Stats** box illustrates the most popular forms of contraception reported by college students.

Cost-Free Methods

Three methods of contraception are always available, and are cost-free. They are intimacy without intercourse, fertility awareness, and withdrawal. Note that none of them are 100% reliable.

Intimacy without intercourse. Some couples who desire a sexual relationship yet want to avoid the risks of pregnancy and sexually transmitted infections opt for non-intercourse sexual activities like kissing, "making out," manual stimulation of the genitals, and mutual masturbation. Because intercourse doesn't occur, the chance of pregnancy or sexually transmitted infection is theoretically zero. However, in reality, this method requires a high level of commitment, self-discipline, and mutual cooperation and trust.

Fertility awareness (rhythm or calendar method). In this method, a woman tracks on a calendar the day her period begins each month. Ideally, she also logs the days on which she had copious, slippery cervical mucus, because its presence indicates that she is fertile (the mucus occurs as ovulation approaches). Finally, if possible, she makes a note of the day on which she experienced mid-cycle pain (indicating ovulation). **Figure 10.5** provides an example of fertility tracking over the course of a month. Because most women's cycles vary somewhat from month to month, it's essential that a woman using the

fertility awareness (rhythm or calendar method) The tracking of a woman's monthly menstrual cycle; may be used as a method of preventing pregnancy if the woman tracks carefully and has regular periods, though is not fail-safe.

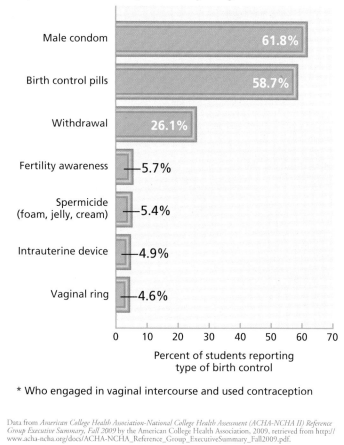

Start of period: ◯   Avoid sex: ✕

Figure 10.5 Fertility awareness. Jotting down key events in the menstrual cycle can help couples identify which dates to avoid sex.

fertility awareness method track her cycles for several months (a full year is ideal) before relying on this method. Also, keep in mind that this method is not fail-safe, and that women with irregular menstrual cycles should rely on other methods of contraception.

Using the data from several months, the woman next calculates her average cycle length (for example, 28 days, 32 days, etc.). Because sperm can survive for 5 days in the vagina—possibly more, and an egg is viable for up to 2 days, a woman is theoretically able to conceive as many as 5 days before she ovulates, and as many as 2 days afterward. However, to be on the safe side, women should avoid intercourse for 7 days prior to ovulation, and for 4 days afterward.

Some women also track their body temperature, which typically rises slightly after ovulation. However, because the temperature increase is so slight—usually less than 1 degree—and must be recorded at the same time every morning before getting out of bed, many women do not have success with this method.

In addition to the careful planning required, the fertility awareness method requires couples to abstain from sexual intercourse for 11 days out of each cycle. If couples also abstain during the first few days the woman is having her period, this can eliminate half of all days each month. During that time, the couple can use other forms of contraception, or engage in non-intercourse sexual activity. Also note that when the couple does engage in unprotected intercourse, both partners may be at risk for sexually transmitted infection.

Withdrawal. Also called *coitus interruptus,* the withdrawal method requires the man to withdraw his penis from his partner's vagina before he ejaculates. Often the man is unable to do this, and withdrawal is associated with a very high failure rate (see Table 10.1). Even if the man can exert the required self-control, pregnancy can still occur because the pre-ejaculate fluid may contain sperm. This

withdrawal The withdrawal of the penis from the vagina before ejaculation.

condom (male condom) A thin sheath typically made of latex, polyurethane, or lambskin that is unrolled over the erect penis prior to vaginal penetration.

method also provides no protection against sexually transmitted infection, and can be unsatisfying for both partners.

Over-the-Counter Methods

Over-the-counter methods are available without a prescription or examination. They include condoms, which may be available from campus health clinics and other sources free of charge; the contraceptive sponge; spermicides; and emergency contraceptives.

Condoms. The male condom is a thin sheath, typically made of latex, polyurethane, or lambskin, which is unrolled over the erect penis prior to vaginal penetration **(Figure 10.6).** If used correctly and consistently, it offers excellent protection against pregnancy and sexually transmitted infection. Either can occur, however, if the condom breaks or comes off during sex. Most condoms are lubricated. However, note that lambskin condoms do not provide as much protection against infection as do latex and polyurethane.

Some men feel that wearing a condom decreases their level of stimulation and pleasure. Experimenting with different sizes, types, and brands, as well as using a water-based personal lubricant, may help.

When using condoms, it's important to check the expiration date on the packet. Discard a condom if the expiration date has passed. When the penis is erect, squeeze the air out of the tip of the condom and place it over the glans (head) of the penis. Roll the condom down over the shaft of the penis as far as possible. After ejaculation, but before the penis has become flaccid, grasp the condom at the base of the penis and withdraw. Throw the condom away.

The female condom is a lubricated latex or polyurethane sheath with flexible rings on either end **(Figure 10.7).** Using a special applicator, the woman inserts it into the vagina until the inner ring rests against the cervix. The outer ring remains outside the body, partly

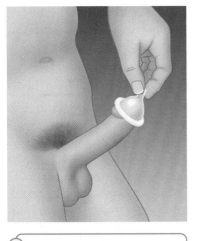 ① Pinch the tip of the condom to expel any air.

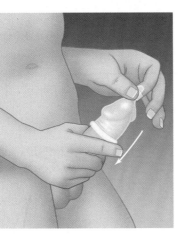 ② Keep the tip pinched with one hand. Use the other hand to roll the condom onto the penis.

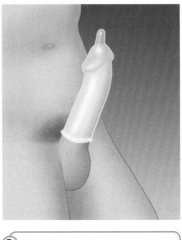 ③ Make sure the condom smoothly covers the entire penis.

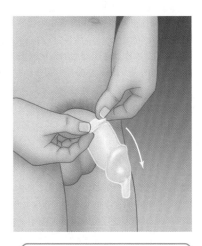 ④ After ejaculation, hold on to the base of the condom as you withdraw. Remove the condom carefully so that semen does not spill.

Figure 10.6 Applying a male condom.

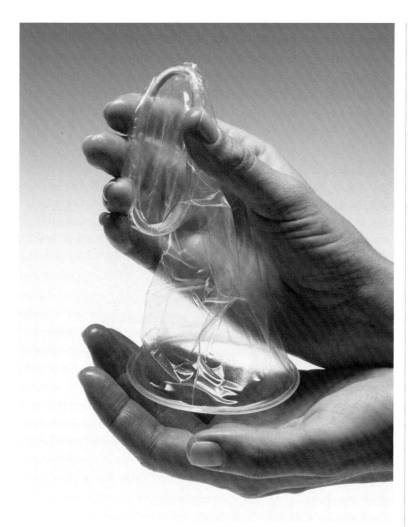

Figure 10.7 The female condom.

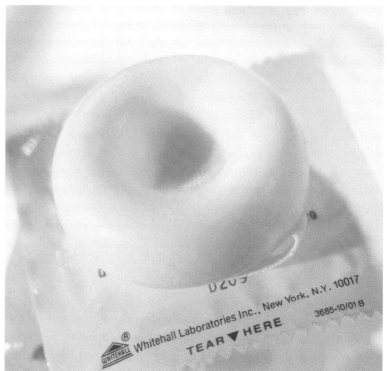

Figure 10.8 A contraceptive sponge.

covering the labia. The female condom can be inserted several hours before sex, and provides protection against both pregnancy and sexually transmitted infection. However, some women find it awkward to insert, and it can cause some discomfort during sex. It can also get pushed upward into the vagina. Finally, it is associated with a higher pregnancy rate than is the male condom.

Contraceptive sponge. A flexible foam disk **(Figure 10.8)** containing spermicide, the contraceptive sponge is moistened with water and inserted into the vagina until it rests against the cervix. The sponge can cause irritation and dryness. It does not protect against sexually transmitted infection; in fact, it slightly increases the risk of contracting one. It must be left in place for 6 hours after intercourse, and is associated with an increased risk for a urinary tract infection, vaginal infection, and toxic shock syndrome.

Spermicides. A spermicide is a substance containing nonoxynol-9, a chemical that kills or immobilizes sperm. Spermicides are available as foams, gels, film, and suppositories. They are not very effective in preventing pregnancy and don't

contraceptive sponge A flexible foam disk containing spermicide that is inserted in the vagina prior to sex.

spermicide A substance containing chemicals that kill or immobilize sperm.

emergency contraception (EC; "morning after" pill) A pill containing levonorgestrel, a synthetic hormone that is used to prevent pregnancy after unprotected sex.

diaphragm A flexible silicone cup filled with spermicide and inserted in the vagina prior to sex to prevent pregnancy.

prevent sexually transmitted infection when used alone (see Table 10.1). In fact, spermicide use can increase a woman's chance of developing a urinary tract infection.

Emergency contraception (EC). Also called the "morning after" pill, EC is currently available over-the-counter under the brand name Plan B. Plan B is a pill containing levonorgestrel, a synthetic hormone similar to those found in birth control pills. It is effective up to 72 hours after unprotected sex. However, it is most effective within the first 24 hours after intercourse.[40] It prevents pregnancy by tricking the body into believing that pregnancy has already occurred, preventing ovulation, fertilization, or implantation. It should not be confused with *RU-486,* the so-called "abortion pill." If a woman is already pregnant, Plan B will do nothing to stop the pregnancy.

See page 229 for a discussion of ella, a recently approved, prescription-only form of emergency contraception that can be effective 120 days after intercourse.

Methods Available by Prescription

Many more sophisticated methods of contraception are available by prescription. Prescription barrier methods include the diaphragm, cervical cap, and IUD. Prescription hormonal methods are available in various delivery methods. Notice that all of these options are for women. Research into such methods for males is ongoing.

Diaphragm and cervical cap. The diaphragm and cervical cap are small, flexible, silicone cups that the woman fills with spermicide and inserts into the vagina **(Figure 10.9).** They must be fitted by the woman's health-care provider, and some

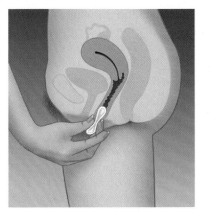

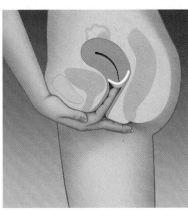

1. After filling the diaphragm with spermicide, hold it dome-side down and squeeze the opposite sides of the rim together.

2. Insert the diaphragm into the vagina, pushing it along the vaginal floor as far back as it will go. Make sure the diaphragm completely covers the cervix (the bump at the back of your vagina.) Tuck the front rim of the diaphragm up against your pelvic bone.

Figure 10.9 Inserting a diaphragm.

devices must be replaced annually. These devices must be left in place for at least 6 hours following intercourse, and may be left in place for up to 24 hours. However, they do not reliably protect against sexually transmitted infection, and are associated with an increased risk of urinary tract infection and toxic shock syndrome.

IUD. An **intrauterine device (IUD)** is a plastic, T-shaped device that is inserted by a health-care provider into the uterus for long-term pregnancy prevention. There are two types, both of which are highly effective in preventing pregnancy:

- The ParaGard copper IUD continually releases copper, which works either by preventing sperm from reaching the fallopian tubes, or by preventing implantation of a fertilized egg, should conception occur. It can be effective for up to 10 years. Side effects include cramps, nausea, severe menstrual pain and bleeding, painful sex, and anemia.[41]

- The Mirena hormonal IUD releases progestin, which works either by thickening the cervical mucus—blocking sperm transit—or by suppressing ovulation. It can be effective for up to 5 years. Side effects include weight gain, acne, headaches, ovarian cysts, and abdominal pain.[42]

Neither of these devices guards against sexually transmitted infection, and both can be expelled from the uterus.

Pharmaceutical hormones. Synthetic hormones, including estrogen and progestin, are combined in **birth control pills,** typically referred to simply as "the pill." A progestin-only "mini-pill" is also available. However, synthetic hormones don't only come in pill form: they're also available as a skin patch that is replaced weekly, a vaginal ring replaced monthly, injections given monthly or quarterly, and an under-the-skin implant that can last for up to 3 years. To compare these hormonal methods, see Table 10.1.

intrauterine device (IUD) A plastic, T-shaped device that is inserted in the uterus for long-term pregnancy prevention.

birth control pills Pills containing combinations of hormones that prevent pregnancy when taken regularly as directed.

Bear in mind that, although all of the hormonal methods are convenient and highly effective at preventing pregnancy, they do not protect against sexually transmitted infection; thus, condom use is still important. Also, because they release reproductive hormones into the body, these methods can provoke symptoms that mimic those of early pregnancy, including nausea, weight gain, breast tenderness, and moodiness.

In addition, women who have taken the pill for several months can experience long-term adverse effects. These include post-pill amenorrhea that can last for 3–6 months, as well as increased blood pressure and an increased risk of cardiovascular disease, especially in smokers. Long-term use can also increase a woman's risk for cervical and liver cancer. On the upside, pill use can decrease a woman's risk for ovarian and endometrial cancer. The relationship between pill use and breast cancer is not clear.[43]

Other forms of hormonal contraceptives can have similarly serious adverse effects. For example, the skin patch can increase the risk for blood clots, heart attack, and stroke, whereas the injection form can lead to loss in bone mineral density. Thus, anyone considering the hormonal methods should carefully weigh the risks and benefits with her health-care provider.

In 2010, the FDA approved a new emergency contraception pill called ella. Unlike Plan B, which begins to lose effectiveness within 24 hours after sexual intercourse, ella is effective for up to 120 hours (5 days) after unprotected sex, and its effectiveness does not diminish with time. As this book went to press, ella was scheduled to become available by prescription in the U.S. by fall 2010.

Surgical Methods

The surgical methods discussed here are classified as *sterilization;* that is, they permanently prevent conception by involving surgical manipulation of the reproductive organs.

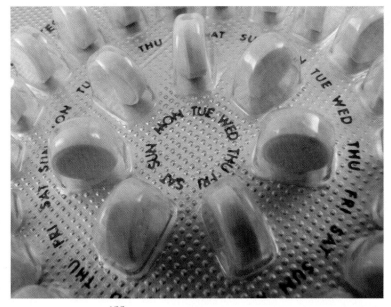

Birth control **pills**.

Tubal ligation is a surgical procedure in which a woman's fallopian tubes are tied off or sealed to prevent the egg from traveling toward the uterus. Sperm also cannot reach the egg; thus, fertilization cannot occur. Tubal ligation can sometimes be reversed, but should not be undertaken if a woman thinks she may change her mind.

A *hysterectomy* is a procedure in which a woman's uterus is surgically removed, sometimes along with her ovaries and fallopian tubes. It is considered a method of permanent, absolute, irreversible sterilization and is not an option for women who merely desire contraception. However, if a woman has other factors, such as excessive menstrual bleeding, or benign or malignant tumors in the uterus, and she desires to permanently cease childbearing, then the procedure may be considered.

A *vasectomy* is a surgical procedure in which a man's vas deferens is tied off and cut on both sides of the scrotum. This makes it impossible for sperm—which are manufactured in the testes—to make their way upward and into the semen. The man typically notices no difference in the quantity of semen he ejaculates, and although there

failure rate The percentage of women who typically get pregnant after using a given contraceptive method for one year.

continuation rate The percentage of couples who continue to practice a given form of birth control.

abortion A medical or surgical procedure used to terminate a pregnancy.

is some swelling, bruising, and discomfort immediately after the surgery, long-term complications are rare. The procedure is nearly 100% effective at preventing pregnancy; however, it is difficult to reverse. Thus, men who choose vasectomy should consider the procedure permanent.[44]

Which Method Is the Best?

The answer to this question depends on each individual couple. When deciding which type of birth control to use, couples should consider how comfortable they are with the method, how many side effects it has, how well it works, and how likely they are to use it correctly. It is important to note that although every method has a published **failure rate** (indicating the percentage of women who typically get pregnant after using that method for one year), the figures are a bit misleading. That's because failure rates indicate pregnancy rates if the method is used exactly as directed, a concept known as "perfect use." In reality, couples do not always use birth control perfectly. Women forget to take their pills. Men put condoms on improperly. The end result is what is known as "typical use," which has substantially higher pregnancy rates. Another critical factor is the **continuation rate,** or the percentage of couples who continue to practice that form of birth control. Often, couples will stop using one method and, before choosing a new method, will have unprotected sex.

Which contraceptive method is right for you? To find out, log onto www.plannedparenthood.org/all-access/my-method-26542.htm and take the MyMethod quiz. It's written for women, but men can take it as well, by answering the questions from the perspective of their partner.

Abortion

Birth control failure—and the failure to use birth control—combine to create a large number of unintended pregnancies, as we noted at the beginning of this chapter, about 3 million in the United States every year.[45] Many women experiencing an unplanned pregnancy decide to keep their baby. Some—typically fewer than 2%—maintain the pregnancy but relinquish the baby for adoption. About 14% miscarry, and about 42% choose abortion each year.[46]

Abortion is a medical or surgical procedure used to terminate a pregnancy, and involves removing the embryo or fetus from the uterus. The number of abortions performed has been declining in recent years, and the abortion rate is at its lowest level since 1974. Nevertheless, 1.2 million abortions were performed in 2005, indicating that more needs to be done to help couples avoid unintended pregnancy.[47]

Methods of Abortion

There are two types of procedures for terminating a pregnancy: medical and surgical abortion. *Medical abortion,* which involves the administration of medications (via pill or injection) to end a pregnancy, has been gaining in popularity since its approval by the U.S. Food and Drug Administration in 2000. About 13% of women who underwent an abortion in 2005 used the medical method, up from 1% just a few years before. Moreover, 22% of abortions performed in the first 9 weeks of pregnancy used the medical method.[47] *Surgical*

Deciding to Get on the Pill

"Hi, I'm Betty. When discussing contraceptives with my mom, she gave me so many options. She works in maternal health care, so she had this huge planner out and she was like 'this is a female condom and this is this and that'—and it was just like, I don't even want to know all the other stuff. I didn't want an IUD and I didn't want a female condom or anything like that . . . I was like, let me go to the simplest form. That way if I decide 'OK, if I don't want to take this anymore, then I can get rid of it.' I ended up deciding to get on the pill. The pros are that you always know when your period is going to arrive, it lessens PMS and cramping, and you won't get pregnant. The cons—you have to continuously stay on it. You have to keep it as a ritual: like, get in the shower, brush your teeth, and before you brush your teeth, take your pill. Sometimes it can make you nauseous. That's another con, but other than that, it's great."

1: Given what you've learned in this chapter, do you think birth control pills alone are enough to protect you (or your partner) against pregnancy? How about STIs? Explain your answer.

2: Betty was able to turn to her mom for advice on what contraceptive was right for her. Think about the resources available to you. Where will you go to learn more about contraceptive options and decide which one is right for you?

Do you have a story similar to Betty's? Share your story at www.pearsonhighered.com/choosinghealth.

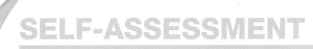

Are You and Your Partner Ready for Sex?

Maybe you've only been on two dates. Maybe you've been "just friends" for two years. But sooner or later, the question is going to demand an answer: Are the two of you ready for your relationship to become sexual? Here are some questions that can help you decide.

1. Is your decision to have sex completely your own? (that is, you feel no pressure from others, including your partner)
   yes   no

2. Is your decision to have sex based on the right reasons? (The **wrong reasons** are peer pressure, a need to fit in or make your partner happy, or a belief that sex will make your relationship with your partner better, or closer. If you decide to have sex, it **should be** because you feel emotionally and physically ready and your partner is someone you love, trust, and respect.)
   yes   no

3. Do you feel your partner would respect any decision you made about whether to have sex or not?
   yes   no

4. Do you trust and respect your partner?
   yes   no

5. Are you able to comfortably talk to your partner about sex and your partner's sexual history?
   yes   no

6. Do you know how to prevent pregnancy and STIs?
   yes   no

7. Are you and your partner willing to use contraception to prevent pregnancy and STIs?
   yes   no

8. Have you and your partner talked about what both of you would do in the event of pregnancy or if one of you were to develop an STI?
   yes   no

9. Do you feel completely comfortable with the idea of having sex with this partner?
   yes   no

HOW TO INTERPRET YOUR SCORE

If you answered **No** to **any** of these questions, you are not really ready for sex. If you think you should have sexual intercourse because others want you to or everyone else is doing it, these are not the right reasons. You should only decide to have sex because you trust and respect your partner, you know the possible risks, you know how to protect yourself against the risks, and most importantly, because you know that you are ready!

abortion has a much longer history in the United States, and remains the prevailing option, with 87% of women who sought an abortion in 2005 ultimately selecting it.[47]

Which method is advised? The World Health Organization has stated, "There is little, if any, difference between medical and surgical abortion in terms of safety and efficacy. Thus, both methods are similar from a medical point of view and there are only very few situations where a recommendation for one or the other method for medical reasons can be given."[48]

Medical Abortion

Medical abortions are intended for women in the earliest stages of pregnancy, within 7 weeks of the start of their last menstrual period (9 weeks of pregnancy). There is no surgery, and no anesthesia. The medical route is recommended if the woman has health risks that make surgery unadvisable, such as obesity or uterine malformations.

Some women opt for surgical abortion because the medical method is more time-consuming. The process starts with the administration—either by pill or injection—of the medication *mifepristone,* also known as *RU-486.* The medication blocks progesterone, which is needed to support a pregnancy. Two days later, the woman takes a pill containing the drug *misoprostol,* which causes the uterus to contract and expel the fertilized egg along with the endometrial lining. The pregnancy usually terminates within hours after the second drug is ingested, but sometimes can take up to 2 days. Two weeks after the process is initiated, women are instructed to return to their physician's office for a follow-up exam. The procedure successfully terminates pregnancy in more than 96% of cases.[49] If the pregnancy was not successfully terminated, a surgical abortion is then recommended.

The expulsion of the pregnancy from the uterus can cause severe cramping pain, nausea, heavy bleeding, fever, and diarrhea. Nevertheless, many women choose medical abortion because it allows them to end an unwanted pregnancy in privacy at home, and without the trauma of an invasive surgical procedure.

Surgical Abortion

Suction curettage, or vacuum aspiration, is the surgical abortion method most commonly chosen. Typically used in the first 6 to 12 weeks of pregnancy, it involves an injection to numb the cervix, followed by the insertion of a series of rods of increasing thickness to dilate (widen) the opening of the cervix. Once the cervix is adequately dilated, the physician inserts a hollow tube through the cervix into the uterus. The tube is attached to a pump, which generates suction to remove tissue from the uterine walls. Usually performed in a doctor's office or outpatient clinic, suction curettage is a relatively quick procedure, often taking just minutes to complete.

Manual vacuum aspiration is similar to suction curettage, but can be performed much earlier in the pregnancy. Doctors use thin flexible tubing attached to a handheld syringe and insert it through the cervix into the uterus. The syringe—rather than a machine—creates enough suction needed to strip the uterine lining and terminate the pregnancy.

For pregnancies that have progressed beyond 12 weeks, **dilation and evacuation (D&E)** may be performed. This procedure requires multiple trips to the health-care provider. During the first visit, the health-care provider performs an ultrasound scan to determine the status of the pregnancy and eligibility for the procedure. Then, 24 hours before the surgery, the cervix is numbed and a medication administered that will dilate it slowly. At the final appointment, either at a clinic or a hospital, the woman is given a local anesthetic, or in some cases spinal or general anesthesia, and the physician uses instruments and suction to remove the pregnancy. The procedure can produce pain and heavy bleeding, and is

suction curettage A method of surgical abortion characterized by vacuum aspiration; typically used in the first 6 to 12 weeks of pregnancy.

dilation and evacuation (D&E) A multistep method of surgical abortion that may be used in pregnancies that have progressed beyond 12 weeks.

associated with a variety of possible complications. Follow-up care is important.

Physical and Psychological Complications of Abortion

As with any medical procedure, abortion has some risks. One analysis of abortions in New York City found that for every 1,000 women terminating a pregnancy, 9 experienced complications, usually a minor infection.[50] Rarely, excessive bleeding, a serious blood infection, or injury to the uterus or cervix can occur. Another risk is that the abortion will be incomplete.

Deaths due to abortion are rare. For example, of the more than 820,000 legally induced abortions performed in the United States in 2004, there were 7 known fatalities—1 from a medical abortion and 6 from surgical procedures.[51]

For the vast majority of women who get an abortion, physical complications are not an issue. But what about psychological ones? Abortion critics have argued that women who undergo an abortion are at risk for a constellation of mental health problems they call *postabortion traumatic stress syndrome*. Yet this is not recognized as a legitimate mental health condition by either the American Psychological Association or the American Psychiatric Association. Still, recognizing that abortion can be stressful for some women, causing feelings of sadness or guilt, an American Psychological Association convened a task force on abortion and mental health. In 2008, it concluded that there is no credible evidence that terminating a single unwanted pregnancy creates mental health problems for adult women.[52] The risk, they found, was no greater than if the women had opted to give birth.

Legal Status of Abortion

Abortion has long been a contentious issue in the United States. Despite largely being legal during the nation's founding years, both abortion and contraception gradually fell out of favor. The Federal Comstock Act of 1873 criminalized the distribution or possession of devices, medication, or even information used for abortion or contraception. For an entire century, many women who wanted to terminate an unwanted pregnancy resorted to "back-alley" abortions, performed in unsterile locations, often by untrained personnel using rudimentary instruments. These procedures were dangerous, and many women died attempting to end an unwanted pregnancy.

In 1973, the U.S. Supreme Court made a landmark decision in the case of *Roe v. Wade* that all women had a constitutional right to an abortion in the first 6 months of their pregnancy. The legislation trumped all state laws limiting women's access to an abortion, and stipulated that individual states could only ban abortions during the final 3 months of pregnancy, when a fetus would have a chance at surviving outside the womb. From the fourth through the sixth month of pregnancy, however, states could regulate the abortion procedure in the interest of maternal health.

Abortion continues to be legal in the United States, but a number of rulings have chipped away at *Roe v. Wade,* placing new restrictions on who can get an abortion, and when. More than 30 states now require that minors notify their parents before getting an abortion, often needing parental permission to continue with the procedure. Others impose a mandatory waiting period on women, requiring them to read information on alternatives to abortion before being allowed to terminate their pregnancy. The U.S. Congress has also blocked the use of federal Medicaid funds to pay for elective abortions except when a pregnancy would endanger a woman's life, or in cases of rape or incest.

Pregnancy and Childbirth

Among the milestones in life that people cherish the most is the journey to becoming a parent and the birth of their child. The following sections provide an overview of the stages of pregnancy and childbirth, as well as an examination of the choices available to couples struggling with infertility.

Pregnancy

For young, healthy couples having unprotected sex, there is about a 20% chance the woman will get pregnant during any given menstrual cycle.[53] Pregnancies are divided into three trimesters, each lasting about 3 months. Women may experience vastly different symptoms during each phase of their pregnancy, with the second trimester often being referred to as the "golden age" because women tend to have more energy and less nausea at this point.

A woman who suspects she might be pregnant can find out for certain with the use of a simple pregnancy test. There are two types on the market, a urine test available over the counter, and a blood test offered only in physicians' offices. Both look for the presence of human chorionic gonadotropin (hCG), a hormone that is only made in the body during pregnancy.

The blood test can detect hCG about a week after ovulation. But many women opt for a home urine test, which is painless, inexpensive, and private. It's able to detect hCG levels about 2 weeks after ovulation—approximately the day a woman's period is due. For the most accurate results, however, health experts recommend waiting until a few days later before taking a home pregnancy test. In one study of 18 popular home pregnancy kits, researchers found that only one, the First Response Early Result Pregnancy Test, was consistently able to provide correct results the day a woman's period was due.[54]

Because home pregnancy tests are not 100% accurate, women who get a negative result are encouraged to test again one week later if they still have not started menstruating.

Preconception Care

Many women recognize that **prenatal care,** including nutritional counseling and regular medical screenings throughout pregnancy, is important for the growth and development of the unborn baby. So, too, is preconception care, initiated before a woman has even gotten pregnant. Obstetricians encourage their patients who are attempting to start a family to first take care of any health problems that could affect the pregnancy, including type 2 diabetes and high blood pressure. Prenatal vitamins containing a sufficient amount of folic acid are also recommended as they significantly reduce the risk of birth defects.

During a preconception visit, a doctor may also suggest changes in a woman's nutrition or exercise patterns, and will instruct women not to use

prenatal care Nutritional counseling and regular medical screenings throughout pregnancy to aid the growth and development of the fetus.

tobacco, alcohol, or illegal drugs, or take certain medications while they attempt to conceive. Because women do not learn they are pregnant until several weeks after conception, it is critical to make positive lifestyle changes long before that faint positive sign first appears on a home pregnancy test.

Early Signs of Pregnancy

At one time in their lives, most women will find themselves asking "Am I pregnant?" If they listen closely, their bodies may tell them the answer. Pregnancy symptoms can begin to surface before a woman even misses her period, although the first signs could also be indicative of an illness or even impending menstruation. Still, women who begin to experience many of these symptoms should consider taking a home pregnancy test or visiting their gynecologist:

- A skipped period
- An extremely light "period" known as implantation bleeding that occurs when a fertilized egg implants itself in the uterus
- Frequent urination
- Nausea
- Swollen breasts
- Fatigue
- Food aversions or cravings
- Mood swings
- Abdominal bloating or pressure
- Dizziness

Some women will experience none of these symptoms in the early weeks of their pregnancy. Others may notice a few signs but not right away.

Changes in a Pregnant Woman's Body

A woman's body undergoes a series of physical changes throughout the course of pregnancy **(Figure 10.10).** Some go unnoticed by the mother-to-be. For example, the heart begins to work harder, and a physician may notice fluctuations in the woman's blood pressure. Breathing patterns change slightly, with breaths becoming deeper and faster. The kidneys kick into high gear, filtering an increasing volume of blood. Ligaments and muscles stretch. The cervix becomes thinner and softer.

Myriad other changes, however, are difficult for women to miss. Hormone changes, especially in the first trimester, can cause bouts of nausea and vomiting called "morning sickness," a misnomer because women afflicted with it often find it persists throughout most of the day. Breasts become fuller and tender to the touch as they get ready for milk production. The uterus enlarges as the fetus grows, ultimately extending up to the woman's rib cage. The growing uterus presses on the bladder, creating the constant urge to urinate. It also shifts the woman's center of gravity, exaggerating the curve in her lower back and giving her a characteristic "waddling" walk. The skin stretches to accommodate the growing breasts and abdomen, and sometimes darkens at points on the face and in a thin line near the navel. As the pregnancy draws near a close, women may also develop heartburn or hemorrhoids. By the time the baby is born, the average woman will have gained between 25 and 30 pounds—or more if she is carrying twins or triplets. Not surprisingly, as a result of all these physical changes, many women report experiencing significant fatigue during their pregnancy.

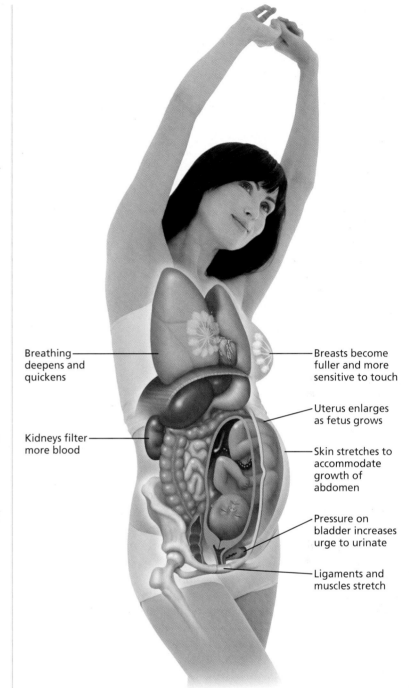

Figure 10.10 Changes in a pregnant woman's body.

Development of the Fetus

The fetus also undergoes significant physical changes as it transforms from a microscopic fertilized egg into an average 7.5-pound newborn.

First trimester. The first trimester, which accounts for the first 13 weeks of pregnancy, is the most critical period in the baby's development. At this stage, it is most susceptible to any substances a woman ingests, including drugs, alcohol, and certain medications, and any environmental toxins, from pesticides to the chemicals in cigarette smoke.

Recall that when an egg and sperm combine, they form a single-celled organism known as a zygote. As the zygote makes its way from a woman's fallopian tube to her uterus, it rapidly divides and becomes a cluster of dozens of cells called a *blastocyst*. The blastocyst, which is no larger than a pinhead, implants itself in the uterine wall, where it begins to receive nourishment. About 2 weeks after fertilization—around the time a woman first misses her period—the growing collection of cells is known as an **embryo** and is already beginning to differentiate into three tissue layers. One layer becomes the fetal nerves, brain, and spinal cord. The second layer becomes bone, muscle, and skin. The third develops into the fetal respiratory, digestive, and urinary organs.

The growing embryo has a powerful support system. It receives its nutrients and oxygen—and gets rid of its waste products—from the **placenta,** the tissue that connects mother and baby. The **umbilical cord** also plays a key role, linking the bloodstream of the placenta to that of the embryo and enabling the exchange of gases, nutrients, and wastes. The embryo is surrounded and protected by **amniotic fluid,** which keeps the baby's temperature regulated and allows it to move freely.

At 8 weeks after fertilization, the embryo is called the **fetus,** a name it will keep until childbirth. By the time the first trimester comes to a close, the fetus is much larger than the pinhead it once was, measuring 3 to 4 inches in length. Still, it weighs only the equivalent of two dozen paper clips. The bulk of the fetus's growth will occur in the trimesters to come.

Second trimester. The second trimester is an exciting time for many women. Fatigue and nausea tend to dissipate, and the fetus provides them with a few welcome signs of the life developing within. During this trimester, the woman begins to feel the fetus moving and kicking, and the fetal heartbeat can be heard through an obstetrician's stethoscope. All major organs and physiological systems become fully formed. The fetus continues its rapid growth, measuring 13 to 16 inches by the end of the second trimester and weighing around 2 or 3 pounds. A fetus might survive if born at the end of this trimester, but would require a lengthy hospitalization and could suffer long-term health effects.

Third trimester. During the last 3 months of pregnancy, the fetus gains most of its weight, including a layer of fat needed for insulation during the first weeks of life outside the womb. Its organs continue to mature, and it moves into position—head down—as it gets ready for birth. Throughout the last trimester, the mother may experience *Braxton Hicks contractions,* irregular movements of the uterus that may be confused with the signs of premature labor. Braxton Hicks contractions, however, are simple tightenings of the uterus, nothing more than false labor.

While a standard pregnancy lasts about 40 weeks, babies are considered full term if they are born between 37 and 42 weeks. Babies born before 37 weeks gestation are considered preterm and are at risk for developmental delays and other complications. Babies born after 42 weeks gestation are postterm and may stop growing in the uterus. In some instances, postterm pregnancies result in stillbirth.

embryo The growing collection of cells that ultimately become a baby.

placenta The tissue that connects mother and baby.

umbilical cord A vessel linking the bloodstream of the placenta to that of the baby and enabling the exchange of gases, nutrients, and wastes.

amniotic fluid Fluid that surrounds the developing fetus that aids in temperature regulation and allows the baby to move freely.

fetus The name given to the developing embryo 8 weeks after fertilization.

ectopic pregnancy A pregnancy that occurs when a fertilized egg implants within one of the fallopian tubes instead of the uterus; considered a medical emergency.

Figure 10.11 illustrates the various stages of fetal development.

Prenatal Care
The health of the baby depends in part on the health of the mother and the measures she takes during pregnancy to protect them both. Prenatal care, which includes regular checkups during pregnancy and counseling about nutrition, exercise, sleep, and other topics, should be an integral part of every pregnancy. Babies born to mothers who receive no prenatal care are five times more likely to die than those whose mothers do get regular care.[55] As soon as a woman learns she is pregnant, she is encouraged to:

- **Get regular checkups.** Select an obstetrician or certified nurse midwife and schedule an initial appointment. This is followed by regularly scheduled appointments at which the woman is monitored for many factors, including blood pressure, blood sugar, weight gain, and fetal well-being.
- **Follow good nutrition advice.** It is commonly said that a pregnant woman is "eating for two," but that is only partially accurate. During pregnancy, the body only needs an extra 300 calories per day—not exactly a doubling of food. Yet what is true is that what a woman consumes, her growing fetus consumes, be it fruits, vegetables, lean meats, and whole grains—or cake, cookies, drugs, and alcohol.
- **Exercise regularly.** Fitness is important to the health of the mother and her growing baby. Exercise can help relieve some of the symptoms of pregnancy and may prevent gestational diabetes. It can also help prepare a woman for labor and childbirth. Kegel exercises are recommended for strengthening the muscles of the pelvic floor, which support the uterus and bladder. By repeatedly contracting the muscles used to stop the flow of urine, women can reduce their risk of incontinence, a common complaint during and after pregnancy.
- **Avoid drugs, including alcohol and tobacco.** These substances, including some prescription and over-the-counter medications, can be harmful to the growth and development of the unborn fetus. A pregnant woman should always check with her physician before taking any medications. The same holds true for dietary supplements, including herbs.

Complications
Most pregnancies progress without a hitch, with the fetus developing properly and the birth being trouble-free. For some women, however, there are complications, problems that pose a risk to the health of the mother or baby, or both.

Ectopic pregnancy. An **ectopic pregnancy** occurs when a fertilized egg implants within one of the fallopian tubes. It can also implant in the cervix or an ovary, although much less frequently. About 2% of all pregnancies in the United States are ectopic.[56]

As the improperly located embryo begins to grow, the woman may experience severe pain, and the fallopian tube may rupture. An

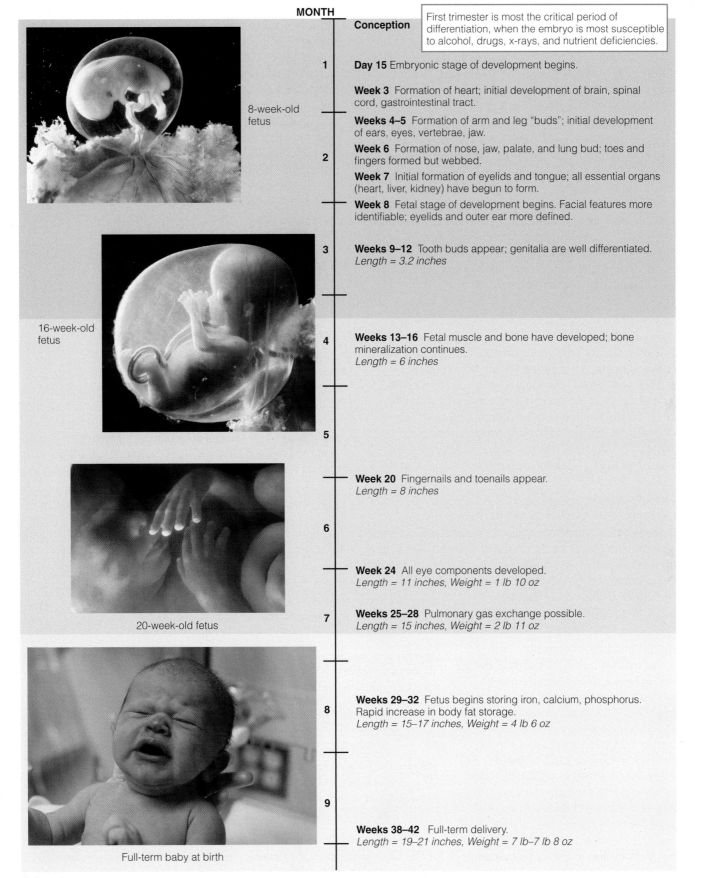

MONTH

Conception

First trimester is most the critical period of differentiation, when the embryo is most susceptible to alcohol, drugs, x-rays, and nutrient deficiencies.

8-week-old fetus

1

Day 15 Embryonic stage of development begins.

Week 3 Formation of heart; initial development of brain, spinal cord, gastrointestinal tract.

Weeks 4–5 Formation of arm and leg "buds"; initial development of ears, eyes, vertebrae, jaw.

2

Week 6 Formation of nose, jaw, palate, and lung bud; toes and fingers formed but webbed.

Week 7 Initial formation of eyelids and tongue; all essential organs (heart, liver, kidney) have begun to form.

Week 8 Fetal stage of development begins. Facial features more identifiable; eyelids and outer ear more defined.

3

Weeks 9–12 Tooth buds appear; genitalia are well differentiated. *Length = 3.2 inches*

16-week-old fetus

4

Weeks 13–16 Fetal muscle and bone have developed; bone mineralization continues. *Length = 6 inches*

5

Week 20 Fingernails and toenails appear. *Length = 8 inches*

6

Week 24 All eye components developed. *Length = 11 inches, Weight = 1 lb 10 oz*

20-week-old fetus

7

Weeks 25–28 Pulmonary gas exchange possible. *Length = 15 inches, Weight = 2 lb 11 oz*

8

Weeks 29–32 Fetus begins storing iron, calcium, phosphorus. Rapid increase in body fat storage. *Length = 15–17 inches, Weight = 4 lb 6 oz*

9

Full-term baby at birth

Weeks 38–42 Full-term delivery. *Length = 19–21 inches, Weight = 7 lb–7 lb 8 oz*

Figure 10.11 Stages of embryonic and fetal development.

ectopic pregnancy can never develop normally and survive, and is a threat to the mother's life. It is the leading cause of maternal mortality during the first trimester, accounting for 10–15% of all maternal deaths.[57] Ectopic pregnancies can also cause scarring in the fallopian tubes, creating future fertility problems. Risk factors include smoking, having endometriosis, and having been infected with the sexually transmitted infections gonorrhea or chlamydia.

Miscarriage. A **miscarriage**, or *spontaneous abortion,* is a pregnancy that suddenly ends on its own before the 20th week. An estimated 10–15% of known pregnancies end this way, but because many losses occur before a woman realizes she is pregnant, experts believe the true number could be closer to 40%.[58] Exactly what causes a pregnancy to terminate is not always clear, but the majority of miscarriages are thought to be caused by chromosomal problems in the fetus. The risk is higher in women who are over age 35, have a history of diabetes or thyroid disease, or have a history of miscarriages. Smoking, drinking alcohol, or using illicit drugs while pregnant may also increase a woman's risk of miscarriage.

Hypertension. A pregnant woman's blood pressure is normally checked at every prenatal visit to screen for hypertension (high blood pressure), which is the most common medical disorder in pregnancy.[59] If left untreated, hypertension during pregnancy can progress to **preeclampsia,** a serious health condition that can threaten the life of both mother and fetus. Characterized by high blood pressure and protein in the urine, preeclampsia typically develops after the 20th week of pregnancy. Women may begin experiencing headaches, swelling of the hands and face, excessive weight gain, abdominal pain, and even vision changes. Without skilled medical care, preeclampsia can result in seizures and multiple organ failure, as well as fetal death.

About 5–7% of pregnant women develop preeclampsia.[60] Unfortunately, there is no way to prevent it, and the only cure is childbirth. Physicians will often admit a woman with preeclampsia to the hospital so she and her fetus can be closely monitored. Although it can be harmful to the baby to be born prematurely, often it can be even more dangerous for a preeclamptic pregnancy to go full term. Doctors may decide to induce labor early in an effort to save both mother and child.

Low birth-weight and infant mortality. We noted earlier that the average birth-weight in the U.S. is about 7.5 pounds. Newborns weighing less than 5 pounds, 8 ounces at birth are called **low birth-weight** babies and are at risk for serious health problems, including death. About 1 in every 12 babies born in the United States falls into this category, and the number has been on the rise for the past few decades.[61] Preterm labor is the leading cause, with two out of three low birth-weight babies arriving before the 37th week of pregnancy.[61] Low birth-weight babies are vulnerable to a host of health problems and disabilities, including learning disabilities, cerebral palsy, hearing loss, and vision problems. Women are more likely to have a low birth-weight baby if they smoke, drink alcohol, or use illicit drugs during pregnancy.

miscarriage A pregnancy that suddenly terminates on its own before the 20th week.

preeclampsia A serious health condition characterized by high blood pressure in the pregnant woman.

low birth-weight The term given to birth-weights less than 5 pounds, 8 ounces.

infant mortality rate A calculation of the ratio of babies who die before their first birthday to those who survive until their first birthday.

sudden infant death syndrome (SIDS) The sudden death of a seemingly healthy infant while sleeping.

labor The physical processes involved in giving birth.

Low birth-weight and prematurity are two factors influencing the **infant mortality rate,** a calculation of the ratio of babies who die before their first birthday to those who survive until their first birthday. In 2008, the infant mortality rate in the U.S. was 6.7 per 1,000 births.[62] Congenital abnormalities, pregnancy complications, and **sudden infant death syndrome (SIDS)** are also to blame. SIDS is the sudden death of a seemingly healthy infant while sleeping. Although researchers still do not entirely understand the phenomenon, they recognize that putting a baby to sleep on its stomach or side increases its risk for the condition. In 1992, public health experts and advocates launched the "Back to Sleep" campaign to encourage parents to place babies on their backs at bedtime. After the first decade of this program, the National Center for Health Statistics noted that SIDS deaths had dropped by more than 50%.[63]

Childbirth

For expectant parents longing to meet their unborn baby, pregnancy and its 40 weeks of waiting can seem like an eternity. Childbirth is a moment they await with anticipation—and sometimes apprehension—knowing that their lives are about to change forever.

Childbirth Options

Pregnant women have many choices about where to give birth, ranging from hospitals to alternative birthing centers to their own home. They must also decide who will be their care provider—e.g. an obstetrician, a certified nurse midwife, or a lay midwife. Some parents-to-be even draft birth plans, documents that spell out their preferences on everything from the use of pain relievers during labor to the number of people they would like in the birthing room.

Even with so many choices, 99% of women still opt to have their baby in a hospital, attended by a physician or certified nurse midwife.[64] Fortunately, many U.S. hospitals today have birthing rooms designed to resemble a bedroom in a home, with comforting wall colors, pictures, a rocking chair, soft lighting, and even music.

Women whose pregnancies are considered high-risk because of their age, health problems, or concerns about the health of the baby may be encouraged to give birth in a medical center that has a neonatal intensive care unit. This is also true of women carrying twins, triplets, or quadruplets.

Labor and Birth

Anywhere from several hours to several days before labor begins, many women experience a discharge of copious, red-tinged mucus commonly called the "bloody show." This mucus plug has been blocking the cervix throughout the pregnancy, protecting it from bacteria and other harmful agents, and its discharge signals that the cervix is beginning to dilate in preparation for labor.

Onset of labor. The precise events signaling the onset of **labor** differ for every woman and every pregnancy. Some women begin to experience regular, mild contractions—caused by the release of a hormone called oxytocin—that become more frequent and intense over several hours. Other women don't experience contractions until their "water breaks"; that is, until the sac holding the amniotic fluid ruptures and amniotic fluid flows out from the vagina. Some women may experience vague abdominal cramps and lower back pain that do not go away. Such symptoms are a sign that a woman is experiencing the first of three stages of the birth process **(Figure 10.12)**.

First stage of labor. First-time mothers spend an average of 12 to 14 hours in labor, although some progress much more quickly and others more slowly.[65] The first stage of labor is the longest: 9 or more hours. Those who have already had one vaginal birth tend to experience a faster first stage during subsequent pregnancies.

During early labor, contractions of the uterus begin to move the fetus toward the birth canal. Contractions also cause the cervix to begin to open—or dilate—and thin out, a process known as *effacement*. Between each contraction, the pain typically abates completely and the woman can rest. If the sac holding the amniotic fluid has not already broken, it may do so now. During active labor, the cervix dilates further and contractions strengthen, lengthen, and become more frequent. Many women request pain medication during this time. The final phase of this first stage of labor is known as **transition.** Amidst strong and prolonged contractions, the cervix dilates to about 10 centimeters, usually large enough for the baby's head to fit through. A woman may begin to feel shaky, sweaty, and weak. Physical and emotional support from care providers and the woman's partner are important during this phase.

Second stage of labor. Once the cervix has dilated to 10 centimeters, the woman will be encouraged to help move the fetus further into the birth canal by actively pushing; that is, bearing down with each contraction. Many women find this stage of labor, which can last an average of 30 minutes to 3 hours, more rewarding than the first stage because they can feel that their efforts help the birth to progress.[65] Others, however, view this as the hardest stage of labor. When the baby's head "crowns," or appears at the vaginal opening, labor is almost over. The woman stops pushing, and after one or two further contractions, the baby is born, slick and sticky from the amniotic fluid. The birth attendant removes mucus and fluid from the newborn's mouth and nose, and dries him or her off with a towel. The umbilical cord, which still attaches the newborn to the placenta, is clamped and cut.

Third stage of labor. Although the baby has been born, the body still has one important task to do: expel the placenta. This is typically accomplished by a few more contractions. The woman continues to bleed, but massaging the abdomen or breast-feeding the newborn can control the bleeding within about 5 to 15 minutes. The final stage of labor is over.[65]

---

transition The final phase of the first stage of labor, characterized by the dilation of the cervix and strong, prolonged contractions.

Apgar score A measurement of how well a newborn tolerated the stresses of birth, as well as how well he or she is adapting to the new environment.

For the baby, the work has just begun. Just one minute after birth, the baby is given its first test, a measurement of how well it tolerated the stresses of birth.[66] This test is known as the APGAR and the resulting score, from 1 to 10, is an **Apgar score.** Babies are assessed on five characteristics: their muscle tone, their heart

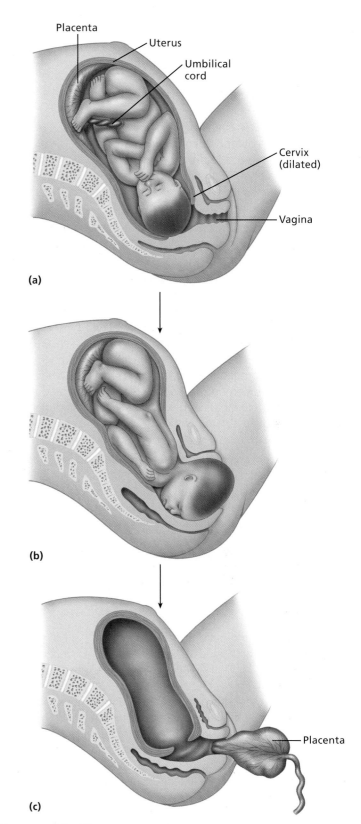

(a)

(b)

(c)

Figure 10.12 Stages of childbirth. (a) The first stage is characterized by cervical dilation and contractions of the uterus that begin to move the baby toward the birth canal. (b) In the second stage, the woman pushes until the baby is born. (c) In the third stage, the placenta is expelled.

rate, their reflexes, their skin coloration, and their breathing. Five minutes after birth, the test is repeated to see if the baby's score has improved. A final score between 7 and 10 is considered normal. Babies who receive a lower rating may need additional medical assistance.

Doctors will also take a sample of blood from the infant's heel to test for hidden disorders that are not always apparent at birth. Rare metabolic disorders such as phenylketonuria, or PKU, can be successfully controlled if detected early, but can cause mental retardation or even death if left undiagnosed.

Cesarean birth. In consultation with their health-care provider, some women decide during pregnancy to give birth via a scheduled **cesarean section** (or C-section).

This surgery involves making an incision through the woman's abdominal and uterine walls in order to deliver the baby. A C-section may be necessary if the mother is experiencing hypertension or another disorder, if the placenta is covering the cervix, or if the fetus is very large or in the wrong position in the birth canal. Also, women who have had a prior C-section may be encouraged to have one during subsequent pregnancies to avoid the small but serious risk of uterine rupture. An emergency C-section may be warranted if labor is not progressing, if the fetus appears to be in distress during labor, or if there is a problem with the umbilical cord or placenta, putting the baby's life in jeopardy.

The rate of C-sections doubled between 1996 and 2006, according to national statistics.[67] Nearly one in three babies, 31.1%, are now delivered via C-section, a statistic that has troubled critics, some of whom argue that the increase is caused by financial incentives and fear of malpractice suits rather than concern for the patients. Although the surgery is relatively safe, it has a higher rate of complications and involves a longer recovery time for mothers than a vaginal birth.

Infertility

Many couples attempt to get pregnant only to find that it is not always easy to do. An estimated 12% of couples in the United States—including 7.3 million American women—experience **infertility,** or the inability to conceive after trying for one year.[68] The problem becomes more prevalent with age, and so doctors recommend that a woman in her 30s get checked for underlying health issues if she has been trying unsuccessfully to get pregnant for more than 6 months. Doctors will also examine her partner, as infertility can be due to a low sperm count or other factors involving the male. Fortunately, there are many treatment options available, and about two-thirds of couples who have difficulty conceiving ultimately go on to have their own biological children.[69]

Causes of Infertility

Roughly one-third of infertility cases are due to health problems in the woman; another third are due to problems in the man, and the final third are either caused by problems in both partners or simply cannot be explained.[69]

cesarean section (C-section) A surgical procedure involving the incision of a woman's abdominal and uterine walls in order to deliver the baby.

infertility The inability to conceive after trying for at least a year.

For women, the most common causes of infertility are:

- A failure of ovulation prompted by hormonal problems, advanced age, premature menopause, or scarred ovaries.
- Blocked fallopian tubes, stemming from a prior ectopic pregnancy, surgery, or, most commonly, an untreated sexually transmitted infection such as chlamydia or gonorrhea that caused scarring in the fallopian tubes and/or progressed into pelvic inflammatory disease (PID). Endometriosis, discussed earlier, also can block the tubes.
- A deformed uterus, which can not only cause infertility but may lead to miscarriage.
- Uterine fibroids and other noncancerous growths, which can obstruct both the uterus and the fallopian tubes.

The most common causes of infertility in men include:

- A low sperm count, defined as less than 10 million sperm per milliliter of semen. This can be caused by smoking cigarettes or marijuana.
- Incorrectly formed sperm, which are not able to penetrate the egg.
- Poor sperm motility, or the inability of sperm to move quickly and effectively.
- Prior infection. Contracting mumps during adulthood is a common culprit. Sexually transmitted infections such as gonorrhea can also cause scarring that hinders sperm movement.
- Environmental exposure to pesticides, lead, and other substances that disrupt hormones in the body.

Options for Infertile Couples

The type of medical treatment ultimately used by couples to get pregnant depends to a large degree on the root cause of their troubles. Options for infertile couples include:

- Surgery to repair blocked fallopian tubes, remove scarring or uterine growths, and treat endometriosis in women. Occasionally, surgery may be indicated if there is a problem with a man's sperm.
- Fertility drugs, which promote ovulation in women. Side effects can include headaches, nausea, hot flashes, and breast tenderness. Because the medications can spur the body to release more than one egg at a time, couples using fertility drugs have a higher chance of having twins, triplets, or quadruplets.
- Intrauterine insemination, to boost the odds that an egg will be fertilized. Sperm are collected from a woman's partner or a donor and processed in a laboratory, enabling a higher concentration of sperm to be injected into the vagina or uterus through a syringe.
- *In vitro fertilization (IVF),* a procedure that dramatically transformed the field of fertility treatment when the first "test-tube baby" was born in 1978. Egg and sperm are retrieved from a woman and a man and combined in a laboratory dish (*in vitro* means "in glass"), where fertilization may occur. If eggs do become fertilized, they are implanted in the uterus. When multiple eggs are transferred, multiple births may occur.

- *Gamete intrafallopian transfer (GIFT)*, a process similar to IVF. The egg is not fertilized in a laboratory, however. Instead, sperm and several eggs are placed in a woman's fallopian tube. There is no guarantee, though, that the sperm will penetrate at least one of the eggs.
- *Zygote intrafallopian transfer (ZIFT)*, fertilization of an egg or eggs in a laboratory setting. Unlike IVF, however, the fertilized eggs are transferred to a fallopian tube rather than the uterus.
- *Intracytoplasmic sperm injection (ICSI)*, the direct injection of a single sperm into an egg. The fertilized egg is then implanted in the uterus through normal IVF technology. ICSI may be considered when men have low sperm counts or when fertilization failed to occur in previous IVF attempts.
- Surrogate motherhood, which requires an agreement with a third party—a fertile woman—to carry a pregnancy to term. In some cases the surrogate's egg is fertilized through intrauterine insemination with the prospective father's sperm. In other cases, she is impregnated through IVF with the couple's embryo. The woman is paid for her service to the couple, and immediately following the baby's birth, she relinquishes the infant to them.

Not all couples choose medical treatment. Many opt for adoption, either domestically or internationally. In 2008, there were 55,000 adoptions in the United States involving public child-welfare agencies.[70] Statistics on adoptions involving private agencies do not have to be reported by states and are therefore not available. The adoption experience can be as satisfying to parents as pregnancy and childbirth. It can also cost less—or much more. Adoptions from foster-care agencies typically cost very little or are free of charge. Domestic adoptions using private agencies can cost several thousand dollars, and costs for international adoptions can reach $30,000 or more and take several years to be approved. Not all couples that want to adopt a baby are successful.

Prevention remains one of the best options for infertility. Although many couples in their late teens and early 20s are more interested in *avoiding* pregnancy, steps should be taken to preserve fertility for the years to come. Practicing safe sex can reduce the spread of sexually transmitted infections, which are often the cause of fertility problems. Getting timely treatment for a sexually transmitted infection is also important. Because fertility drops and the risk of birth defects and miscarriages rises when a woman is in her 30s, couples who want to have a child are encouraged to start their family planning before the woman turns 35.

Watch videos of real students discussing sexuality, contraception, and reproductive choices at www.pearsonhighered.com/choosinghealth.

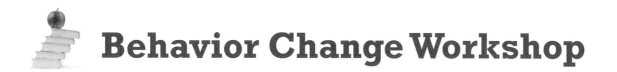

Behavior Change Workshop

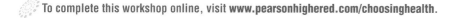 To complete this workshop online, visit **www.pearsonhighered.com/choosinghealth.**

Consider the facts about sex and excessive drinking on campus:

- Approximately 70% of college students have engaged in sexual activity primarily because they had been drinking and indicate that they wouldn't have done so had they been sober.
- Twenty percent of the college students who use safer sex practices when they are sober abandon them when they are intoxicated.
- Up to 60% of college women who contract STIs report that they were intoxicated at the time they were infected.
- More than half of female students and three-quarters of male students involved in acquaintance rape admit that they were intoxicated at the time of the incident.

Data from "Facts on Tap," www.factsontap.org/factsontap/risky/the_facts.htm.

If you have sex while intoxicated, especially with a first-time partner, you may be putting yourself at considerable risk.

Part I. Identify Emotional or Situational "Triggers"

1. What are your top five "triggers"? Think back on past situations when you had sex while drinking. What particular factors or emotions provoked that situation?

_____

_____

_____

_____

_____

2. Target one of the above triggers. Ask yourself honestly: How ready are you to commit to a behavior change that will help you deal with that trigger in a way that doesn't result in having sex while intoxicated? What stage of behavior change are you in?

Target trigger: _____

_____

Current stage of behavior change: _____

_____

Part II. Take Action

1. Assuming you are truly committed to changing your behavior, describe what you might do to deal with your target trigger instead of resorting to having sex while intoxicated.

Next step: _____

_____

Example: Instead of drinking before I have sex with a new partner, I will commit to getting to know them first. Consequently, I will be less likely to feel anxiety, embarrassment or guilt and to resort to alcohol to deal with these feelings.

Next step: _____

_____

_____

_____

2. Describe how you will fight the temptation to have sex while intoxicated.

_____

_____

_____

_____

● Chapter Summary

- Good sexual health requires knowledge, effort, and appropriate medical care.
- Male and female sexual anatomy includes both external and internal organs. Among the female organs are the paired ovaries, one of which releases an egg cell monthly, and the uterus, where a fertilized egg implants and grows. Among the male organs are the paired testes, which constantly manufacture sperm—the male reproductive cells—which travel through a series of ducts to contribute to the man's semen.
- The menstrual cycle is an approximately monthly series of events in a nonpregnant woman of childbearing age. These events, which include the buildup and shedding of the uterine lining, are controlled by hormones, which simultaneously coordinate the maturation and release of an egg cell from a woman's ovary.
- The sexual response cycle consists of a series of phases from arousal to orgasm to resolution.
- Sexual dysfunction is fairly prevalent in the United States, with a sizable portion of men and women having difficulty enjoying sex at some point in their lives.
- Abstinence is the avoidance of sexual intercourse.

- Sexual behavior includes much more than just sexual intercourse, with hugging, kissing, masturbation, and other forms of non-intercourse sexual activity all being a healthy part of a sexually active lifestyle.
- About half of all pregnancies in the United States are unplanned, despite the wide variety of contraceptive options available.
- Among the choices in contraceptive methods, only male and female condoms provide protection against sexually transmitted infections.
- Pregnancy involves three trimesters, each with unique stages of development for a fetus and physical effects for the mother.
- Women planning a pregnancy need preconception health care.
- Regular prenatal care can lead to a healthier pregnancy and a healthier baby.
- The first stage of labor is characterized by uterine contractions and cervical dilation. The fetus descends into the birth canal. During the second stage, the woman bears down with each contraction until the baby is born. The third stage of labor is expulsion of the placenta.
- Fertility declines with increasing age. Males and females have about an equal rate of infertility.

● Test Your Knowledge

1. What is a woman's first period called?
   a. menstruation
   b. ovulation
   c. menarche
   d. menopause

2. Which of the following is/are not part of the internal male genitals?
   a. glans penis
   b. epididymis
   c. vas deferens
   d. testes

3. What is the name for the last phase of the sexual response cycle?
   a. finality
   b. resolution

   c. conclusion
   d. climax

4. What is a transgendered individual?
   a. a person whose assigned sex differs from the gender he or she identifies with
   b. a person born with both male and female genitalia
   c. a person who is about equally attracted to both males and females
   d. a person who is only attracted to people of the opposite sex

5. Where must a fertilized egg implant in order to survive and thrive?
   a. ovary
   b. fallopian tube
   c. endometrium
   d. cervix

6. Of the following methods of birth control, which provide(s) protection against sexually transmitted infection?
   a. diaphragm
   b. female condom
   c. cervical sponge
   d. spermicides

7. What is the average annual percentage of unplanned pregnancies in the United States?
   a. 20%
   b. 30%
   c. 40%
   d. 50%

8. What is the approximate chance of getting pregnant in any given month for young, healthy couples who are having unprotected sex?
   a. 5%
   b. 10%
   c. 20%
   d. 30%

9. What is the developing baby called after the first 8 weeks of a pregnancy?
   a. embryo
   b. blastocyst
   c. fetus
   d. zygote

10. Which of the following is not an infertility treatment?
    a. ZIFT
    b. ICSI
    c. GIFT
    d. PIXY

Get Critical

What happened:

On September 22, 2010, 18-year-old Tyler Clementi leapt to his death from the George Washington bridge connecting New York and New Jersey. Clementi, a talented violinist, was a freshman at Rutgers University. Shortly before his death, Clementi learned that two of his classmates had secretly videotaped him having a sexual encounter with another man and streamed live footage of the encounter over the internet. The case received national attention, sparking debates about online privacy, the social pressures felt by gay teens, and whether Clementi's classmates' actions should be considered a hate crime.

What do you think?

- What can communities do to provide more support for gay, bisexual or questioning teens?
- Do you consider Clementi's classmates' filming and streaming of Clementi's private life a hate crime? Why or why not?

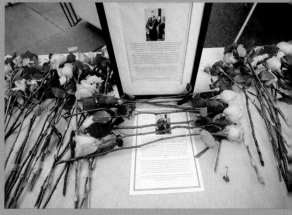
A memorial for Tyler Clementi.

Get Connected

References

i. American College Health Association. (2009). *American College Health Association National College Health Assessment (ACHA-NCHA II) reference group executive summary, Fall 2009*. Retrieved from www .acha-ncha.org/docs/ACHA-NCHA_ Reference_Group_ExecutiveSummary_ Fall2009.pdf

ii. National Campaign to Prevent Teen and Unplanned Pregnancy and CosmoGirl.com. (2009). *Sex and tech: Results from a survey of teens and young adults*. Retrieved from http://www.thenationalcampaign.org/sextech/ PDF/SexTech_Summary.pdf

iii. National Campaign to Prevent Teen and Unplanned Pregnancy. (2010). *National data*. Retrieved from http://www .thenationalcampaign.org/national-data/ default.aspx

1. American College Health Association. (2009). *American College Health Association National College Health Assessment (ACHA-NCHA II) reference group executive summary, Fall 2009*. Retrieved from http://www .acha-ncha.org/docs/ACHA-NCHA_ Reference_Group_ExecutiveSummary_ Fall2009.pdf

2. American Cancer Society. (2010). *Learn about cancer: Cervical cancer*. Retrieved

from http://www.cancer.org/Cancer/ CervicalCancer/DetailedGuide/ cervical-cancer-risk-factors

3. National Cancer Institute. (2008). *What you need to know about prostate cancer*. Retrieved from http://www.cancer.gov/ cancertopics/wyntk/prostate/page4

4. National Women's Health Information Center. (2009). *Menstruation and the menstrual cycle*. Retrieved from: http://www .womenshealth.gov/faq/menstruation.cfm#f

5. American Congress of Obstetricians and Gynecologists. (2008). *Premenstrual syndrome*. Retrieved from http://www.acog.org/ publications/patient_education/bp057.cfm

6. Dickerson, L. M., Mazyck, P. J., & Hunter, M. H. (2003). Premenstrual syndrome. *American Family Physician, 67*(8), 1743–1752. Retrieved from http://www.aafp.org/ afp/20030415/1743.html

7. National Women's Health Information Center. (2010). *Premenstrual syndrome frequently asked questions*. Retrieved from http://www.womenshealth.gov/faq/ premenstrual-syndrome.cfm

8. National Women's Health Information Center. (2008). *Premenstrual syndrome frequently asked questions*. Retrieved from http://www.womenshealth.gov/faq/ premenstrual-syndrome.cfm

9. American Congress of Obstetricians and Gynecologists. (2006). *Dysmenorrhea.* Retrieved from: http://www.acog.org/publications/patient_education/bp046.cfm

10. French, L. (2005). Dysmenorrhea. *American Family Physician, 71*(2), 285–291.

11. American Congress of Obstetricians and Gynecologists. (2008). Endometriosis. Retrieved from http://www.acog.org/publications/patient_education/bp013.cfm

12. National Women's Health Information Center. (2009). *Menstruation and the menstrual cycle.* Retrieved from http://www.womenshealth.gov/faq/menstruation.cfm#e

13. Farley, D. (1991). On the teen scene: TSS—Reducing the risks. *FDA Consumer,* October 1991.

14. Masters, W. H., & Johnson, V. E. (1966). *Human sexual response,* 1st ed. New York: Bantam.

15. American Society for Reproductive Medicine. (2008). *Patient fact sheet: Sexual dysfunction and infertility.* Retrieved from http://www.asrm.org/FactSheetsandBooklets

16. MedlinePlus. (2010). *Female sexual dysfunction.* Retrieved from http://www.nlm.nih.gov/medlineplus/sexualproblemsinwomen.html

17. Mayo Foundation for Medical Education and Research. (2009). *Painful intercourse (dyspareunia).* Retrieved from http://www.mayoclinic.com/health/painful-intercourse/DS01044

18. Mayo Foundation for Medical Education and Research. (2009). *Low sex drive in women.* Retrieved from http://www.mayoclinic.com/health/low-sex-drive-in-women/DS01043

19. Mayo Foundation for Medical Education and Research. (2009). *Anorgasmia.* Retrieved from http://www.mayoclinic.com/health/anorgasmia/DS01051/DSECTION=symptoms

20. National Kidney and Urologic Diseases Information Clearinghouse. (2005). *Erectile dysfunction* (NIH Publication No. 06-3923). Retrieved from http://kidney.niddk.nih.gov/kudiseases/pubs/impotence

21. MedlinePlus. (2008). *Premature ejaculation.* Retrieved from http://www.nlm.nih.gov/medlineplus/ency/article/001524.htm

22. Mayo Foundation for Medical Education and Research. (2009). *Premature ejaculation.* Retrieved from http://www.mayoclinic.com/health/premature-ejaculation/DS00578/DSECTION=alternative%2Dmedicine

23. Rosenbaum, J. E. (2009). Patient Teenagers? A comparison of the sexual behavior of virginity pledgers and matched nonpledgers. *Pediatrics, 123*(1), 110–120.

24. Higgins, J. A., Trussell, J., Moore, N. B., & Davidson, J. K. (2010). Young adult sexual health: Current and prior sexual behaviours among non-Hispanic white U.S. college students. *Sexual Health, 7*(1), 35–43.

25. National Campaign to Prevent Teen and Unplanned Pregnancy and CosmoGirl.com. (2009). *Sex and tech: Results from a survey of teens and young adults.* Retrieved from http://www.thenationalcampaign.org/sextech

26. Lenhart, A. (2009). *Teens and sexting.* Retrieved from http://www.pewinternet.org/Reports/2009/Teens-and-Sexting.aspx

27. Newman, A. (2010. March 23). Senate passes Arizona sexting law. *Arizona Daily Wildcat.* Retrieved from http://wildcat.arizona.edu/news/senate-passes-arizona-sexting-law-1.1276167

28. Brigham Young University. (2010). *National pornography statistics.* Retrieved from https://wsr.byu.edu/content/national-pornography-statistics

29. O'Reilly, S., Knox, D., & Zusman, M. E. (2007, June). College student attitudes toward pornography use. *College Student Journal,* (41), 402–404.

30. Jaishankar, K. (2009, January–June). Editorial: Sexting: A new form of victimless crime? *International Journal of Cyber Criminology, 3*(1), 21–25.

31. Centers for Disease Control and Prevention. (2009). Key statistics from the National Survey of Family Growth. Retrieved from http://www.cdc.gov/nchs/nsfg/abc_list_s.htm

32. American Pregnancy Association. (2010). *Statistics.* Retrieved from http://www.americanpregnancy.org/main/statistics.html

33. Pew Research Center. (2009). *Majority continues to support civil unions.* Retrieved from http://pewforum.org/Gay-Marriage-and-Homosexuality/Majority-Continues-To-Support-Civil-Unions.aspx#4

34. Joyce, A. (2006, June 30). Majority of large firms offer employees domestic partner benefits. *Washington Post.* Retrieved from http://www.washingtonpost.com/wp-dyn/content/article/2006/06/29/AR2006062902049.html

35. Massachusetts Department of Education. (2001). *2001 Massachusetts Youth Risk Behavior Survey results.* Retrieved from http://www.doe.mass.edu/cnp/hprograms/yrbs/01/results.pdf

36. Kosciw, J. G. (2004). *The 2003 National School Climate Survey: The school-related experiences of our nation's lesbian, gay, bisexual and transgender youth.* New York: GLSEN.

37. Federal Bureau of Investigation. (2009). *2008 hate crime statistics.* Retrieved from http://www.fbi.gov/ucr/hc2008/data/table_01.html

38. Diamond, L. M. (2008). Female bisexuality from adolescence to adulthood: Results from a 10-year longitudinal study. *Developmental Psychology, 44*(1), 5–14.

39. American Psychological Association. (2010). *Answers to your questions about transgendered individuals and gender identity.* Retrieved from http://www.apa.org/topics/sexuality/transgender.aspx

40. McGuire, L. (2010). *New emergency contraceptive.* Mayo Foundation for Medical Education and Research. Retrieved from: http://www.mayoclinic.com/health/emergency-contraceptive/MY01365

41. Mayo Foundation for Medical Education and Research. (2010*). ParaGard (copper IUD).* Retrieved from http://www.mayoclinic.com/health/paragard/MY00997/DSECTION=risks

42. Mayo Foundation for Medical Education and Research. (2010). *Mirena (hormonal IUD).* Retrieved from http://www.mayoclinic.com/health/mirena/MY00998

43. Mayo Foundation for Medical Education and Research. (2010). *Birth control pill FAQ: Benefits, risks and choices.* Retrieved from http://www.mayoclinic.com/health/birth-control-pill/WO00098/NSECTIONGROUP=2

44. Mayo Foundation for Medical Education and Research. (2009). *Vasectomy: Risks.* Retrieved from http://www.mayoclinic.com/health/vasectomy/MY00483/DSECTION=risks

45. National Campaign to Prevent Teen and Unplanned Pregnancy. (2010). *National data.* Retrieved from http://www.thenationalcampaign.org/national-data/default.aspx

46. National Campaign to Prevent Teen and Unplanned Pregnancy. (2008). Policy Brief: Thoughts for Elected Officials About Teen and Unplanned Pregnancy. Retrieved from http://www.thenationalcampaign.org/resources/pdf/Briefly_PolicyBrief_Thoughts_Elected_Officials.pdf

47. Guttmacher Institute. (2008). *U.S. abortion rate continues long-term decline.* Retrieved from http://www.guttmacher.org/media/nr/2008/01/17/index.html

48. World Health Organization. (2006). *Frequently asked clinical questions about medical abortion.* Retrieved from http://whqlibdoc.who.int/publications/2006/9241594845_eng.pdf

49. Jones, R. K., Zolna, M. R. S., Henshaw, S. K., & Finer, L. B. (2008). Abortion in the United States: Incidence and access to services, 2005. *Perspectives on Sexual and Reproductive Health, 40*(1), 6–16.

50. Hakim-Elahi, E., Tovell, H. M. M., & Burnhill, M. S. (1990). Complications of first-trimester abortion: A report of 170,000 cases. *Obstetrics & Gynecology, 76,* 129–135.

51. Gamble, S. B., Strauss, L. T., Parker, W. Y., Cook, D. A., Zane, S. B., & Hamdan, S. (2007). Abortion surveillance—United States, 2004. *Morbidity and Mortality Weekly Report Surveillance Summaries, 56*(9), 1–33.

52. American Psychological Association, Task Force on Mental Health and Abortion. (2008). *Report of the APA Task Force on Mental Health and Abortion.* Washington, DC: American Psychological Association. Retrieved from http://www.apa.org/pi/wpo/mental-health-abortion-report.pdf

53. American Congress of Obstetricians and Gynecologists. (2007). *Treating infertility.* Retrieved from http://www.acog.org/publications/patient_education/bp137.cfm

54. Cole, L. (2004). Accuracy of home pregnancy tests at the time of missed menses. *American Journal of Obstetrics and Gynecology, 190*(1), 100–105.

55. U.S. Department of Health and Human Services, Health Resources and Services Administration, Maternal and Child Health Bureau. (2009). *A healthy start: Begin before baby's born.* Retrieved from http://mchb.hrsa.gov/programs/womeninfants/prenatal.htm

56. Tenore, J. L. (2000). Ectopic pregnancy. *American Family Physician, 61*(4), 1080–1088.

57. Centers for Disease Control and Prevention. (1995). Ectopic pregnancy—United States, 1990–1992. *Morbidity and Mortality Weekly Report, 44,* 46–48.

58. March of Dimes. (2009). *Miscarriage.* Retrieved from http://www.marchofdimes.com/professionals/14332_1192.asp

59. American Congress of Obstetricians and Gynecologists. (2004). *High blood pressure during pregnancy.* Retrieved from http://www.acog.org/publications/patient_education/bp034.cfm

60. Wagner, L. K. (2004). Diagnosis and management of preeclampsia. *American Family Physician, 70*(12), 2317–2324.

61. Martin, J. A., Hamilton, B. E., Sutton, P. D., Ventura, S. J., Menacker, F., Kirmeyer, S., & Munson, M. L. (2007). Births: Final data for 2005. *National Vital Statistics Reports, 56*(6), 1–103.

62. World Bank. (2010). *Mortality rate, infant (per 1,000 live births).* Retrieved from http://data.worldbank.org/indicator/SP.DYN.IMRT.IN

63. U.S. Department of Health and Human Services. (2004). *Birth, infant mortality, and life expectancy, 1980–2002.* Retrieved from http://www.hhs-stat.net/scripts/topic.cfm?id=738

64. Martin, J. A., Hamilton, B. E., Sutton, P. D., Ventura, S. J., Menacker, F., Kirmeyer, S., & Munson, M. L. (2007). Births: Final data for 2005. *National Vital Statistics Reports, 56*(6), 1–104. Retrieved from http://www.cdc.gov/nchs/data/nvsr/nvsr56/nvsr56_06.pdf

65. American Congress of Obstetricians and Gynecologists. (2007). *You and your baby: Prenatal care, labor and delivery, and post-partum care.* Retrieved from http://www.acog.org/publications/patient_education/ab005.cfm

66. MedlinePlus. (2009). *APGAR.* Retrieved from http://www.nlm.nih.gov/medlineplus/ency/article/003402.htm

67. Martin, J. A., Hamilton, B. E., Sutton, P. D., Ventura, S. J., Menacker, F., Kirmeyer, S., & Mathews, T. J. (2009). Births: Final data for 2006. *National Vital Statistics Reports, 57*(7), 1–104. Retrieved January 17, 2009, from http://www.cdc.gov/nchs/data/nvsr/nvsr57/nvsr57_07.pdf

68. Centers for Disease Control and Prevention. (2002). *National Survey of Family Growth.* Retrieved from http://www.cdc.gov/nchs/nsfg/abc_list_i.htm#infertility

69. MedlinePlus. (2009). *Infertility.* Retrieved from http://www.nlm.nih.gov/medlineplus/infertility.html

70. U.S. Department of Health and Human Services, Administration for Children & Families. (2009). *Trends in foster care and adoption—FY 2002–FY 2008.* Retrieved from http://www.acf.hhs.gov/programs/cb/stats_research/afcars/trends.htm

71. Phoenix House. (n.d.). *Facts on Tap: Just the Frightening Facts, Ma'am.* Retrieved from http://www.factsontap.org/factsontap/risky/the_facts.htm

11

- Each year in the U.S. 5%–20% of the population gets the seasonal flu, resulting in 200,000 hospitalizations and, on average, 36,000 deaths.[i]

- About 19 million people in the U.S. are infected each year with a sexually transmitted infection and almost half occur in young people aged 15–24.[ii]

- Approximately 25% of the people in the United States infected with HIV do not realize it.[iii]

Preventing Infectious Diseases and Sexually Transmitted Infections

LEARNING OBJECTIVES

IDENTIFY the causes of infectious diseases and recognize how they are transmitted.

DESCRIBE how the body's immune response works against infections.

UNDERSTAND how immunization prevents infectious disease, both in individuals and in communities.

DISCUSS the most common infectious diseases, how they affect the body, and how they can be treated.

LIST common sexually transmitted infections (STIs), their causes, risk factors, symptoms, and treatment.

UNDERSTAND how to prevent infectious diseases and sexually transmitted infections.

 Health Online icons are found throughout the chapter, directing you to web links, videos, podcasts, and other useful online resources.

The air we breathe, the food we eat, and even everyday items we handle constantly—

like door handles and cell phones—carry tiny microorganisms. They may be small, but microorganisms have a large impact on human health. Some of these microbes are harmless or even helpful, but others are capable of causing disease. Millions of people die each year from infectious diseases such as influenza, malaria, tuberculosis, and acquired immunodeficiency syndrome (AIDS).

Knowing how to protect yourself from infection is critical to your health. This chapter will help you understand what causes infections, how they spread, and how your body defends itself. We will discuss common infectious diseases and their symptoms and treatments. Finally, the chapter will cover the human immunodeficiency virus (HIV) and other sexually transmitted infections (STIs), and walk you through the steps of how to protect yourself from these types of infection.

How Are Infections Spread?

Despite our best intentions to stay free of illness, it is impossible to make it to adulthood without ever having battled an infection. An **infection** is an invasion of body tissues by microorganisms that use the body's environment to multiply. In the process, these organisms damage and weaken the body and make us sick.

Pathogens are agents that cause disease. Common pathogens are harmful bacteria, viruses, fungi, protozoa, and parasitic worms. The natural environment for any particular pathogen, where it accumulates in large numbers, is called a **reservoir.** Pathogens move from a reservoir to a **host**—a person, plant, or animal in which or on which they can live and reproduce. The mode of transmission, or the way a pathogen moves from reservoir to host or from host to host, depends on the pathogen. Some of the ways infections are transmitted include:

Direct Transmission

- **Contact with infected people.** Close person-to-person contact with someone who has an infection is a common mode of disease transmission. Even if a person does not have any symptoms, he or she can still be infectious and considered a **carrier.** Many infections are spread sexually or even through simple touch. Contact with blood, saliva, or other bodily fluids can directly transmit infection from one person to another as well. Follow safe sex practices, avoid kissing sick people or direct contact with blood, and thoroughly wash your hands often to reduce your risk of infection. See the **Spotlight** on page 246 for tips on hand washing and hand sanitizer use.

infection The invasion of body tissues by microorganisms that use the body's environment to multiply and cause disease.

pathogen An agent that causes disease.

reservoir The natural environment for any particular pathogen, where it accumulates in large numbers.

host A person, plant, or animal in which or on which pathogens live and reproduce.

carrier A person infected with a pathogen who does not show symptoms but who is infectious.

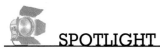
Hand Washing and Hand Sanitizers

Keeping your hands clean is one of the best ways to prevent infections. The most effective method is to wash your hands with soap and water. Be sure to wash them thoroughly and frequently, especially during cold and flu season. Wet your hands with running water, lather up to your wrists with soap, and scrub for at least 20 seconds. Dry your hands on a clean towel or disposable paper towel.

You do not need to use antibacterial soap when washing your hands; regular soap is just as effective, and antibacterial soaps can lead to antibiotic resistance (discussed later in the chapter).[1]

Unlike antibacterial soaps, alcohol-based hand sanitizers will not cause antibiotic resistance. If you don't have access to a sink, using hand sanitizer that contains at least 60% alcohol is a good backup. When using a hand sanitizer, apply enough to wet your hands completely and rub them together until dry. If your hands are ever visibly dirty, however, you should opt for hand washing instead.

You should clean your hands:

- before and after handling food, eating, treating wounds, or touching a sick person.
- after using the toilet, changing a diaper, touching an animal or animal waste, blowing your nose, coughing, sneezing, or handling garbage or anything that could be contaminated with dirt or germs.

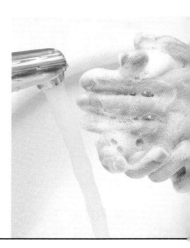

*Reference:*1. *Hand Washing: Do's and Don'ts* by Mayo Clinic staff, 2009, retrieved from http://www.mayoclinic.com/health/hand-washing/HQ00407.

- **Contact with infected animals.** The recent outbreaks of avian influenza showed us that people living and working closely with certain animals can risk catching infections from them. The CDC estimates that approximately 60% of human pathogens originated in animals and that 75% of emerging diseases involve transference from animals to humans.[1] It doesn't take an exotic animal to spread disease either. Pets can carry rabies, meningitis, salmonella, or other infections that can be passed on to humans. Vaccinating your pets, washing your hands after handling animals, and avoiding contact with animal feces greatly reduce the risks of transmission.

Indirect Transmission:

- **Touching contaminated objects.** If you have an infection and then cough or sneeze on an object—or touch it with your dirty hands—you leave pathogens behind for the next unwitting person to pick up. Some bacteria can survive on solid surfaces for days.[2] Telephones, doorknobs, steering wheels, and computer keyboards are common hotspots for infectious microorganisms. Touching a contaminated object, then touching your mouth, nose, or eyes, can move pathogens into your body. Think twice before sharing cups, straws, utensils, and toothbrushes with others. Wash your hands and disinfect your cell phone, keyboard, or dorm room doorknob from time to time.

- **Breathing airborne pathogens.** When you cough and sneeze, tiny droplets of mucus tainted with pathogens waft in the air, which can be inhaled by another person. Viruses and bacteria that cause colds, influenza, and tuberculosis are commonly spread in this manner.

- **Bites from infected insects.** Pathogens can hitch a ride to a host onboard a **vector,** an animal or insect that transports pathogens from one point to another. A classic example of a vector is the mosquito, which transmits the malaria parasite and the West Nile virus. Other examples include deer ticks, which transport the bacteria that cause Lyme disease, and fleas, which are the vector for the plague. Protecting yourself from insect bites is one way to protect yourself from infectious disease.

- **Drinking or eating contaminated water or food.** Viruses, protozoa, and bacteria from animal or human feces can get into lakes, rivers, oceans, swimming pools, hot tubs, water slides, and public fountains. Chlorine can help kill pathogens, but not entirely. Avoid swallowing water while in pools or other bodies of water and stay out of them whenever you have diarrhea. When traveling in foreign countries that may lack reliable sources of clean water, opt for bottled water, even when brushing your teeth. Food can also become contaminated with pathogens when handled or processed in unsanitary ways.

Protecting Against Infections

Your body is not defenseless against infectious microorganisms. Even if you are exposed to pathogens, your body's defenses may protect you.

The Body's First Line of Defense

One of the most powerful barriers between you and pathogens is your skin. Your skin keeps the millions of bacteria that live on it from entering your body. Breaches can occur, however, if you get a cut, bad scrape, or puncture wound—one of the reasons why doctors encourage you to thoroughly cleanse and cover a wound immediately after sustaining it.

Skin doesn't shield your entire body, of course. Openings such as your mouth and nose need other forms of protection. Mucous membranes line the mouth, airways, vagina, and digestive tract, trapping many unwanted microorganisms. *Cilia,* tiny hairlike projections, line the airways and help sweep away tiny pathogens. Bodily fluids such as saliva, tears, earwax, vaginal fluid, and digestive acid trap and kill or expel many potential invaders. Coughing, sneezing, vomiting, and diarrhea are other ways the body expels foreign intruders.

vector An animal or insect that transports pathogens from one point to another.

If any of the systems that provide these first defenses becomes damaged, for instance if your skin is severely burned or your cilia are damaged from smoking, you become more susceptible to infection. Even with healthy first defenses, however, pathogens can occasionally enter your body and infect you, at which point your immune response kicks in.

The Body's Immune Response

The **immune system** is the set of your body's cellular and chemical defenses against pathogens. Key players in the immune system are white blood cells, which patrol the circulatory system and body tissues looking for microscopic enemies **(Figure 11.1).**

Nonspecific Response

Some white blood cells respond to a broad range of foreign invaders and attack and destroy them, in what is called a *nonspecific response*. These cells are neutrophils, natural killer (NK) cells, and macrophages. Neutrophils, the most common type of white blood cells, conquer bacteria and other foreign invaders traveling in the blood by ingesting and destroying them. NK cells eliminate body cells that are infected by viruses. Macrophages survey our tissues and gobble up bacteria and wounded and dead cells.

Another essential component of nonspecific response is the **inflammatory response.** If body tissue is damaged, the inflammatory response kicks in. Neutrophils and macrophages migrate to the area of damage. They release chemical signals, called cytokines, which attract additional white blood cells to the location, increase blood flow to the area (promoting the delivery of immune cells), and induce fever. This response is designed to kill any pathogens that reside in the damaged tissue, promote healing, and prevent the spread of infection to other parts of the body.

immune system Your body's cellular and chemical defenses against pathogens.

inflammatory response A response to damaged body tissues designed to kill any pathogens in the damaged tissue, promote healing, and prevent the spread of infection to other parts of the body.

antigen Tiny regions on the surface of an infectious agent that can be detected by B cells and T cells.

antibodies Proteins released by B cells that bind tightly to infectious agents and mark them for destruction.

acquired immunity The body's ability to quickly identify and attack a pathogen that it recognizes from previous exposure. In some cases acquired immunity leads to life-long protection against the same infection.

Specific Response

Other white blood cell types, the lymphocytes, mount a *specific response* in which they recognize and attack specific pathogens. The lymphocytes consist of B cells and T cells and are mostly found in the body's lymph fluid, lymph nodes, and other lymph organs such as the spleen. Both B cells and T cells bear surface receptors that detect **antigens,** tiny regions on the surface of a pathogen.

In response to an antigen, B cells release **antibodies,** proteins that bind tightly to invaders and mark them for destruction. In fact, the term *antigen* is a contraction of *anti*body-*gen*erator. Antibodies are highly specialized, with each type targeting only one specific antigen, just as a key will only fit one lock.

How T cells respond to an antigen depends on the T cell

STUDENT STORY

How I Avoid Infections

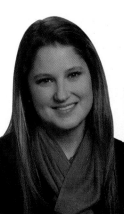

"Hi, I'm Jessica. As a germaphobe, I'm constantly sanitizing my hands after touching doorknobs, ATMs, or anything in a store. I absolutely have to keep clean everywhere I go. I always have little hand sanitizer bottles in my bag, and I have a gigantic one in my room. I use it when I don't have access to a sink to wash my hands. It's really easy just to dab some on your hand and just go and it's quick. I also get the seasonal flu vaccine every year.

Living on campus, you're always around people and touching everything everyone else touches. Your chance of getting sick is always way higher than if you were to live on your own somewhere. So I'm just really careful to keep my hands clean—it's the best solution to prevent getting a cold every other week."

1: Will using hand sanitizer and getting a flu vaccine prevent Jessica from getting all infections? What other ways might Jessica get an infection?

2: Do you think Jessica is right that living on campus increases your chances of getting sick? Why?

Do you have a story similar to Jessica's? Share your story at **www.pearsonhighered.com/choosinghealth.**

type. There are three types of T cells. Cytotoxic T cells (CD8 T cells) kill virus-infected cells. Helper T cells (CD4 T cells) secrete cytokines that help activate B cells, cytotoxic T cells, and NK cells. Regulatory T cells help turn down the specific immune response once the infection is under control.

The antigen-activated B cells and T cells also create long-lived *memory B cells* and *memory T cells*. These cells stay in the body and quickly identify and attack that specific pathogen should it enter the body again in the future. This is why successfully defeating an infection leaves us with **acquired immunity,** which in some cases leads to life-long protection against the same infection. For example, if you have ever had chicken pox, you are unlikely to get it again.

Immunization

Acquired immunity can protect you against infections that your immune system recognizes, but what about diseases that your body has never seen before? In the past, the primary way people developed immunity was by contracting a disease and surviving it, a process known as *naturally acquired immunity*. Many diseases such as polio, whooping cough, measles, mumps, and rubella commonly killed or crippled victims before their bodies could fight them off. Widespread adoption of immunizations turned that tide. The advent of immunizations has been recognized as one of the most monumental

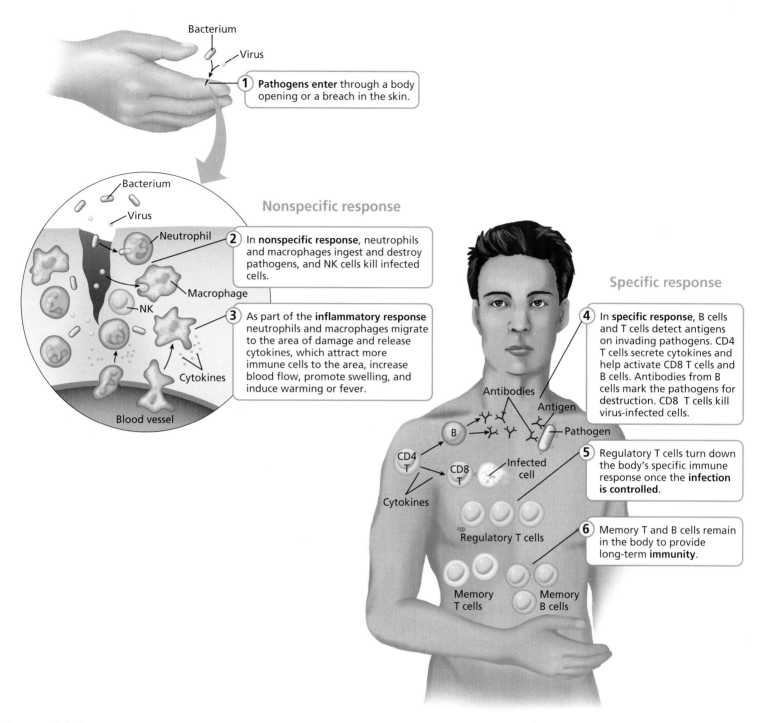

1 **Pathogens enter** through a body opening or a breach in the skin.

Nonspecific response

2 In **nonspecific response**, neutrophils and macrophages ingest and destroy pathogens, and NK cells kill infected cells.

3 As part of the **inflammatory response** neutrophils and macrophages migrate to the area of damage and release cytokines, which attract more immune cells to the area, increase blood flow, promote swelling, and induce warming or fever.

Specific response

4 In **specific response**, B cells and T cells detect antigens on invading pathogens. CD4 T cells secrete cytokines and help activate CD8 T cells and B cells. Antibodies from B cells mark the pathogens for destruction. CD8 T cells kill virus-infected cells.

5 Regulatory T cells turn down the body's specific immune response once the **infection is controlled**.

6 Memory T and B cells remain in the body to provide long-term **immunity**.

Figure 11.1 Your body's immune response.

developments in modern medical history, effectively eradicating some diseases such as smallpox and limiting others significantly.

Immunization often involves exposing a person to a pathogen through a vaccine, which allows the body to develop immunity to the pathogen without actually falling ill. This is called *artificially acquired immunity*. Vaccines are composed of pathogens—or parts of pathogens—that have been killed or weakened. When they are introduced into the body, these dead or weakened microbes pose little threat, yet the body believes it is under attack and sounds the alarm to battle them. The immune system then produces memory B cells and memory T cells that can stave off that particular type of infectious disease for years to come, perhaps for a lifetime. This is known as *active immunity* because it induces an immune response.

In other instances, injections can provide temporary *passive immunity*, when ready-made antibodies specific to a particular pathogen are introduced into the body to fight off an infection. Passive immunity is used, for example, in the case of exposure to the hepatitis A virus. The injected antibodies immediately target the virus for destruction. Passive immunity lasts

immunization Creating immunity to a pathogen through vaccination or through the injection of antibodies.

herd immunity The condition where greater than 90% of a community is vaccinated against a disease, giving it little ability to spread through the community, providing some protection against the disease to members of the community who are not vaccinated.

only as long as the injected antibodies survive, a few months at most.

The Centers for Disease Control has developed recommended immunization schedules for children, teens, and adults **(Table 11.1)** and all states require certain immunizations before children can enter school. Exemptions to immunization laws can be given if a child has certain medical conditions, for religious reasons, and sometimes for other beliefs. In addition, some people are not immunized because they don't know or understand the recommendations, don't have access to health care, or cannot afford the shots. When groups of people are not immunized it can compromise **herd immunity.** Herd immunity occurs when greater than 90% of people in a community or group are fully vaccinated against a disease, leaving that disease with little ability to spread through the population. Herd immunity is important because it offers some protection against the disease for individuals who cannot be vaccinated (due to medical conditions) or who haven't been vaccinated yet (such as newborns).

Immune Disorders

Not all immune systems are strong. Newborns do not yet have fully developed immune systems, and seniors tend to have weak ones, which grow less and less effective as they age. This leaves these

Table 11.1: Vaccines Recommended for College Students[a]

Vaccine	Number of Doses
Tetanus, diphtheria, pertussis (Tdap, Td)[a]	Single dose of Tdap then boost with Td every 10 years
Measles, mumps, rubella (MMR)[a]	2 doses recommended for college students
Polio (IPV)[a]	4 doses if given in childhood; 3 doses if given in adulthood
Varicella (Var) (chicken pox)[a]	2 doses
Human papillomavirus (HPV)][a, b]	3 doses
Hepatitis B (Hep B)[a]	3 doses
Meningococcal disease[c]	1 dose
Pneumococcal polysaccharide (PPV)[d]	1 dose with revaccination after 5 years for those with elevated risk factors.
Hepatitis A (Hep A)[d]	2 doses
Annual influenza (and H1N1)[d]	1 dose annually

[a]Recommended for those who lack documentation of past vaccination with all recommended doses and have no evidence of prior infection.
[b]Recommended for those ages 26 and under.
[c]Recommended for previously unvaccinated college freshmen living in dormitories.
[d]Recommended if some other risk factor is present
Source: Vaccines Needed by Teens and College Students by the U.S. Department of Health and Human Services, Centers for Disease Control and Prevention, 2010, retrieved from http://www.cdc.gov/vaccines/recs/schedules/teen-schedule.htm.

MYTH OR FACT?

Do Vaccines Cause Autism?

In 1998, an article appeared in the British medical journal *The Lancet* that claimed that autism—a developmental brain disorder that causes problems in communication, social

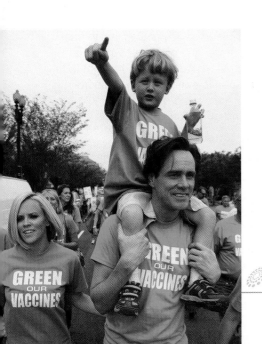

interaction, and behavior—was caused by the childhood vaccine for measles, mumps, and rubella (MMR).[1] In response, some parents' groups began a movement against vaccinations, and more and more parents stopped vaccinating their children.

Anti-vaccine groups claim autism is linked to the recommended number and schedule of childhood vaccinations and the use of thimerosal, a preservative that contains mercury, in some vaccines. As evidence of the damage of vaccinations, parents of autistic children publicized "before" and "after" home videos of their children displaying autistic characteristics only after the date of

vaccination. Celebrities such as Jenny McCarthy and Holly Robinson Peete advocated for vaccination reform.

However, after much research, there is no evidence of a link between autism and vaccines.[2] Thimerosal, which was never present in the MMR vaccines most blamed for autism, was removed from most common childhood vaccines by 2001 and autism rates did not decline.[3,4] And in February of 2010 *The Lancet* retracted the original paper linking autism to the MMR vaccine, citing a recent British medical panel ruling that the lead author had been deceptive and violated basic research ethics in his study.

The causes of autism remain unknown. However one thing is clear: It is dangerous to become infected with a disease that could be prevented by a vaccine.

References: 1. "Ileal-Lymphoid-Nodular Hyperplasia, Non-Specific Colitis, and Pervasive Developmental Disorder in Children," by A. J. Wakefield, S. H. Murch, A. Anthony, J. Linnell, D. M. Casson, M. Malik, . . . J. A. Walker-Smith, 1998, *The Lancet, 351*(9103), pp. 637–641. 2. *Vaccine Studies: Examine the Evidence* by the American Academy of Pediatrics, retrieved from http://www.aap.org/immunization/families/faq/VaccineStudies.pdf. 3. Thimerosal Content of Vaccines Routinely Recommended for Children 6 Years of Age and Younger," Table 1 in "Thimerosal in Vaccines," in *Vaccines, Blood & Biologics* by the U.S. Food and Drug Administration, 2010, retrieved from http://www.fda.gov/BiologicsBloodVaccines/SafetyAvailability/VaccineSafety/ucm096228.htm#t1. 4. "Prevalence of Autism Spectrum Disorders—Autism and Developmental Disabilities Monitoring Network, United States, 2006," by Catherine Rice for the Centers for Disease Control and Prevention, 2009, *Morbidity and Mortality Weekly Report Surveillance Summaries* December 18, 2009/58(SS10), pp. 1–20, retrieved from http://www.cdc.gov/mmwr/preview/mmwrhtml/ss5810a1.htm.

Frontline: The Vaccine War explores both sides of the vaccine debate: www.pbs.org/wgbh/pages/frontline/vaccines/view.

groups more vulnerable to infection and disease. Chronic stress can also impair the immune system, a topic discussed in more detail on page 49 of Chapter 3. In addition, the immune system can sometimes develop disorders that are difficult to control. Two common problems are allergies and asthma.

Allergies

More than 50 million people in the U.S. have **allergies,** abnormal immune system reactions to substances that are otherwise harmless. Allergies are widespread on college campuses, with almost 20% of students in one survey stating that they had been treated for allergies in the last year.[3]

Allergies are due to a hypersensitive immune system, which mistakenly perceives substances such as pollen, peanuts, pet dander, and pest droppings to be serious threats.[4] If you have allergies, you may suffer from itching, sneezing, coughing, watery eyes, difficulty breathing, and congestion. When allergic people come into contact with substances they are sensitive to, their immune systems begin to produce antibodies called immunoglobulin E, or IgE. IgE molecules bind simultaneously to the allergen and to a **mast cell,** a type of cell in the skin and mucous membranes. As a result of these interactions, the mast cell releases powerful chemicals such as histamine into the bloodstream. It is these chemicals—and not the allergens themselves—that make allergy sufferers miserable.

In some instances, allergens cause a rare, serious allergic reaction known as *anaphylaxis*. In this case, the wave of histamine and chemicals released by mast cells occurs throughout the body, and can cause **anaphylactic shock.** Blood pressure drops and airways swell. If not treated immediately with an injection of epinephrine, a person can lapse into unconsciousness and even death.

Fortunately, there are strategies for coping with allergies. Allergists recommend you steer clear of the things you are allergic to whenever possible, staying indoors on high-pollen days and keeping your room clear of dust and dander. Your doctor may recommend prescription or over-the-counter medications that can help alleviate symptoms. Immunotherapy, in which patients are given repeated shots containing increasing amounts of the allergen to desensitize them, is also an option.

The incidence of allergies has increased steadily in recent years. Ironically, this increase may be the unintended result of our antiseptic, health-conscious lifestyle. A possible explanation, the *hygiene hypothesis*, contends that early childhood exposure to microbes can prevent the development of allergies, and conversely, reduced exposure to microbes can increase the chances of developing allergies. Many factors in developed countries today reduce exposure to microbes: smaller family size (fewer siblings means fewer family members bringing microbes into the home); less exposure to animals, specifically farm animals; use of vaccines and antibiotics; and less exposure to general dirt and microorganisms.

The hygiene hypothesis may also contribute to the increasing rates of asthma, a condition that we'll look at next.

> This video explores the hygiene hypothesis of developing allergies: www.pbs.org/wgbh/evolution/library/10/4/l_104_07.html.

Asthma

Asthma occurs when the airways of the lungs become constricted and inflamed, making breathing difficult. The symptoms and severity of asthma range from shortness of breath and wheezing (a whistling-type noise produced during exhalation), to the life-threatening inability to effectively move air in and out of the lungs. There are two general types of asthma. *Allergic asthma* is caused by exposure to allergens such as those in the air (e.g., pollen), in the blood (e.g., bee venom), or in food (e.g., peanuts). *Intrinsic asthma*, on the other hand, can be induced by exercise or cold temperatures, and is not associated with an allergy. It isn't clear why some people have asthma and others do not, but it is likely a combination of genetics (if one of your parents has asthma, you are more likely to have it) and the environment in which you live.

An asthma attack is the result of three main physiological changes: the constriction of the airway muscles, known as *bronchoconstriction;* the overproduction of mucus in the airway; and inflammation of the airway lining. All of these changes can lead to a terrifying result—the inability to breathe. Prevention of asthma includes avoiding known triggers and, in some cases, taking regular doses of medicines that prevent bronchoconstriction and inflammation. Once an attack has begun, fast-acting bronchodilators, administered through inhalers, and oral anti-inflammatory medicines help open the airways and ease breathing.

Nearly 1 in 10 school-aged children in the U.S. suffers from asthma, reflecting a doubling of asthma rates over the last 30 years.[5] Also notable is the racial disparity in asthma rates. Whereas 8% of Caucasian children have asthma, 13% of African American children have the disease. This is thought to reflect socioeconomic conditions, with poorer children more likely to be exposed to mold, diesel soot, and air pollution.

> The American Lung Association provides more information on how to manage asthma and minimize triggers of an asthma attack: www.lungusa.org/lung-disease/asthma/.

Infectious Diseases

Even with advances in modern medicine, infections remain the world's leading killer of children and young adults. The burden on society from even minor infections is immense. Infectious disease costs the U.S. more than $120 billion per year.[6]

Infections can be categorized by the types of pathogens that cause them: viruses, bacteria, fungi, protozoa, and parasitic worms **(Table 11.2).**

---

allergies Abnormal immune system reactions to substances that are otherwise harmless.

mast cell A type of cell in the skin and mucous membranes that releases histamine and other chemicals into the bloodstream during an allergic reaction.

anaphylactic shock A result of anaphylaxis where the release of histamine and other chemicals into the body leads to a drop in blood pressure, tightening of airways, and possible unconsciousness and even death.

asthma Chronic constriction and inflammation of the airways, making breathing difficult and causing shortness of breath, wheezing, coughing, and chest tightness.

Table 11.2: **Pathogens and the Diseases They Cause**

Pathogen	Description	Examples	Diseases Caused
Viruses Influenza viruses (32,000 ×).	Microscopic organisms that cannot multiply without invading body cells	Rhinoviruses, coronaviruses	Common cold
		Influenza viruses	Flu
		Epstein-Barr virus	Mononucleosis
		Hepatitis A, B, C	Hepatitis
		Human immunodeficiency virus (HIV)	Acquired immunodeficiency syndrome (AIDS)
		Herpes simplex virus type 1 (HSV-1)	Herpes (usually oral)
		Herpes simplex virus type 2 (HSV-2)	Herpes (usually genital)
		Human papillomavirus	Cervical cancer, warts, genital warts
Bacteria Mycobacterium tuberculosis bacteria (15,549 ×).	Single-celled microorganisms that invade a host and reproduce inside, releasing toxic enzymes and chemicals	*Neisseria meningitidis*	Meningitis
		Staphylococcus aureus	Staph infection, food poisoning, toxic shock syndrome
		Group A *streptococcus*	Strep throat
		Streptococcus pneumoniae	Pneumonia, meningitis
		Borrelia burgdorferi	Lyme disease
		Mycobacterium tuberculosis	Tuberculosis
		Chlamydia trachomatis	Chlamydia
		Neisseria gonorrhoeae	Gonorrhea
		Treponema pallidum	Syphilis
Fungi Histoplasma capsulatum (400 ×).	Organisms that must get their food from organic matter, including human tissue	*Candida albicans*	Candidiasis (yeast infections), thrush, diaper rash, infections of nail beds
		Histoplasma capsulatum	Histoplasmosis
		Trichophyton	*Tinea pedis* (athlete's foot), jock itch, ring worm, nail infections
Protozoa Trichomonas vaginalis (9,000 ×).	Single-celled parasites that rely on other living things for food and shelter	*Plasmodium*	Malaria
		Toxoplasma gondii	Toxoplasmosis
		Trichomonas vaginalis	Trichomoniasis
Parasitic worms (helminths) Tapeworm (*Taenia* sp.) (15 ×)	Multicellular parasitic creatures that are ingested as eggs or burrow through the skin and compete with a host body for nutrients	*Taenia solium, Taenia saginata, Hymenolepis nana, Enterobius vermicularis, Ancylostoma duodenale*	Tapeworm, pinworm, hookworm infection

Viral Infections

Viruses are microscopic organisms that can not multiply without invading body cells. They hijack the cellular machinery and force it to crank out duplicate viruses at the expense of the cells' normal functions—and at the expense of your health. Viruses can not survive for long periods outside of a host, but once inside a host cell they can multiply very quickly. For example, a cell infected with the common flu virus begins to release new flu viruses only six hours after the virus enters the cell, and it produces enough new viruses to infect another 20 to 30 cells. In the process, the infected cell dies about 11 hours after the virus entered.[7]

Colds

More than 200 different viruses cause cold symptoms. Common culprits are groups of viruses called rhinoviruses and coronaviruses. They are typically spread by touching contaminated objects, through personal contact, or by breathing airborne pathogens. Symptoms appear about two or three days after infection and can include a runny nose or congestion, sneezing, cough, sore throat, headache, and mild fever. There is no known cure, but over-the-counter pain relievers, antihistamines, and decongestants may provide some relief from symptoms.

If it seems like you are always sick, you may not be imagining it. Adults get about two to four colds a year, usually during the fall and winter, and children average three times as many. Women in their 20s get more colds than men of the same age.[8] Colds generally end in about a week and can not be treated with antibiotics, since antibiotics are designed to fight bacteria, not viruses. However, sometimes viral infections leave the body susceptible to secondary bacterial infections of the sinuses, ears, or respiratory tract, in which case antibiotics would be prescribed. Wash your hands frequently, keep your hands away from your face, and stay away from people who have colds to keep from getting one yourself.

Influenza

The flu is a contagious respiratory condition caused by a number of **influenza** viruses. Between 5% and 20% of the U.S. population get the flu every year, suffering from high fever, body aches, fatigue, and a dry cough. Although it often is a moderate illness, lasting a little longer and making people a little more miserable than the common cold, the flu can cause a medical emergency in some infants, seniors, or people with weakened immune systems. The flu can also lead to bacterial pneumonia, dehydration, sinus infections, and ear infections and tends to exacerbate underlying medical conditions such as asthma and diabetes. Every year, more than 200,000 people in the U.S. are hospitalized with flu complications, and at least 36,000 die from an influenza infection.[9]

As with colds, influenza viruses are spread through personal contact, airborne pathogens, or touching inanimate objects covered with a virus. There is no known cure—although antiviral medications may be prescribed to reduce symptoms—and so prevention remains the best medicine. In addition to proper hand washing and coughing and sneezing into the bend of your arm rather than your hand, federal health officials recommend that children, pregnant women, health workers, people over age 65, and people of all ages with

virus A microscopic organism that can not multiply without invading body cells.

influenza A group of viruses that cause the flu, a contagious respiratory condition.

pandemic A worldwide epidemic of a disease.

mononucleosis A viral disease that causes fatigue, weakness, sore throat, fever, headaches, swollen lymph nodes and tonsils, and loss of appetite.

chronic medical conditions such as asthma and diabetes get an influenza vaccine annually. "Flu shots" are available at many campus health centers, doctors' offices, pharmacies, and even grocery stores every fall. You can receive influenza vaccines as injections into the arm or as a nasal-spray.

When a flu is able to pass quickly from person-to-person unchecked and eventually spreads worldwide, it is called a **pandemic.** Pandemics can occur when a new influenza virus emerges that humans have not been exposed to before. This lack of exposure leaves people with no acquired immunity to help defend against the virus, and it can become very contagious. Often, animals are the reservoir for flu viruses that mutate into new strains that cause pandemics. The most recent pandemic, the 2009 H1N1 flu pandemic, was caused by a virus that started in pigs. When a pandemic virus is also deadly the casualties can be staggering. In 1918 an influenza pandemic killed approximately 40 million people.

> **This CDC video explains how to "Take 3" to avoid catching or spreading influenza: www.cdc.gov/CDCTV/IR_Take3/index.html.**

Mononucleosis

Infectious **mononucleosis,** or *"mono,"* is often called "the kissing disease" and is caused by the Epstein-Barr virus. It is transmitted through contact with an infected person's saliva, mucus, or tears. Sharing drinking glasses or straws, eating utensils, or toothbrushes can expose you to the Epstein-Barr virus. Common among teens and young adults, mono causes fatigue, weakness, sore throat, fever, headaches, swollen lymph nodes and tonsils, and loss of appetite. The condition usually is not serious, although some people may experience complications such as hepatitis or jaundice or enlargement of the spleen. Most symptoms dissipate within 2 or 3 weeks, but the fatigue, weakness, and swollen lymph nodes can persevere for months. Blood tests may be used to diagnose mononucleosis, and

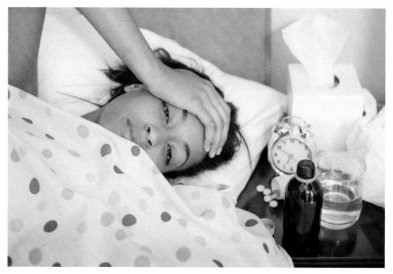

Many infections cause **fatigue**.

the primary treatments are as basic as getting lots of rest and drinking plenty of fluids.

Hepatitis

Hepatitis is an inflammation of the liver. It causes **jaundice,** fatigue, fever, nausea, abdominal pain, and muscle and joint pain. In some cases it can be deadly. Viral infections are the primary cause of hepatitis, though alcohol, drugs, and some underlying medical conditions can be to blame. There are several types of hepatitis. Hepatitis A, hepatitis B, and hepatitis C are the most common forms in the United States, but there are also rarer hepatitis viruses, known as D and E. Hepatitis B is transmitted mostly through sexual contact and is discussed on page 261.

Hepatitis A is the most widespread form of hepatitis. It is contracted through consuming microscopic amounts of feces that can lurk on contaminated fruits, vegetables, and ice cubes. The virus can also be spread during oral-anal sexual contact, or by changing dirty diapers and failing to thoroughly wash your hands afterward. Symptoms can last for weeks or months, although some people never feel ill. Although the virus can cause liver failure and death in a small portion of the population, most people make a full recovery, sustaining no permanent liver damage. Rates of hepatitis A have decreased in recent years. A vaccine for hepatitis A was introduced in 1995, and doctors recommend that children, travelers to certain countries, and other at-risk individuals get the vaccine, which has led to a reduction in infections.

Hepatitis C is the primary reason for liver transplants in the United States. More than three-fourths of those who are infected with this highly destructive virus go on to develop chronic infections that can last a lifetime, scarring the liver or triggering liver cancer. Unfortunately, early symptoms of this form of hepatitis are mild or nonexistent, and many people do not realize they have it until liver damage has occurred. Hepatitis C kills between 8,000 and 10,000 people in the U.S. every year, and typically is spread through sharing syringes and other drug-related paraphernalia.[10] It can also be passed on by unsterilized tattoo needles and piercing equipment or sexual contact. Before screening tests were developed and made available in the United States, it was also spread through blood transfusions and organ transplants. It is still possible to pick up the infection from needles or other medical instruments in other parts of the world where sterilization practices may not be as rigorous.

People with hepatitis may not be aware that they have the disease, since their symptoms can be so mild, but they can still spread it to others. Blood tests can determine whether you have hepatitis. Treatment is usually nothing more than rest, fluids, and proper nutrition for acute cases of hepatitis, but chronic cases sometimes benefit from medications. If you have chronic hepatitis, your doctor should regularly screen you for liver disease.

Bacterial Infections

Bacteria are single-celled microorganisms that are found throughout nature. They can exist independently or as parasites, drawing their nourishment from other forms of life. Harmful bacteria release toxins

hepatitis Inflammation of the liver that affects liver function.

jaundice A yellowing of the skin, mucous membranes, and sometimes the whites of the eyes often caused by liver malfunction.

bacteria (singular *bacterium*) Single-celled microorganisms that invade a host and reproduce inside. Harmful bacteria release toxic enzymes and chemicals.

antibiotic resistance When a bacterium is able to overcome the effects of an antibiotic through a random mutation, or change in the bacterium's genetic code.

or damaging enzymes that disrupt the body. However, less than 1% of the many types of bacteria are actually harmful.[11] Some bacteria are even beneficial, helping us digest food, synthesize vitamins, and fight off disease. Manufacturers even add the *Lactobacillus acidophilus* bacteria to many yogurt and cheese products because of their healthful properties.

Unlike viruses, bacteria are able to replicate on their own without the help of a host cell, by dividing in two. Antibiotics help defeat bacteria by blocking key steps in this process. However, bacteria can also develop **antibiotic resistance** to these important drugs. This occurs when a random mutation, or change in a bacterium's genetic code, enables the bacterium to overcome the effects of the antibiotic. Perhaps only 1 bacterium in 10 million gains this advantage, but that cell rapidly grows and divides, even in the presence of the antibiotic, and the resistant bacteria take over. This is why it is very important to take antibiotics only when they have been prescribed by a physician, to take them for the full course, and only for bacterial infections!

Meningitis

Meningitis is an infection of the meninges, the thin membranes that surround both the spinal cord and brain. The infection can be caused by a number of viral and bacterial strains, and is characterized by high fever, stiff neck, headaches, and even confusion or seizures. When caused by a virus, meningitis tends to be much less severe and dissipates on its own. Bacterial meningitis, however, can be life-threatening, and may cause hearing loss, brain damage, and other disabilities. The bacteria that most commonly cause meningitis are *Streptococcus pneumoniae* and *Neisseria meningitidis*; most often, meningitis occurs when these bacteria have infected another part of the body and then enter the bloodstream and migrate to the meninges. Even when treated promptly with the proper antibiotics, bacterial meningitis kills between 5% and 10% of patients worldwide, usually within a day or two of the onset of symptoms.[12]

Adolescents and young adults account for nearly one-third of all cases of bacterial meningitis in the United States, and college students—especially those living in dormitories—are at moderately increased risk. The American College Health Association estimates that between 100 and 125 cases arise on college campuses every year, and that between 5 and 15 students die as a result. To reduce their risk, the Centers for Disease Control and Prevention recommends that all youths between the ages of 11 and 18 receive the meningococcal vaccine, an inoculation that protects against some but not all of the bacterial strains that cause meningitis.

Staphylococcal Infections

There are more than two dozen types of *Staphylococcus* bacteria, but one—*Staphylococcus aureus*—is responsible for the bulk of all "staph" infections. It causes boils and other minor skin ailments, especially in people with eczema (a chronic, itchy skin rash) or burned skin. Sometimes staph can cause more serious infections of the blood, lungs, heart, or urinary tract, most often in those whose immune system is compromised because of illness or other conditions.

Staphylococcus aureus also releases toxins that can trigger food poisoning and **toxic shock syndrome.** Toxic shock syndrome is a rare yet serious disease that resembles a bad cold or flu in the first few hours but can quickly progress to a medical emergency. Fever, chills, nausea, and diarrhea give way to seizures, low blood pressure, and organ failure and, in about 5% of cases, death.[13] In 1980, more than 800 menstruating women developed the condition, and 38 died from it. Federal investigators linked the cases to use of a highly absorbent tampon that was subsequently taken off the market. Menstruating women can avoid toxic shock syndrome by changing their tampons every 4 to 8 hours, using the lowest absorbency tampon possible, and alternating between tampons and pads.

Some staph bacteria are resistant to the antibiotics typically used to treat them. Known as **methicillin-resistant *Staphylococcus aureus* or MRSA,** these bacteria cause skin infections and are responsible for many cases of pneumonia. See the **Spotlight** on MRSA below.

toxic shock syndrome A rare, serious illness caused by staph bacteria that begins with severe flu symptoms but can quickly progress to a medical emergency.

methicillin-resistant *Staphylococcus aureus* (MRSA) A strain of staph that is resistant to the broad-spectrum antibiotics commonly used to treat staph infections.

Streptococcus Infections

Chances are you or someone you know has been infected with the bacteria *Streptococcus*, perhaps more than once. Group A *Streptococcus* is behind all bouts of strep throat, a relatively mild illness that causes throat pain, swollen tonsils, fever, headache, and stomachache. Particularly common in children and teens, strep throat is highly contagious through airborne droplets or touching contaminated objects. Strep throat usually requires a course of antibiotics to treat. If left untreated, it can lead to scarlet fever or rheumatic fever.

Lyme Disease

If you have ever been hiking in the northwestern, midwestern, or northeastern states, you may have seen warning signs about Lyme disease. The infection is caused by the bacterium *Borrelia burgdorferi* and is transmitted to people through the bite of infected deer ticks and blacklegged ticks. Early symptoms are headache, fatigue, fever, and muscle or joint pain. Within 4 weeks of infection, 70–80% of victims also experience a bull's-eye-shaped skin rash that starts

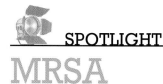

SPOTLIGHT

MRSA

MRSA, or methicillin-resistant *Staphylococcus aureus*, is a strain of staph that is resistant to the broad-spectrum antibiotics commonly used to treat staph infections. MRSA is responsible for serious skin infections, which first appear as painful, red, pus-filled lesions, but it can also cause other infections, including pneumonia. Because it is not treatable with many antibiotics, it poses a threat to anyone who is infected. The Centers for Disease Control and Prevention estimates that nearly 100,000 people in the U.S. develop a serious MRSA infection in any given year and that about one-fifth of them die from it. These statistics reflect a drastic rise in MRSA: in 1974, 2% of all staph infections were MRSA, in 1995, 22%, and in 2004 MRSA accounted for 64% of all staph infec-

tions.[1] It is thought that the development of bacteria like MRSA, which are resistant to multiple antibiotics, is in part due to the misuse of antibiotics.

The infection can be spread by direct skin-to-skin contact or by touching something that has been touched by an infected person. Most people with MRSA become infected when in the hospital or in other health-care settings such as dialysis centers and nursing homes. However, MRSA is becoming more common in schools and on college campuses. School athletes are especially susceptible, due to frequent skin-to-skin contact with others, the higher possibility of cuts or abrasions on the skin, and the use of facilities like locker rooms that may harbor MRSA.

Frequent hand washing, especially when in a clini-

cal setting, is critical to limiting the spread of this serious infection. The following steps will also help you avoid catching or spreading MRSA.

- In addition to hand washing, keep open wounds covered with dry, sterile bandages.
- Shower immediately after exercise or participating in a close contact sport.
- Do not share personal items such as towels or razors with others.
- If you have a skin infection that does not appear to be getting better after a day or so, see a doctor and request that you be tested for MRSA.

Early detection is important, especially since some MRSA strains, at least for now, respond to the antibiotic vancomycin, and small

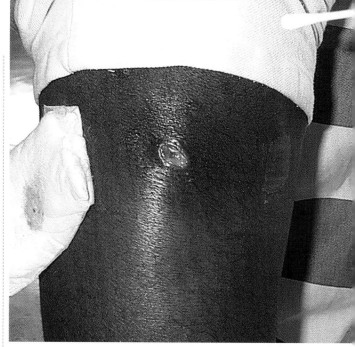

A sore due to MRSA.

skin infections can be treated by draining and cleaning the lesion.

*Reference:***1.** "Overview of Healthcare-Associated MRSA," in *Healthcare-Associated Methicillin Resistant Staphylococcus aureus (HA-MRSA)* by the Centers for Disease Control and Prevention, 2010, retrieved from http://www.cdc.gov/ncidod/dhqp/ar_mrsa.html.

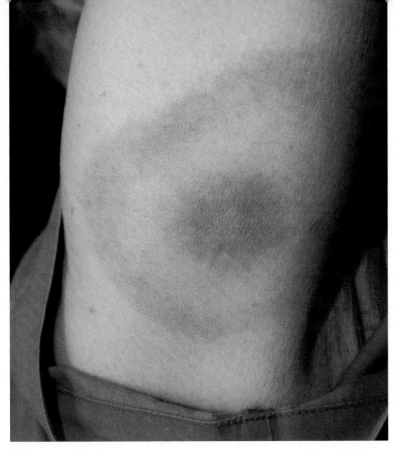

Figure 11.2 Lyme disease "bull's-eye" rash.

small and grows larger **(Figure 11.2).** If the infection goes untreated, it can cause swelling and pain in the joints, rapid heartbeat or other heart problems, partial facial paralysis, and neurological problems such as memory loss, which can last for years. Antibiotics are usually successful at treating Lyme disease if used in the early stages, but some people will have recurring symptoms of the disease for years. Prevention remains the best medicine. Hikers should avoid wooded areas and overgrown grass and brush, and wear long pants, long sleeves, and long socks to help keep ticks off their skin. Checking your body for ticks after being outdoors is also advised, and should you ever find one, pull it straight out with a pair of tweezers. Ticks normally will not transmit the bacterium until after they have fed, which can take anywhere from 36 to 48 hours.

Pneumonia

Pneumonia ranks as the eighth leading cause of death in the United States, and the number-one cause of death for children worldwide.[14, 15] It is an inflammation of the lungs that can be caused by bacteria, viruses, fungi, or parasites. Pneumonia can vary from mild to deadly. Bacterial pneumonias are the most common in adults, and usually the most severe, causing high fever, chest pain, shortness of breath, chills, and a cough with green, yellow, or bloody mucus. Pneumonia tends to occur in conjunction with a cold or flu, and is often mistaken by patients for these lesser infections. You should see a doctor immediately if you suddenly experience pneumonia symptoms.

The most common bacterial cause of pneumonia is the *Streptococcus pneumoniae* bacterium. Antibiotics are used to treat bacterial pneumonia infections, but as antibiotic-resistant strains have

fungi Multicellular or single-celled organisms that obtain their food from organic matter, in some cases human tissue.

become more common, these drugs are less effective. Prevention remains the best measure. Health-care experts recommend that people get an annual flu shot to reduce their risk. Seniors and infants are at higher risk for pneumonia, as are younger people with asthma and other chronic respiratory problems, impaired immune systems, or who have been exposed to certain chemicals and environmental pollutants. High-risk individuals are encouraged to get the pneumococcal pneumonia vaccine.

Tuberculosis

Tuberculosis, or TB, is a serious disease caused by the bacterium *Mycobacterium tuberculosis* that is spread through the air. The bacteria typically attack the lungs, where they create holes in the airways and hinder breathing. They can also settle into the brain, spine, or kidneys, and without proper treatment can prove fatal.

Symptoms of TB include weight loss, fatigue, fever, night sweats, and a persistent cough that does not go away after 3 weeks. But not everyone with a TB infection will become ill from it. Many have what is called a *latent* TB infection that does not cause any symptoms, is not infectious, and may never progress to active TB disease. In fact, only about 5–10% of people with TB develop the active form of the disease.[16] Medication, taken for many months, can help keep latent TB infections from evolving into active TB disease, although drug-resistant strains of TB are emerging.

Once the leading cause of death in the United States, TB cases have been declining in recent years and reached an all-time low in 2008. Infection rates continue to be highest among immigrants and racial and ethnic minorities, the poor, the homeless, and those infected with HIV. Although there were only 12,898 new cases reported in 2008, millions of people in the U.S. are estimated to be living with a TB infection. Worldwide, about 2 billion people are infected.[17, 18]

Fungal Infections

Fungi are organisms that obtain their food from organic matter, in some cases human tissue. Common examples of fungi are multicellular mold, mildew, and mushrooms, and single-celled yeast. Fungi can be found in soil, on plants, in water, and even in the air we breathe. Some fungi reproduce as microscopic spores, which can become airborne and come into contact with skin or surfaces you touch, opening the door to infection.

Some of the thousands of fungi that exist are quite beneficial. Penicillin, the powerful antibiotic used to treat a number of bacterial infections, is made from fungi. Yeast is used in making bread and cheese. Other types are not so helpful. Fungi are behind many minor infections of the skin, scalp, and nail beds, but can also cause life-threatening systemic infections, especially for people with weakened immune systems.

Yeast infections are some of the most common types of fungal infections. Small amounts of a yeast called *Candida albicans* are always present in a person's body, but if imbalances occur—after taking antibiotics, for example, or, for women, during the normal hormonal changes that come with menstrual periods—this fungus is able to multiply out of control. It can cause infections in various parts of the body, such as the intestinal tract or vagina. Yeast infections, although uncomfortable and unpleasant, are usually not serious. In women, they are

Emerging INFECTIOUS Diseases

Although some diseases have plagued humankind for as long as records have been kept, others have only become a human health threat in recent years or have reemerged as worldwide travel has spread them. Some of the more troubling emerging infections are described here.

H1N1 ("Swine flu"). H1N1 is a new influenza virus first detected in the United States in April 2009. The virus contains genes not only from pigs, but also from birds and humans. H1N1 spreads from person to person similarly to the seasonal flu and in June 2009 the World Health Organization declared it a worldwide pandemic. The virus causes cough, sore throat, congestion, body aches, headaches, chills, and fatigue. Most people recover on their own without treatment, but in some cases the illness can cause severe respiratory problems and even death.

H5N1 (Avian influenza or "bird flu"). H5N1 has been diagnosed in hundreds of people in more than a dozen countries since November 2003. Most of them contracted the serious infection after coming into direct contact with infected poultry. It causes conjunctivitis (pink eye), pneumonia, and for more than half its victims, death. The virus has, in a few rare instances, spread from person to person, and it would only take a slight mutation for it to spread very easily. If that were to occur, H5N1 would have the potential of becoming the next influenza pandemic.

SARS (severe acute respiratory syndrome). SARS is caused by a type of coronavirus. It emerged in southeastern China in 2003, and within a matter of months spread to more than two dozen countries throughout the world, including the United States. The virus, which causes pneumonia in most of those who are infected with it, is believed to have made the jump to humans through animals that were sold in Asian food markets. The respiratory illness killed hundreds and sickened thousands worldwide during the outbreak of 2003. It is spread through close person-to-person contact.

West Nile Virus. This infectious disease is spread through the bite of an infected mosquito. Although it appeared in other parts of the world earlier, it was not discovered in the United States until 1999. Since then it has spread rapidly, infecting tens of thousands of people across the country, and killing more than 1,000.[1] Although 80% of infected people experience no effects, about 1 in every 150 people infected go on to experience severe symptoms ranging from muscle weakness and disorientation to vision loss, paralysis, coma, and death. The only way to avoid getting the virus is to avoid mosquito bites.

Hantavirus. Hantavirus is a disease transmitted by rodents. The respiratory illness causes fatigue, fever, muscle aches, coughing, shortness of breath, and a buildup of fluid in the lungs. Symptoms appear after exposure to the urine, droppings, or saliva of infected rodents.

Reference: 1 "Statistics, Surveillance, and Control Archive" in *West Nile Virus* by the Centers for Disease Control and Prevention, retrieved from http://www.cdc.gov/ncidod/dvbid/westnile/surv&control.htm#maps.

Close contact with poultry or other animals can pass new diseases to humans.

marked by itching in the vagina and around the genitals, and are often accompanied by an abnormal vaginal discharge that can resemble cottage cheese. Sexual intercourse can also be painful. Treatment involves inserting a cream or suppository into the vagina, or taking an oral medication. Other *Candida* infections include thrush (an overgrowth in the mouth), diaper rash, and infections of the nail beds.

Protozoan Infections

Protozoa are single-celled organisms that, like fungi, obtain nutrients from feeding on organic matter. While some are free-living, and even helpful—consuming harmful bacteria or serving as food for fish and other animals—protozoan parasites rely on other living things, such as humans, for food and shelter. These protozoa are capable of causing serious diseases in humans, especially in people living in developing countries. In the United States, where sanitation and food-handling standards have reduced our exposure to them, protozoan infections are less common.

One of the protozoan diseases of most concern is **malaria,** which kills nearly one million people every year, primarily infants, children, and pregnant women.[19] The infection is caused by the protozoa *Plasmodium,* and is typically transmitted to humans through the bites of infected mosquitoes. Malaria is a serious threat throughout much of sub-Saharan Africa and parts of Latin America, Asia, and the Middle East, and fully 50% of the world's population is at risk of contract-

protozoa Single-celled parasites that rely on other living things for food and shelter.

malaria A serious disease that causes fever and chills that appear in cycles. In some cases malaria can be life-threatening.

parasitic worms (helminths) Multicellular creatures that compete with a host body for nutrients.

ing it.[19] Although it was controlled in the United States more than five decades ago, occasional outbreaks still occur here. As global temperatures rise, malaria rates might increase if malaria-carrying mosquitoes move into areas that historically have not been affected by the disease.

Initial symptoms include fever, chills, vomiting, and headache. If not treated with antimalarial drugs promptly, the infection can be fatal. Some strains of malaria have become resistant to drugs, making treatment much more difficult. Malaria can be prevented by preventing mosquito bites through the use of insecticides, wearing long pants and long-sleeved shirts, and using mosquito netting imbued with insecticides. Antimalarial drugs can also be taken during trips to malaria-rich areas to reduce the risk of contracting the disease.

Parasitic Worm Infections

Parasitic worms (helminths) are creatures that compete with a host body for nutrients. Some tiny worms burrow through the skin, while others are contracted from eating microscopic eggs in undercooked foods. Once inside the body, some can grow up to 10–15 feet in length. Others can live for up to 15 years. They are most frequently found in tropical regions and are a problem in areas with poor sanitation. Infections are most common in travelers, refugees, migrant workers, children, and the homeless. Two of the more common parasitic worms in the U.S. are tapeworms and pinworms.

☺ *Practical Strategies for Health*

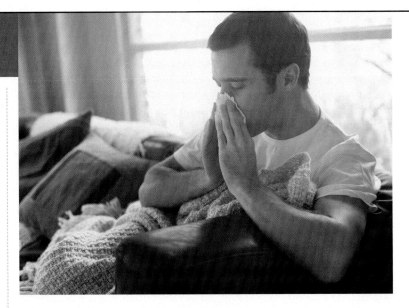

Protecting Yourself Against Infectious Diseases

To avoid contracting an infection:

- Wash your hands often, or use hand sanitizer with at least 60% alcohol.

- Keep your hands away from your eyes, nose, and mouth. Touching your face is a common way to transmit pathogens from your hands into your body.

- Avoid close contact with people who are sick.

- Routinely clean and disinfect surfaces, including keyboards, phones, and kitchen counters.

- Keep up-to-date on your vaccinations and get an annual flu shot.

- Avoid contact with wild animals. Rodents, bats, raccoons, skunks, and foxes can all spread harmful bacteria or viruses. Make

sure your pets are up-to-date on their vaccinations as well.

- Avoid mosquito bites. In mosquito-dense areas, wear insect repellent when you are outdoors, particularly at dusk and dawn; eliminate standing water in flower pots, bird baths, or other containers left outdoors; make sure you have intact window screens; and wear long-sleeved shirts and pants to avoid bites.

- Avoid walking barefoot in locker rooms or on dirt.

- Don't smoke, and avoid secondhand smoke.

- Don't drink alcohol or drink only in moderation.

- Get enough sleep. Lack of sleep can impair the immune system.

- Eat well. Proper nutrition supports your immune system.

If you are feeling under the weather, take steps to prevent infecting others. Stay home when you are sick, cover your mouth or nose with a tissue when you cough or sneeze, or cough or sneeze into the bend of your elbow, and wash your hands after coughing or sneezing.

The tapeworm, the largest of the parasitic worms, is usually spread through poorly cooked beef, pork, or fish. The pork tapeworm is the most dangerous, because its eggs can invade tissues and even the central nervous system, resulting in seizures. The dwarf tapeworm, which only grows to about 2 inches, is the variety most commonly found in the United States, and has been linked to food contaminated with mouse droppings. Oral medications can usually treat tapeworm infections.

Pinworm infections are the most common worm infections in the U.S. They are generally not serious and are often caught in day cares, schools, and summer camps. Infection occurs when the eggs of pinworms are inadvertently swallowed, often by placing dirty fingers in or near the mouth. The eggs then travel to the intestines where they hatch. Female worms, which have pin-shaped tails, travel at night through the anus and deposit their eggs on the skin. Infections can be treated with oral medications, and topical ointments are often used to relieve anal itching.

Sexually Transmitted Infections

Sexually transmitted infections (STIs) are commonplace. It is estimated that worldwide nearly a million people acquire a sexually transmitted infection *every day,* and there are approximately 19 million new cases of STIs every year in the United States.[20–22]

> **sexually transmitted infections (STIs)** Infections transmitted mainly through sexual activity, such as vaginal, anal, or oral sex.

The CDC estimates that while 15- to 24-year-olds represent only 25% of the sexually active population, they account for nearly half of all new STI cases.[23] Among sexually active U.S. teens, the STI prevalence is 40% and those with three or more partners have a prevalence of more than 50%. Even among girls aged 14 to 19 reporting only one lifetime partner, approximately 20% have at least one STI.[24] As many as one in two sexually active people will have an infection by age 25.[25]

There are more than 30 different sexually transmissible bacteria, viruses, and parasites.[22] Bacterial STIs include gonorrhea, chlamydia, and syphilis, and can be successfully treated with antibiotics if detected early enough. Viral STIs such as HIV, hepatitis B, herpes, and the human papillomavirus have no cure, although they can often be controlled with prompt medical treatment.

This interactive tutorial gives an overview of STIs: www.nlm.nih.gov/medlineplus/tutorials/sexuallytransmitteddiseases/htm/_yes_50_no_0.htm.

These videos discuss STIs: www.cdc.gov/std/Be-Smart-Be-Well/default.htm.

Risk Factors for STIs

The college years can be a time of elevated risk for contracting an STI. Your likelihood of contracting a sexually transmitted infection depends a lot on your behaviors. Some activities that increase risk are:

- Having unprotected vaginal, anal, or oral sex.
- Having sex with multiple partners, especially strangers, and not discussing STIs before sex.
- Exchanging sex for drugs or money.
- Participating in sex while drunk or high on drugs.

- Coming into direct skin-to-skin contact with someone who has infections such as HPV, herpes, pubic lice, or scabies.
- Injecting drugs or steroids with dirty needles or syringes—or having unprotected sex with someone who has.
- Sharing needles for tattoos and body piercings.
- Failing to be vaccinated against human papillomavirus (HPV) or hepatitis B.

Are you at risk for a sexually transmitted infection? Take the **Self-Assessment** on the next page to find out.

Sexual Conduct and Risk

Only abstinence provides 100% protection from STIs. If you choose to have sex, the safest sex is between two completely monogamous partners who have been tested and are uninfected with any STIs. Although condoms are not 100% effective against STIs, when used correctly and consistently they significantly reduce risk and make sex safer. If you or your partner is not monogamous or has not been tested, it is considered high-risk to have vaginal, anal, or oral sex with that person without a condom. Unprotected anal sex carries the highest risk, especially for the receiving partner. Unprotected vaginal sex is next highest risk. Unprotected oral sex is also considered high risk, although it is less risky than unprotected anal or vaginal sex.

Talking About Safer Sex

It may feel awkward or embarrassing to talk about sexual history or STIs with a new partner, but it's important. Before you have sex with a new person, you should ask him or her:

- Does he or she have any STIs?
- Has he or she participated in risky activities in the past?
- Has he or she been tested for STIs in the past? If so, has he or she participated in any risky activities since then?
- Is he or she prepared to use a condom? Are there any other safer sex measures he or she wants to take?

Be prepared to answer these questions yourself as well. In many cases, you will find that your partner is concerned about these issues too. If your partner is unwilling to discuss safe sex or does not want to participate in the same level of safe sex that you do, reconsider sex with that person.

HIV and AIDS

Accounting for more than 1.5 million deaths worldwide every year, the human immunodeficiency virus (HIV) is the most serious of all sexually transmitted pathogens.[26] Worldwide, there are more than 33 million people with the infection, with infection rates in sub-Saharan Africa, India, southeast Asia, and Russia especially high **(Figure 11.3)**. In 2008, 68% of new HIV infections in adults and 91% of new HIV infections in children were in sub-Saharan Africa; 20% of all new cases occurred in Asia.[26] First identified in the United States in 1981, today more than 1.4 million people in the U.S. live with HIV infection and the condition it causes, acquired immunodeficiency syndrome or AIDS (also called advanced HIV disease). African Americans are disproportionately infected, as are sex workers, intravenous drug users, and men who have sex with other men.

Scientists believe that HIV infections in humans can be traced back to chimpanzees in West Africa. It is thought that the virus

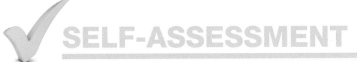

SELF-ASSESSMENT

To complete this self-assessment online, visit www.pearsonhighered.com/choosinghealth.

Are You at Risk for an STI?

If you engage in sexual activity, then you are at risk for contracting an STI. However, your level of risk depends on certain behaviors.

"Sex" includes oral, vaginal, or anal sex, and a sexual partner is somebody with whom you have had oral, vaginal, or anal sex.

1. In the past 12 months, have you been diagnosed with any STI?*
   yes   no

2. In the past 12 months, have you had more than one sexual partner?
   yes   no

3. In the past 12 months, do you think your sexual partner(s) had any other partners?
   yes   not sure   no

4. In the past 12 months, have you had sex with a new partner?
   yes   no

5. Are you currently planning on having sex with a new partner?
   yes   not sure   no

6. In the past 12 months, how often have you used condoms during vaginal or anal intercourse or latex barriers during oral sex?
   aways   some of the time   most of the time   never

7. Do you discuss sexual history and testing with your partner(s)?
   always   sometimes   never

HOW TO INTERPRET YOUR SCORE

If you answered "yes" or "not sure" to questions 1–5, you may be at higher risk for STIs. If you answered anything other than "always" to questions 6 and 7, you may be at higher risk for STIs.

Consider making an appointment at your campus health center for STI screening and/or to discuss prevention strategies.

*Having had an STI recently may put you at higher risk for other STIs.

Source: Adapted from *UC Berkeley Sexually Transmitted Infection (STI) Risk Assessment* by UC Berkeley University Health Services Tang Center, no date, retrieved from http://uhs.berkeley.edu/students/pdf/Patient%20Self-assessment.pdf.

jumped from primates to people when hunters seeking monkeys as bush meat came into contact with the infected blood of their prey. The virus spread across Africa and then to other parts of the world. There are two forms of the virus: HIV-1, which is responsible for most of the infections in Europe, Asia, the Middle East, and the Americas, and HIV-2, the cause of most of the infections in Africa.

HIV infection severely damages the body's immune system. In particular, the virus infects and destroys helper T cells (CD4 T cells), important players in the body's specific immune response. HIV enters CD4 T cells and multiplies within them, generating millions of new HIV viruses and destroying the CD4 T cells in the process. The new viruses go on to infect more CD4 T cells and begin the replica-

North America
Living with HIV/AIDS:
1.4 million
Deaths: 25,000

Western & Central Europe
Living with HIV/AIDS:
850,000
Deaths: 13,000

Eastern Europe & Central Asia
Living with HIV/AIDS:
1.5 million
Deaths: 87,000

East Asia
Living with HIV/AIDS:
850,000
Deaths: 59,000

Caribbean
Living with HIV/AIDS:
240,000
Deaths: 12,000

North Africa & Middle East
Living with HIV/AIDS:
310,000
Deaths: 20,000

South & Southeast Asia
Living with HIV/AIDS:
3.8 million
Deaths: 270,000

Latin America
Living with HIV/AIDS:
2.0 million
Deaths: 77,000

Sub-Saharan Africa
Living with HIV/AIDS:
22.4 million
Deaths: 1.4 million

Oceania
(Australia, New Zealand, Polynesia, Micronesia, Melanesia)
Living with HIV/AIDS:
59,000
Deaths: 2,000

Figure 11.3 HIV/AIDS around the world.

Source: Data from *AIDS Epidemic Update December 2009* by the Joint United Nations Programme on HIV/AIDS (UNAIDS) and World Health Organization (WHO), 2009, UNAIDS/09.36E / JC1700E.

tion process all over again. The immune system mounts a vigorous response, with B cells mulitplying and secreting antibodies, and CD4 T cells multiplying and secreting cytokines. After years or decades, however, CD4 T cell levels begin to decline, the immune system is progressively weakened, and the body loses its ability to fight off illness.

The first few weeks after contracting HIV are called the primary infection stage. During that period, some—but not all—people experience initial symptoms that resemble those of a cold or flu. Fatigue, fever, headache, sore throat, swollen lymph glands, and muscle aches are reported, as are diarrhea, yeast infections, rashes, and mouth sores. The primary infection is followed by an asymptomatic stage and new symptoms may not occur for another 8 to 10 years. However, during this period the virus is still reproducing rapidly and the immune system is fighting it. Eventually, with the loss of CD4 T cells, the person will become more vulnerable to **opportunistic diseases**—infections and other disorders that take advantage of a weakened immune system—like pneumonia, tuberculosis, eye infections, yeast infections, and cancer, including Kaposi's sarcoma. An HIV-positive person is diagnosed with AIDS when at least one opportunistic disease has developed or when that person's CD4 T cell count drops below 200 cells per microliter of blood (a healthy CD4 count is between 450 and 1200 cells per microliter). Once AIDS develops, additional complications can arise, including severe weight loss, dementia, brain tumors, and a protozoan infection called toxoplasmosis.

opportunistic diseases Infections and other disorders that take advantage of a weakened immune system.

Transmission of HIV

Once infected with HIV, people can transmit it to others regardless of the stage of the disease or whether or not they have experienced symptoms. HIV can be found in blood, seminal fluid, vaginal secretions, and breast milk. It can be transmitted during unprotected vaginal, oral, or anal sex, or when sharing needles for intravenous drug use, tattoos, or piercing **(Figure 11.4).** You can not catch the virus through sneezing, handshakes, insect bites, sharing food, or any other type of casual contact. If you already have another STI, such as herpes or syphilis, your risk of becoming infected with HIV increases significantly. In the past, HIV was occasionally transmitted to recipients of blood transfusions; however, due to reforms, all donated blood in the United States is now screened for the virus and is considered safe.

Infected mothers are at risk of giving the virus to their infants, which is called *mother-to-child-transmission* (MTCT). This can occur during pregnancy, childbirth, and breastfeeding. The World Health Organization estimates that worldwide 430,000 children are newly infected each year, 90% through MTCT.[27] Untreated, approximately 50% of these infected children will die before age two. The risk of MTCT of HIV ranges from 20% to 45%; however, with targeted prevention interventions, this risk can be reduced to less than 5%.[28]

This interactive tutorial discusses HIV infection and AIDS: **www.nlm.nih.gov/medlineplus/tutorials/aids/htm/index.htm.**

HIV Testing and Treatment

The Centers for Disease Control and Prevention estimates that about one-fourth of the people in the U.S. infected with HIV do not realize it. Because early HIV infections can have no or few symptoms, HIV screening is very important. Early diagnosis of HIV and prompt treatment is critical to slowing the virus's progression to AIDS. Knowing you have the virus can also help you take measures to avoid giving it to others.

The HIV test looks for the presence of antibodies to the virus rather than the virus itself—the presence of antibodies to HIV indicates that HIV is present in the body. The most common test is the EIA or enzyme immunoassay, which is used to examine blood, saliva, or urine for antibodies to HIV. If an EIA test is positive, it is followed by an additional test such as the Western blot before a positive diagnosis of HIV infection is made. HIV antibody tests only work after a person's immune system has begun to develop antibodies to HIV. Because this can take up to 6 months in some people, testing too quickly after potential exposure to the virus is considered ineffective.

The CDC recommends that all people between the ages of 13 and 64 be tested for HIV at least once during a routine doctor's visit. People at high-risk for HIV (intravenous-drug users, people engaging in unprotected sex or with multiple sex partners) should be tested annually, and pregnant women should be tested as part of their routine prenatal testing. Despite these recommendations, only 24.3% of college students report having ever been tested for HIV.[3]

HIV and AIDS are not curable, but they are treatable. Treatments called antiretroviral therapies can dramatically slow the deterioration of a person's immune system, and are responsible for a dramatic decrease in AIDS deaths in recent years. There are three main types of antiretroviral drugs: reverse transcriptase inhibitors, protease inhibitors, and fusion inhibitors. The medications are frequently prescribed in combinations of three or four in a regimen often referred to as *highly active antiretroviral therapy*, or HAART. For many living with HIV, HAART has changed the condition from a life sentence to a chronic manageable disease. The average life expectancy of a per-

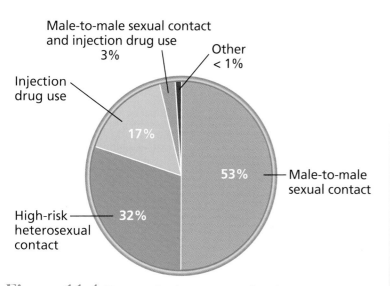

Male-to-male sexual contact and injection drug use 3%

Other < 1%

Injection drug use

17%

Male-to-male sexual contact

53%

High-risk heterosexual contact

32%

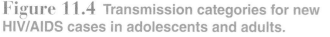

Figure 11.4 Transmission categories for new HIV/AIDS cases in adolescents and adults.

Source: "HIV/AIDS in the United States" by the U.S. Department of Health and Human Services, Centers for Disease Control and Prevention. (2009). *CDC HIV/AIDS Facts*, CS201851-D, retrieved from www.cdc.gov/hiv/resources/factsheets/us.htm

son newly diagnosed with HIV is approaching that of most uninfected people. Recent projection models suggest that a 39-year-old entering HIV care can expect to live until 63.[29]

However, HIV drugs are very expensive, have toxic side effects, and do not work for everyone. For some, they may work for only a limited period of time. Doctors may also prescribe other medications such as antibiotics in an effort to prevent opportunistic infections like pneumonia, toxoplasmosis, or tuberculosis.

Preventing HIV Infection

To avoid getting HIV and AIDS, you need to keep the blood, seminal fluid, vaginal fluids, or breast milk of an infected person from entering your vagina, penis, anus, mouth, or breaches in your skin. The surest way to protect yourself from HIV or any other STI is to avoid any sexual behavior that could transmit the disease. See **Practical Strategies for Health: Reducing Risk of STIs** for information on how to avoid STIs.

Intravenous drug users are at very high risk of contracting HIV if they share needles or syringes with other users. Efforts to sterilize equipment, including washing with bleach, are not always successful at killing HIV. Having intercourse while high on drugs is also risky, as you are less likely to think clearly and practice safe sex.

> These podcasts discuss HIV testing and prevention: www.cdc.gov/hiv/resources/podcasts/index.htm.

Hepatitis B

Hepatitis B—which is more than 50 times as infectious as the virus that causes HIV—is most commonly spread through unprotected sex.[30] It can also be caught through sharing needles, razors, or syringes with an infected person. Symptoms generally occur 2–3 months after infection and involve abdominal and joint pain, nausea, dark urine, weakness and fatigue, and jaundice. Although the virus can cause immediate symptoms that go away on their own, for some people it can also remain in the body forever, resulting in long-term health problems ranging from liver damage to liver cancer and death. If you know you have been exposed to hepatitis B, contact your doctor right away. An injection of hepatitis B immune globulin (antibodies specific for hepatitis B; a passive immunization) within 24 hours of exposure may reduce your risk of developing hepatitis B. Since health-care providers began to routinely immunize children against hepatitis B in 1991, infection rates have dropped by an estimated 80%.[30] However, for as many as 1.4 million people in the U.S. currently living with a chronic hepatitis B infection, the vaccine became available too late.[30]

Genital Herpes

Genital herpes affects 16.2% of adults in the United States.[31] More than 80% of infected people do not realize they have the condition because they don't have symptoms or their symptoms are mild or mistaken for something else, such as jock itch, a yeast infection, or even insect bites. There are two types of herpes simplex virus: herpes simplex virus type 2 (HSV-2) and herpes simplex virus type 1 (HSV-1). Genital herpes is usually caused by HSV-2, while HSV-1 is the virus most often responsible for cold sores around the mouth. Herpes is extremely contagious. Genital herpes most often results from direct skin-to-skin contact, usually through vaginal,

☺ *Practical Strategies for Health*

Reducing Risk of STIs

A few simple steps can dramatically reduce your risk of contracting an STI.

- **Consider abstinence.** Abstinence from sexual intercourse is the most effective method for avoiding STIs.

- **Be faithful.** If you have sex, do it with one uninfected partner who is not having sex with others.

- **Be picky.** Limit the number of sex partners you have in your lifetime.

- **Use a condom or latex barrier.** Use latex or polyurethane condoms correctly and consistently for all vaginal or anal sexual encounters. Condoms, dental dams, or latex squares should be used for oral sex.

- **Talk with your partner.** Discuss STIs and prevention before you ever have sex. If you or your partner does not feel comfortable having that conversation, consider it a sign that you may not want to have sex with that person.

- **Get tested.** If you are sexually active, the only way to know for sure whether you have an infection is to be tested by a health practitioner. Many STIs have no noticeable symptoms and can go undetected for years, when treatment may be too late. It is a good idea for both partners to be tested before beginning a new sexual relationship.

- **Get annual checkups.** Annual checkups are a good time to discuss your sexual practices with your doctor.

- **Get vaccinated.** Ask your doctor about vaccines for HPV and hepatitis B. Men who have sex with other men should be vaccinated for hepatitis A as well.

- **Be alert to symptoms.** Should you develop any signs of an STI, get checked out by a physician right away. Prompt treatment can make all the difference between an effective treatment and long-term problems.

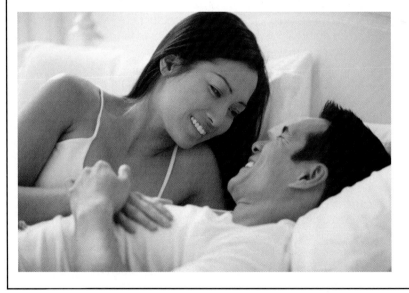

oral, or anal sex. Oral sex can pass both types of herpes virus back and forth between the mouth and the genitals. HSV-2 is almost always transmitted through sexual contact so most people do not contract it until they have become sexually active, whereas many people are exposed to HSV-1 in childhood, through nonsexual kisses by family members or friends. HSV-1 is very common;

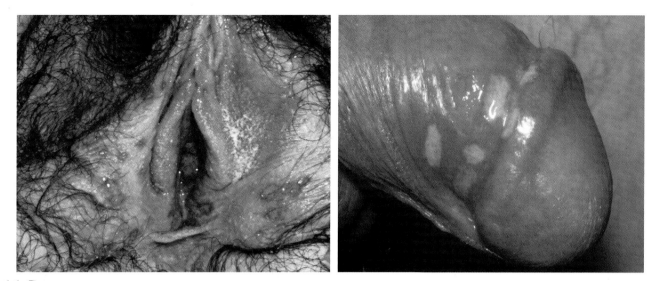

Figure 11.5 Genital herpes sores.

50–80% of people in the U.S. have it, and as many as 90% of people have it by age 50.[32]

The hallmark of genital herpes is small, painful blisters or sores in the genital or anal area, although some people do not experience any symptoms at all **(Figure 11.5).** The first outbreak usually occurs within 2 weeks of infection, is accompanied by flu-like symptoms, and takes about 3 weeks to heal. Outbreaks can recur, but tend to become less severe and less frequent over time. Stress, illness, poor diet, inadequate rest, and friction in the genital area can trigger outbreaks. The virus usually stays in the body forever, lying dormant in nerve cells, until the next recurrence. Herpes is most infectious when blisters or sores are present on an infected person. However, the herpes virus can be shed and passed on to others even when a person shows no symptoms. If you have ever had an outbreak of genital herpes, you should consider yourself contagious even if you have not had an outbreak for years. It is important to tell any potential partners that you have genital herpes.

Genital herpes can leave the body vulnerable to other sexually transmitted infections. The risk to a herpes patient of becoming infected with HIV if exposed to it is two to three times that of people who do not have herpes.[32] It can also make people with an HIV infection more infectious. Genital herpes can be fatal to a newborn baby if passed along during childbirth.

To diagnose herpes, a doctor takes a swab from a blister within the first 48 hours after it appears. If there is a sufficient amount of virus in the blister it is possible to distinguish it as either HSV-1 or HSV-2. Tests are also available that look for antibodies to the herpes virus in the blood. Many of the older tests can not differentiate between infection with HSV-1 or HSV-2, but newer blood tests are much more accurate and are capable of differentiating between the two.

Treatments for genital herpes are targeted toward alleviating symptoms. Antiviral medications such as acyclovir can reduce pain, hasten the healing of sores, and reduce the number of recurrences. Sex should be avoided when one partner has visible herpes sores, but the partner can still be contagious even when the sores have healed. Condoms or dental dams should always be used if a partner

has genital herpes. They can reduce the risk of passing on the virus but are not foolproof, since contagious sores can appear on areas not covered by the barrier. When taken daily to suppress herpes outbreaks and viral shedding, antiviral medications can also reduce the risk of transmitting herpes to a sexual partner, although condoms or dental dams should still be used.

Human Papillomavirus

Human papillomavirus (HPV) causes all types of warts, wherever they may be on your body. There are over 100 types of HPV. More than 40 types can infect the genitalia, although only 4 are responsible for most genital HPV infections. HPV is the most reported STI on college campuses. Most sexually active Americans will become infected with HPV at some point in their lives.[33] An estimated 20 million people in the U.S. are currently infected with HPV, and an additional 6 million develop the infection every year.[34] The infection is spread through skin-to-skin contact, usually during vaginal, oral, or anal sex.

Most people do not realize they are infected with HPV. With the exception of the few HPV types that cause genital warts, HPV does not have any symptoms. For those who do experience warts, they can arise weeks or even months after infection. Warts can be raised or flat, pink or flesh-toned, and there may be only a single one or multiple **(Figure 11.6).** These warts can be treated with topical medications that are applied directly to the skin. They can also be frozen off through cryotherapy, burned off through electrocauterization, or removed by laser surgery. Warts can return even after treatment because these treatments do not cure HPV infection, they just help symptoms.

In about 90% of cases, the body's immune system overcomes an HPV infection naturally. However, some infections linger and cause cells to become abnormal or even cancerous. The types of HPV that cause cancer of the cervix, vagina, throat, penis, and anus are called "high-risk" strains of HPV. These strains do not cause warts and must be tested for. Cervical cancer is the biggest concern. Highly treatable when detected early, it can be fatal when left undetected. That is why the Pap smear, which is used to screen for abnormal and potentially cancerous cervical cells, now typically

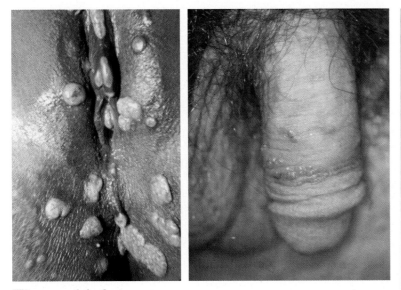

Figure 11.6 Genital warts.

includes a test for HPV. More than 11,000 women are diagnosed with cervical cancer every year.[35]

In 2006, the FDA approved the first vaccine for HPV, Gardasil®, for females aged 9–26. A second brand, Cervarix®, has recently been added to the market as well. The vaccines protect against the two most common types of HPV associated with high-risk cervical cancer (types 16 and 18) and the two most common types of HPV associated with genital warts (types 6 and 11). The vaccine is highly effective in women who were previously uninfected with those types of HPV. In October 2009, the FDA also approved the use of Gardasil® for the prevention of genital warts due to HPV types 6 and 11 in males, aged 9–26.[36]

Chlamydia

Chlamydia, which is caused by the bacterium *Chlamydia trachomatis*, is extremely common in the United States. Young women are especially at risk, with an estimated 1 in 10 adolescent girls testing positive for the infection.[37] The infection can be spread during vaginal, anal, or oral intercourse, and can be passed from mother to newborn baby during childbirth. Chlamydia can infect the vagina, penis, anus, cervix, urethra, and even the eyes or throat. Chlamydia is called the "silent disease" because the majority of those infected with it do not notice any unusual signs. Men, however, are more likely to show symptoms, often a burning sensation while urinating, as well as a discharge from their penis. Women who develop symptoms often notice an abnormal vaginal discharge and pain during urination. Symptoms usually develop within 1–3 weeks of infection.

If left untreated, chlamydia can have serious health consequences and lead to infertility. In 10–15% of the women whose chlamydia is not treated promptly, pelvic inflammatory disease occurs.[38] This condition damages the fallopian tubes and uterus, resulting in pelvic pain, infertility, and **ectopic pregnancies** that can be

ectopic pregnancy A pregnancy where the embryo implants outside of the uterus, often in the fallopian tubes.

deadly to mother and fetus. Chlamydia can also leave men infertile, inflaming the prostate gland and epididymis and scarring the urethra.

The U.S. Preventive Services Task Force recommends that all sexually active women aged 24 or younger undergo regular screening for chlamydia.[39] As a result, many pediatricians offer routine testing to their adolescent patients. Women who are 25 and older and at increased risk because of unsafe sex practices or intercourse with multiple partners are also encouraged to get screened regularly. A simple urine test or swab taken from the penis or cervix can detect a chlamydia infection. Chlamydia can be cured with antibiotics. All sexual partners should be treated at the same time to avoid reinfection. Doctors recommend that anyone with a chlamydia infection avoid sex during treatment.

Gonorrhea

Gonorrhea, sometimes referred to as "the clap," is a common and highly contagious sexually transmitted infection. It is caused by the bacteria *Neisseria gonorrhoeae*, and most often afflicts teenaged girls and men aged 20–24.[40] The bacteria are spread through intimate contact with an infected penis, vagina, anus, or mouth, and can be passed on to a newborn baby during childbirth. Most women infected with gonorrhea experience no symptoms at all. Those that do may mistake the painful urination or increased vaginal discharge for a bladder or yeast infection. Men are more likely to have noticeable signs of the condition, including sore testicles, colored penile discharge or a burning sensation while urinating. Symptoms usually occur within the first week after infection.

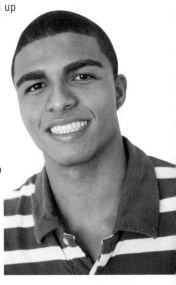

Rates of STIs for Different
Sexes, Ages, Races, and Sexual Orientations

STIs may affect people of different sexes, ages, races, and sexual orientations differently. Certain groups are at higher risk for particular STIs or STIs in general.

Sex

- Women are biologically more susceptible to becoming infected with STIs than men are. Young women, especially, are at high risk because the cells lining the cervix are more immature and vulnerable to infection.

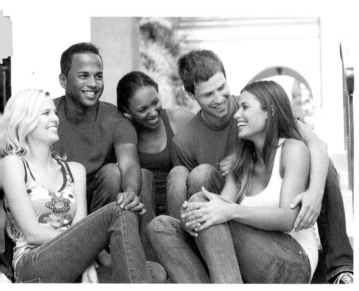

Young people are one of the groups at elevated risk for STIs.

- Women are less likely than men to experience symptoms of STIs, which can postpone detection and treatment.
- Women are more likely than men to experience long-term, severe side effects of STIs, such as infertility and cervical cancer.
- Women report 2.8 times as many cases of chlamydia as men.[1]
- Men accounted for 74% of new HIV/AIDS cases in 2007; women accounted for 26%.[2]
- Men reported 5.1 times as many cases of syphilis as women.[1]

Age

- People aged 15–24 have five times the reported rate of chlamydia as people aged 25 and older.[1]
- People aged 15–24 have four times the reported rate of gonorrhea as the rest of the population.[1]
- People aged 20–29 made up 25% of new HIV/AIDS cases in 2007.[2]

Race

- African Americans continue to experience an epidemic of HIV/AIDS, comprising 46% of the people living with HIV in the U.S.[2]

- African Americans—especially young African American women—are at disproportionately high risk for other STIs as well.
- Hispanics are disproportionately affected by HIV/AIDS, gonorrhea, chlamydia, and syphilis.[1] Although Hispanics make up 15% of the U.S. population, they comprise 18% of new HIV/AIDS cases in the U.S.[2]
- Native Americans/Alaska Natives are at a disproportionately high risk for gonorrhea and chlamydia.[1]
- Asian and Pacific Islander groups are experiencing growing rates of HIV/AIDS in the U.S.[2]

Sexual Orientation

- Young men who have sex with men, especially those of minority races or ethnicities, are at high risk for HIV infection, syphilis, and other STIs.
- The risk of female-to-female HIV transmission is low but possible, especially if one or both partners have sores on their genitals, if partners share sex toys, or if they participate in rough sex. Women can pass other STIs to one another as well.

Data from **1.** *STD Health Disparities* by the Centers for Disease Control and Prevention, 2010, retrieved from http://www.cdc.gov/std/health-disparities/default.htm. **2.** *HIV/AIDS* by the Centers for Disease Control and Prevention, 2010, retrieved from http://www.cdc.gov/hiv.

Without proper treatment, the bacteria can spread to the blood or joints, which can be life threatening. Pelvic inflammatory disease can also occur, causing pain and infertility. Women are at risk of having an ectopic pregnancy. Men can be left sterile. People with gonorrhea are also at greater risk of getting HIV.

Several laboratory tests can be used to diagnose gonorrhea, including a urine test or swab samples taken of the cervix, urethra, rectum, or throat. If you have the condition, your sexual partners should also be tested and treated. Antibiotics can often cure gonorrhea, but drug-resistant strains have been on the rise, making treatment more complicated. Because many people who have gonorrhea are infected with chlamydia at the same time, treatment often includes antibiotics for both. Avoid sexual contact until treatment is finished.

Pelvic Inflammatory Disease

Pelvic inflammatory disease, or PID, is an infection of a woman's uterus, fallopian tubes, and other reproductive organs that occurs when bacteria travel up from the vagina and spread. It affects an estimated 750,000 women in the U.S. every year, causing infertility in about 10%.[41] PID is caused by bacteria, most often from the bacteria associated with two of the most common sexually transmitted infections, chlamydia and gonorrhea.

With PID, bacteria infect the fallopian tubes, turning normal tissue into scar tissue. This can cause chronic abdominal pain. It also may block eggs from moving into the uterus, causing ectopic pregnancies or leaving a woman infertile.

Women may have no idea that they have PID, even as their reproductive system is being damaged. When symptoms do occur, they

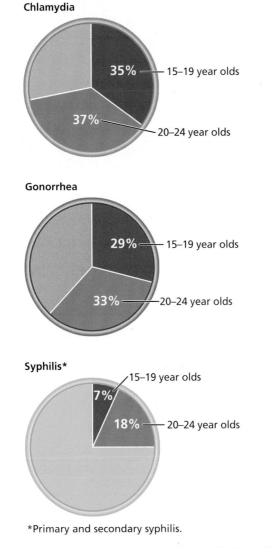
STIs in People Aged 15–24

Of the total new STI cases in 2008, these graphs show what percentages were in 15–19 year olds and 20–24 year olds.

Chlamydia

35% — 15–19 year olds

37% — 20–24 year olds

Gonorrhea

29% — 15–19 year olds

33% — 20–24 year olds

Syphilis*

15–19 year olds

7%

18% — 20–24 year olds

*Primary and secondary syphilis.

Source: Data from Centers for Disease Control and Prevention, National Center for HIV, STD, and TB Prevention (NCHSTP), Division of STD/HIV Prevention. (2009). *Sexually transmitted disease morbidity for selected STDs by age, race/ethnicity, and gender 1996–2008.* CDC WONDER On-line Database.

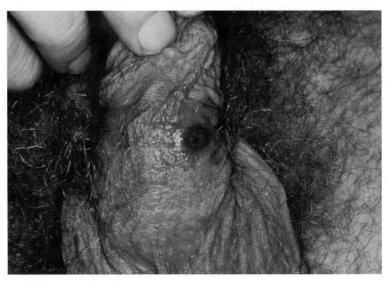

Figure 11.7 A syphilis chancre.

otics can cure the infection, but can not undo any of the damage already done to a woman's reproductive organs. For that reason, prompt treatment is always critical. A woman's sex partners also should be treated—even if they have no symptoms—to keep from spreading the bacteria that cause PID back and forth. In some cases, a woman may need surgery to reduce the scarring. However, she may still remain infertile.

Avoiding sexually transmitted infections—or getting immediate medical care should one occur—will help protect women from developing pelvic inflammatory disease. Because chlamydia and gonorrhea often have no noticeable symptoms, young sexually active women should undergo regular pelvic examinations and annual chlamydia testing. Sexually active women under the age of 25 have a higher risk of PID. In addition, women increase their risk of PID by douching, having recently had an IUD for birth control inserted, and having multiple sex partners.

Syphilis

Although syphilis is less widespread than other STIs, more than 46,000 cases of syphilis were reported in the United States in 2008, and the number of cases rose seven years in a row during the 2000s.[42] Syphilis is especially prevalent in parts of the South and in urban areas, with men who have sex with men disproportionately affected. The infection can be transmitted from mother to child during pregnancy or childbirth. Syphilis is caused by the bacterium *Treponema pallidum*, which enters the body through irritated skin or mucous membranes, including the vagina, anus, penis, lips, and mouth.

If left untreated, syphilis can progress through three different stages. In the first stage, 10 days to 3 months after infection, primary syphilis appears. A painless sore called a *chancre* appears where the bacteria entered the body, around the genitals, inside the vagina or rectum, or on the lips or mouth **(Figure 11.7).** The chancre will go away without treatment, but the infection itself will not. During the

may be subtle or vague, including fever, irregular menstrual bleeding, painful intercourse, or lower abdominal pain. The condition often goes unrecognized by patients and physicians alike.

No single test detects the presence of PID. Doctors typically perform a pelvic examination and test for chlamydia and gonorrhea. However, an abdominal ultrasound and even laparoscopy (minimally invasive surgery) may be needed to confirm the diagnosis. Antibi-

next stage, secondary syphilis, symptoms may include a rash on the hands or feet, neck, head, or torso, wart-like growths around the genitals, and grayish sores in the mouth. Hair loss may occur. The infection will then enter a latent stage, which lacks symptoms, and can last for years. If syphilis isn't treated, about 15% of people will develop the late or tertiary stage, where small tumor-like growths called *gummas* appear on internal organs and damage to the nervous system occurs. Tertiary syphilis can also cause severe problems with the heart, brain, and eyes, causing blindness, paralysis, brain damage, dementia, and even death. Syphilis also increases the chances of contracting HIV.

Examination of a fluid sample taken from a chancre or swollen lymph nodes can confirm infection during primary or secondary syphilis. Two types of blood tests are also available to detect the bacteria during any of its stages. Antibiotics are the first line of defense against syphilis. If treatment is not initiated until the final stage, the bacteria can be killed but the internal damage that has already occurred can not be reversed.

Pubic Lice and Scabies

Pubic lice, or *Pthirus pubis*, are tiny six-legged creatures that infest pubic hair **(Figure 11.8).** Commonly known as "crabs," they can also attach themselves to eyebrows, eyelashes, beards, mustaches, or chest hair. Scabies is caused by tiny, eight-legged mites that burrow into the top layer of a person's skin and lay eggs. Scabies generally occurs in and around folds of skin, but can affect other parts of the body as well. Pubic lice and scabies are usually transmitted through sexual contact but occasionally are spread through contact with clothing, towels, sheets, or toilet seats that have been used by an infected person.

The most common symptom of pubic lice and scabies is itching, especially during the night. In some instances, the infested area also becomes inflamed, and scabies can sometimes cause allergic reactions. The pests themselves do not spread disease, but excessive scratching of the skin can cause a bacterial infection.

A pubic lice or scabies infestation can be easily diagnosed with a doctor's visit. Prescribed creams or lotions can usually clear up these conditions, although an oral medication may be used for cases that are harder to treat.

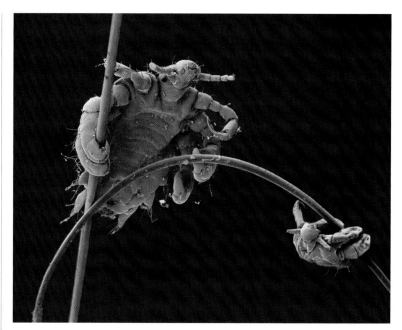

Figure 11.8 Pubic lice.

Trichomoniasis

Trichomoniasis, or "trich," is caused by a protozoa called *Trichomonas vaginalis*. It is a very common STI in young women, although men can be infected as well. More than 7.4 million infections occur annually in the U.S.[43] Fortunately, women often experience symptoms, so they seek medical treatment. Symptoms include painful urination, pain during intercourse, vaginal itching and irritation, and a greenish-yellow, strong-smelling vaginal discharge. Men often do not experience symptoms, but if they do they include irritation inside the penis and slight discharge. Trich can be cured with oral antibiotics.

Watch videos of real students discussing STIs and other infections at: **www.pearsonhighered.com/choosinghealth.**

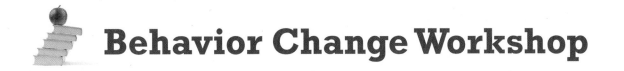

Behavior Change Workshop

To complete this workshop online, visit **www.pearsonhighered.com/choosinghealth**.

The research findings are clear: Certain behaviors put you at greater risk for STIs. Are there sexual behaviors that you can change to reduce your risk? Are you willing to make some changes?

Part I. Assessing Your Personal STI Risk

1. What are your risk factors for contracting an STI? List both ones you can change and ones you can't.

_____

_____

_____

_____

_____

_____

2. Ask yourself honestly: How ready am I to commit to a behavior change that will help me reduce or eliminate one of these risks? What stage of behavior change am I in?

_____

_____

_____

_____

3. Keeping your current stage of behavior change in mind, describe what you might do or think about as a next step to reduce or eliminate one of your STI risks.

_____

_____

_____

_____

_____

4. What might be some barriers to making your next step and how could you overcome them?

Barrier	**Strategy for Overcoming Barrier**
Example: My partner doesn't want to wear a condom.	_I will explain to him why it is important to wear one and how I feel about his lack of wanting to use one._
_____	_____
_____	_____
_____	_____

Part II. Taking Action to Reduce STI Risk

You can take responsibility for your sexual health and reduce your STI risk in several key areas. For each of the risk reduction guidelines listed below, indicate one action you can take (or have already taken) to meet that guideline in your own life. Be specific.

Reducing Your Personal STI Risk

STI Risk Reduction Guideline	Specific Action to Meet Guideline
Become more educated about the risks, symptoms, treatment, and prevention of STIs.	
For STIs with an available vaccine (HPV and hepatitis B) get vaccinated! (HPV vaccine is now available for males too.)	
Be alert for signs or symptoms of STIs.	
Get tested.	
Communicate with sexual partners about your sexual histories, including histories of STIs.	
Don't impair your judgment before participating in sexual activity by using drugs or alcohol.	
Always use a condom.	
Practice safe oral sex by using condoms, dental dams, or latex squares.	
Limit your number of sexual partners.	

Chapter Summary

- Pathogens are the agents that cause infections. Pathogens include viruses, bacteria, fungi, protozoa, and parasitic worms.

- Infectious diseases can be spread by personal contact with an infected person, touching inanimate objects that are contaminated with pathogens, inhaling airborne pathogens, or contact with infected animals, insects, water, or food.

- Your body's first line of defense against infection is your skin, mucous membranes, cilia, and bodily fluids, which prevent pathogens from entering the body or trap and expel them if they do.

- Your immune system, a powerful network of cellular and chemical defenses, fights pathogens that enter the body. Neutrophils, natural killer cells, and macrophages are key nonspecific defenders. B cells and T cells work with precision and focus to produce antibodies and kill specific pathogens. Memory B cells and T cells sometimes provide long-term immunity to an infection, which makes getting the same infection again unlikely.

- Sometimes the immune system mistakes common substances, such as nuts, pet dander, or pollen, as harmful agents, triggering allergies. Allergies can cause asthma.

- HIV/AIDS is the most serious of the sexually transmitted infections. It targets and destroys the immune system and eventually leads to death. Early detection is important because proper treatment can significantly prolong life.

- Other common sexually transmitted infections are genital herpes, human papillomavirus (HPV), chlamydia, gonorrhea, syphilis, pubic lice, and scabies.

- It is up to you to help protect yourself from infections by keeping up to date on your immunizations, properly washing your hands, and engaging in safe sexual practices.

- Prevention is the best medicine for sexually transmitted infections. Many may not show symptoms until irreparable damage has been done. Among other things, certain sexually transmitted infections can cause infertility or death.

Test Your Knowledge

1. Pathogens
   a. can not be stopped by your body's first line of defense.
   b. are agents that cause disease.
   c. infect animals but not humans.
   d. die once they enter your body.

2. A person who spreads infectious disease to others is called a
   a. reservoir.
   b. carrier.
   c. contaminator.
   d. pathogen.

3. Your first line of defense against infection is
   a. your immune system.
   b. antibiotics.
   c. immunization.
   d. your skin.

4. What type of organism takes over the body's cells, forcing them to make replicas of it?
   a. viruses
   b. fungi
   c. bacteria
   d. protozoa

5. Lyme disease is spread by
   a. fleas.
   b. ticks.
   c. mosquitoes.
   d. mice.

6. Antibiotics are appropriate treatments against
   a. bacteria.
   b. viruses.
   c. fungi.
   d. none of the above.

7. The most commonly reported sexually transmitted infection among college students is
   a. genital warts/HPV.
   b. genital herpes.
   c. chlamydia.
   d. HIV/AIDS.

8. What percentage of sexually active people in the U.S. get a sexually transmitted infection by age 25?
   a. 15%
   b. 25%
   c. 30%
   d. 50%

9. Which of the following practices will NOT reduce risk of contracting HIV?
   a. correct use of condoms
   b. abstinence
   c. avoiding multiple partners and getting tested with new partners
   d. avoiding partners who look sick

10. Cervical cancer is caused by
    a. pelvic inflammatory disease.
    b. chlamydia.
    c. human papillomavirus (HPV).
    d. gonorrhea.

Get Critical

What happened:

A month into her freshman year, Indiana State University student Ashley Lee came home for a weekend visit. Feeling sick, she assumed she was coming down with the flu and went to bed early. The next morning she was so weak she couldn't walk to the bathroom on her own. Her family took her to the hospital, where doctors and nurses struggled to identify the mystery illness that left her weak, in excruciating pain, and with a rash that covered her body. Ashley was finally diagnosed with bacterial meningitis and given powerful antibiotics. Although lucky to survive, the meningitis did not leave Ashley unscathed. Doctors had to amputate her left foot and three of her fingers and remove much of the flesh from her right leg; leaving Ashley with a long and painful recovery. Despite the physical and emotional trauma of her meningitis infection, a year later Ashley returned to school with the hopes of becoming a doctor and specializing in treating infectious diseases.

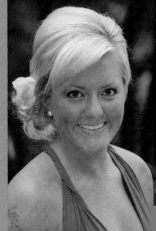

What do you think?

- Why was Ashley at increased risk for contracting bacterial meningitis?
- What can you do to reduce your risk of contracting bacterial meningitis?
- Would it have been better or worse for Ashley to have contracted viral meningitis?

Watch a video of Ashley's story at www.msnbc.msn .com/id/21134540/vp/20538897.

Get Connected

i. Centers for Disease Control and Prevention. (2008). *Seasonal influenza (flu)*. Retrieved from http://cdc.gov/flu/about/disease/index.htm

ii. Centers for Disease Control and Prevention. (2009). *Sexually transmitted diseases in the United States, 2008: National surveillance data for chlamydia, gonorrhea, and syphilis*. Retrieved from http://www.cdc.gov/std/stats08/trends.htm

iii. Centers for Disease Control and Prevention. (2008). *It helps to know*. [Audio podcast]. Retrieved from http://www.cdc.gov/hiv/topics/testing/podcasts.htm

1. Centers for Disease Control and Prevention, National Center for Zoonotic, Vector-Borne, and Enteric Diseases. (2009). *Did you know . . .* Retrieved from http://www.cdc.gov/nczved

2. Rusin, P., Maxwell, S., & Gerba, C. (2002). Comparative surface-to-hand and fingertip-to-mouth transfer efficiency of gram-positive bacteria, gram-negative bacteria, and phage. *Journal of Applied Microbiology, 93*(4), 585–592.

3. American College Health Association. (2009). *American College Health Association National College Health Assessment (ACHA-NCHA II) reference group executive summary, Fall 2009*. Linthicum, MD: American College Health Association.

4. American Academy of Allergy, Asthma & Immunology. (n.d.). *Tips to remember: Allergic reactions* Retrieved from http://www.aaaai.org/patients/publicedmat/tips/whatisallergicreaction.stm

5. American Lung Association Epidemiology and Statistics Unit, Research and Program Services. (2007). *Trends in asthma morbidity and mortality*. Retrieved from http://www.aaaai.org/media/statistics/asthma-statistics.asp

6. Directors of Health Promotion and Education. *Addressing infectious disease threats*. Retrieved from http://www.dhpe.org/infect/infectintro.html

7. Baccam, P., Beauchemin, C., Macken, C., Hayden, F., & Perelson, A. (2006). Kinetics of influenza A virus infection in humans. *Journal of Virology, 80*(15), 7590–7599.

8. National Institute of Allergy and Infectious Diseases. (n.d.). *Common cold*. Retrieved December 20, 2008, from http://www3.niaid.nih.gov/topics/commonCold/overview.htm

9. Centers for Disease Control and Prevention. (2008). *Seasonal influenza (flu)*. Retrieved from http://cdc.gov/flu/about/disease/index.htm

10. Centers for Disease Control and Prevention. (2009). *Hepatitis C FAQs for the public*. Retrieved from http://www.cdc.gov/hepatitis/C/cFAQ.htm#cFAQ04

11. National Institutes of Health, National Institute of Allergy and Infectious Diseases. (2006). *Understanding microbes in sickness and in health*. NIH Publication No. 06-4914. Retrieved from http://www.speit.org/monografias/microbesbook.pdf

12. World Health Organization. (2010). *Meningococcal meningitis*. Fact sheet No. 141. Retrieved from http://www.who.int/mediacentre/factsheets/fs141/en/print.html

13. Centers for Disease Control and Prevention. *Toxic shock syndrome*. Retrieved from http://www.cdc.gov/ncidod/dbmd/diseaseinfo/toxicshock_t.htm

14. Centers for Disease Control and Prevention, National Center for Health Statistics. *Leading causes of death*. Retrieved from http://www.cdc.gov/nchs/FASTATS/lcod.htm

15. World Health Organization. (2009). *Pneumonia*. Fact Sheet No. 331. Retrieved from http://www.who.int/mediacentre/factsheets/fs331/en/index.html

16. Centers for Disease Control and Prevention. (2009). *The difference between latent TB infection and active TB disease*. Retrieved from http://www.cdc.gov/tb/publications/factsheets/general/ltbiandactivetb.htm

17. Centers for Disease Control and Prevention. (2009). Trends in tuberculosis–United States, 2008. *Morbidity and Mortality Weekly Report, 58*(10), 249–253.

18. National Institutes of Health. *TB still declining in U.S., but at slower rate*. Retrieved from http://www.nlm.nih.gov/medlineplus/news/fullstory_81946.html

19. World Health Organization. (2010). *Malaria*. Fact sheet No. 94. Retrieved from http://www.who.int/mediacentre/factsheets/fs094/en/print.html

20. World Health Organization. (2007). *Global strategy for the prevention and control of sexually transmitted infections: 2006–2015. Breaking the chain of transmission*. Geneva, Switzerland: WHO Press.

21. Weinstock, H., Berman, S., & Cates, Jr., W. (2004). Sexually transmitted diseases among American youth: Incidence and prevalence estimates, 2000. *Perspectives on Sexual and Reproductive Health 2004, 36*(1), 6–10.

22. World Health Organization. (2007). *Sexually transmitted infections*. Fact sheet No. 110. Retrieved from http://www.who.int/mediacentre/factsheets/fs110/en/index.html

23. Centers for Disease Control and Prevention. (2009). *Sexually transmitted diseases in the United States, 2008: National surveillance data for chlamydia, gonorrhea, and syphilis*. Retrieved from http://www.cdc.gov/std/stats08/trends.htm

24. Forhan, S. E., Gottlieb, S. L., Sternberg, M. R., Fujie, X., Datta, S. D., McQuillan, G. M., . . . Markowitz, L. E. (2009). Prevalence of sexually transmitted infections among female adolescents aged 14 to 19 in the United States. *Pediatrics, 124*(6), 1505–1512. doi: 10.1542/peds.2009-0674

25. Cates, J. R., Herndon, N. L., Schulz, S. L., & Darroch, J. E. (2004). *Our voices, our lives, our futures: Youth and sexually transmitted diseases*. Chapel Hill, NC: University of North Carolina at Chapel Hill School of Journalism and Mass Communication.

26. Joint United Nations Programme on HIV/AIDS (UNAIDS) and World Health Organization. (2009). *AIDS epidemic update 2009*. UNAIDS/09.36E / JC1700E. Retrieved from http://www.unaids.org/en/KnowledgeCentre/HIVData/EpiUpdate/EpiUpdArchive/2009/default.asp

27. World Health Organization. (n.d.). *Mother-to-child transmission of HIV*. Retrieved from http://www.who.int/hiv/topics/mtct/en/index.html

28. Word Health Organization. (2009). *Rapid advice: Use of antiretroviral drugs for treating pregnant women and preventing HIV infection in infants*. Geneva, Switzerland: WHO Press.

29. World Health Organization. (2009). Love in the era of HAART. *HIV/AIDS Prevention and Care Newsletter, 2*(1): 1. Retrieved from http://www.wpro.who.int/NR/rdonlyres/48B1DC54-F2CC-4704-8199-1E7FBEA002EA/0/ARVnewsletter_vol2issue1_July2009.pdf

30. Centers for Disease Control and Prevention. (2009). *Hepatitis B FAQs for the public*. Retrieved from http://www.cdc.gov/hepatitis/B/bFAQ.htm

31. Centers for Disease Control. (2010). *CDC study finds U.S. herpes rates remain high* [Press release]. Retrieved from http://www.cdc.gov/nchhstp/Newsroom/hsv2pressrelease.html

32. American Social Health Association. (n.d.). *Treatment for oral herpes*. Retrieved from http://www.ashastd.org/herpes/herpes_learn_treatment.cfm#2

33. Centers for Disease Control and Prevention. (2007). *CDC fact sheet: HPV and men*. Retrieved from http://www.cdc.gov/STD/HPV/HPV&Men-Fact-Sheet.pdf

34. Centers for Disease Control and Prevention. (2009). How common are HPV and related diseases?, *CDC fact sheet: Genital HPV infection*. Retrieved from http://www.cdc.gov/STD/HPV/STDFact-HPV.htm#common

35. American Cancer Society. (2009). *Overview: Cervical cancer. How many women get cancer of the cervix?* Retrieved from http://www.cancer.org/docroot/CRI/content/CRI_2_2_1X_How_many_women_get_cancer_of_the_cervix_8.asp?sitearea=

36. U.S. Food and Drug Administration. (2009, October 16). *FDA approves new indication for Gardasil to prevent genital warts in men and boys* [News release]. Retrieved from http://www.fda.gov/NewsEvents/Newsroom/PressAnnouncements/ucm187003.htm

37. American Social Health Association. (n.d.). *Chlamydia: Questions & answers*. Retrieved from http://www.ashastd.org/learn/learn_chlamydia.cfm

38. Centers for Disease Control and Prevention. (2010). What are the symptoms of chlamydia?, *CDC fact sheet: Chlamydia*. Retrieved from http://www.cdc.gov/std/chlamydia/STDFact-Chlamydia.htm#symptoms

39. U.S. Preventive Services Task Force. (2007). Screening for chlamydial infection: U.S. Preventive Services Task Force recommendation statement. *Annals of Internal Medicine, 147*(2), 128–134.

40. Mayo Clinic. (2009). *Gonorrhea*. Retrieved from http://www.mayoclinic.com/print/gonorrhea/DS00180

41. Centers for Disease Control and Prevention. (2010). *CDC fact sheet: Pelvic inflammatory disease*. Retrieved from http://www.cdc.gov/std/PID/STDFact-PID.htm

42. Centers for Disease Control and Prevention. (2009). *Sexually transmitted diseases surveillance, 2008: Syphilis*. Retrieved from http://www.cdc.gov/std/stats08/syphilis.htm

43. Centers for Disease Control and Prevention. (n.d.). How common is trichomoniasis?, *CDC fact sheet: Trichomoniasis*. Retrieved from http://www.cdc.gov/std/trichomonas/stdfact-trichomoniasis.htm#Common

12

- Statistics suggest that 1 out of every 3 children born in the U.S. in 2000 will eventually develop diabetes.[i]

- Cardiovascular disease is the number 1 cause of death in both men and women in the U.S.[ii]

- More than 1 million people develop skin cancer every year.[iii]

Preventing Cardiovascular Disease, Diabetes, and Cancer

IDENTIFY four key behaviors that influence an individual's risk for chronic disease.

DESCRIBE the difference between type 1 and type 2 diabetes.

COMPARE and contrast the four major types of cardiovascular disease.

DEFINE cancer and identify the factors involved in its initiation and spread.

ASSESS your personal risk factors for developing a chronic disease, and develop a plan for reducing your risk.

Health Online icons are found throughout the chapter, directing you to web links, videos, podcasts, and other useful online resources.

College is all about preparing for your future.

Where will your major take you? Will you go to graduate school? What will your career be like? How will the friendships and relationships you make on campus shape your life in your post-college years?

To that list of questions, we'd like to add one more: Will the behaviors you practice today help maintain your health or lead you to chronic disease?

It's an important question because, when it comes to your risk of developing a chronic disease—like diabetes, cardiovascular disease, or cancer—the odds are against you. If 100 students were enrolled in your health course, and you all were to follow current U.S. health trends, here is where national statistics suggest you would wind up:

- About 27 of you would experience either diabetes or prediabetes over the course of your lifetime.[1]
- About 32 of you would die of diseases of the heart or blood vessels, such as coronary artery disease, heart attack, sudden cardiac arrest, or stroke.[2]
- About 26 of you would die of cancer.[2]

These numbers are sobering. But they do not necessarily predict your fate. Just as you can use your time in college to shape your career, you can also use these years to start beating the odds of developing a chronic disease.

Overview of Chronic Diseases

A **chronic disease** is one that comes on gradually and lasts for a long time, causing either continual symptoms or recurring bouts of illness. The first two chronic diseases discussed in this chapter—diabetes and cardiovascular disease—usually resist complete cure, and instead are typically managed by a combination of lifestyle changes, medications, and other treatments. Cancer, the third disease we'll focus on, can be cured, in some cases allowing decades of healthy living after successful treatment.

Scope of the Problem

Chronic diseases are the leading causes of death and disability in the United States.[3] Just two of the chronic diseases discussed in this chapter—cardiovascular disease and cancer—are responsible for more than half of all deaths in the U.S. every year.[4]

Many of the deaths due to chronic disease occur prematurely; that is, at an earlier than expected age. But chronic diseases not only deprive us of years of life; they reduce our *quality* of life because of their accompanying discomfort, pain, psychological distress, and activity limitations. If you've ever seen someone with advanced diabetes walking with crutches because of an amputated foot, or heard someone struggling to speak because of the effects of a stroke, then you've witnessed some of the severe limitations that can accompany chronic disease.

Finally, the financial burden of chronic disease is tremendous: about 75% of health-care expenditures in the United States are for treatment of chronic disease.[5] Moreover, the economy of the United States loses

chronic disease A disease with a gradual onset of symptoms that last a long time or recur.

more than $1 trillion annually to medical care and lost productivity due to chronic disease.[6]

Influence of Four Key Behaviors

Diabetes, cardiovascular disease, and cancer might seem unrelated, but in fact they share some underlying physiological mechanisms and risk factors. That's because the functions of the chemicals, cells, and tissues of our bodies are densely interrelated, and certain factors that initiate disease in one body organ or system can initiate disease in another. For example, smoking can cause inflammation, reduced circulation, genetic changes, and other problems that in turn are factors in diabetes, cardiovascular disease, and cancer—as well as chronic respiratory diseases.[7]

In fact, the more we have learned about chronic disease, the more we have come to appreciate the role of just four key health-risk behaviors in promoting it **(Figure 12.1).** These four behaviors, which we have discussed throughout this text, are:

- Poor nutrition, especially a diet high in saturated and *trans* fats and low in fruits and vegetables.

The Centers for Disease Control and Prevention have a comprehensive website covering chronic diseases, including strategies for prevention, statistics, fact sheets, and more: **www.cdc.gov/ chronicdisease/index.htm.**

- Lack of physical activity.
- Tobacco use—the single most avoidable cause of disease, disability, and death in the United States.
- Excessive alcohol consumption.[8]

In addition, people in the U.S. are consuming more total calories than they expend, and as a result experiencing increased rates of overweight and obesity. The Centers for Disease Control and Prevention link obesity to an increased risk for the more common form of diabetes, cardiovascular disease, and certain cancers.[8]

Diabetes, cardiovascular disease, and cancer are all serious diseases. But by making healthful choices each day—eating a nutritious diet, exercising, avoiding tobacco, and limiting your alcohol intake—you can increase your chances of beating the odds of developing a chronic disease.

Reducing Your Risk for Diabetes

Do you know someone with diabetes? Do you have it yourself? Your answer is far more likely to be "Yes" than was your parents' reply at your age.

Once a condition seen mostly in children and older adults, diabetes is now one of the most common serious illnesses in the United States, and the number of cases continues to grow rapidly **(Figure 12.2).** About 8% of the population has some form of diabetes, and another 19% is on its way to developing it.[1] As of 2008, the number of people in the U.S. with diabetes had more than doubled in 15 years.[1] At this rate of growth, health experts anticipate that one out of every three U.S. children born in the year 2000 will develop diabetes.[9]

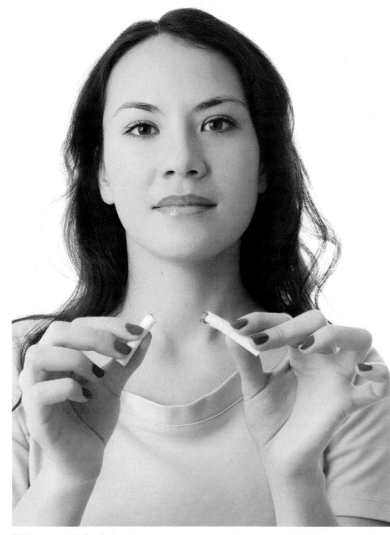

Figure 12.1 Live a healthy lifestyle. Not smoking is one of the best things you can do to reduce your risk of developing a chronic disease.

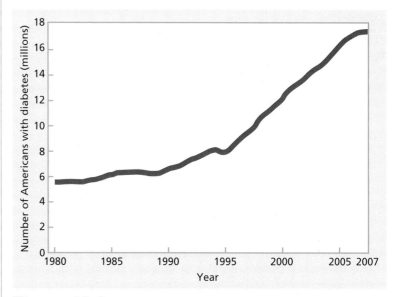

Figure 12.2 Diabetes is on the rise. From 1980 to 2007, the number of people in the U.S. with diabetes tripled.

Source: Number (in Millions) of Civilian/Noninstitutionalized Persons with Diagnosed Diabetes, United States, 1980–2007 by the Centers for Disease Control and Prevention, retrieved from http://www.cdc.gov/diabetes/statistics/prev/national/figpersons.htm.

What Is Diabetes?

Diabetes, known formally as **diabetes mellitus,** is a broad term that covers a group of diseases characterized by high levels of sugar, or *glucose,* in the blood. In fact, the word *mellitus* is derived from the Latin word for honey. These high levels of blood glucose arise from problems with **insulin,** a hormone produced by the **pancreas** that is necessary for transportation of glucose into the body's cells. Some people with diabetes simply don't make enough insulin. Others make enough, but their body cells can't use insulin effectively. In either case, glucose from the breakdown of carbohydrates in food builds up in the bloodstream, while the body's cells—unable to take in glucose—suffer from lack of nourishment.

Type 1 Diabetes

Type 1 diabetes arises when the body's own immune system destroys the cells in the pancreas that make insulin. Type 1 diabetes usually appears in childhood or adolescence, and researchers are investigating the role of specific genes in its development, as well as the possible role of external factors such as viruses. People with type 1 diabetes must monitor their blood sugar level throughout each day, and take supplemental insulin through injections or a pump implanted in their bodies. For this reason, type 1 diabetes is often known as *insulin-dependent diabetes.* Insulin can't be taken by mouth because it is a protein, and would be digested in the gastrointestinal tract.

Type 1 diabetes accounts for the majority of diabetes in children and up to 10% of diabetes cases in adults.[10] There is no cure for type 1 diabetes, but the condition is the focus of intense research, including studies into the use of stem cell therapy to replace the pancreas's insulin-making beta cells.

Type 2 Diabetes

Once known as *adult-onset diabetes,* **type 2 diabetes** is more common than type 1, accounting for about 90–95% of all adult diabetes cases.[10] Although it is still most common after age 60, the incidence of type 2 diabetes has surged among all age groups, including teenagers. One study of prescription medication use found that preteen and teenage use of type 2 diabetes drugs more than doubled between 2002 and 2005.[11] Type 2 diabetes cases also tend to occur in higher numbers in certain parts of the country, with regions of the South and Southwest showing the highest concentrations of adult cases.[1]

In type 1 diabetes, the cells of the pancreas stop making insulin, whereas most cases of type 2 diabetes begin as *insulin resistance.* The pancreas makes normal amounts of insulin, but the body's cells don't respond to it properly—they resist its effects. One factor in this resistance is an overabundance of fatty acids concentrated in fat cells. This explains why type 2 diabetes is linked not only to age but also to obesity. If the body's cells can't respond to insulin, they can't take up glucose, and it remains in the bloodstream. The resulting **hyperglycemia** (persistent high blood glucose) signals the pancreas

diabetes mellitus A group of diseases in which the body does not make or use insulin properly, resulting in elevated blood glucose.

insulin A hormone necessary for glucose transport into cells.

pancreas An abdominal organ that produces insulin as well as certain compounds helpful in digestion.

type 1 diabetes A form of diabetes that usually begins early in life and arises when the pancreas produces insufficient insulin.

type 2 diabetes A form of diabetes that usually begins later in life and arises when cells resist the effects of insulin.

hyperglycemia A persistent state of elevated levels of blood glucose.

prediabetes A persistent state of blood glucose levels higher than normal, but not yet high enough to qualify as diabetes.

to produce more insulin to get more glucose into the cells. As the demand for insulin continues to rise, the cells of the pancreas begin to fatigue and eventually lose their ability to produce it. Blood glucose levels rise and remain dangerously elevated: the person has diabetes.

Figure 12.3 illustrates the differences between type 1 and type 2 diabetes.

Other Forms of Diabetes

Less common varieties of diabetes resemble type 2, but also have differences that set them apart:

- *Gestational diabetes* develops in a woman during pregnancy, and affects up to 5% of pregnant women. The condition usually disappears after childbirth, but researchers have learned that women who develop gestational diabetes are at greater risk for type 2 diabetes later in life.[12]

- *Type 1.5* is a general term for several varieties of diabetes that blend aspects of type 1 and type 2 diabetes. For instance, a physician may suspect a type 1.5 variety when a newly diagnosed adult diabetic is not overweight. Research suggests that perhaps as many as 10% of people diagnosed with type 2 diabetes have type 1.5, and the number of cases may be growing.[13]

Detecting Diabetes

The physical signs and symptoms of diabetes include:

- Frequent urination
- Excessive thirst
- Hunger
- Tendency to tire easily
- Numbness or tingling in the hands and feet
- In women, a tendency to develop vaginal yeast infections

These symptoms, while common across all types of diabetes, can develop differently from person to person. Keep in mind, too, that early stages of diabetes may not be accompanied by any symptoms at all.

Simple laboratory tests can reveal whether or not you have—or are developing—diabetes. One of the most common is the *fasting plasma glucose test* (*FPG*), which requires you to fast (consuming nothing other than plain water) overnight. A technician then draws a blood sample, and the level of glucose in your blood is measured. Here is what the measurement values mean:

- A blood glucose level below 100 mg/dL is normal.
- A blood glucose level between 100 and 125 mg/dL means that you have **prediabetes.** That is, your blood glucose is higher than normal but not high enough to warrant a diagnosis of diabetes. Prediabetes indicates that your body is struggling to regulate your blood glucose, and you are at significant risk for developing diabetes.
- A blood glucose level 126 mg/dL or higher indicates true diabetes.

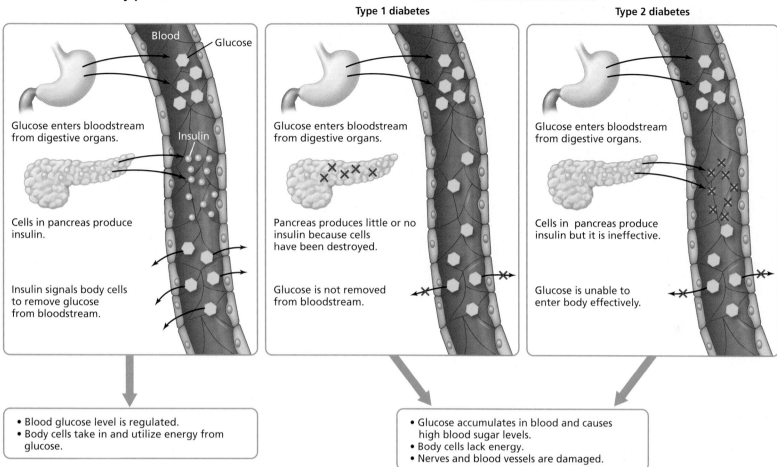

Healthy person

Blood

Glucose

Glucose enters bloodstream from digestive organs.

Insulin

Cells in pancreas produce insulin.

Insulin signals body cells to remove glucose from bloodstream.

- Blood glucose level is regulated.
- Body cells take in and utilize energy from glucose.

Person with diabetes

Type 1 diabetes

Glucose enters bloodstream from digestive organs.

Pancreas produces little or no insulin because cells have been destroyed.

Glucose is not removed from bloodstream.

Type 2 diabetes

Glucose enters bloodstream from digestive organs.

Cells in pancreas produce insulin but it is ineffective.

Glucose is unable to enter body effectively.

- Glucose accumulates in blood and causes high blood sugar levels.
- Body cells lack energy.
- Nerves and blood vessels are damaged.

Figure 12.3 Two types of diabetes. In type 1 diabetes, the pancreas stops producing or produces insufficient insulin. In type 2 diabetes, the body is unable to use insulin properly. In either case, the body's cells are unable to take in glucose from the bloodstream.

Fortunately, you can take steps to bring your blood glucose levels back down. We'll discuss these shortly.

Long-Term Effects of Diabetes

Persistent high blood glucose (hyperglycemia, discussed earlier) causes damage throughout the body, especially to blood vessels. This damage in turn can lead to a variety of complications:

- Damage to the blood vessels that supply the heart and brain raises the risk of heart attack and stroke.
- The kidneys have microscopic blood vessels that filter wastes from the blood into urine. Hyperglycemia stresses this delicate filtration system, leading to kidney disease, a common and serious complication of diabetes.
- Hyperglycemia also damages blood vessels that serve nerves, causing loss of sensation and tissue breakdown, especially in the feet, ankles, and lower legs. This contributes to the high risk of non-healing wounds, which may require surgical amputation, among people with diabetes.
- When hyperglycemia damages the tiny blood vessels serving the retina of the eye, vision deteriorates. In fact, diabetes is a leading cause of blindness among U.S. adults.[14]

Overall, diabetes is now the seventh most common cause of death in the United States, and shaves 10 to 15 years off a person's life.[9]

Risk Factors for Type 2 Diabetes

Did you grab an apple or a bag of fries for your last snack? When you had some free time over the weekend, did you opt for an activity like going for a bike ride, or crash on the couch to play a video game? Your answers have something to say about your risk for type 2 diabetes **(Figure 12.4)**.

In addition to age, the risk factors for type 2 diabetes include:

- **Overweight.** Being overweight or obese increases your risk, and the more overweight you are, the more that risk goes up at a young age. In one national study that gauged lifetime diabetes risk according to body mass index (BMI), 18-year-old men who were very obese had a 70% risk of developing diabetes, while the risk for very obese women of the same age was 74%.[15]
- **Disproportionately large waist.** As you learned in Chapter 6, people who carry more of their excess weight around their abdominal area are at greater risk for diabetes. Greater amounts of abdominal fat have been linked to insulin resistance.

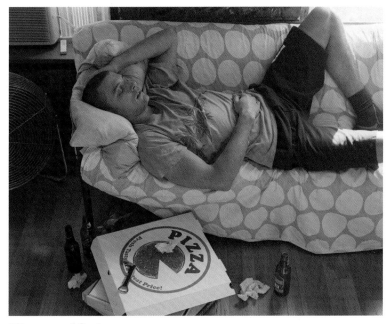

Figure 12.4 **A sedentary lifestyle puts you at risk.** Risk factors for type 2 diabetes include lack of physical activity and being overweight.

- **Lack of exercise.** Exercise helps control weight, burns glucose, and makes your body cells more receptive to insulin. Physical activity also builds up muscle mass, and muscle cells absorb most of the glucose in your blood.

- **Genetic factors.** Do members of your family have type 2 diabetes? If so, you are at higher risk. A variety of common genetic variants can increase a person's risk of type 2 diabetes. This inherited risk is seen both within families and within ethnic groups. African Americans, Hispanics, and Native Americans develop diabetes at higher rates than other U.S. population groups.[16] Although the cause of these population differences is probably a mix of inherited and environmental factors, researchers say genetics clearly play a role.[13]

In addition, a cluster of conditions collectively known as **metabolic syndrome** increases an individual's risk for type 2 diabetes and cardiovascular disease. The characteristics of this syndrome include abdominal obesity (that is, a waist measurement of more than 40 inches in men or more than 35 inches in women), elevated levels of fat in the blood, low levels of "good" cholesterol, high blood pressure, and high blood glucose. Having three or more of these characteristics constitutes the diagnosis of metabolic syndrome.

metabolic syndrome A set of unhealthy physical and metabolic characteristics linked to type 2 diabetes, cardiovascular disease, and other serious diseases.

Are you at risk for prediabetes or diabetes? Take this online quiz from the American Diabetes Association to find out: www.diabetes.org/diabetes-basics/prevention/diabetes-risk-test.

Changing Behaviors to Reduce Your Risk for Type 2 Diabetes

Although the statistics on type 2 diabetes can sound alarming, the list of risk factors above also points out how you can take control. Several large-scale research initiatives, including the National Institutes of Health's Diabetes Prevention Program, offer proven steps to reduce your risk:

- **Watch your weight, and lose weight if necessary.** If you are overweight or obese or are carrying extra weight around your midsection, losing just 5–10% of your body weight can make a significant difference in your risk. Aim for a waist measurement of less than 40 inches if you are a man or less than 35 inches if you are a woman. For more discussion of weight management, see Chapter 6.

- **Get moving.** Exercise at least 30 minutes a day, at least 5 days a week. Aim for a mix of activities that build cardiorespiratory endurance and muscle strength. For more information on physical activity, see Chapter 5.

- **Eat a healthy diet.** Go for food choices that include complex carbohydrates, lots of fiber, and low levels of sodium and saturated fat. In one study of more than 80,000 women, researchers found that following a diet low in red meat and processed meats, high in produce and whole grains, and moderate in plant-based fats and alcohol reduced diabetes risk by 36%.[18] For a detailed discussion of nutrition, see Chapter 4.

- **Get a physical exam.** Find out your fasting blood glucose level and your measurement of other factors related to metabolic syndrome. Talk to your health-care provider about reducing your risk.

- **Be aware of the risks in your background.** Do you know your family's history of diabetes? If not, ask. Awareness of your family history is especially important if your ethnicity puts you at increased risk. Becoming aware of inherited risks is important because it allows you to discuss them with your health-care provider and to take steps, such as improving your diet and exercise habits, to reduce those risks.[17]

Controlling Diabetes

If you do develop diabetes, your doctor will work with you toward one central goal—stabilizing your body's use of glucose. The approach you take will depend on the type of diabetes you have.

People with type 1 diabetes require urgent intervention. To stay healthy, they must measure their blood glucose levels several times a day and receive regular doses of insulin to keep their bodies functioning. Fortunately, new technologies have made diabetes control easier. For example, in the past, blood glucose monitoring required pricking the finger several times a day. Now, devices are available that can read glucose levels through the skin, or from a small needle implanted in the body. For insulin delivery, instead of giving themselves injections, diabetics can wear an insulin infusion pump that delivers insulin into the body through a thin tube **(Figure 12.5)**. Most of the new devices are about the size and weight of an MP3 player, and some are even free of tubing, delivering insulin via skin absorption from a "pod" attached to the skin with a gentle adhesive.

For people with type 2 diabetes, treatments are more varied. If you have prediabetes or are a diabetic whose blood glucose levels are not extremely high, you may be able to get your blood glucose under control by improving your diet and exercise habits and thus losing weight. As noted earlier, weight loss of just a few pounds can significantly improve your cells' ability to respond to insulin. If you are not successful in losing weight, or weight loss doesn't reduce

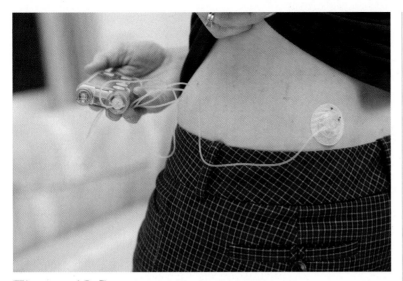

Figure 12.5 Controlling diabetes. Insulin pumps allow many people to control their blood glucose levels throughout the day without painful injections.

your blood glucose significantly enough, your doctor may prescribe oral medications that help lower blood glucose. If the condition deteriorates, however, your doctor is likely to recommend a type 1 approach involving insulin therapy.

Controlling diabetes requires consistent attention to diet, exercise, blood glucose levels, and prescribed therapies. But the rewards, including more years of healthy life and reduced risk of other serious conditions, are worth it.

A Family History of Diabetes

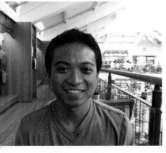

"Hi, I'm Andrew and I have a father with diabetes. It's always been a subject of health in my family. I can remember watching my father inject insulin ever since I was a young child. Having a family history of diabetes has really encouraged me to try to stay healthy—not only eating right, but also keeping active on a daily basis. It not only keeps my body going and reduces the likeliness of diabetes, but also keeps my mind alert. I do this in hopes that one day my children won't have to see me inject insulin."

1: Why do some people with diabetes have to inject insulin?

2: Andrew is paying attention to his diet and trying to stay physically active. What else could he do to lower his risk for developing diabetes?

Do you have a story similar to Andrew's? Share your story at **www.pearsonhighered.com/choosinghealth**.

Reducing Your Risk for Cardiovascular Disease

Every so often, a sad piece of news arrives. A favorite teacher from high school has died of a heart attack. A friend's grandmother has had a stroke. You take note of these losses, but you may not see any direct connection to your own health. After all, these people were a lot older than you, right? Their health issues are altogether different—aren't they?

The answer to that last question is a resounding "No." Although both heart attacks and strokes typically occur later in life, the conditions that lead to these events often begin to develop far earlier. As the rates of obesity and type 2 diabetes rise in children and adolescents, researchers are becoming increasingly concerned about an accompanying rise in cardiovascular disease. For instance, a 2006 study involving more than 2000 youth with diabetes, aged 3 to 19, revealed that 21% already had at least two risk factors for cardiovascular disease.[19]

Cardiovascular disease, or **CVD,** is actually a group of disorders that includes high blood pressure, coronary heart disease (including heart attacks), congestive heart failure, and stroke. It is the leading cause of adult mortality in the United States, responsible for more than 3 in 10 deaths.[8] **(Figure 12.6).**

cardiovascular disease (CVD)
Diseases of the heart or blood vessels.

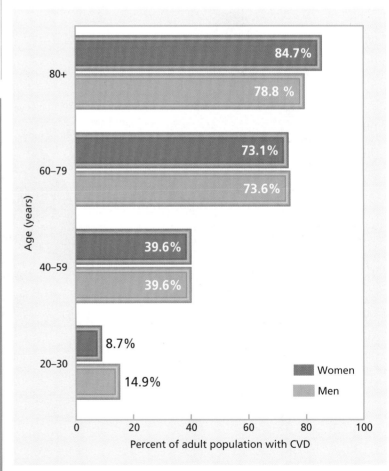

Figure 12.6 Prevalence of cardiovascular disease in U.S. adults. By age and gender.

Source: Heart Disease and Stroke Statistics: 2010 Update by the American Heart Association. Used with permission.

Research shows that many college students don't realize their risks of joining this epidemic. One survey of undergraduates found that most rated their own risk as lower than that of their peers, an indication of thinking that CVD is "someone else's problem."[20] Another study found that female students tended to overestimate their risk of breast cancer but underestimate their risk of CVD.[21] Rethinking your real risks may seem depressing, but it can actually be empowering. As with diabetes, cardiovascular disease is closely linked to lifestyle. By choosing to live healthfully now, you can reduce your risk for many forms of CVD.

A meaningful understanding of CVD requires that you become familiar with the structures and activities of the cardiovascular system.

The Normal Cardiovascular System

The cardiovascular system is made up of blood vessels and the heart, which together form the delivery network that keeps the body functioning. Blood, circulating through blood vessels, ferries oxygen, nutrients, and wastes to and from cells through **arteries,** which carry blood away from the heart, and **veins,** which carry blood back to the heart **(Figure 12.7a).**

arteries Blood vessels that flow away from the heart, delivering oxygen-rich blood to the body periphery and oxygen-poor blood to the lungs.

veins Blood vessels that flow toward the heart, delivering oxygen-poor blood from the body periphery or oxygen-rich blood from the lungs.

myocardium The heart's muscle tissue.

atria The two upper chambers of the heart, which receive blood from the body periphery and lungs.

ventricles The two lower chambers of the heart, which pump blood to the body and lungs.

At the center of this system is the heart, which is only about the size of a fist, but is surprisingly strong. That's because it's almost entirely made up of a thick layer of muscle called the **myocardium.** The contractions of the myocardium keep blood moving, ensuring that it transports oxygen and nutrients to, and eliminates wastes from, every region of the body.

Although the heart is a single organ, it's surprisingly complex, consisting of four hollow, muscular chambers **(Figure 12.7b).** The two upper chambers are the **atria.** Each atrium is connected by a valve to a corresponding lower chamber. These are the two **ventricles.** A thick wall of tissue divides the right-hand pair of chambers from the pair on the left, creating two side-by-side pumps. This division lets each side of the heart focus on a different task—either sending oxygen-poor blood to the lungs for replenishment or carrying that reoxygenated blood back to the body. On the cleanup side, the right atrium receives oxygen-depleted blood from the superior and inferior vena cava, the largest veins in the body, and then pushes it to the right ventricle, which sends it into the pulmonary arteries, which take it to the lungs. There, blood cells collect

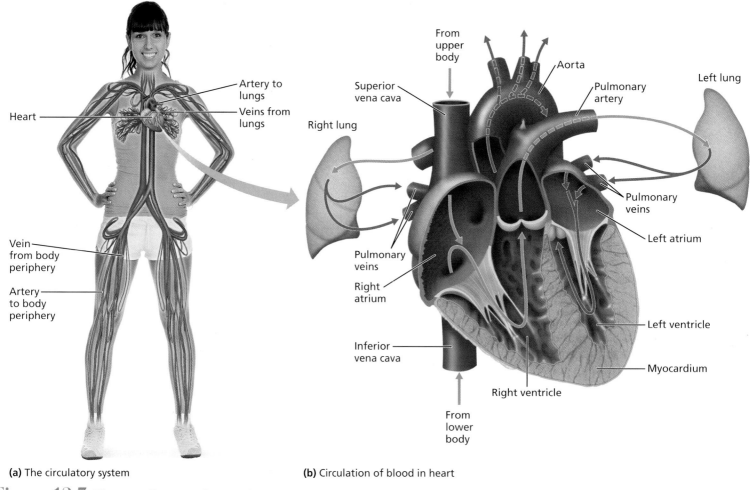

(a) The circulatory system

- Artery to lungs
- Veins from lungs
- Heart
- Vein from body periphery
- Artery to body periphery

(b) Circulation of blood in heart

- From upper body
- Aorta
- Pulmonary artery
- Left lung
- Superior vena cava
- Right lung
- Pulmonary veins
- Left atrium
- Pulmonary veins
- Right atrium
- Left ventricle
- Inferior vena cava
- Myocardium
- Right ventricle
- From lower body

Figure 12.7 The cardiovascular system.

freshly inhaled oxygen and dispense with carbon dioxide (a metabolic waste), which we exhale. On the delivery side, the pulmonary veins bring oxygen-rich blood to the left atrium and ventricle. They receive this blood and pump it out into the body via the aorta, a large artery that branches off into smaller arteries. The first two of these are the right and left **coronary arteries,** which sustain the heart muscle itself.

The body's blood vessels divide into a network of smaller and smaller branches, eventually fanning out into **capillaries,** tiny blood vessels that deliver oxygen and nutrients to individual cells and collect their wastes. Once blood in the capillaries has exchanged oxygen and nutrients for wastes, it is returned to the heart via the veins. As with any system of pipes or tubes, the arteries, capillaries, and veins do this work best when they are free of blockage or damage, allowing blood to flow smoothly.

This entire process is complex—yet remarkably quick. The average person has about five to six quarts of blood, all of which is pumped by the heart in a single minute. At rest, the heart typically beats 60–120 times per minute, pumping a few ounces of blood with each beat until all the blood has been circulated. To keep up this rapid rhythm, the heart relies on electricity. A bundle of specialized cells in the heart's **sinus node,** located in the right atrium, generate electrical impulses and transmit them throughout the myocardium at a steady, even rate, setting the heart to beat about 100,000 times a day.

If your cardiovascular system is healthy, this delivery network runs smoothly. Your heart pumps strongly, and your blood vessels deliver blood efficiently. Your heartbeat thumps at the steady, even pace required for healthy blood flow through all parts of your body. But if damage occurs to even one part of this interconnected system, the rest of the network begins to struggle to do its job.

Next, we'll look at the mechanisms that most commonly damage the cardiovascular system, and the cascade of disorders they can cause. Then we'll follow with a look at how cardiovascular disease is detected and treated. Once you've learned the basics, we'll move on to the part you can do something about—reducing your risk.

What Is Cardiovascular Disease?

Although CVD can strike any part of the cardiovascular system, the individual cardiovascular diseases described below rarely happen in isolation. One condition often contributes to or occurs simultaneously with another, reflecting the complex interrelationship of your heart and blood vessels. In addition, as noted earlier, the damage to the body's blood vessels caused by diabetes also contributes to CVD.

As shown in **Figure 12.8,** the form of CVD responsible for the greatest percentage of deaths is coronary heart disease. Stroke is second, followed by congestive heart failure and hypertension (high blood pressure). Before we can distinguish between these disorders, we need to explore a disease mechanism underlying them: a process called atherosclerosis.

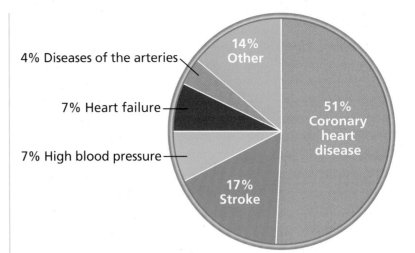

Figure 12.8 Deaths from cardiovascular disease in the U.S. The majority of deaths resulted from coronary heart disease.

Source: *Heart Disease and Stroke Statistics: 2010 Update* by the American Heart Association. Used with permission.

Atherosclerosis

Atherosclerosis is an arterial condition characterized by inflammation, scarring, and the buildup of mealy deposits along artery walls. In fact, the word's root, *athere,* is Greek for porridge! Together, these factors cause a narrowing of arteries, which restricts blood flow to cells and tissues "downstream" of the narrowed area. Cells starved of oxygen and nutrients cannot function; thus, when atherosclerosis affects the coronary arteries, the person can suffer a heart attack. When it affects arteries in the brain (cerebral arteries), the person can suffer a stroke.

Let's take a closer look at how atherosclerosis develops. The condition begins when the delicate inner lining of an artery becomes damaged. Although the cause of this damage is not always known, in some cases, it is thought to result when **blood pressure**—the force of blood pulsating against the artery walls—is excessive. In others, it reflects the lining's encounter with irritants: high levels of blood glucose, cholesterol, or triglycerides. The toxins in tobacco smoke are also known to injure the lining, and even certain types of infection may promote this initial damage.

The body responds to injury with inflammation, and at injured arterial sites, the resulting inflammation spreads into the artery wall. This leaves it weakened, scarred, and stiff (sclerotic). As a result, two types of lipids circulating in the bloodstream—triglycerides and cholesterol—can seep between the damaged lining cells and become trapped within the artery wall. Soon they are joined by white blood cells, calcium, and other substances. Eventually, this buildup, called *plaque*, narrows arteries significantly enough to impair blood flow **(Figure 12.9).** When this occurs in a coronary artery, the person may experience chest pain (called *angina*), weakness, shortness of breath, and other symptoms.

coronary arteries The blood vessels that feed the heart.

capillaries The smallest blood vessels, delivering blood and nutrients to individual cells and picking up wastes.

sinus node A group of cells in the right atrium that generate the electricity that keeps the heart beating evenly.

atherosclerosis Condition characterized by narrowing of the arteries because of inflammation, scarring, and the buildup of fatty deposits.

blood pressure The force of the blood moving against the arterial walls.

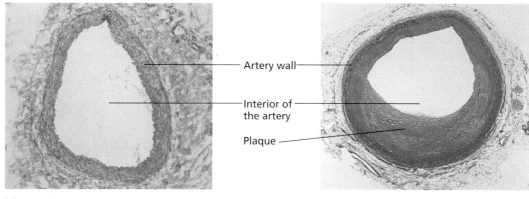

(a) Normal artery   **(b)** Artery partially blocked with plaque

Figure 12.9 **Atherosclerosis.** These light micrographs show a cross section of (a) a normal artery allowing adequate blood flow and (b) an artery that is partially blocked with plaque, which can lead to a heart attack or stroke.

Plaque may build up to the point where it significantly blocks or even stops the flow of blood through an artery. This causes death of the "downstream" tissue. Sometimes plaque can become hardened and rupture, causing microscopic tears in the artery wall that allow blood to leak into the tissue on the other side. When this happens, blood platelets rush to the site to clot the blood. This clot can obstruct the artery and—if it occurs in a coronary or cerebral artery—cause a sudden heart attack or stroke. Alternatively, softer plaque can break off and travel through the bloodstream until it blocks a distant artery.

As noted earlier, cholesterol, a lipid made by the body and found in the food you eat, is a major component of plaque. We all need cholesterol for our bodies to function, but excessive amounts can be a key contributor to atherosclerosis. We'll look more closely at types of cholesterol, and what levels are considered healthful, when we talk about CVD detection and prevention later in this chapter.

Atherosclerosis is difficult to detect without specific medical tests, and most people who are developing the condition are unaware it is occurring. But researchers have found that the condition can start early in life, especially in people with known risk factors. For example, in one study of young adults (most were in their early 30s) who had metabolic syndrome but otherwise appeared healthy, participants showed significant development of atherosclerosis in their cerebral arteries.[22]

Although we said that high blood pressure can cause the arterial damage that leads to atherosclerosis, it's also true that atherosclerosis can contribute to high blood pressure! How? First let's look at what high blood pressure really is.

Hypertension (High Blood Pressure)

Hypertension, more commonly known as *high blood pressure,* is a chronic condition characterized by consistent blood pressure readings above normal. (We'll define normal and hypertensive readings shortly.) Hypertension in and of itself is considered a form of CVD. In addition, it's also a risk factor for other forms of CVD, including coronary heart disease, congestive heart failure, and stroke.

The level of your blood pressure is typically measured in an artery in your upper arm, but it's determined, in part, by the pumping actions of your heart. When your heart contracts, an action called

---

hypertension (high blood pressure)
A persistent state of elevated blood pressure.

---

systole, the pressure of the blood in your arteries momentarily increases. When it relaxes, an action called *diastole,* your blood pressure drops. But the force of your heart isn't the only actor. Blood pressure is also affected by the *compliance*—the ability to stretch and recoil—of your arteries.

We noted earlier that atherosclerosis can lead to both narrowing and stiffening of the arteries. When it does, blood pressure rises. To appreciate why, imagine the difference between trying to pump a pulsing stream of water into a network of wide, soft rubber tubes versus narrow, stiff metal pipes. The wide rubber tubing would stretch and bounce back with each pulsation, absorbing some of the pressure and allowing the turbulence to quickly settle down and the water to flow. In contrast, the narrow metal pipes would not accommodate the pulsating flow. This means the pump would have to work harder to propel the water against their resistance. Now imagine that atherosclerosis has stiffened your arteries and narrowed them with plaque! The more stiff and narrow your arteries become, the more they impede blood flow and drive your blood pressure up.

What readings constitute hypertension? Blood pressure is measured using a stethoscope and a device called a *sphygmomanometer.* Readings are recorded in millimeters of mercury (mm Hg). The systolic pressure—the pressure in your arteries as your heart contracts—is given first, and the diastolic pressure—the pressure when the heart is momentarily relaxed—is given second. As with diabetes, three values are important: normal, prehypertension, and true hypertension **(Table 12.1).**

Although atherosclerosis contributes to hypertension in many people, usually the causes aren't entirely clear. But your age, weight, ethnic background, and diet all play a role, with a high-sodium diet putting you at especially significant risk. In the United States, the prevalence of hypertension is rising, especially among women. One study found that almost 30% of the U.S. adult population, or about 73 million people, have hypertension, with increased body weight emerging as a key factor in this trend.[23] African Americans have the condition at an even higher rate, about 40% of the adult population.[23] Though risk for everyone rises with age, more and more young people are also developing the condition. One study of hypertension in young people found that as many as 1.5 million children

Table 12.1: **Blood Pressure Classification**

Classification	Systolic Reading (mm Hg)		Diastolic Reading (mm Hg)
Normal	<120	and	<80
Prehypertension	120–139	or	80–89
Hypertension			
Stage 1	140–159	or	90–99
Stage 2	≥160	or	≥100

Source: The Seventh Report of the Joint National Committee on Prevention, Detection, Evaluation, and Treatment of High Blood Pressure (NIH Publication No. 03-5233) by the National Heart, Lung, and Blood Institute, 2005 (Bethesda, MD: National Institutes of Health).

and teenagers in the U.S. may have the condition, and many of them don't know it.[24]

Later in this chapter, we'll discuss steps you can take to lower your risk of hypertension. Awareness is an important first step, since hypertension is often silent, with no outward symptoms. If left undetected or uncontrolled, high blood pressure can drive up your risk for other forms of CVD, including coronary heart disease, which we'll look at next.

Coronary Heart Disease

The arteries that feed your heart are especially vulnerable to atherosclerosis. **Coronary heart disease,** also called *coronary artery disease,* arises when plaque in the coronary arteries builds up to the point that it impairs your heart's ability to function. Coronary heart disease is the single leading cause of death in the United States, and the American Heart Association estimates that the condition kills more than 425,000 people each year.[25]

Partial coronary artery blockages can cause *angina,* or chest pain that occurs when the heart muscle doesn't get enough blood. Larger or even total blockages can trigger a *heart attack* or a disruption in heart rhythm known as *sudden cardiac arrest.* We'll look at these conditions next.

Angina. If your coronary arteries have been narrow or obstructed, they can still deliver some blood to your heart—but not necessarily as much as this powerful muscle needs. If your heart's need for nutrients and oxygen exceeds what your coronary arteries can provide, you may feel chest pain, or **angina pectoris.** Angina can feel like pressure or like a squeezing pain in the chest. These sensations can also radiate out to your shoulders, arms, neck, jaw, or back, or even resemble indigestion.

Nearly 7 million people in the United States suffer from angina. Once considered more of a health concern for men, recent research has found that angina is equally common in women.[26]

Angina itself may not be life-threatening, but it signals that a person is at greater risk of a life-threatening cardiac event. If angina isn't correctly

recognized or treated, the arterial narrowing behind it may progress to a full blockage, leading to the next condition we'll discuss—heart attack.

Heart attack. When blockage of a coronary artery deprives a region of the myocardium of its blood supply, that region can stop working effectively. Its cells can even die if they go too long without blood and the oxygen and nutrients it carries. During a heart attack, or **myocardial infarction,** the more time that passes without treatment to restore blood flow, the greater the damage. Symptoms of a heart attack include angina, discomfort in the chest or other parts of the upper body, shortness of breath, and sweating, nausea, or dizziness. Chest pain, which is a hallmark symptom in men, often doesn't occur (or is experienced differently) in women. Because of this, women are often misdiagnosed and released from emergency rooms with unrecognized acute myocardial infarctions.

When a heart attack strikes, it may seem sudden. But as you are learning in this chapter, a heart attack is actually the end result of a steady, silent buildup of heart disease, often over many years or even decades. According to the American Heart Association, more than 1 million people in the U.S. have a heart attack each year, and more than 140,000 die as a result.[25] Those who survive often continue to face significant health risks and functional impairment as they try to recover. The good news is that the U.S. death rate from heart attack has dropped in recent years. We'll discuss the prevention and control of CVD shortly.

If the heart is starved of blood, muscle function isn't the only aspect of the heart's work at risk. The nerve cells that set the pace of the heart's pumping can also be affected, resulting in a dangerously irregular heartbeat. We'll look at this and other types of uneven heartbeats, or *arrhythmias,* next.

Arrhythmia. An **arrhythmia** is an irregularity in the speed or rhythm of the heart. As you learned earlier, your heartbeat is regulated by your sinus node, which sets a series of electrical currents flowing through your heart in a steady, even pattern. If this electrical conduction is disrupted, your heart can beat too slowly, too quickly, or unevenly. More than 2 million people in the U.S. live with some form of arrhythmia.[27]

Arrhythmias come in many forms that affect different aspects of the heart's function, and some are more serious than others. A slow heart rate of less than 60 beats per minute is called **bradycardia.** A fast heart rate—more than 100 beats per minute—is called **tachycardia.** An especially dangerous type of tachycardia is *fibrillation.* In fibrillation, an improper electrical signal causes either your atrium or your ventricles to contract so quickly and unevenly that they quiver rather than pump, unable to move blood effectively.

In heart attacks that damage the heart's electrical system, a person may go into **ventricular fibrillation,** an extremely dangerous situation that stops the heart from functioning, leading to loss of consciousness. In these cases of **sudden cardiac arrest,** the person's heart must be restarted within 6 minutes via electrical shock to prevent death.

coronary heart disease (coronary artery disease) Atherosclerosis of the arteries that feed the heart.

angina pectoris Chest pain due to coronary heart disease.

myocardial infarction (heart attack) A cardiac crisis in which a region of heart muscle is damaged or destroyed by reduced blood flow.

arrhythmia Any irregularity in the heart's rhythm.

bradycardia A slow arrhythmia.

tachycardia A fast arrhythmia.

ventricular fibrillation A life-threatening arrhythmia marked by ineffective pumping of the ventricles.

sudden cardiac arrest A life-threatening cardiac crisis marked by loss of heartbeat and unconsciousness.

Many factors increase the risk for arrhythmias. These include stress, smoking, genetic factors, heavy alcohol use, strenuous exercise, certain medications, and even air pollution. But atherosclerosis and coronary heart disease, which affect how well your heart is nourished, are especially important factors.

Congestive Heart Failure

All of the conditions we've just discussed can be serious on their own. But they can also contribute to a gradual loss of heart function. In **congestive heart failure,** the heart can no longer pump enough blood to meet the body's needs. As a result, blood may pool—or become congested—in other areas of the body, such as the lungs, the abdomen, or the arms and legs. This pooled blood quickly becomes depleted of oxygen and nutrients, so the affected regions become damaged and unable to function properly. More than 5 million people in the U.S. live with congestive heart failure.[25]

A common cause is coronary heart disease, which damages heart muscle, reducing its ability to beat strongly. Persistent tachycardia may also cause your heart to work too hard, slowly wearing it out. However, a landmark heart health study found that hypertension, which forces the heart to work harder than it should to pump blood against resistance, is the most common risk factor for congestive heart failure. Less than one-third of adults found to have hypertension-related heart failure are still alive 5 years after their diagnosis.[28] Other factors, including having diabetes or a viral infection that triggers inflammation of your heart muscle, can also cause heart failure.

Regardless of the cause, a failing heart results in a failing body. When congestion occurs in the arms and legs, they swell with fluid. Fluid pooling in the lungs makes it difficult to breathe. Heart failure also typically causes weakness and exhaustion, and an inability to concentrate or stay alert. Thus, the individual may find it difficult to perform everyday tasks.

Stroke

As you've learned in this chapter, a blockage in an artery that feeds the heart can cause angina, a heart attack, or even sudden cardiac arrest. What would happen if a similar obstruction or serious damage hit an artery serving the brain?

The answer is a **stroke,** a medical emergency in which the blood supply to a part of the brain ceases. Strokes can take either of two forms **(Figure 12.10)**. In **ischemic stroke,** either a cerebral artery or one of the carotid arteries that run through the neck into the brain is blocked. Ischemic strokes represent about 80% of the more than 700,000 strokes that occur each year in the United States.[29] In **hemorrhagic stroke,** a cerebral artery ruptures, spilling blood into brain tissue and depriving oxygen and nutrients to regions downstream of the broken vessel. Hypertension and *aneurysm* (a bulge in an artery wall that may weaken or rupture) are the main causes.

Brain cells deprived of blood quickly die. The outward signs of stroke often portray this damage as it unfolds. A person having a stroke may suddenly feel numb or weak in the arm, leg, or face, especially on one side of the body. The person may suddenly seem confused, or have trouble

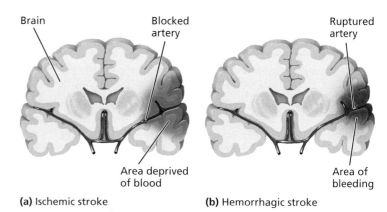

(a) Ischemic stroke **(b)** Hemorrhagic stroke

Figure 12.10 Two types of stroke. (a) In an ischemic stroke, a blocked artery damages brain tissue by depriving it of blood. (b) In a hemorrhagic stroke, a ruptured artery damages brain tissue by flooding it with too much blood.

speaking, seeing, and walking. A sudden and severe headache is also common. Some people at risk for stroke may experience a fleeting episode of a milder version of these symptoms days, weeks, or months before having a full stroke. Such a mini-stroke, known as a **transient ischemic attack** or TIA, isn't always easy to recognize, but it is a clear warning sign of an impending stroke.

Anyone showing signs of a TIA or stroke requires immediate medical attention. CT and other scanning technologies may reveal damaged blood vessels and signs of brain damage. In an ischemic stroke, drugs and surgical procedures are used to open blocked cerebral arteries. In a hemorrhagic stroke, drugs are used to reduce the force of blood moving into the damaged area, and surgery can sometimes repair the ruptured vessel. If stroke treatment doesn't start quickly, however, permanent brain damage often results. People who have suffered a stroke may experience paralysis, difficulty speaking or swallowing, or loss of memory and the ability to understand. Rehabilitation efforts can help restore some of these lost abilities, but most people who survive a stroke must usually learn to live with some level of disability.

Other Forms of Cardiovascular Disease

Less common types of CVD in the United States include:

- **Congenital heart disease.** About 9 in every 1000 babies is born with some type of heart defect.[30] Some of the more frequent forms these defects take include holes in the walls that divide the chambers of the heart, abnormal narrowing of the coronary arteries, and malformations of the arteries that connect the heart and lungs. Most congenital heart defects can now be accurately diagnosed and treated with drugs or surgery.

- **Heart valve disorders.** Blood flows through your heart in only one direction, from atrium to ventricle, because the chambers of your heart are gated with valves. These flaps of connective tissue swing open and shut like one-way doors, allowing blood to pass from atrium to ventricle but preventing it from pooling or

congestive heart failure A gradual loss of heart function.

stroke A medical emergency in which blood flow to or in the brain is impaired.

ischemic stroke A stroke caused by a blocked blood vessel.

hemorrhagic stroke A stroke caused by a ruptured blood vessel.

transient ischemic attack (TIA) A temporary episode of stroke-like symptoms, indicative of high stroke risk.

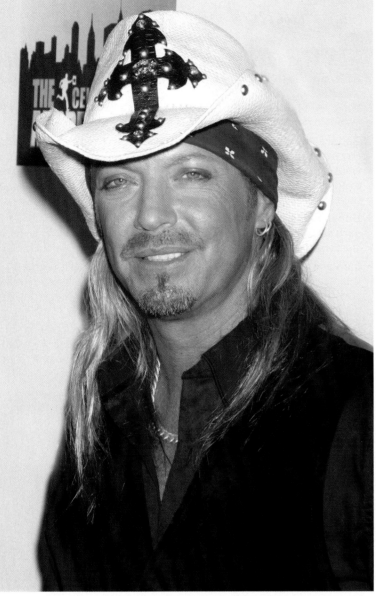

Singer Bret Michaels suffered a series of health problems in 2010, including a **transient ischemic attack (TIA)**.

illness causes inflammation of connective tissues throughout the body. Sometimes, that damage includes the heart valves. Rheumatic heart disease is easily prevented by taking antibiotics in the early stages of a strep infection, stopping it before it can progress to rheumatic fever.

Along with the heart and brain, other parts of the body can suffer from blood vessel damage due to atherosclerosis and hypertension. For instance, *peripheral artery disease* is a narrowing and stiffening of the arteries that serve the legs and feet. This causes pain, aching, burning, and tingling sensations that are sometimes severe, and increases the risk for non-healing wounds, tissue death, and surgical amputation of the leg or foot.

Detecting Cardiovascular Disease

Although CVD can develop silently, showing few outward symptoms until it is quite serious, medical care can help you assess the health of your heart and blood vessels. Some of these detection methods are fairly simple:

- **Measuring blood pressure.** At a doctor's visit or health fair, have your blood pressure measured. As noted earlier, hypertension in adults is defined as blood pressure equal to or greater than 140 over 90. For more detailed guidelines, see Table 12.1 on page 281.
- **Measuring levels of blood lipids.** A simple blood test can give you a variety of data about your blood lipid levels, which are an indication of your risk of coronary heart disease. These include your total cholesterol score as well as your readings for two cholesterol-carrying compounds: LDL and HDL. LDL, short for **low-density lipoprotein,** is often dubbed "bad" cholesterol because excess LDLs degrade over time, releasing their cholesterol load into your bloodstream. This circulating cholesterol can then become trapped in injured blood vessels. HDL, an abbreviation of **high-density lipoprotein,** is often called "good" cholesterol because it transports excess cholesterol back to your liver for recycling. The same blood test also measures your levels of triglycerides. For a detailed look at these guidelines, see **Table 12.2.**

Other detection methods are more complex:

- **Electrocardiogram.** An **electrocardiogram,** also called an *ECG* or *EKG,* measures the heart's electrical activity. This test can detect not only arrhythmias, but other problems such as restricted blood flow. You can take an ECG while sitting quietly, which will give you a baseline measurement, or have the test done while you are exercising. This more vigorous form, called a **stress test,** shows how your heart performs under increased physical demands.
- **Exercise thallium test.** Also called a *nuclear stress test,* this test tracks a radioactive substance that is injected into your bloodstream to see how blood is flowing through your arteries.
- **Non-invasive imaging technologies.** Various diagnostic tools provide views of different aspects of heart function without the need for invasive procedures. An *echocardiogram,* for

streaming backward. Congenital defects, infections, or heart disease can damage these. In some cases, a valve may let too little blood pass. In others, a valve may leak. Medications can ease some valve problems, whereas more serious malfunctions may require surgical repair or replacement.

- **Rheumatic heart disease.** Although it is rare in the United States, around the globe, rheumatic heart disease is the leading cause of cardiovascular death among people younger than age 50.[31] It begins when a bacterial infection—caused by the same *Streptococcus* bacterium that causes strep throat—flares into rheumatic fever. Along with an elevated temperature, the

low-density lipoprotein (LDL) A cholesterol-containing compound that, as it degrades, releases its cholesterol load into the bloodstream; often referred to as "bad cholesterol."

high-density lipoprotein (HDL) A cholesterol-containing compound that removes excess cholesterol from the bloodstream; often referred to as "good cholesterol."

electrocardiogram A test that measures the heart's electrical activity.

stress test An analysis of heart function during monitored exercise.

Table 12.2: **Classification of Blood Lipid Levels for Adults**

LDL Cholesterol	
<100	Optimal
100–129	Near optimal/above optimal
130–159	Borderline high
160–189	High
≥190	Very high

HDL Cholesterol	
<40	Low
≥60	High

Total Cholesterol	
<200	Desirable
200–239	Borderline high
≥240	High

Triglycerides	
<150	Normal
150–199	Borderline high
200–499	High
≥500	Very high

Source: Third Report of the Expert Panel on Detection, Evaluation, and Treatment of High Blood Cholesterol in Adults. (NIH Publication No. 05-3290) by the National Heart, Lung, and Blood Institute, 2005, retrieved from www.nhlbi.nih.gov/health/public/heart/chol/wyntk.htm.

example, uses sound waves to produce an image of the heart and its ability to work. A different scan detects calcium in the arteries, which is a marker of atherosclerosis.

- **Invasive imaging.** This category of diagnostic tool, usually used only when doctors suspect serious heart problems, provides a detailed picture of any serious arterial blockages. The most common technique, *coronary angiography,* relies on a dye injected into your bloodstream to track the flow of blood through your heart and coronary arteries.

These detection methods can also be used to look for more unusual types of CVD, which occur less often but carry equally significant health risks.

Changing Behaviors to Reduce Your Risk for Cardiovascular Disease

Diseases of the heart and blood vessels may be common, but that doesn't mean they are inevitable. As we've discussed, many of the factors leading up to these conditions are within your control. Believing in your ability to make healthy choices and lower your risk is an important first step. One study of college students found that higher self-efficacy, or a belief in your own ability to control events in your life, indicated a better likelihood of making healthy choices.[32]

Not sure how to begin reducing your risks of CVD? Try starting with what you eat for lunch.

Eat a Healthy Diet
Few aspects of your life matter more for your risk of heart disease and stroke. Diet is closely tied to weight, waist size, blood sugar lev-

---

Practical Strategies for Change

Heart-Healthy Food Choices

Making heart-healthy diet choices can substantially reduce your risks for developing cardiovascular disease. Here are a few suggestions:

- **Reduce your fat and cholesterol intake.** Eat less red meat, and avoid processed meats like pepperoni and sausage. Choose skim milk over whole milk, and consume less cheese. Replace butter with *trans*-fat–free margarine, nut butters, and plant oils. Snack on fruits and nuts instead of potato chips.

- **Boost your consumption of omega-3 fatty acids.** Choose fatty fish such as salmon, which provides heart-protective omega-3 fatty acids, at least twice a week.

- **Increase your fiber intake.** Fiber not only helps you feel full and eat less, but can reduce the amounts of fat and cholesterol absorbed by your digestive system. Whole grain bread and fresh fruits and vegetables are good sources.

- **Decrease your sodium intake.** Cut back on processed foods, which tend to contain a great deal of sodium. Regular canned soup, for example, can contain almost a full day's recommended allowance of sodium in a single can. Opt for fresh foods when possible, or choose low-sodium versions of prepared foods.

- **Put some color in your diet.** Brightly colored fruits and vegetables, such as blueberries, raspberries, red grapes, tomatoes, black beans, and parsley, contain compounds called *flavonoids,* which have been associated with reduced CVD risk[1]. You don't need to carry around a detailed list of foods to find those higher in flavonoids—just focus on choosing colorful fruits and vegetables, and aim for a mix of colors to consume a wide variety of these compounds.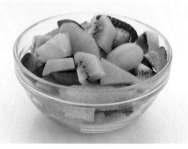

Reference: 1. Hertog, M., Kromhout, D., Aravanis, C., Blackburn, H., Buzina, R., Fidanza, F.... Nedeljkovic, S. (1995). Flavonoid intake and long-term risk of coronary heart disease and cancer in the seven countries study. *Archives of Internal Medicine, 155*(11), pp. 1184–1192.

---

els, blood lipid levels, and high blood pressure. See **Practical Strategies for Change** for suggestions on how to make your diet more heart-healthy.

If you're motivated to reduce your risk for hypertension, download the National Institutes of Health free guide to the DASH eating plan, which has been shown in two key studies to reduce blood pressure. DASH, short for Dietary Approaches to Stop Hypertension, can help you increase your consumption of fruit and vegetables, and control your sodium and saturated fat intake. **www.nhlbi.nih.gov/health/public/heart/hbp/dash/new_dash.pdf**

Get Enough Exercise
Physical activity helps control blood sugar, burn calories, control weight, and tone your heart. This fact holds true throughout your life—one study of elementary schoolchildren found that those with low levels of physical activity already showed more risk factors for

cardiovascular disease.[33] If you aren't exercising right now, aim for at least 30 minutes of physical activity a few days a week. If you already meet that level, start exercising every day, and work on slowly increasing the intensity and duration of your workouts. Remember to balance cardiorespiratory fitness, or activities that build heart and lung capacity, with strength training.

Maintain a Healthy Weight
Remember to watch more than the number on the scale. See Chapter 6 for a refresher on BMI and waist circumference. Find a range of weight, BMIs, and waist sizes that are healthy for you, and rely on a healthy diet and exercise to keep you within that range. We can't all hit an ideal weight or body shape and freeze ourselves there. But you can work to stay within a range that is healthy for you, right for your body type, and good for your cardiovascular system.

Don't Smoke
We all know that tobacco smoke damages the lungs. But as you've learned in this chapter, it also drives up your risk for heart disease and stroke. Studies suggest that the ingredients in tobacco smoke irritate the lining of your arteries and trigger inflammation.[34] If you don't smoke, don't start. If you do, talk to your campus health center about quitting.

Limit Alcohol Intake
Excessive drinking is bad for your health and your heart. This holds true even at a young age. One study of college students found that those on their way to developing hypertension were also far more likely to drink heavily.[35]

Manage Stress and Anger
People who carry stress, anger easily, and are prone to hostility are more likely to suffer a heart attack. Just as physical factors such as cholesterol or excess weight put the heart under stress, so do angry or tense emotions. Is whatever caused your bad mood now worth CVD later in life?

Get Enough Sleep
Long-term sleep deprivation, usually defined as sleeping 6.5 hours a night or less, is linked to increases in high blood pressure, heart rate, and other heart disease risk factors, One study of teenagers between the ages of 13 and 16 found that those sleeping less than 6.5 hours a night were 2.5 times more likely to have elevated blood pressure.[36] Aim for 8 hours of sleep a night.

Maintain Good Oral Hygiene
Brush and floss daily, and visit the dentist regularly. The health of your mouth and your heart may not seem connected, but scientists have found clear links between dental problems and cardiovascular disease.[37] Periodontal disease, or disorders of the gums and bones that surround your teeth, are a prime concern. Researchers are still trying to nail down why, but suspect that the pathogens involved in gum disease trigger an inflammatory reaction that can cascade throughout the body and contribute to atherosclerosis.

Monitor Your Blood Pressure and Blood Lipids
Take advantage of annual physicals and health fairs to have your blood pressure and blood lipids monitored. Because your body's functioning changes as you age, don't assume that the numbers you show now will last a lifetime. Get checked regularly.

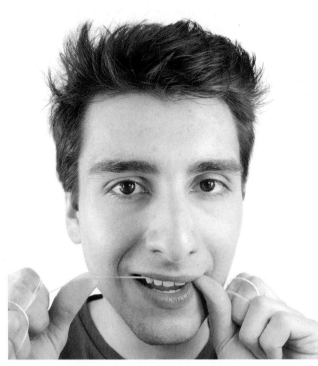

Good **dental hygiene** can help keep your heart healthy.

If You Have Diabetes, Control It
Having diabetes is one of the top risk factors for developing cardiovascular disease. If you have diabetes or prediabetes, take steps to keep your condition under control: Watch your blood glucose level, eat nutritiously, exercise, maintain a healthy weight, and do not smoke.

Offsetting Other Risk Factors

Taking the above steps can't control all your risks for heart disease and stroke. Some factors behind these conditions can't be changed. But by focusing on the risks you can control, you can offset some of the following inherent links to CVD:

- **Your age.** Most cases of heart attack, sudden cardiac arrest, and stroke occur in people older than 65. You can't stop yourself from aging, but you can work to make sure every year of life is as healthy as possible.

- **Your sex.** Men face greater heart attack risks than women, and they tend to have heart attacks earlier in life. However, CVD is still the top killer of women in the United States over the course of their lifetime, and women need to pay attention to CVD risks as well. The **Diversity & Health** box on the next page explores some of the factors behind sex differences in CVD rates.

- **Your genetic inheritance.** Children of parents with hypertension, stroke, and heart disease are more likely to develop these conditions themselves. Some ethnic groups, especially African Americans, are also at increased risk for these conditions.[38] You can't change your genetics. But when it comes to CVD, your DNA isn't destiny. By reducing the CVD risks you can control, you can help make sure that your genes don't equal your fate.

Why Do Men
Have Greater CVD Risk?

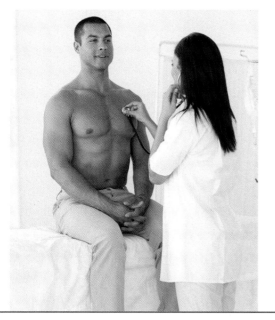

Although cardiovascular disease is the leading killer of both men and women in the United States, men typically develop heart disease and suffer cardiac crises about 10 to 20 years earlier than women.[1]

When this disparity first became apparent, some researchers theorized that the differences were due to lifestyle factors. Men, they assumed, experienced more stress, drank more, smoked more, and ate more heavily than women. But scientists have since realized that other factors are at play. Men and women often actually share these lifestyle factors. Instead, it's hormones that appear to make the difference.

Estrogen, the female hormone, appears to have a protective effect against heart disease, largely by helping the blood vessels guard against atherosclerosis and other forms of damage.[2] This theory fits with general patterns of heart disease in men and women. Whereas men are at greater risk earlier in life, women's risks increase greatly after menopause, when estrogen production drops.

This doesn't mean, however, that women should be any less vigilant about lowering their CVD risks. Both men and women can benefit from adopting heart-healthy behaviors as early in life as possible.

References: 1. Wilson, P., D'Agostino, R., Levy, D., Belanger, A., Silbershatz, H., & Kannel, W. (1996). Prediction of coronary heart disease using risk factor categories. *Circulation. 97*(18), pp. 1837–1847. 2. Packer, C. (2007). Estrogen protection, oxidized LDL, endothelial dysfunction and vasorelaxation in cardiovascular disease: New insights into a complex issue. *Cardiovascular Research, 73*(1), pp. 6–7.

Controlling Cardiovascular Disease

If you develop clear signs of cardiovascular disease but haven't yet had a serious event such as a heart attack, your doctor will likely talk to you about changing your diet and exercise habits, just as we have described in this chapter. If your cholesterol levels are high and don't respond to lifestyle changes, cholesterol-lowering medications, called **statins,** may help. Millions of people in the U.S. use statins to control cholesterol levels, but their use must be monitored for rare but dangerous side effects. Prescription drugs can also help control hypertension, although many doctors prescribe a medication straight off the drugstore shelf: low-dose aspirin. Although better known as a pain reliever, aspirin also works as a mild blood thinner and appears to lower CVD risk.

In patients whose arteries are already dangerously obstructed, procedures are available to open them. One common artery procedure, called a **balloon angioplasty,** involves threading a catheter through the artery and inflating a small balloon at the obstructed spot, flattening plaque against the arterial walls and opening the vessel. To keep the vessel open, the physician may place a *stent,* a small metal tube that keeps the plaque flat. Some stents contain slow-release medication to further reduce the risk of blockage.

statins A group of cholesterol-lowering prescription medications.

balloon angioplasty An arterial treatment that uses a small balloon to flatten plaque deposits against the arterial wall.

bypass surgery A procedure to build new pathways for blood to flow around areas of arterial blockage.

If a blockage is extremely dangerous, especially if it involves coronary arteries, **bypass surgery** may be recommended. This procedure circumvents the blocked vessel rather than opening it. Using a healthy blood vessel from another part of your body, the surgeon builds an alternative route for blood to flow around the arterial obstruction. If more than one artery is blocked, multiple bypasses can be performed.

If you've worked to reduce your CVD risks, you may never need a bypass. And by taking steps that reduce your risks of CVD, you'll also be reducing your risk for another common chronic disease, cancer.

Reducing Your Risk for Cancer

Although more people die of heart disease than cancer, few diseases evoke more worry and fear. Many people are understandably afraid of getting cancer, and apprehensive about the treatments involved if they do. But recent developments in our understanding of cancer can also evoke another emotion—hope. Our ability to detect and treat cancer is improving rapidly, as is our understanding of how to prevent it.

To be sure, cancer remains a health priority for good reason. In a given year, about 1.5 million new cases of cancer will be diagnosed in the U.S., and more than 500,000 people will die from the disease.[39] Cancer is the second leading cause of death in the U.S. Statistics on cancer cases and deaths by body site are illustrated in **Figure 12.11.**

Helping Someone in a
CVD Emergency

We all know that someone showing signs of a heart attack, cardiac arrest, or stroke needs to head for the nearest hospital. But before the person is under medical care, you can take steps to help.

- If you see someone showing the signs of a heart attack, cardiac arrest, or stroke, the first thing you should do is call 9-1-1. If possible, make this call from a land line, not a cell phone. Land line calls to 9-1-1 are usually routed straight to local emergency dispatch centers, whereas calls from cell phones are often routed to local highway safety agencies, who must then reroute the call to the correct dispatch center, sometimes costing valuable time.

- Once you call 9-1-1, wait with the person until emergency medical services arrive rather than driving to the hospital yourself. Paramedic and ambulance units have life-saving equipment and skills that they can deploy immediately and sustain during the trip to the hospital. If you drive the person to the hospital, he or she can't benefit from this faster access to medical help.

In addition, here are ways you can help in specific types of emergencies.

Heart Attack

- Although the symptoms of a heart attack aren't always clear-cut, don't hesitate to call 9-1-1 if you suspect one is occurring. Trying a "wait and see" approach could cost the person important time and even raise his or her risk of cardiac arrest.

- Have the person chew an aspirin, unless he or she is allergic to aspirin or is under medical orders to avoid it. Aspirin has blood-thinning properties that can help in a heart attack. The drug used must be aspirin, not another type of pain reliever.

- Have the person take nitroglycerin, but only if already prescribed. This drug is often used in people with CVD.

- If the person falls unconscious, begin CPR. If you've never received CPR training, let the 9-1-1 dispatcher know. She can instruct you on the proper procedures until help arrives.

Sudden Cardiac Arrest

- If you suspect cardiac arrest, call 9-1-1 immediately. People in cardiac arrest need their heart restarted within 6 minutes or they will die.

- Check the unconscious person for a pulse *after* you call 9-1-1. The side of the neck is a more reliable place to look for a pulse than the wrist.

- If you don't find a pulse, begin CPR. If you don't know how, the 9-1-1 dispatcher will instruct you on the proper procedures until help arrives.

- If you are in a public place such as an airport, shopping mall, or office building, ask someone nearby to look for a device called an *automated external defibrillator*, or AED. AEDs are electrical heart-starting machines, and they are designed for anyone to use. Just open the box and follow the instructions. Don't worry about shocking someone unnecessarily—AEDs are designed to scan for a heartbeat and not deliver a shock if a heartbeat is detected.

Stroke

- The signs of stroke aren't always obvious, but if you suspect a stroke, call 9-1-1 immediately. The faster medical help arrives, the more permanent brain damage can be avoided.

- Make note of the time you first noticed the symptoms. This information is vital for paramedics and doctors trying to provide treatment as fast as possible.

- While you wait for help, don't administer cardiac aid such as mouth-to-mouth resuscitation or CPR unless the person goes into cardiac arrest. A person having a stroke may be disoriented or have trouble moving, but CPR should be reserved for people who are unconscious and have no pulse. Otherwise, it could be harmful.

References: 1. Mayo Clinic (2010). Cardiopulmonary resuscitation (CPR): First aid. retrieved from http://www.mayoclinic.com/health/first-aid-cpr/FA00061. 2. Medline Plus. (2010). Heart attack first aid, retrieved from http://www.nlm.nih.gov/medlineplus/ency/article/000063.htm. 3. National Heart, Lung, and Blood Institute. (n.d.). How to use an automated external defibrillator, retrieved from http://www.nhlbi.nih.gov/health/dci/Diseases/aed/aed_use.html. 4. Harvard Health Publications. (n.d.). Stroke: Preventing and treating "brain attack," retrieved from http://www.harvardhealthcontent.com/70,BA0908?Page=Section1. 5. American Stroke Association. (2010). Learn to recognize a stroke, retrieved from http://www.strokeassociation.org/presenter.jhtml?identifier=1020.

Estimated new cases of cancer*

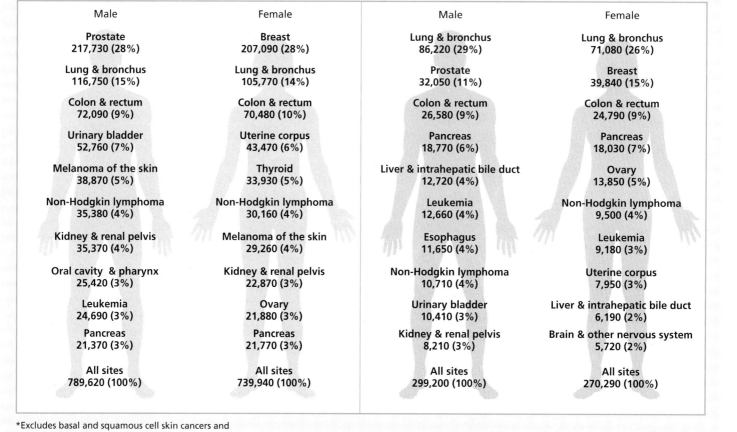

Male	Female
Prostate 217,730 (28%)	**Breast** 207,090 (28%)
Lung & bronchus 116,750 (15%)	**Lung & bronchus** 105,770 (14%)
Colon & rectum 72,090 (9%)	**Colon & rectum** 70,480 (10%)
Urinary bladder 52,760 (7%)	**Uterine corpus** 43,470 (6%)
Melanoma of the skin 38,870 (5%)	**Thyroid** 33,930 (5%)
Non-Hodgkin lymphoma 35,380 (4%)	**Non-Hodgkin lymphoma** 30,160 (4%)
Kidney & renal pelvis 35,370 (4%)	**Melanoma of the skin** 29,260 (4%)
Oral cavity & pharynx 25,420 (3%)	**Kidney & renal pelvis** 22,870 (3%)
Leukemia 24,690 (3%)	**Ovary** 21,880 (3%)
Pancreas 21,370 (3%)	**Pancreas** 21,770 (3%)
All sites 789,620 (100%)	**All sites** 739,940 (100%)

Estimated deaths from cancer

Male	Female
Lung & bronchus 86,220 (29%)	**Lung & bronchus** 71,080 (26%)
Prostate 32,050 (11%)	**Breast** 39,840 (15%)
Colon & rectum 26,580 (9%)	**Colon & rectum** 24,790 (9%)
Pancreas 18,770 (6%)	**Pancreas** 18,030 (7%)
Liver & intrahepatic bile duct 12,720 (4%)	**Ovary** 13,850 (5%)
Leukemia 12,660 (4%)	**Non-Hodgkin lymphoma** 9,500 (4%)
Esophagus 11,650 (4%)	**Leukemia** 9,180 (3%)
Non-Hodgkin lymphoma 10,710 (4%)	**Uterine corpus** 7,950 (3%)
Urinary bladder 10,410 (3%)	**Liver & intrahepatic bile duct** 6,190 (2%)
Kidney & renal pelvis 8,210 (3%)	**Brain & other nervous system** 5,720 (2%)
All sites 299,200 (100%)	**All sites** 270,290 (100%)

*Excludes basal and squamous cell skin cancers and in situ carcinoma except urinary bladder.

©2010, American Cancer Society, Inc., Surveillance and Health Policy Research

Figure 12.11 Leading sites of new cancer cases and deaths.

Source: Cancer Facts and Figure 2010 by the American Cancer Society. Used with permission.

Despite these disturbing figures, more people are surviving cancer than ever before. The 5-year survival rate for cancer is now 68%, an increase of 50% over the rate 30 years ago.[39] However, significant health disparities persist in cancer rates, especially for African Americans, who are more likely to develop and die of cancer than any other ethnic group.[39] Eliminating this disparity is a key focus of national cancer prevention efforts.

To reduce your own risk for cancer, it helps to have a basic understanding of how the disease arises and—in some cases—spreads. You'll also need to know about risk factors, early detection, and warning signs to watch for. After that, we'll provide a quick look at some common cancers, and discuss treatment—and survival.

What Is Cancer?

Cancer is a group of diseases characterized by uncontrolled reproduction of abnormal cells and, in some cases, the spread of these cells to other sites in the body. These cells often don't start as abnormal, but for a variety of reasons, they undergo changes in their operating instructions that turn them into rogue agents of abnormal growth.

Understanding how this happens starts with a look at *DNA*. We'll talk more about human genet-

ics and DNA in Chapter 13. But for now, it's important to note that just about every cell in the body is operated by DNA, the genetic code for the cells, tissues, organs, and biochemical substances that enable the body to function. DNA enables cells to divide and replicate, ensuring that the body's tissues are as fresh and vital as possible. For instance, the cells lining your digestive tract are replaced every few days, and your skin cells are continually being shed and replaced. If you're injured, the replacement process speeds up to help you heal. If you burn your hand, for example, your DNA issues instructions for new cells to be produced more quickly than normal until the injury is healed.

The genes in your DNA that control this cell growth normally operate a bit like the accelerator and brakes on a car. If you need lots of new cells quickly, growth-related genes accelerate their production. Once enough new cells are in place, the same genes slow the process back down to normal. As you can imagine, if something damages these genes, they will no longer be able to regulate cell reproduction appropriately.

The genes that control cell reproduction can be damaged by a variety of external hazards. These include the toxins in tobacco and tobacco smoke, alcohol, many chemicals used in industry,

cancer A group of diseases marked by the uncontrolled multiplication of abnormal cells.

carcinogen A substance known to trigger DNA mutations that can lead to cancer.

oncogene A mutated gene that encourages the uncontrolled cell division that results in cancer.

tumor An abnormal growth of tissue with no physiological function.

benign tumor A tumor that grows slowly, does not spread, and is not cancerous.

malignant tumor A tumor that grows aggressively, invades surrounding tissue, and can spread to other parts of the body; all cancers are malignant.

metastasis The process by which a malignant tumor spreads to other body sites.

radiation from sunlight, sunlamps or sunbeds, and even certain viruses.[40] When we come into contact with such agents—whether by absorbing them via our skin, or breathing or ingesting them—they can cause dangerous *mutations*, or DNA changes, that can lead to cancer. These cancer-generating agents are known as **carcinogens.** Our body's defenses seek out cells with such mutations and either repair the damage, cause the cells to self-destruct, or kill them. But some mutations are more severe than the body can fix, or the encounter with the carcinogen is so frequent that the body's defenses become overwhelmed. And, in some people, other features of their DNA actually diminish their body's ability to protect and repair its cells. We'll look at these genetic risks for cancer more closely a little later in this chapter.

If these growth-control genes are irreparably damaged, they become cancer-causing **oncogenes,** issuing faulty orders for accelerated cell growth. As cells begin reproducing out of control, they form clusters of immature cells that serve no purpose. Their only function is to keep multiplying. Such clusters of cells eventually form clumps of abnormal tissue called **tumors.**

Not all tumors are cancerous. Many are **benign tumors**—that is, they grow only very slowly, do not invade surrounding tissues, and do not spread to other parts of the body. In contrast, **malignant tu-** mors are by definition cancerous **(Figure 12.12).** They invade surrounding tissue, and their cells can break away and enter the bloodstream or lymphatic system, where they circulate and find new places to take root. This aggressive spreading process, called **metastasis,** makes malignant tumors far more dangerous. When malignant cells have metastasized throughout the body, the cancer is far more challenging to treat.

It's important to note that, whereas cancer can spread throughout the body, it can not be spread from person to person. Though certain cancer-associated viruses, such as HIV or hepatitis, are contagious, cancer itself is not.

Risk Factors for Cancer

Given the complex series of interactions involved in cancer, it's no surprise that many different factors can influence cancer risk. These include genetic and biological factors, lifestyle factors, environmental exposure to carcinogens, and exposure to infectious agents.

Genetic and Biological Factors

As you've learned, cancer is fundamentally a disease of the DNA. It involves not only the genes that become damaged in cancer, but other genes involved in preventing this damage.

Many types of cancer run in families or are more common in certain ethnic groups. These include breast, colon, prostate, stomach, skin, and lung cancers. But researchers are learning that these cancers are rarely caused by a single cancerous gene passed through the family bloodline. Instead, in many cases, such as some forms of breast cancer, inherited risks for cancer are more closely related to genes involved in protecting the body from DNA damage.[41] If a weaker version of a protective gene is passed from parent to child, an affected person is more prone to developing cancer if he or she encounters carcinogens.

Cancer can also be related to biological factors, such as the body's hormones. This is especially true for women. The age at

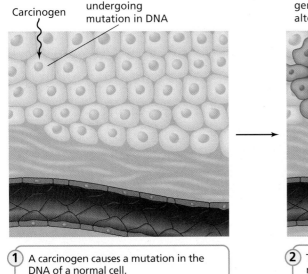

Carcinogen

Normal cell undergoing mutation in DNA

1 A carcinogen causes a mutation in the DNA of a normal cell.

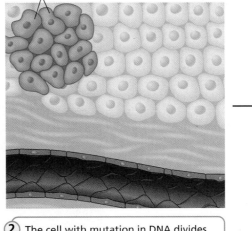

Rapidly dividing genetically altered cells

2 The cell with mutation in DNA divides repeatedly.

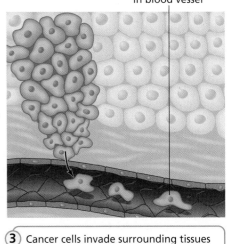

Cancer cell transported in blood vessel

3 Cancer cells invade surrounding tissues and spread to other sites in the body.

Figure 12.12 Progression of cancer.

which a woman had her first period and entered menopause, along with whether she used hormonal birth control, had children (and if so, at what age) all factor into her risk for breast cancer.

Lifestyle Factors

When you think about the vegetables you eat, do you picture a colorful salad or a bag of fries? How often do you exercise? Are your BMI and waist size within a healthful range? Do you smoke, or spend time with someone who does? Do you drink alcohol, and if so, how much?

The same basic lifestyle choices that are important in diabetes and cardiovascular disease also affect your risk of cancer. Although a healthier lifestyle offers no guarantee against cancer, it significantly reduces your risk. **Practical Strategies for Health: Ways to Lower Your Risk for Cancer** summarizes simple steps you can take to lower your risk.

Environmental Exposure to Carcinogens

Do you like to tan? Do you have a job that involves working with chemicals or radiation, or live in an area with high levels of air pollution?

If so, you may be exposing your body—and your DNA—to carcinogens on a regular basis. Some of these risks are more a matter of personal choice and are easier to control. For instance, you can opt to avoid sunbathing or visiting the tanning salon. But reducing your exposure to carcinogens in your workplace or neighborhood can be more challenging.

Many jobs involve working with chemicals or radiation, or produce airborne particles, such as wood dust from sanding, that are known carcinogens. Be sure you are aware of all safety procedures used at your workplace and follow them. If you aren't sure about these safety procedures, talk to your boss or human resources department. State and federal laws lay out clear occupational safety requirements that

☺ Practical Strategies for Health

Ways to Lower Your Risk for Cancer

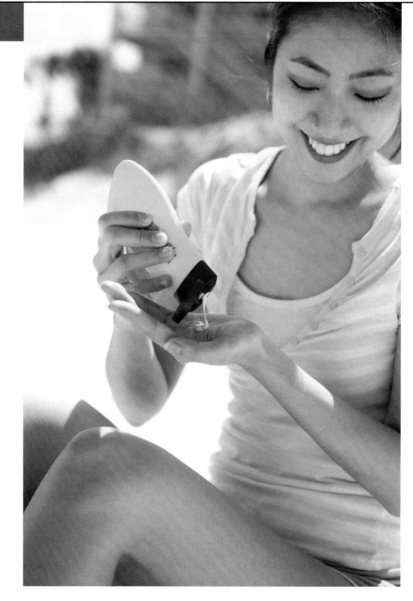

1. Don't smoke or use any tobacco products.

2. Eat a nutritious diet. Aim for five or more servings of fresh fruits and vegetables each day.

3. Exercise at least 30 minutes a day, as many days a week as possible.

4. Maintain a healthful weight.

5. Limit your alcohol consumption.

6. Wear sunscreen when you are outdoors, with a sun protection factor (SPF) of at least 30. Wear clothing to cover as much of your skin as possible, including a hat. Wear sunglasses that block UV rays. Avoid tanning salons, and limit your exposure to the sun between the hours of 10 a.m. and 4 p.m.

7. Practice safe sex. Use condoms, even if you rely on other methods for birth control. Safe sex dramatically reduces your risk of HPV and other STIs linked to cancer.

8. If you are female, consider an HPV vaccine to reduce your chances of developing cervical cancer. Also, begin cervical cancer screening no later than age 21 with a regular Pap test.

9. Check your home for radon, a carcinogen linked to lung cancer. Visit www.epa.gov/radon/healthrisks.html for more information.

10. If you have a family history of cancer, talk to your doctor about steps you can take to lower your risk.

11. Find out if your ethnicity puts you at higher risk for some cancers. Certain cancers are more common among specific ethnic groups, such as prostate cancer in African American men, hepatitis-related liver cancer in Asians, or certain types of breast cancer in Jewish women of European descent. Simply being aware that you may be at an elevated risk can prompt you to take active steps to lower your risk.

12. Talk to your doctor about whether he or she advises breast self-exams or testicular self-exams. Though self-exams cannot prevent cancer per se, they may be able to aid in early detection.

13. If you are a female over 40, talk to your doctor about whether he or she advises yearly mammograms for breast cancer detection.

companies must follow. If you devise your own summer job that requires you to work with chemicals—for instance, house painting, house cleaning, or landscaping—research the appropriate safety measures, such as wearing gloves and mask, and follow them!

If you live in an area known for air pollution, you can start reducing your risks by being aware of the ebbs and flows in pollution levels. For example, pay attention to public service announcements identifying days when pollution levels are especially high, and avoid outdoor exercise during those times. If pollutants from nearby industry or a landfill or other waste site are a concern, or the safety of your public water supply is uncertain, consider getting involved in public pollution-reduction efforts. Many communities have environmental and health advocacy groups dedicated to reducing pollution and the diseases connected to it.

Exposure to Infectious Agents

Certain infectious microorganisms are now known to be linked to some forms of cancer, and researchers are looking for others. They theorize that these disease-causing agents trigger cancer by causing persistent inflammation, suppressing a person's immune system, or stimulating cells into extended periods of growth. In the United States, some of the more common cancer-causing infectious agents include the following viruses:

- **Hepatitis B and C.** These forms of the hepatitis virus can lead to liver cancer. In people from certain countries in Asia, such as China, where Hepatitis B is common, virus-related liver cancer is a top health concern.[40]

- **HIV.** This virus, in suppressing the immune system, can lead to certain types of cancer that are otherwise rare. These are called *opportunistic* cancers because they occur when reduced immune defenses allow them the opportunity to develop.[40]

- **HPV.** The human papilloma virus, or HPV, is usually transmitted through sexual contact. Nearly all women with cervical cancer have evidence of HPV, although not all cervical HPV infections turn into cancer. Young women are now also able to receive a vaccine against certain dangerous strains of HPV. You'll find more information on cervical cancer later in this chapter, and more information on the HPV vaccine in Chapter 11. HPV is also linked to a rise in cases of throat cancer, most likely due to transmission during oral sex.[42]

Detecting Cancer

Since cancer can occur in sites as varied as lungs, bones, and blood, no single test can detect all cancers. But an increasing variety of detection methods are allowing more cancers to be caught earlier, when they are easier to treat.

Some types of cancer can be found even before they cause any symptoms. Tests that "screen" large numbers of people to check for the presence of disease or conditions associated with disease are called *screening tests*. For instance, mammograms are a form of x-ray test used to detect breast cancer. A colonoscopy is an examina-

How safe is the environment at your summer job? Visit www.osha.gov/SLTC/youth/summerjobs.

biopsy A test for cancer in which a small sample of the abnormal growth is removed and studied.

carcinoma Cancer of tissues that line or cover the body.

sarcoma Cancer of muscle or connective tissues.

central nervous system cancer Cancer of the brain or spinal cord.

tion of the colon (the large intestine) with a tiny camera. It allows a physician to find and remove precancerous growths called *polyps*. Screening tests are also used for many other types of cancer.

When cancer is suspected, either following the results of a screening test or because a patient has detected a suspicious mass, the physician may perform a **biopsy,** removing a small sample of the abnormal growth so that it can be studied for signs of cancer. In addition, lab tests of blood or other body fluids can check for the presence of substances called *tumor markers* that suggest cancer. Other detection methods rely on imaging technologies. These include ultrasound (US), magnetic resonance imaging (MRI), computed tomography (CT), and positron emission tomography (PET), each of which has advantages and disadvantages for different types of tissues.

Newer methods analyze body fluids for signs of cancer-related DNA. A test being developed for oral cancer, for example, analyzes a saliva sample for the cancer's DNA "signature." If proven effective, this test will allow for earlier detection and treatment.[43]

In addition to these clinical detection methods, you should also be aware of 10 general symptoms that can warn you of cancer. Most often, these symptoms *are not due to cancer*. However, if you notice any of them, and don't see an apparent reason for them, make an appointment with your doctor:[44]

- A thickening or lump in the breast or any other part of the body
- A new mole or a change in an existing mole
- A sore that does not heal
- Hoarseness or a cough that does not go away
- Changes in bowel or bladder habits
- Discomfort after eating
- Difficulty swallowing
- Weight gain or loss with no known reason
- Unusual bleeding or discharge
- Feeling weak or very tired

Types of Cancer

Cancers can be grouped into five broad categories according to the type of tissue in which the cancer arises:

- **Carcinomas** begin in the body's epithelial tissues, which include the skin and the tissues that line or cover internal organs. These are the most common sites for cancer, and cancers that occur here usually come in the form of solid tumors.

- **Sarcomas** start in the muscles, bones, fat, blood vessels, or other connective or supporting tissue. Sarcomas also take the form of solid tumors.

- **Central nervous system cancers** begin in the tissues of the brain and spinal cord. These form solid tumors, and do damage both by directly altering nerve function and by growing large enough to interfere with the function of surrounding tissue.

Surviving Cancer

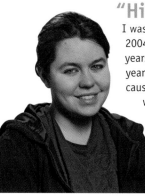

"Hi, my name is Amanda. I'm 19. I was diagnosed with acute lymphocytic leukemia in 2004 at the age of 13. I was on chemo for about three years, had two surgeries, and had to miss about two years of school. The surgeries affected me socially because I basically had plastic tubes in my chest, so it was hard to give people hugs. People didn't understand, you know, when they would try to hug me—I'd be like, 'Oh you can't hug me, I'm a little bit fragile right here.' I've been in remission since 2007. I go for blood tests all the time just to make sure it hasn't come back.

My mother had breast cancer and shortly after she was in remission, she was diagnosed with ovarian cancer. Also, my mother's mother died of breast cancer, and her sister, my great-aunt, died of leukemia. So we have a lot of cancer in the females in our family.

I get a bi-yearly pelvic exam and I go for mammograms fairly regularly. I would say at least once a year. I am pretty young to be getting mammograms but I probably should be going about twice a year because the frequency of cancer in my family is so high."

1: How does leukemia differ from other types of cancer?

2: Do you have a family history of cancer? If so, are you taking extra precautions such as scheduling regular cancer screenings?

Do you have a story similar to Amanda's? Share your story at www.pearsonhighered.com/choosinghealth.

---

lymphoma Cancer of the lymph system.

myeloma Cancer of the bone marrow.

leukemia Cancer of blood-forming tissue.

malignant melanoma An especially aggressive form of skin cancer.

- **Lymphomas** and **myelomas** begin in the cells of the immune system. These cancers first infect the disease-fighting parts of your body, and take the form of solid tumors.
- **Leukemias** start in the tissues that make your blood. This type of cancer does not cause solid tumors, instead filling the blood with abnormal blood cells.

Common Cancers in Men and Women

Although cancer can arise in hundreds of different sites in your body, some sites are far more prone to cancer than others. We'll start with a look at cancers that affect both men and women, and follow with a separate overview of common sex-specific cancers.

Skin cancer. More than 2 million people develop skin cancer each year.[39] Many of these cases are treatable, about 68,000 of these cases are **malignant melanomas,** the most deadly form of skin cancer.[39]

Risk Factors Risk factors for skin cancer include:

- Fair skin and light hair or eyes.
- Skin that sunburns easily.

- Personal or family history of skin cancer.
- Sun exposure with no or low-SPF sunscreen.

What should you watch for? Less serious forms of skin cancer look like bumps, colored spots, or scaly patches on the skin. These may bleed, itch, or ooze. In contrast, melanoma may arise as a new mole or changes to an existing mole **(Figure 12.13).** When examining any mole, use the ABCDE acronym to remember to look for these signs:

- **A**symmetry, where one side does not match the other.
- **B**order irregularity, where edges are uneven or scalloped.
- **C**olor changes, where pigmentation is not uniform.
- **D**iameter, where the size is more than 6 millimeters (about the size of a pea).
- **E**volving, where the mole looks different from others nearby or is changing in size, shape, or color.

If you notice any of these changes, see your doctor as soon as possible.

If you don't have a history of skin cancer in your family, doctors don't recommend regular screenings for melanoma. But everyone's risk begins to increase at age 20, so it's a good idea to check your skin periodically for signs of change.

If you do have a family or personal history of skin cancer, many doctors recommend augmenting your own checks with a yearly skin exam from a dermatologist.

Reducing Your Risk Especially for people with fair skin, lots of unprotected sun exposure equals higher risks. Avoid extended time in the sun without a hat, protective clothing, and/or high-SPF sunscreen. Avoid tanning. The skin cancer risks of sustained, repeated exposure to UV light have been widely documented by medical researchers. Especially in fair-skinned people, tanning is linked to an increased risk of melanoma and other forms of skin cancer. Some tanning beds emit doses of UV radiation far more powerful than those that come from the sun. And though some people like to tan because they think it makes them look better now, they overlook the fact that sun exposure actually ages your skin later on.

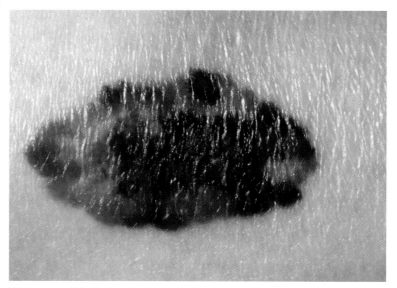

Figure 12.13 Malignant melanoma.

Lung cancer. With more than 200,000 new cases diagnosed each year, lung cancer is the second most common malignancy in the United States—and the most deadly.[39]

Risk Factors   Risk factors for lung cancer include:

- A history of smoking or being exposed to second-hand smoke. The longer you've smoked or been exposed to tobacco smoke, the higher your risk.
- Genetic factors.
- Exposure to radon. In some areas, this naturally occurring radioactive gas exists in high concentrations in the soil and, over time, seeps into people's homes or water supplies.
- Exposure to other cancer-causing substances, such as asbestos or arsenic.

What should you watch for? By the time any of the following symptoms have appeared, a case of lung cancer is usually fairly advanced:

- Spitting up blood-streaked mucus.
- Chest pain.
- A persistent cough.
- Recurrent attacks of pneumonia or bronchitis.

So far, this cancer has proven very difficult to detect early, and there are no established general screening guidelines. CT scans have been found effective at catching the disease early in people at higher risk, but it is not yet clear if this helps patients live longer.[45]

Reducing Your Risk.   Smoking or regular exposure to second-hand smoke remain the single largest risk factors for lung cancer. If you smoke, get started on a plan to quit and, in the meantime, keep your smoke away from others. In addition, check your home for radon. According to the U.S. Environmental Protection Agency, nearly 1 in 15 U.S. homes has elevated radon levels.[46] You can purchase an inexpensive test kit to check the air in your home. You can also talk to campus officials about radon testing in campus buildings, and ask your employer for test results from your workplace.

Colon and rectal cancers. Approximately 102,000 cases of colon cancer and 39,600 cases of rectal cancer are diagnosed each year in the U.S.,[39] resulting in the deaths of about 51,300 people annually.[39]

Risk Factors   Risk factors for colorectal cancer include:

- A family history of colorectal cancer.
- A family history of polyps, or precancerous growths, in the colon or rectum.
- Being over the age of 50.
- Presence of an inflammatory bowel disorder, such as colitis or Crohn's disease.

What should you watch for? In its early stages, when it is easiest to treat, colorectal cancer often has no outward symptoms. As the cancer progresses, warning signs include bleeding from the rectum, blood in the stool, and changes in bowel habits.

Screening is recommended for everyone once they reach the age of 50, using methods that include:

- A yearly test that detects blood in the stool.
- Every 5 to 10 years, an internal imaging test that looks for polyps, such as a colonoscopy.

- For people at higher risk, such as those with a family history of colorectal cancer, doctors usually recommend a more frequent screening schedule.

Reducing Your Risk   The following measures may help to prevent colorectal cancer:

- Engaging in regular exercise.
- Consuming a diet rich in fiber and plant-based foods.
- Maintaining a healthy weight.
- Limiting alcohol consumption.
- Avoiding smoking.
- Following recommended screening guidelines, as precancerous polyps can be removed during colonoscopy, and cancerous tumors can often be surgically removed if caught at earlier stages.

Pancreatic cancer. Pancreatic cancer is the fourth leading cause of cancer death in the United States. Approximately 43,000 cases are diagnosed each year, and about 36,800 people die from it.[39] Much remains to be learned about pancreatic cancer, which often goes undetected in its early stages and has a low survival rate.

Risk Factors   Risk factors for pancreatic cancer include:

- Obesity.
- Diabetes.
- Smoking.
- Physical inactivity.
- Genetic factors.

What should you watch for? Signs of pancreatic cancer rarely appear until the disease is advanced. These include:

- Upper abdominal pain.
- Jaundice, or a yellowing of your skin and the whites of your eyes.
- Loss of appetite.
- Unexplained weight loss.

Currently, no standard screening guidelines exist for pancreatic cancer. Researchers are looking for ways to detect this cancer early and determine who would benefit most from screening.

Reducing Your Risk   Reduce your risk by following basic health guidelines, which include:

- Not smoking.
- Eating a healthy diet high in fiber and plant-based fats and low in sugar, processed foods, and saturated fats.
- Maintaining a healthy weight.
- Exercising regularly—at least 30 minutes a day on most days.

Leukemia. Approximately 43,000 cases of leukemia—cancer of the blood—are diagnosed in the U.S. each year, and about 21,800 people die from it.[39] Although commonly thought of as a childhood cancer, most cases actually occur in older adults. The disease arises in one of two primary forms: acute and chronic. Research into the genetics of cancer has revealed that these broader categories actually contain dozens of subtypes, each with unique DNA features.

Risk Factors   Risk factors for leukemia include:

- Being male.
- Having an inborn genetic disorder, such as Down syndrome.
- Exposure to carcinogens such as tobacco smoke, certain chemicals, or radiation.

What should you watch for? The symptoms of leukemia resemble those of many other, less serious illnesses, making this disease difficult to diagnose early. Signs include:

- Fatigue.
- Nosebleeds.
- Pallor.
- Repeated infections.
- Unexplained fever.
- Bruising.
- Weight loss.

There are currently no general recommendations for leukemia screening. Doctors are most likely to spot the disease early when they order a routine blood test to check for a variety of risk factors and notice abnormal levels of white blood cells or other signs of leukemia.

Reducing Your Risk   Much remains to be learned about the causes of leukemia, so specific preventions are not yet clear. However, recommendations include avoiding carcinogens known to increase leukemia risk, such as tobacco smoke.

Oral cancer. About 36,500 malignancies of the lips, tongue, mouth, and throat are diagnosed each year, and about 7,800 deaths result from oral cancers.[39]

Risk Factors   Risk factors include:

- Smoking.
- Use of "smokeless" or chewing tobacco.
- Excessive drinking. A mix of heavy drinking and smoking is linked to a significant increase in risk.

What should you watch for? Symptoms include:

- A sore that doesn't heal.
- Red or white patches that don't heal or go away.
- An unexplained lump or thickening.
- Ear pain.
- A lump in the neck.
- Coughing up blood.

Although there are no general screening guidelines, doctors and dentists usually make checking for oral cancer a routine part of any regular exam. As you learned earlier in this chapter, scientists are also trying to develop a screening test that would detect oral cancer's DNA signatures in a person's saliva.

Reducing Your Risk   The best strategies are to avoid all types of tobacco products and excessive drinking.

Common Cancers in Men

Cancers affecting the male reproductive system include prostate cancer and testicular cancer. Although both are common, prostate cancer tends to occur in older men, whereas testicular cancer more commonly develops in younger men.

Prostate cancer. The **prostate** is a gland in the male reproductive system that secretes a fluid that assists in the movement of sperm. It is located below the bladder. Prostate cancer is the most commonly diagnosed malignancy among men in the United States, and the second most deadly.

---

prostate A gland in the male reproductive system that is prone to malignancy.

About 217,000 cases are diagnosed each year, and about 32,000 deaths each year are caused by it.[39]

Risk Factors   Risk factors include:

- Age. Most cases arise in men over 65.
- Genetic inheritance. Family history and ethnicity strongly affect your risk. African American men are more likely to be diagnosed with prostate cancer and are more likely to have an aggressive form.
- Diet. A high-fat diet translates into higher risk.
- Being overweight. Less physical activity and higher weight increase risk.

What should you watch for? Detecting prostate cancer in its early stages can be difficult, so talk to your doctor if you have any questions. Symptoms are less noticeable in the disease's early stages, but later may include:

- Difficulty urinating.
- The urge to urinate frequently.
- Blood in the urine.
- Pain in the low back, thighs, or pelvis.

Reducing Your Risk   To lower your risk, head for the produce aisle. Fruits and vegetables high in lycopene, a pigment found in tomatoes and other red produce, may lower risk. You can also keep yourself healthier by following a diet low in saturated fats and by maintaining a healthful weight.

Testicular cancer. Brought to public attention by cycling champion Lance Armstrong (see page 300), testicular cancer is one of the most common malignancies in young men. About 8,400 men are diagnosed with it each year, and about 350 will die from it.[39]

Risk Factors   The risk factors for testicular cancer include:

- Being a male between the ages of 20 and 39.
- Having a family history of cancer.
- A history of an undescended testicle; that is, a testicle that did not descend from the abdomen into the scrotum before birth. The risk of cancer is increased for both testicles, and remains whether or not the individual has had surgery to move the testicle into place.

Reducing Your Risk   Because researchers still haven't uncovered the cause of testicular cancer, the most effective preventions aren't yet clear. Testicular self-exams can aid in detection (see the **Spotlight** on page 295), but there is no definitive evidence that they lead to a reduction in deaths from testicular cancer. If you are concerned about testicular cancer or have a family history of it, consult your doctor for advice on what to do.

Common Cancers in Women

Cancers affecting the female reproductive system include breast cancer, ovarian cancer, and cervical and uterine cancers.

Breast cancer. With more than 200,000 new cases and 40,000 deaths each year, breast cancer is the most common cancer among women in the United States and the second leading cause of cancer death.[39] Though more women are surviving breast cancer, prevention, detection, and treatment remain a top health concern.

Risk Factors   Risk factors include:

- A family history of breast cancer, on either side of your family.
- Ethnicity. Certain ethnic groups, such as Jews of European descent, are at higher risk of inherited forms of breast cancer, such

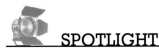
Testicular Self-Exam

The American Cancer Society advises men to be aware of testicular cancer and to see a doctor right away if a lump is found. Regular testicular self-exams have not been studied enough to show whether they reduce the death rate from this cancer. Because of this, the ACS does not make recommendations about regular testicular self-exams for all men. Still, some doctors recommend that all men do monthly testicular self-exams after puberty.

Men with risk factors, such as an undescended testicle, previous testicular can- cer, or a family member who has had this cancer should seriously think about monthly self-exams. If you have risks, talk it over with a doctor. Each man has to decide for himself whether to examine his testicles each month. Here are instructions on how to do it if you decide it's right for you.

How to Do a Testicular Self-Exam

The best time to do the self-exam is during or after a bath or shower, when the skin of the scrotum is relaxed. To do a testicular self-exam:

- Hold your penis out of the way and check one testicle at a time.
- Hold the testicle between your thumbs and fingers of both hands and roll it gently between your fingers.
- Look and feel for any hard lumps or smooth rounded bumps or any change in the size, shape, or consistency of the testes.

You should know that each normal testis has an epididymis, which feels like a small "bump" on the upper or middle outer side of the testis. Normal testicles also contain blood vessels, supporting tissues, and tubes that conduct sperm. Other noncancerous problems can sometimes cause swellings or lumps around a testicle. It's easy to confuse these with cancer. If you have any doubts, see a doctor.

If you choose to check your testicles, you will learn what is normal for you and be able to tell when something is different. Always report any changes to a doctor right away.

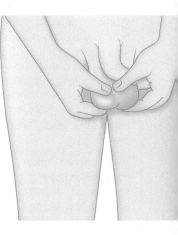

---

as those linked to mutations in genes called *BRCA1* and *BRCA2*. Normal versions of these genes appear to offer protection from cancer, whereas the mutated versions are far less protective.

- Menstrual periods that started early and ended late in life.
- Use of hormonal medications, such as birth control pills or hormone replacement therapy.
- Being overweight.
- Never having children, or having your first child after age 30.
- Having two or more drinks a day on a regular basis.

What should you watch for? Symptoms usually include changes in breast tissue, such as:

- A lump or thickening in your breast or in the lymph nodes under your arm.
- Dimpling, skin distortion, or skin irritation.
- Unusual nipple appearance or discharge.

Reducing Your Risk A healthy lifestyle—including maintaining a healthful weight, limiting alcohol use, and regularly exercising—is a great starting point for any woman who wants to reduce her risk. Women who breast-feed for several months may have added protection, and women who do not use postmenopausal hormone therapy may also lower their risk.[47]

Women whose family histories put them at increased risk should talk to their doctors about what to do. A doctor may advocate mammograms or other screenings at an earlier age, or even genetic testing that can determine whether a woman has genes linked to cancer. Women at especially high risk may consider *chemoprevention* (the use of drugs to reduce cancer risk), or in the most extreme cases, surgical mastectomies to reduce their cancer risk.

The American Cancer Society (ACS) recommends that women in their 20s and 30s have a clinical breast exam at least once every 3 years, and at least once a year once they are over 40.[48] The ACS also recommends mammograms every year for women age 40 and older. Breast self-exams are optional and have both benefits and limitations. See the **Spotlight** on page 296 for instructions on how to perform a breast self-exam.

Ovarian cancer. An estimated 21,880 women are diagnosed with ovarian cancer each year, and 13,850 die from it.[39]

Risk Factors Risk factors for ovarian cancer include:

- A family history of ovarian cancer or breast cancer
- Mutations in genes, such as *BRCA 1* or *BRCA 2*, which are also associated with breast cancer
- Age. Ovarian cancer most often develops in women after menopause.
- Never having children
- Infertility
- Obesity
- Participation in hormone replacement therapy

Symptoms of ovarian cancer are non-specific and mimic other common conditions, like bladder and digestive disorders, which can make diagnosis difficult. Women with ovarian cancer are more likely to have a feeling of abdominal pressure, swelling, or bloating; urination urgency; and pelvic discomfort or pain that is persistent and continues to gradually worsen over time.

Reducing Your Risk Women between the ages of 35 to 40 who have gene mutations and a strong history of cancer may elect to have their ovaries removed. This, however, is a very important

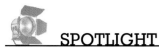
Breast Awareness and Self-Exam

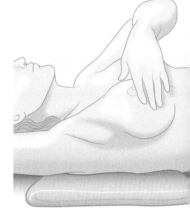

Women should be aware of how their breasts normally look and feel and report any new breast changes to a health professional as soon as they are found. Finding a breast change does not necessarily mean there is a cancer.

A woman can notice changes by knowing how her breasts normally look and feel and feeling her breasts for changes (breast awareness), or by choosing to use a step-by-step approach and using a specific schedule to examine her breasts.

If you choose to do breast self-exam (BSE), the following information provides a step-by-step approach. The best time for a woman to examine her breasts is when the breasts are not tender or swollen. Women who examine their breasts should have their technique reviewed during their periodic health exams by their health-care professional.

It is acceptable for women to choose not to do BSE or to do BSE occasionally. Women who choose not to do BSE should still know how their breasts normally look and feel and report any changes to their doctor right away.

How to Examine Your Breasts

Lie down on your back and place your right arm behind your head. The exam is done while lying down, not standing up. This is because when lying down the breast tissue spreads evenly over the chest wall and is as thin as possible, making it much easier to feel all the breast tissue.

Use the finger pads of the three middle fingers on your left hand to feel for lumps in the right breast. Use overlapping dime-sized circular motions of the finger pads to feel the breast tissue.

Use three different levels of pressure to feel all the breast tissue. Light pressure is needed to feel the tissue closest to the skin; medium pressure to feel a little deeper; and firm pressure to feel the tissue closest to the chest and ribs. It is normal to feel a firm ridge in the lower curve of each breast, but, you should tell your doctor if you feel anything else out of the ordi-

nary. If you're not sure how hard to press, talk with your doctor or nurse. Use each pressure level to feel the breast tissue before moving on to the next spot.

Move around the breast in an up-and-down pattern starting at an imaginary line drawn straight down your side from the underarm and moving across the breast to the middle of the chest bone (sternum or breast-bone). Be sure to check the entire breast area going down until you feel only ribs and up to the neck or collar bone (clavicle).

There is some evidence to suggest that the up-and-down pattern (sometimes called the vertical pattern) is the most effective pattern for covering the entire breast without missing any breast tissue.

Repeat the exam on your left breast, putting your left arm behind your head and using the finger pads of your right hand to do the exam.

While standing in front of a mirror with your hands pressing firmly down on your hips, look at your

breasts for any changes of size, shape, contour, or dimpling, or redness or scaliness of the nipple or breast skin. (The pressing down on the hips position contracts the chest wall muscles and enhances any breast changes.)

Examine each underarm while sitting up or standing and with your arm only slightly raised so you can easily feel in this area. Raising your arm straight up tightens the tissue in this area and makes it harder to examine.

This procedure for doing breast self-exam is different from previous recommendations. These changes represent an extensive review of the medical literature and input from an expert advisory group. There is evidence that this position (lying down), the area felt, pattern of coverage of the breast, and use of different amounts of pressure increase a woman's ability to find abnormal areas.

Source: Breast Awareness and Self-Exam by the American Cancer Society, 2009. Modified and reprinted by the permission of the American Cancer Society, Inc. from www.cancer.org. All rights reserved.

---

personal decision and the pros and cons should be discussed in depth with a physician.

Cervical and uterine cancers. About 80% of the approximately 55,600 cases of these cancers each year arise in the lining of the uterus, or endometrium.[39] The rest arise in the cervix, at the base of the uterus. Uterine cancer results in approximately 7,900 deaths each year, and cervical cancer results in approximately 4,200 deaths.[39]

Risk Factors   Risk factors for cervical cancer include:

- HPV infection, which you learned about earlier in this chapter and in Chapter 11.
- Other sexually transmitted infections, such as herpes simplex type 2.

- Cigarette smoking.
- Having multiple sexual partners, which increases the risk of HPV and other infections.

The risk factors for endometrial cancer are less well understood.

What should you watch for? Signs include unexplained vaginal bleeding or discharge. Cervical cancer can also cause pain during sex. However, in most cases, it develops silently. That's why a Pap test, performed during a woman's pelvic exam, is the most effective way to check for cervical cancer. This swab of the cervix is used to look for precancerous cell changes.

Are You At Risk for Developing a Chronic Disease?

Are you at risk for developing diabetes, cardiovascular disease, or cancer? Answer the following questions to determine your risk. Circle your answer.

1. Are you overweight or obese? — yes no
2. Do you live a sedentary lifestyle? — yes no
3. Do you drink excessive amounts of alcohol? — yes no
4. Do you smoke or use smokeless tobacco products? — yes no
5. Do you eat a high-fat diet? — yes no
6. Do you eat few fruits and vegetables? — yes no
7. Do you have excess weight around your abdominal area? — yes no
8. Do you spend a lot of time in the sun without sunscreen or protective clothing? — yes no
9. Do you practice unsafe sex? — yes no
10. Do you have a family history of diabetes, cardiovascular disease, or cancer? — yes no

HOW TO INTERPRET YOUR SCORE

Answering "Yes" to any of the questions above means that you should modify your lifestyle to reduce the risk of chronic disease.

To take this self-assessment online, visit www.pearsonhighered .com/choosinghealth.

Watch videos of real students discussing cardiovascular disease, diabetes, and cancer at www.pearsonhighered.com/choosinghealth.

The American Cancer Society recommends the following screening schedule:

- Have your first Pap test within 3 years after you begin having vaginal intercourse, or no later than age 21.
- Continue getting tested every year (if using the regular Pap test) or every two years (if using the newer liquid-based Pap test).[49]

Reducing Your Risk After the age of 30, talk to your doctor about getting an HPV test. The best way to lower your risk of cervical cancer is to protect your sexual health and reduce your risk of HPV and other STDs. If you have male partners, use a condom, even if you rely on another birth control method as well. This is especially important if you or your partner have other partners. Young women may also choose to receive a vaccine against certain strains of HPV.

Treating Cancer

Over many decades, cancer treatment has evolved into a variety of methods that attempt to remove or shrink malignant tumors, stop or slow metastasis, or even confront cancerous DNA. More established cancer-treatment methods include surgery to remove tumors whenever possible. In some cases, however, surgery is not an option because tumor removal would risk the life of the patient. *Radiation therapy* directs wavelengths of energy at a tumor to kill cancer cells or damage their DNA so that they can no longer reproduce. *Chemotherapy* uses one or more drugs to eradicate cancer cells.

Newer techniques focus on cancer's DNA, often relying on drugs that disrupt a tumor's ability to grow. Some researchers are now analyzing cancerous DNA itself, looking for identifying genetic features that enable them to classify tumors into subtypes and develop targeted drug and treatment plans.

DIVERSITY & HEALTH

Racial Disparities in
Incidences of Chronic Disease

Even as broad public health efforts focus on reducing the risks of chronic diseases such as cancer, heart disease, and diabetes, significant racial and ethnic disparities remain. Consider the following:

- African-Americans die of cancer, heart disease, and diabetes at significantly higher rates than Caucasians or members of other racial and ethnic groups.[1,2] Socioeconomic factors such as inequities in income, education, standard of living, and access to health care are believed to play a role in these disparities, more so than any biological differences associated with race.[3]

- Rates of stomach cancer are 70% higher among Hispanics than among

non-Hispanic whites.[4] Higher rates of infection with *Helicobacter pylori* are believed to play a role, as well as higher consumption of certain kinds of food, such as salted meat or fish and pickled vegetables.[4]

- Native Americans have the highest rates of diabetes in the world.[5] African-Americans and Hispanics also have disproportionately higher rates of diabetes.[6] Obesity, less nutritious diets, and economic barriers to health care are all believed to play a role.

If you are at higher risk for a certain disease, talk to your doctor or a health counselor to find out what you can do to reduce

your risk. Remember that maintaining a healthy weight, exercising, eating a nutritious diet, not smoking, and limiting alcohol intake can go a long way toward keeping you healthy—regardless of your race/ethnicity.

References: **1.** "Health, United States, 2009: With Special Feature on Medical Technology," by the National Center for Health Statistics, 2009, retrieved from http://www.cdc.gov/nchs/data/hus/hus09 .pdf#032. **2.** "Diabetes Death Rate by Race/Ethnicity," by the Kaiser Family Foundation, 2010, retrieved from http://www.statehealthfacts .org/comparemaptable.jsp?cat=2&ind=76. **3.** "Cancer Facts and Figures for African Americans, 2009-2010," by the American Cancer Society, 2009. **4.** "Cancer Facts & Figures for Hispanics /Latinos, 2006-2008," by the American Cancer Society, 2006. **5.** "Health Disparities Experienced by American Indians and Alaska Natives," by the Centers for Disease Control and Prevention, 2003, *Morbidity and Mortality Weekly Report, 52*(30), pp. 697. **6.** "Diabetes Disparities Among Racial and Ethnic Minorities," by the U.S. Department for Health and Human Resources and Agency for Healthcare Research and Quality (AHRQ), retrieved from http://www.ahrq.gov/research/diabdisp.htm.

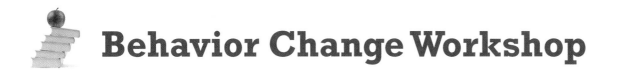

Behavior Change Workshop

To complete this workshop online, visit **www.pearsonhighered.com/choosinghealth**.

Remember that just four key behaviors can have a tremendous influence in increasing your risk for developing diabetes, cardiovascular disease, or cancer. They are (1) poor nutrition, (2) lack of physical activity, (3) tobacco use, and (4) excessive alcohol consumption. In addition, the following factors can play a significant role in increasing your risk of disease: being overweight or obese, spending a lot of time outdoors without sunscreen or protective clothing, and practicing unsafe sex.

Unlike genetics, all of the above behaviors are controllable! It is within your power to change your behavior and reduce your risk of disease.

At this point in the course, it's likely you have already completed Behavior Change Workshops for improving your nutrition (Chapter 4), increasing your physical activity (Chapter 5), maintaining a healthy weight (Chapter 6), quitting smoking (Chapter 8), reducing your alcohol consumption (Chapter 8), and practicing safer sex (Chapter 10). If not, turn to those chapters for targeted workshops on any of these key topics.

In this workshop, assess your progress overall. What did your behavior look like at the beginning of this course? What does it look like today? What are your goals for the future? Answer the questions below.

1. Diet. What changes have you made to your daily meals in order to improve your overall nutrition?

_____

_____

_____

2. Physical activity. What changes have you made to your daily routine in order to incorporate more physical activity into your life?

_____

_____

_____

3. Tobacco use. At the beginning of this course, did you smoke or use other tobacco products? If so, what steps have you taken to reduce or stop your use of tobacco products?

_____

_____

_____

4. Alcohol use. At the beginning of this course, how many alcoholic beverages (if any) did you consume per week? How many alcohol beverages (if any) do you consume per week today?

_____

_____

_____

5. Weight maintenance. At the beginning of this course, were you overweight, obese, or underweight? If so, what steps have you taken to get closer to achieving a healthy weight?

_____

_____

_____

6. Protecting yourself from skin cancer. At the beginning of this course, did you regularly wear protective clothing and sunscreen when you spent time outdoors in the sun?

_____

Do you regularly wear protective clothing and sunscreen outdoors today?

_____

7. Practicing safer sex. If you are sexually active, did you take measures to always protect yourself from sexually transmitted diseases and unwanted pregnancy, at the beginning of this course?

_____

Do you take measures to always protect yourself from sexually transmitted diseases and unwanted pregnancy today?

_____

8. Review your responses to the questions above. Are there aspects of your behavior that you are still working on, in order to reduce your risk for developing a major disease? If so, what are they?

_____

_____

What steps can you take to begin adjusting your behavior?

_____

_____

_____

Chapter Summary

- Four lifestyle choices—eating a nourishing diet, engaging in regular physical activity, not smoking, and limiting alcohol—can significantly reduce your risks of developing a chronic disease.

- Diabetes is a disorder in which blood glucose levels are consistently elevated above normal.

- The cardiovascular system consists of the heart and blood vessels. This network supplies your body with oxygen and nutrients and hauls away wastes.

- The four most common forms of cardiovascular disease are coronary heart disease, stroke, congestive heart failure, and hypertension. Cardiovascular diseases are the top killer of men and women in the United States.

- Atherosclerosis is the development of plaque along the lining of an artery.

- Coronary heart disease is characterized by atherosclerosis affecting a coronary artery. It can lead to angina (chest pain) and/or a heart attack or arrhythmia.

- Hypertension is a blood pressure consistently higher than normal.

- Stroke is a blockage or rupture of a cerebral artery. Permanent brain damage or death can result.

- Congestive heart failure is an inability of the heart to pump blood effectively throughout the circulatory system, causing blood to back up (congest) in the lungs, abdomen, or other body regions.

- Cancer is the second most common cause of death in the United States. The term covers a wide group of diseases marked by uncontrolled growth of abnormal cells.

Test Your Knowledge

1. What are common characteristics of diabetes?
   a. high levels of glucose in the blood
   b. the inability to manufacture or use insulin properly
   c. undernourished cells
   d. all of the above

2. Risk factors for diabetes include all of the following except
   a. obesity.
   b. excess weight around the abdominal area.
   c. a high-fiber diet.
   d. a sedentary lifestyle.

3. What is atherosclerosis?
   a. a rupture in a blood vessel
   b. the buildup of plaque in arteries
   c. a clot in a cerebral artery
   d. widened arteries

4. What is the term for chest pain that is the result of coronary arteries being narrowed or obstructed?
   a. arrhythmia
   b. angina pectoris
   c. hypoglycemia
   d. hypertension

5. What is myocardial infarction another term for?
   a. atherosclerosis
   b. hypertension
   c. heart attack
   d. angina pectoris

6. What kind of cholesterol is considered "good" cholesterol?
   a. low-density lipoprotein (LDL)
   b. high-density lipoprotein (HDL)
   c. both LDL and HDL
   d. none of the above

Get Critical

What happened:

At the age of 25, Lance Armstrong was already a top cyclist when he was diagnosed with testicular cancer. His cancer was in an advanced stage by the time it was caught, and had even spread to his brain. Armstrong searched the country for treatments, and through a combination of superior medical care, lifestyle changes, and spiritual resolve, managed to recover from his cancer. He went on to win seven Tour de France cycling championships, and founded the LiveStrong program, which helps promote cancer survival and awareness. To increase awareness of LiveStrong, the program uses distinctive yellow wristbands, which became an overnight sensation. Millions of the yellow bands have been distributed, and other health awareness causes now issue different colored bands as well. Some people say the wristbands help remind us all to live healthier lives, but others say their widespread use dilutes the message of health, turning it into little more than a fashion statement.

What do you think?

- Have you ever worn a LiveStrong wristband, or another band from a different health-related group? What about a ribbon, such as the pink ribbon for breast cancer awareness? If you have worn a band or ribbon, why?

- Do you think that wearing a band or ribbon helps wearers to live in a more healthy way? If so, how?

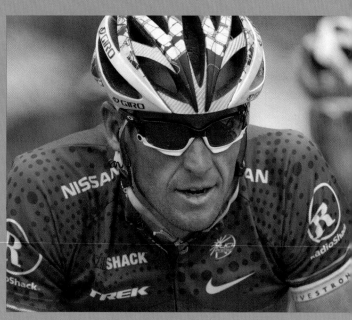

7. Which of the following behaviors can reduce your risk of developing a cardiovascular disease?
   a. eating nutritiously
   b. being physically active
   c. maintaining good oral hygiene
   d. all of the above

8. What is the term for a tumor that grows aggressively and is capable of spreading to other parts of the body?
   a. a benign tumor
   b. a malignant tumor
   c. a carcinogen
   d. an oncogene

9. Which of the following viruses has been linked to causing cancer?
   a. Hepatitis B
   b. HIV
   c. HPV
   d. all of the above

10. Which of the following is a true statement?
   a. Having multiple sexual partners can increase a woman's risk of cervical cancer.
   b. HPV infection can not cause cancer.
   c. Tanning is harmless.
   d. "Smokeless" chewing tobacco can not cause cancer.

Get Connected

Health Online Visit the following websites for further information about the topics in this chapter:

- American Diabetes Association
  www.diabetes.org
- American Heart Association
  www.americanheart.org
- National Cancer Institute
  www.cancer.gov

- American Cancer Society
  www.cancer.org
- My Family Health Portrait, a tool from the U.S. Surgeon General
  https://familyhistory.hhs.gov/fhh-web/home.action

Website links are subject to change. To access updated web links, please visit **www.pearsonhighered.com/choosinghealth.**

References

i. Centers for Disease Control and Prevention, National Center for Chronic Disease Prevention and Health Promotion. (2009). Diabetes: Successes and opportunities for population-based prevention and control. Retrieved from http://www.cdc.gov/nccdphp/publications/aag/pdf/diabetes.pdf

ii. American Heart Association. (2010). *Heart disease and stroke statistics, 2010 update.* Dallas, TX: American Heart Association.

iii. National Cancer Institute. (2010). *Skin cancer.* Retrieved from http://www.cancer.gov/cancertopics/types/skin

1. Centers for Disease Control and Prevention. (2008). State-specific incidence of diabetes among adults, participating states, 1995–1997 and 2005–2007. *Morbidity and Mortality Weekly Report, 57*(43), 1169–1173.

2. Heron, M., Hoyert, D., Xu, J., Scott, C., & Tejada-Vera, B. (2008). Deaths: Preliminary data for 2006. *Centers for Disease Control and Prevention, National Vital Statistics Reports, 56*(16), 1–52.

3. Centers for Disease Control and Prevention. (2009). *Chronic diseases and health promotion.* Retrieved from http://www.cdc.gov/chronicdisease/overview

4. Kung, H. C., Hoyert, D. L., Xu, J. Q., & Murphy, S. L. (2008). Deaths: Final data for 2005. *National Vital Statistics Reports, 56*(10). Retrieved from http://www.cdc.gov/nchs/data/nvsr/nvsr56/nvsr56_10.pdf

5. Kaiser Family Foundation. (2010). *U.S. health care costs.* Retrieved from http://www.kaiseredu.org/topics_im.asp?imID=1&parentID=61&id=358

6. Milken Institute. (2007). An unhealthy America: The economic burden of chronic disease. Retrieved from http://www.milkeninstitute.org/pdf/ES_ResearchFindings.pdf

7. Centers for Disease Control and Prevention. (2004). 2004 Surgeon General's report: The health consequences of smoking. Retrieved from http://www.cdc.gov/tobacco/data_statistics/sgr/2004/pdfs/executivesummary.pdf

8. Centers for Disease Control and Prevention. (2009). The power of prevention: Chronic disease... the public health challenge of the 21st century. Retrieved from http://www.cdc.gov/chronicdisease/pdf/2009-Power-of-Prevention.pdf

9. Centers for Disease Control and Prevention, National Center for Chronic Disease Prevention and Health Promotion. (2009). Diabetes: Successes and opportunities for population based prevention and control. Retrieved from http://www.cdc.gov/nccdphp/publications/aag/pdf/diabetes.pdf

10. National Diabetes Information Clearinghouse. (2008). National diabetes statistics, 2007. Retrieved from http://diabetes.niddk.nih.gov/dm/pubs/statistics

11. Cox, E., Halloran, D., Homan, S., Welliver, S., & Mager, D. (2008). Trends in the prevalence of chronic medication use in children: 2002–2005. *Pediatrics, 122*(5), 1053–1061.

12. National Diabetes Information Clearinghouse. (2006). What I need to know about gestational diabetes. Retrieved from http://diabetes.niddk.nih.gov/dm/pubs/gestational

13. Dean, L., & McEntrye, J. (2004). The genetic landscape of diabetes. Published online by the National Center for Biotechnology Information, National Library of Medicine. Retrieved from http://www.ncbi.nlm.nih.gov/bookshelf/br.fcgi?book=diabetes

14. National Diabetes Information Clearinghouse. (2008). Diabetes overview. Retrieved from http://diabetes.niddk.nih.gov/dm/pubs/overview

15. Narayan, K., Boyle, J., Thompson, T., Gregg, E., & Williamson, D. (2007). Effect of body mass index on lifetime risk for diabetes mellitus in the United States. *Diabetes Care, 30*(6), pgs. 1562-1566.

16. American Diabetes Association. (2010). Genetics of diabetes. Retrieved from http://www.diabetes.org/diabetes-basics/genetics-of-diabetes.html

17. National Diabetes Information Clearinghouse. (2008). Diabetes prevention program. Retrieved from http://diabetes.niddk.nih.gov/dm/pubs/preventionprogram

18. Fung, T., McCullough, M., van Dam, R., & Hu, F. (2007). A prospective study of overall diet quality and risk of type 2 diabetes in women. *Diabetes Care, 30,* 1753–1757.

19. Rodriguez, B. L., Fujimoto, W. Y., Mayer-Davis, E. J., Imperatore, G., Williams, D. E., Bell, R. A., . . . Linder, B. (2006, August). Prevalence of cardiovascular disease risk factors in U.S. children and adolescents with diabetes: The SEARCH for diabetes in youth study. *Diabetes Care, 29*(8), 1891–1896.

20. Green, J., Grant, M., Hill, K., Brizzolara, J., & Belmont, B. (2003). Heart disease risk perception in college men and women. *Journal of American College Health, 51*(5), 207–211.

21. Wendt, S. (2005). Perception of future risk of breast cancer and coronary heart disease in female undergraduates. *Psychology, Medicine & Health, 10*(3), 253–262.

22. Tzou, W., Douglas, P., Srinivasan, S., Bond, M., Tang, R., Chen, W., ... Stein, J. (2005). Increased subclinical atherosclerosis in young adults with metabolic syndrome: The Bogalusa heart study. *Journal of the American College of Cardiology, 46*(3), 457–463.

23. Cutler, J., Sorlie, P., Wolz, M., Thom, T., Fields, L., & Roccella, E. (2008). Trends in hypertension prevalence, awareness, treatment, and control rates in United States adults between 1988–1994 and 1999–2004.

Hypertension, 52(5), 818–827. Retrieved from http://hyper.ahajournals.org/cgi/content/abstract/HYPERTENSIONAHA.108.113357v1

24. Hansen, M., Gunn, P., & Kaebler, D. (2007). Underdiagnosis of hypertension in children and adolescents. *Journal of the American Medical Association, 298*(8), 874–879.

25. American Heart Association. (2010). Heart disease and stroke statistics, 2010 update. Dallas, TX: American Heart Association.

26. Hemingway, H., McCallum, A., Shipley, M., Manderbacka, K., Martikanen, P., & Keskimaki, I. (2008). Incidence and prognostic implications of stable angina pectoris among men and women. *Journal of the American Medical Association, 295*(12), 1404–1411.

27. American Heart Association. (2010). *Arrhythmia*. Retrieved from http://www.heart.org/HEARTORG/Conditions/Arrhythmia/Arrhythmia_UCM_002013_SubHomePage.jsp

28. Levy, D., Larson, M., Vasan, R., Kannel, W., & Ho, K. (1996). The progression from hypertension to congestive heart failure. *Journal of the American Medical Association, 275*(20), 1557–1562.

29. American Heart Association. (2010). *Types of stroke*. Retrieved from http://www.strokeassociation.org/presenter.jhtml?identifier=1014

30. American Heart Association. (2010). *If your child has a congenital heart defect – Our guide for parents*. Retrieved from http://www.americanheart.org/presenter.jhtml?identifier=3007586

31. American Heart Association. (2010). *Rheumatic heart disease / Rheumatic fever*. Retrieved from http://www.americanheart.org/presenter.jhtml?identifier=4709

32. Von Ah, D., Ebert, S., Ngamvitorj, A., Park, N., & Kang, D. (2004). Predictors of health behaviors in college students. *Journal of Advanced Nursing, 48*(5), 463–474.

33. Eiberg, S., Hasselstrom, H., Gronfeldt, V., Froberg, K., Cooper, A., & Andersen, L. (2005). Physical fitness as a predictor of cardiovascular disease risk factors in 6- to 7-year-old Danish children: The Copenhagen school-child intervention study. *Pediatric Exercise Science, 17,* 161–170.

34. Bazzano, L., He, J., Munter, P., Vupputuri, S., & Whelton, P. (2005). Relationship between cigarette smoking and novel risk factors for cardiovascular disease in the United States. *Annals of Internal Medicine, 138*(11), 891–898.

35. Jorgensen, R., & Maisto, S. (2008). Alcohol consumption and prehypertension: An investigation of university youth. *Behavioral Medicine, 34,* 21–26.

36. Javaheri, S., Storfer-Isser, A., Rosen, C., & Redline, S. (2008). Sleep quality and ele

vated blood pressure in adolescents. *Circulation, 188,* 1034–1040.

37. Genco, R., Offenbacher, S., & Beck, J. (2002). Periodontal disease and cardiovascular disease. *Journal of the American Dental Association, 133,* 14S–21S.

38. American Heart Association. (2008). *Risk factors and coronary heart disease and stroke*. Retrieved from http://216.185.112.5/presenter.jhtml?identifier=539.

39. American Cancer Society. (2010). *Cancer facts and figures 2010*. Atlanta, GA: American Cancer Society.

40. American Cancer Society. (2008). *Known and probable human carcinogens*. Retrieved from http://www.cancer.org/docroot/ped/content/ped_1_3x_known_and_probable_carcinogens.asp

41. National Cancer Institute. (2009). National Cancer Institute fact sheet: BRCA1 and BRCA2: Cancer risk and genetic testing. Retrieved from http://www.cancer.gov/cancertopics/factsheet/Risk/BRCA

42. D'Souza, G., Kreimer, A., Viscidi, R., Pawlita, M., Fakhry, C., Koch, W.,...Gillison M. (2007). Case-control study of human papilloma virus and oropharyngeal cancer. *New England Journal of Medicine, 356*(19), 1944–1956.

43. Hu, S., Arellano, M., Boontheung, P., Wang, J., Zhou, H., Jiang, J.,...Wong, D. (2008). Salivary proteomics for oral cancer b

iomarker discovery. *Clinical Cancer Research, 14*(19), 6246–6252.

44. National Cancer Institute. (2006). *What you need to know about cancer: Symptoms*. Retrieved from http://www.cancer.gov/cancertopics/wyntk/cancer/page6

45. The International Early Lung Cancer Action Program Investigators. (2006). Survival of patients with stage 1 lung cancer detected on CT screening. *New England Journal of Medicine, 355*(17), 1763–1771.

46. U.S. Environmental Protection Agency. (2010). A citizen's guide to radon. Retrieved from http://www.epa.gov/radon/pubs/citguide.html.

47. American Cancer Society. (2010). *Can breast cancer be prevented?* Retrieved from http://www.cancer.org/Cancer/BreastCancer/OverviewGuide/breast-cancer-overview-prevention

48. American Cancer Society. (2010). *How is breast cancer found?* Retrieved from http://www.cancer.org/Cancer/BreastCancer/OverviewGuide/breast-cancer-overview-diagnosed

49. American Cancer Society. (2006). *Cancer facts for women*. Retrieved from http://www.cancer.org/acs/groups/content/@healthpromotions/documents/document/acsq-020994.pdf

13

Consumer Health

- About 75% of Internet users have sought health information online.[i]

- More than 80% of U.S. adults are taking at least one medication.[ii]

- 70% of college students reported using an herbal or dietary supplement in a given week.[iii]

- An estimated 46 million people in the U.S. have no health insurance.[iv]

DESCRIBE different aspects of *self-care*.

KNOW when it's time to seek professional health care.

DISCUSS strategies for being a smart health-care consumer.

DESCRIBE the differences between *conventional medicine, complementary medicine,* and *alternative medicine.*

IDENTIFY multiple methods of paying for health care.

DISCUSS the genomic revolution and the future of personal health.

Health Online icons are found throughout the chapter, directing you to web links, videos, podcasts, and other useful online resources.

It's near the end of the semester, and you've been feeling physically run-down.

Things got worse this morning, when you woke up with a bad sore throat, a fever, and—most troubling—a skin rash. What should you do?

Maybe you'll go online and do a search on your symptoms to decide whether they are serious enough to seek professional help. You might take an over-the-counter medicine for the sore throat and fever, and ask a parent or friend for advice about the rash. If you decide to consult a doctor, things can quickly get complicated: Should you visit the student health center? What if there isn't one? Should you call your doctor at home? What if you don't have a regular physician? How will you pay for the health care? What if you don't have health insurance?

These are all examples of questions related to **consumer health.** In the United States today, we have more tools and options for taking care of our health than ever before. The Internet makes an unprecedented amount of health information available at our fingertips. We can purchase a wide range of over-the-counter drugs and medications. We can choose to seek care at a traditional hospital, at a drug store clinic, or at a campus health center. We can try alternative therapies like acupuncture or chiropractic, and select from a broad array of health-care professionals and insurance plans.

But this growing world of health choices also requires active and informed decision making. Increasingly, the burden is on you to research information, critically evaluate it, and make educated decisions that are best for you. You need to be a smarter health consumer than ever before. This chapter will help!

Self-Care

There are many things you can do on your own to stay healthy. As you've learned throughout this book, some of the most important health behaviors are preventive, aimed at promoting your overall wellness and reducing the likelihood that you will get sick in the first place. Maintaining basic wellness behaviors, learning how to critically evaluate health information (especially online), educating yourself about over-the-counter medications and supplements, using home health tests, and knowing when it's time to seek professional help are all examples of **self-care.**

Maintaining Basic Wellness Habits

Self-care begins with basic wellness behaviors such as eating nutritiously, exercising, and refraining from unhealthful behaviors like smoking or excessive drinking. Regularly brushing your teeth and flossing, making sure you get enough sleep, keeping your stress level under control, and maintaining good relationships with your friends and loved ones are additional aspects of self-care **(Figure 13.1).**

consumer health An umbrella term encompassing topics related to the purchase and consumption of health-related products and services.

self-care Actions you take to keep yourself healthy.

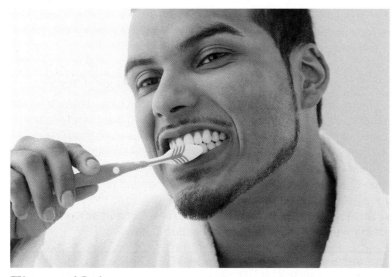

Figure 13.1 Self-care includes basic wellness habits such as regularly brushing your teeth.

Common-sense preventive behaviors—such as wearing a seat belt inside a car, or wearing a helmet while riding a bike—can protect you from serious injuries. Similarly, the simple act of washing your hands with soap and hot water can protect you from contracting infectious diseases.

Evaluating Health Information Online

About 75% of all U.S. adults and about 85% of college students use the Internet.[1] About 75% of Internet users have sought health information online[2], and in one survey of college students, more than 40% said they frequently used the Internet for this purpose.[3] Using the Internet as a health resource has become so common that some health professionals jokingly gripe that they've been replaced by "Dr. Google."

However, finding accurate, credible health information online requires work. As you learned in Chapter 1, online health information comes from a variety of sources, which can vary widely in credibility

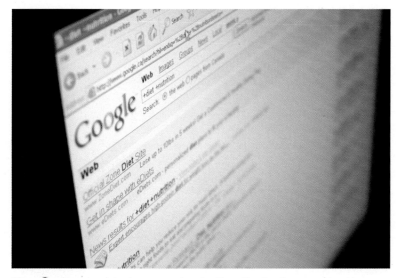

The **Internet** is increasingly the first place people turn for health information.

and scientific validity. Your search results may yield everything from detailed health information in an encyclopedic format to quick advice given by a stranger in an online chat or forum. The "authors" of this content may range from objective experts in their field to advertisers whose main purpose is to persuade you to buy. Most search engines produce a list of websites ranked according to popularity, not necessarily quality. As a result, it can be difficult to know what information to trust.

As you may recall, in Chapter 1, we introduced some basic strategies for evaluating online information (see Consumer Corner: Evaluating Health Information Online in Chapter 1.) In addition to those strategies, ask yourself whether or not the information you find is supported by **evidence-based medicine**—practices which are based on systematic, scientific study. Health topics featured online or in the news often cite scientific studies, but not all studies are equally reliable. To evaluate the validity and reliability of such studies, consider the following questions:

- Is the description of this research specific and detailed? Credible research claims should include who conducted the study and their credentials, the research institutions involved, the question the study was trying to answer, and the dates the research was conducted and/or published.
- Who published this research? Quality science is published in *peer-reviewed journals,* publications where experts screen and evaluate all submissions. Research findings are also sometimes presented at meetings of scientific societies.
- Who were the study participants? Was the research done on microbes, mice, or people? Studies conducted on people usually have the greatest medical validity.
- How many people participated? The larger the pool of participants, the more significant the results. Especially significant studies often involve tens of thousands of people over several years.
- What were the profiles of the participants? How similar were they to you? The results of a health study of breast cancer prevention in 10,000 post-menopausal women may not be relevant to you if you are a young woman in your 20s.
- Is the study the first of its kind? Scientific findings carry more weight if they have been replicated by other researchers.
- Do the people behind the study have any conflicts of interest? Credible studies disclose who paid for the research and whether the scientists involved have any financial or other interest in the outcome.

Credible health information sites highlight this type of information or make it relatively easy to find. If you have trouble finding answers to these types of questions when researching health information or products, think twice about the believability of the information you are viewing.

Evaluating Over-the-Counter Medications

In any given week, more than 80% of U.S. adults are taking at least one type of medication.[4] The most readily available are **over-the-counter (OTC) medications,** which do not require a doctor's pre-

evidence-based medicine Health-care policies and practices based on systematic, scientific study.

over-the-counter (OTC) medication A medication available for purchase without a prescription.

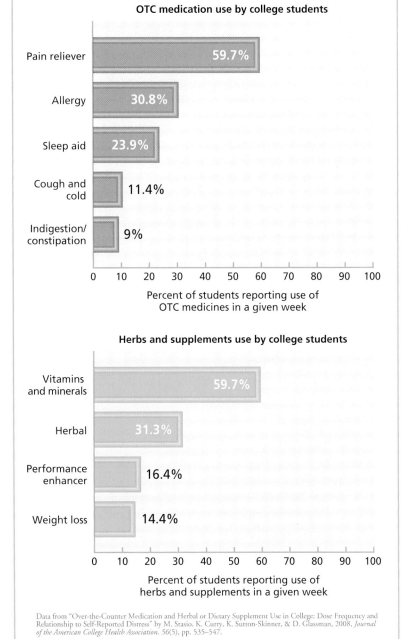

Top Over-the-Counter Medications and Supplements Used by Students

OTC medication use by college students

Medication	Percent
Pain reliever	59.7%
Allergy	30.8%
Sleep aid	23.9%
Cough and cold	11.4%
Indigestion/constipation	9%

Percent of students reporting use of OTC medicines in a given week

Herbs and supplements use by college students

Supplement	Percent
Vitamins and minerals	59.7%
Herbal	31.3%
Performance enhancer	16.4%
Weight loss	14.4%

Percent of students reporting use of herbs and supplements in a given week

Data from "Over-the-Counter Medication and Herbal or Dietary Supplement Use in College: Dose Frequency and Relationship to Self-Reported Distress" by M. Stasio, K. Curry, K. Sutton-Skinner, & D. Glassman, 2008, *Journal of the American College Health Association, 56*(5), pp. 535–547.

- can be adequately labeled.
- do not require consultation with health practitioners for safe and effective use of the product.[5]

About 74% of college students take at least one OTC drug a week, with pain relievers the most common.[6] (See the **Student Stats** box.)

Many OTC drugs are effective, and are often more affordable than prescription medications. One analysis showed that brand-name prescription drugs can cost more than 10 times more than OTC medications.[7] But even though they are widely available, OTC medications can still carry risks and side effects. It is important to read labels carefully, to not exceed the recommended dosage, to use the medications for their intended purposes, and to talk to your doctor or pharmacist if you have any questions. (See **Consumer Corner: Using an Over-the-Counter Medication Safely.**)

Medicines in My Home at **www.mimh-fda-gov.com** is an interactive presentation from the FDA with instruction on how to choose and use OTC medications safely.

Evaluating Herbal and Dietary Supplements

Do you regularly take herbal or vitamin dietary supplements? According to a survey of college students, about 70% used an herbal or dietary supplement in a given week.[6] Although supplements are popular, they are not without risk. Supplements are not legally regulated in the same ways as OTC or prescription medications, and research into the benefits of their use remains controversial and inconclusive.

Supplements are chemical compounds taken for a perceived health benefit **(Figure 13.2).** They are generally not administered by a doctor. Whereas government agencies require extensive evaluations of a prescription drug's safety and efficacy before it can be sold, supplements do not get this same screening. Federal laws bar supplement advertisements from making specific claims about supplement benefits that haven't been proven (supplement advertisements, for example, can not promise to cure a particular type

supplements Chemical compounds taken for a perceived health benefit.

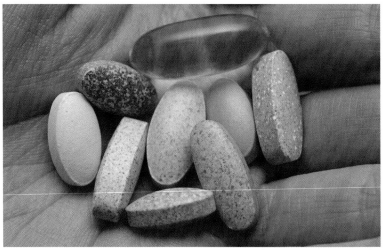

Figure 13.2 Supplements such as multivitamins are popular, but there is no scientific consensus on their health benefits.

scription. The federal Food and Drug Administration defines OTC medications as those that:

- have benefits outweighing their risks.
- have low potential for misuse.
- consumers can use for self-diagnosed conditions.

CONSUMER CORNER

Using an Over-the-Counter Medication Safely

A typical OTC medication label looks like this:

Drug Facts		
Active ingredient (in each tablet)		***Purpose***
Chlorpheniramine maleate 2 mg.......................................Antihistamine		
Uses temporarily relieves these symptoms due to hay fever or other upper respiratory allergies: ■ sneezing ■ runny nose ■ itchy, watery eyes ■ itchy throat		
Warnings Ask a doctor before use if you have ■ glaucoma ■ a breathing problem such as emphysema or chronic bronchitis ■ trouble urinating due to an enlarged prostate gland		
Ask a doctor or pharmacist before use if you are taking tranquilizers or sedatives		
When using this product ■ drowsiness may occur ■ avoid alcoholic drinks ■ alcohol, sedatives, and tranquilizers may increase drowsiness ■ be careful when driving a motor vehicle or operating machinery ■ excitability may occur, especially in children		
If pregnant or breast-feeding, ask a health professional before use. Keep out of reach of children. In case of overdose, get medical help or contact a Poison Control Center right away.		
Directions		
adults and children 12 years and over	take 2 tablets every 4 to 6 hours; not more then 12 tablets in 24 hours	
children 6 years to under 12 years	take 1 tablet every 4 to 6 hours; not more then 6 tablets in 24 hours	
children under 6 years	ask a doctor	
Other Information ■ store at 20–25°C (68–77°F) ■ protect from excessive moisture		
Inactive ingredients D&C yellow no. 10, lactose, magnesium stearate, microcrystalline cellulose, pregelatinized starch		

When you're using an OTC medication, be sure to read the label carefully and note:

- What is its active ingredient? Do you have any allergies to this ingredient? Are you taking any other medications that may interfere with or combine poorly with this ingredient?

- What is the medication's intended purpose or use? Are you using the medication properly?

- What are the warnings accompanying this medication? Could this medication be harmful to you?

- What are this medication's side effects? If it causes drowsiness or sleepiness, think twice before using

it before putting yourself in a situation where it is important to be alert (such as driving a car).

- What is the correct dosage? Keep in mind that dosage amounts can vary depending on age and other factors.

- How should the medication be safely stored? Improperly storing a medication may compromise its effectiveness.

In addition, look for an expiration date on the medication to be sure you are not purchasing or using a medication past its expiration date. Also, keep all medicines out of sight and reach of children.

Source for Drug Label: U.S. Department of Health and Human Services, The U.S. Food and Drug Administration. (2010). *The New Over-the-Counter Medicine Label: Take a Look.*

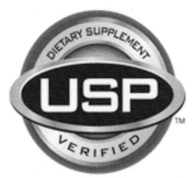

Figure 13.3 The "USP verified" symbol indicates that a product meets minimum safety and purity standards.

of cancer). But there are no regulations for the general claims these ads can make. You may commonly come across supplement advertisements featuring vague statements such as "Stay healthy!" or "Need more energy?" There may be no scientific research to back up such claims. Also, be aware that a supplement may tout itself as free of one risky ingredient, but that doesn't mean it is free of other harmful substances.

Before taking any dietary supplements, consider these guidelines:

- Talk with your doctor first—especially if you are currently taking any medications, are pregnant, are trying to become pregnant, or have any chronic medical conditions. Some supplements can be inappropriate or even harmful for certain populations. Factors such as your diet, age, sex, and health status can all affect whether or not a dietary supplement is appropriate for you.

- Look for the USP verification mark **(Figure 13.3).** This symbol on the label indicates that the product meets minimum safety and purity standards as set forth by U.S. Pharmacopeia, a non-profit organization.

- Choose brands made by nationally known manufacturers. These products likely have higher processing and production standards.

> **For additional tips on evaluating dietary supplements, visit the FDA's website at www.fda.gov/Food/DietarySupplements/default_htm.**

Taking Home Health Tests

Gone are the days when the only health-measuring instrument kept at home was a thermometer. Via drug stores and websites, we now have access to a wide range of medical tests that can be performed at home **(Figure 13.4).** Some of the most common include:

- Pregnancy tests
- Blood pressure tests
- Fertility tests
- Cholesterol tests
- Blood sugar tests
- Colon cancer risk tests
- HIV tests (*Note: If you think you may have been exposed to HIV, consider taking the test in a clinic or hospital setting where on-site counseling will be available. Taking this test at home is not ideal, as there will be no medical professional present to advise you in the event that you have a positive result.*)

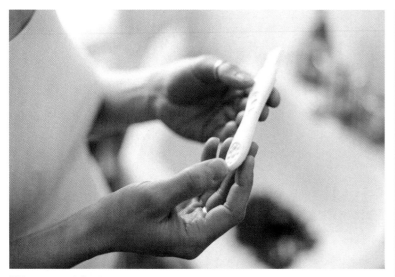

Figure 13.4 Home health tests are now available for everything from fertility testing to HIV detection.

Note that when you take any kind of home health test, it is very important to follow the test instructions precisely. Not doing so can result in erroneous results. Also keep in mind that any number of external factors can also cause test results to be inaccurate. For example, a pregnancy test may yield a "negative" result if the woman takes the test too early on in her pregnancy (before her body has manufactured detectable levels of the hormone that such tests are designed to look for). Drinking copious amounts of fluid or taking prescription medications may also interfere with the accuracy of some home health tests. If your test results indicate that you have a medical issue, consult a doctor immediately to confirm the results.

When to See a Doctor

Smart self-care includes knowing when it's time to seek professional help. Many of us only call a doctor when we are extremely sick. However, it's also important to schedule preventive checkups and exams.

Checkups and Preventive Care

By working with your health-care providers to get regular screenings and checkups, you can prevent problems or catch them early, when they are often far easier to treat. See **Table 13.1** for an overview of

Table 13.1: **Recommended Health Screenings**

Preventive Service	Who Needs It	How Often	Comments
Blood pressure measurement	All adults	Every 2 years for those with normal blood pressure	Those with elevated blood pressure need to be under medical care.
Cholesterol measurement	All adults	At least once every 5 years; more often if results indicate risk	
Pap smear	All women starting at age 18, or earlier if sexually active	At least every 2 years for younger women; check with your health-care provider	
Mammogram	All women age 40 and over; women with a strong family history of the disease may start screenings earlier	Every year	Other tests such as MRI may be suggested, depending on risk factors.
Colorectal cancer screening	Everyone age 50 and over; earlier for those at higher risk, such as those with a family history of the disease	Occult blood test annually; imaging test every 3–10 years on professional advice	
Prostate cancer screening	Men	Check with your doctor	
Thyroid disease screening	People over age 60, especially women, should discuss with their doctor	Check with your doctor	
General vision check	All adults	Every 2 years up to age 60; yearly thereafter	People at risk of vision damage or loss should consider starting yearly exams early in life
Glaucoma screening	People at high risk, including those over 65 who are very nearsighted or diabetic, African-Americans over age 40, and those with a family history of the disease	Talk with your vision care specialist	Many eye specialists advise screening all adults starting at age 40 or 50
Dental checkup	All adults	Check with your dentist	Suggest checkup every six months
Tetanus/diphtheria booster	All adults	Every 10 years	
Influenza vaccine	Everyone 65 and over; people at higher risk, such as those with chronic health conditions	Every year in autumn	
Pneumococcal vaccine	Everyone 65 and over; people at higher risk for complications	Every 5 years	
Rubella vaccine	All women of child-bearing age	Once	Avoid during pregnancy
Hepatitis B vaccine	All young adults, as well as adults at high risk	Check with your doctor	
Meningococcal vaccine (MCV4 or MPSV4)	Includes college freshmen living in a dorm; military recruits; people travelling to or residing in countries where the disease is common	At least once every 5 years, but more often if your results indicate risk	Of special concern to students living in high-density housing situations
Skin and mole exam	All adults	Check with your doctor	Can be done as part of a regular checkup

Data from **1.** "The Wellness Guide to Preventive Care," in *Foundations of Wellness* by the University of California at Berkeley, retrieved from http://www.wellnessletter.com/html/fw/fwL on11PreventiveCare.html. **2.** Vaccines and Preventable Diseases Meningococcal Disease—In Short; Centers for Disease Control and Prevention Vaccines and Immunizations, retrieved from html. **3.** *Recommended Eye Examination Frequency for Pediatric Patients and Adults* by the American Optometric Association, retrieved from http://www.aoa.org/x5502.xml.

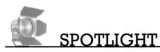
Should You Get Vaccinated?

By the time you are in college, you may think your days of needing vaccinations are behind you. Although it's true that most vaccines are administered during childhood, some are recommended for college-aged students and are worth considering. A few examples:

- If you live in a dorm or other high-density housing situation, consider obtaining a vaccine against *meningitis*, a very contagious illness that mimics symptoms of the flu and can be fatal. National vaccine guidelines call for all freshmen living in dorms to receive this vaccine, but if you are past your freshman year and still living in a dorm with no vaccine protection, talk to your doctor or student health center.

- If you haven't had a tetanus booster shot in the last 10 years, now is the time. Vaccine guidelines for adults call for getting a "booster shot" to protect your immunity once a decade. If you can't remember when you last received such a shot, check with your pediatrician's office. You can usually receive a tetanus booster from your student health center.

- A vaccine is available that protects against human papillomavirus (HPV), a virus that can cause genital warts and cervical cancer. This vaccine is most often recommended for females in their preteen or early teen years, before they become sexually active, but is also recommended for girls and women aged 13–26. An HPV vaccine is also available for males and can protect against genital warts.

- Federal health officials now recommend that everyone over the age of six months receive a flu shot. This is especially important for certain groups, including pregnant women, health-care workers, and people with chronic health conditions such as asthma.

For more information about vaccine recommendations for teenagers and college students, visit the Center for Disease Control's website at **www.cdc.gov/vaccines/ recs/schedules/teen-schedule.htm**.

---

general checkup and screening recommendations. Remember to schedule checkups for all aspects of your health, including oral health, vision, and vaccinations.

Health Problems Beyond Self-Care

Obviously, emergency situations require urgent care. Seek an emergency physician for yourself or someone else if any of the following situations arise:

- Severe injury, such as those sustained in a car accident
- Serious burns
- Sudden, severe pain anywhere
- Adverse reactions to a medication or insect bite
- Other severe allergic reactions
- Heavy bleeding
- Difficulty breathing
- Signs of a heart attack (for details, see Chapter 12)
- Signs of a stroke (for details, see Chapter 12)
- Sudden worsening of a chronic health condition, such as diabetes or asthma[8]

Keep in mind that the above list covers only some of the situations in which people need emergency care. Use your common sense in deciding when a situation requires urgent attention, and consult a health professional whenever you're not sure.

Outside of emergencies, it's not always easy to know when a medical condition warrants professional care. *The Merck Manual,* a reputable guide to common health issues, suggests seeking care if any of the follow situations arise:

- Vomiting or inability to keep fluids down, painful swallowing, coughing that lasts more than two or three weeks, earache, symptoms that last more than seven days
- Black or bloody stools, or more than six to eight watery stools in children (symptomatic of dehydration)
- A feeling that food is stuck in the throat, development of or change in heartburn, especially during exercise, frequent heartburn, persistent or severe abdominal pain, persistent nausea
- Symptoms that prevent participation in usual activities; unexplained weight loss; dizziness; persistent fatigue; sweating, especially heavy or cold sweats
- Severe headache that peaks in intensity within seconds; memory loss or confusion; blurred or double vision; slurred speech; loss of balance or dizziness; seizures; numbness in the arms, face, or legs; nausea
- Rapid or galloping heartbeats (palpitations); chest pain
- Pain in the calves that worsens when walking; swelling in the ankles or legs
- No periods by age 16; sudden stopping of periods; a period that lasts much longer than normal or is excessively heavy; a sudden feeling of illness while using tampons; severe cramps
- Fever of 100.4°F (38°C) or above; a rash that is painful, involves swelling, or oozes

- Swelling or redness in or around an eye; problems with vision
- Moderate or severe abdominal pain; symptoms of dehydration; green, black, or bloody vomit[8,9]

Conventional Medicine

Conventional medicine, also called *allopathic* or *Western medicine*, is the predominant type of care in the U.S. health system. Although conventional medicine includes many complex, fast-developing types of care, a few key features shape its foundation:

- The use of science and the *scientific method.* Evidence-based medicine, which you learned about earlier in this chapter, is just one example of how science underlies all aspects of conventional medicine.
- A focus on physical causes and symptoms. Conventional medicine looks for physical causes of illness, such as injuries or pathogens, and assumes that each illness leads to a set of discernable symptoms similar in most people who suffer from that condition.
- An emphasis on physical exams and treatments. Conventional medicine often relies on physical exams, such as X-rays or blood tests, and physical interventions, such as drugs or surgery, to treat the physical causes of disease.
- A focus on public health. By controlling the spread of the microscopic physical causes of disease through programs such as improved sanitation and vaccination, conventional medicine has vastly improved health and life expectancy in the last century.

Practicing conventional medicine requires many years of education and training and a professional license. Some of the most common types of practitioners of conventional medicine include:

- **Medical doctors,** or M.D.s, who can either serve as *general practitioners* or *specialists* who focus on a particular type of care.
- **Physician Assistants,** or physician associates (P.A.s), are licensed health professionals who practice under the supervision of a physician and provide a broad range of care.
- **Dentists,** who hold either doctor of dental surgery (D.D.S.) or doctor of medical dentistry (D.D.M.) degrees and specialize in care of the teeth, gums, and mouth.
- **Optometrists,** or O.D.s, who examine the eyes and provide vision care.
- **Podiatrists,** or D.P.M.s, who specialize in care of and surgery for the feet.
- **Nurses,** who may hold an R.N. or other degrees, provide a wide range of health services in many types of health-care settings. They often provide detailed or extensive care in times of greater medical need, such as when a patient is recovering from surgery in the hospital.

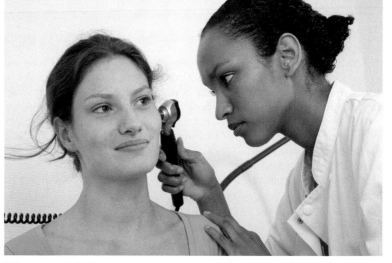

Figure 13.5 Nurse practitioners are an example of conventional health-care providers.

conventional medicine Commonly called Western medicine, this system of care is based on the principles of the scientific method; the belief that diseases are caused by identifiable physical factors and have a characteristic set of symptoms; and the treatment of physical causes through drugs, surgery, or other physical interventions.

medical doctor A physician trained in conventional medicine, with many years of additional formal education and training and a professional license.

physician assistant (P.A.) A licensed health professional who practices under the supervision of a physician and provides a broad range of care.

dentist A conventional medicine practitioner who specializes in care of the teeth, gums, and mouth.

optometrist A licensed professional who provides vision care.

podiatrist A licensed professional who specializes in the care of the feet.

nurse A licensed professional who provides a wide range of health-care services and supports the work of medical doctors.

nurse practitioner Registered nurses who have undergone additional training and can perform some of the care provided by a medical doctor.

- **Nurse practitioners,** R.N.s who have undergone additional training and can perform some of the duties and provide some of the care of a medical doctor **(Figure 13.5).**

Where to Find Conventional Health Care

Conventional medicine was once offered primarily through doctor's offices and hospitals, but its availability has since expanded to better meet the needs of patients. The following are examples of facilities that offer conventional care:

- **Student health centers** serve students on university campuses, and are staffed by doctors, nurses, and nurse practitioners. Some focus on basic primary care and student health needs, such as minor illnesses and contraception. Others feature a wider range of care, including substance abuse counseling, vision care, pharmacy, and dental services. Few offer emergency services. If a center doesn't offer a particular type of care, staff will usually provide referrals to off-campus care providers. On most campuses, student health centers are available to all enrolled students and most of the costs are covered by fees paid as part of student enrollment.
- **Primary care facilities** are the backbone of the health-care system. Staffed by doctors, nurses, nurse practitioners, and medical assistants, primary care centers meet everyday medical needs, seeing patients for checkups, screenings, and minor ailments and providing referrals to more specialized care if needed. Costs are often covered by patient health insurance or a combination of insurance and patient payments.

- **Nonprofit clinics** provide primary care for free or at a reduced cost. Staffed mostly by nurse practitioners and doctors, they often focus on underserved communities and groups who would otherwise have little access to primary care.
- **Corporate wellness centers,** usually staffed by doctors and/or nurses and nurse practitioners, provide care to corporate employees. A few offer a full range of services, but most focus on efforts to help employees live more healthfully by offering programs such as smoking cessation, fitness, or weight loss.
- **Retail clinics,** also known as convenient care clinics or drug store clinics, operate out of large stores and pharmacies **(Figure 13.6).** Usually staffed by nurse practitioners and doctors, these clinics are designed to provide basic primary care, such as screenings and treatment of minor ailments, in a timely manner for people who either don't have a primary care doctor, can't wait for an appointment at a primary care facility, and/or lack health insurance. Costs are lower than they would be at most traditional doctor's offices, and are often paid directly by the patient or through insurance.
- **Urgent care centers,** usually staffed by doctors and nurses, typically see patients with illnesses that need immediate attention but don't require the full resources of an emergency room. These centers often see many patients on evenings and weekends, when primary care centers are closed. Though not as expensive as emergency rooms, urgent care centers often charge a premium for their services, which can either be covered by insurance or paid directly by the patient.
- **Specialists centers,** usually staffed by doctors, nurses, and nurse practitioners, focus on specific categories of medicine, such as obstetrics, cardiac care, or cancer. Most patients access specialists through referrals from a primary care center. Specialty care is an important part of the medical system, but can be quite costly to patients if not covered by insurance.
- **Hospitals,** staffed by doctors, nurses, specialists, and many other types of health professionals, provide the highest level of care.

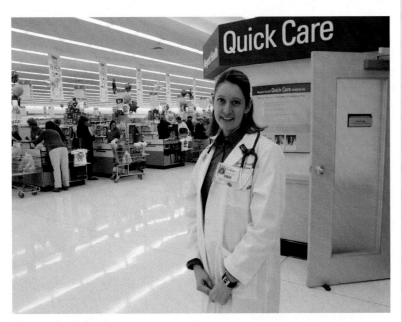

Figure 13.6 Health services are sometimes offered through large retail stores.

Hospitals handle everything from emergencies to surgeries to complex screenings and cancer treatment. Patients can be seen on an *out-patient* basis, in which they visit the hospital but don't stay overnight, or on an *in-patient* basis, where care is provided for an extended period of time and overnight stays are included.

Choosing a Doctor

If you are the age of a traditional college student, you probably haven't had much say in the past over who served as your doctor. Your family probably chose your pediatrician when you were younger, and if you attend your campus health center now, you probably see the first provider with an available appointment.

But at some point, most of us need to choose a physician of our own. This often starts with choosing a primary care doctor, who serves as your everyday contact with the health system. Your primary doctor will see you for checkups and most screenings, answer your basic health questions, treat minor ailments, write prescriptions, and provide referrals for more complex health concerns. Since your primary care doctor will also provide most of your preventive care, it's important to find one before you get sick.

To get started, check two resources—your insurance plan and your friends and family. If your health insurance limits the doctors you can see, start with doctors from the plan's list. Then ask your friends and family for their recommendations.

Once you have a list of doctors to contact, start by calling their offices and ask a few questions of a nurse or other office staff:

- Is this doctor accepting new patients? Some doctors have a full roster and can't take any more patients into their practice.

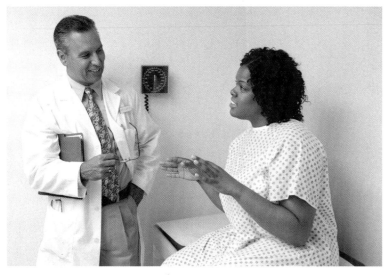

Ask your doctor **questions** to be sure you understand your care needs.

- What insurance plans does this office accept?
- Is this doctor *board-certified,* meaning that he or she has undergone extra training after medical school to specialize in an area such as family practice?
- How does the office handle lab work? Is there a lab in-house or nearby, or will you have to travel to a different location for a procedure such as a blood test?
- Is this a group practice? If so, will you mostly see your doctor, or all the doctors in the group? If so, how many of them are there and what are their specialties?
- Who will care for you if your doctor is unavailable?
- Is this medical practice affiliated with any particular hospitals or specialty centers?
- Does this practice offer newer methods of contacting a doctor, such as email?

When you meet your doctor in person, make sure that he or she listens to you, encourages you to ask questions, answers your questions completely, and treats you with respect. If you don't feel comfortable with a doctor, shop around until you do.

Being a Smart Patient

Once you've chosen a doctor, your visits will be more productive if you think of your doctor as a partner. He or she has the expertise to help you improve your health, but his or her work will be more effective if you are actively and constructively engaged in the process. Here are some suggestions from the American Academy of Family Physicians, a leading group representing primary care doctors, for how to get the most out of a doctor's appointment:

- *Talk* to your doctor. Be sure to tell your doctor any past or current health issues or concerns, even if they are embarrassing. Many medical appointments are only 15 minutes long, so effective communication is key to letting your doctor treat you.

- **Ask questions.** Let your doctor know if you don't understand something. If you need more time to discuss an issue, be vocal about it. If your appointment ends before all your questions have been answered, you can follow up with someone else in the office or schedule another appointment to discuss the issue further.
- **Take information home with you.** Take notes during your appointment, ask your doctor for handouts, or ask the office to supply background or reference materials.
- **Follow up with your doctor.** Follow the instructions you receive, such as getting additional tests or seeing a specialist. If you've been given a new medication and feel worse or have problems with the drug, let your doctor know right away. If you took a test and haven't received the results, let your doctor's office know.
- **Prevent medical errors through active communication.** Let your doctor know all the medicines, supplements, and other substances you may be taking (including alcohol) to help prevent risky drug interactions. Be proactive about sharing information with all members of your medical team, especially if you have more than one caregiver. Make sure you understand the side effects of any medication you are prescribed. If you are being discharged from care, make sure you understand any follow-up treatments to be done at home.[10]

Complementary and Alternative Medicine (CAM)

Conventional medicine can be very effective, but it has its limits. Conventional medicine's focus on physical ailments after they arise may sometimes overlook preventive steps and care that could have warded off illness. Some people are uncomfortable with the way that conventional medicine often treats normal parts of life, such as childbirth or death in old age, as problems that require heavy medical management. Others are interested in health practices that take a broader, more holistic approach, looking beyond the body to include the mind and spirit as well.

These interests have led to the growth of **complementary and alternative medicine (CAM).** The term *alternative medicine* is used to refer to those practices and traditions not typically part of conventional Western medicine, including everything from herbal remedies and meditation to chiropractors and traditional Chinese medicine. *Complementary medicine*, also sometimes referred to as *integrative medicine*, refers to care combining conventional and alternative medicine. Many of us routinely practice complementary medicine without realizing it, perhaps trying an herbal remedy to treat a cold but seeing a traditional doctor for a serious injury.

Alternative medicine has become such a common part of our approach to health that federal health officials now discuss and study it in a scientific way, and many states now require some CAM practitioners to be licensed. The National Center for Complementary and Alternative Medicine (NCCAM) groups CAM into five major domains:

- **Whole medical systems** are built on theories and systems encompassing the totality of a person's health. These systems have typically evolved apart from and earlier than conventional Western

complementary and alternative medicine (CAM) Health practices and traditions not typically part of conventional Western medicine, either used alone (alternative medicine) or in conjunction with conventional medicine (complementary medicine).

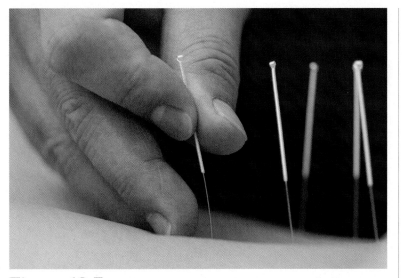

Figure 13.7 Acupuncture, a type of traditional Chinese medicine, is an example of alternative health care.

medicine. Traditional Chinese medicine is a prime example **(Figure 13.7).**

- **Mind-body medicine** uses techniques designed to boost the mind's capacity to affect the body. Some of these techniques are now considered part of Western medicine, such as patient support groups. Others, such as prayer or meditation, are still considered CAM.
- **Biologically based practices** rely on substances found in nature, such as vitamins and herbs.
- **Manipulative and body-based practices** are based on physical manipulation of the body, and typically involve therapies such as chiropractic medicine or massage.
- **Energy therapies** involve interaction with energy fields. These include biofield therapies, believed by practitioners to surround the body, and bio-electromagnetic-based therapies involving the alternative use of electromagnetic fields.[11]

For a more detailed look at some of the better-known CAM practices, please see **Table 13.2** on page 314.

Evaluating Complementary and Alternative Therapies

As you can see in Table 13.2, the effectiveness of many CAM therapies is still being studied, and research is inconclusive for many of these practices. If you are considering a CAM therapy, either on your own or through a practitioner, NCCAM offers the following suggestions:

- Take charge of your health by being an informed consumer. Find out what the scientific evidence is about any therapy's safety and effectiveness.
- Be aware that individuals respond differently to treatments, whether conventional or CAM. How a person might respond to a CAM therapy depends on many things, including the person's state of health, how the therapy is used, or the person's belief in the therapy.
- Keep in mind that "natural" does not necessarily mean "safe." (Think of mushrooms that grow in the wild: some are safe to eat, while others are not.)

- Learn about factors that affect safety. For a CAM therapy that is administered by a practitioner, these factors include the training, skill, and experience of the practitioner. For a CAM product such as a dietary supplement, the specific ingredients and the quality of the manufacturing process are important factors.
- Tell all your health-care providers about any complementary and alternative practices you use. Give them a full picture of what you do to manage your health. This will help ensure coordinated and safe care.[12]

If you are considering using a CAM practitioner, the following guidelines, adapted from NCCAM, may help:

- Speak with your primary health-care provider(s) regarding the therapy in which you are interested. Ask if they have a recommendation for the type of CAM practitioner you are seeking.
- Make a list of CAM practitioners and gather information about each before making your first visit. Ask basic questions about their credentials and practice. Where did they receive their training? What licenses or certifications do they have? How much will the treatment cost? How many treatments will be required to derive a benefit?
- Check with your insurer to see if the cost of therapy will be covered.
- After you select a practitioner, make a list of questions to ask at your first visit.
- Come to the first visit prepared to answer questions about your health history, including injuries, surgeries, and major illnesses, as well as prescription medicines, vitamins, and other supplements you may take.
- Assess your first visit and decide whether the practitioner is right for you. Did you feel comfortable with the practitioner? Could the practitioner answer your questions? Did he or she respond to you in a way that satisfied you? Does the treatment plan seem reasonable and acceptable to you?[13]

Paying for Health Care

In the United States, we are surrounded by highly advanced medical care—but this benefit comes at a steep price. Our system is the most expensive in the world, spending more per person than any other country and spending the most on health as a percentage of gross domestic product.[14] According to the nonprofit National Coalition on Health Care, total health spending reached $2.4 trillion in 2007, or almost $8,000 per person, and costs continue to rise each year.

As a student, you may be not be accustomed to thinking about how your health care is paid for. When you were younger, your family or caregivers probably covered the cost of your care, either through their health insurance or by paying directly out of their own pockets. Now that you are in college, you likely have access to basic care through your student health center, with costs covered by fees you pay as part of student enrollment. You may still be on your family's insurance plan, or your campus may offer a free or low-cost health insurance plan for students. According to one federal study released in 2008, about 80% of college students had some type of health insurance.[15]

But though you may have the luxury of paying little attention to your health-care costs now, it's still worth learning about your options. Once you leave your parents' health insurance plan (assuming

Table 13.2: Common Types of Complementary and Alternative Medicine

Practice	Description	Common Use	Risks	Scientific Evaluation
Acupuncture	This ancient system revolves around the concept of the free flow of qi (pronounced chee), or energy, through the body. Illness is believed to occur when qi is blocked or disrupted. Practitioners restore and rebalance qi not only to treat illness but prevent it and increase overall energy.	Thin needles are inserted at key qi points in the body to balance or restore energy flow. A related technique, acupressure, uses firm touch at key energy points. In addition to being a common part of overall traditional Chinese care, acupuncture has also been used in Western settings for everything from pain relief to reducing nausea during cancer treatment.	Acupuncture appears to have relatively few side effects, although problems can arise when needles are not used or sterilized correctly.	Acupuncture appears to be effective in treating chronic pain, in treating women's health disorders such as PMS or painful periods, and in easing side effects of cancer care.[1]
Homeopathy	Homeopathy is based on the assumption that "like cures like." That is, a substance that produces symptoms or illness is thought to cure or alleviate symptoms of that same illness, if administered in very diluted quantities.	Homeopathy is used in an attempt to treat common health problems such as nausea, sinus infections, and fever.	Given the very diluted levels at which homeopathic substances are usually used, few side effects have been reported.	A large analysis of more than 100 homeopathy studies found that the practice offered no significant effect.[2]
Naturopathy	Naturopathy incorporates traditional therapies and techniques from all over the world, from herbs to dietary changes and exercise, with an emphasis on supporting health rather than treating disease.	Naturopathy is especially popular with some people interested in an overall health approach that promotes wellness and prevents illness.	Some treatments, such as herbs, can have drug interactions and other side effects.	According to NCCAM, scientific studies of the effectiveness of naturopathy are still preliminary.[3]
Ayurveda	One of the world's oldest medical systems, Ayurveda originated in India. It aims to integrate and balance the body, mind, and spirit to help prevent illness and promote wellness.	Ayurvedic medicine uses a variety of products and techniques to cleanse the body and restore balance. People who use Ayurveda, either on its own or in conjunction with conventional medicine, often choose it in the belief that it will help cleanse their body of harmful substances and energies and help restore vitality and overall health.	Some of the herbal and dietary substances, along with other practices meant to cleanse the digestive tract, can have drug interactions if used with conventional medicine, as well as other side effects. One NCCAM study of Ayurvedic medications found that some contained toxins such as mercury or lead.[4]	According to NCCAM, scientific studies of the effectiveness of Ayurveda are still preliminary and more research is needed.[4]
Biologically based practices	These practices focus on using herbs, other plant-derived medicines called *botanicals*, and dietary supplements to treat various conditions.	Botanicals, herbs, and supplements are used in an attempt to treat conditions ranging from the common cold to serious conditions such as depression and cancer. *Echinacea*, or coneflower, for example, is popularly used to treat colds and upper respiratory infections.	This group of alternative therapies is among the most risky, as these substances have the potential for harm if taken in high doses or for long periods of time, or if they interact badly with conventional drugs. For example, one botanical, *ephedra*, is now banned in the United States because of its harmful side effects.	Studies have found that these therapies have limited usefulness at best. But researchers also caution that most such studies are still preliminary and more research is needed.[5]
Mind-body medicine	Mind-body medicines rely on the connection between the mental and physical realms and seek to create a more positive interaction between the two. Guided imagery, yoga, and meditation are popular forms of mind-body medicine.	Mind-body techniques are used to help prevent illness by reducing factors such as stress, and to help treat disorders such as depression, anxiety, and insomnia. These therapies are also sometimes used to support cancer patients by reducing patient anxiety, isolation, and stress.	Most mind-body therapies are considered relatively safe, although more strenuous forms, such as very active yoga, carry some risk of injury.	Some studies show some benefit, but most scientists caution that that research is still preliminary. One study of the efficacy of meditation as a treatment for a variety of illnesses found some benefit, but cautioned that more research remains to be done.[6]
Manipulative therapies	Remedies that focus on moving, stretching, or realigning sections of the body. These therapies focus on restoring overall wellness by correcting parts of the body that are out of alignment.	These techniques are often used to treat stiffness and pain. Chiropractic medicine, which focuses on structure and connections of joints and muscles, is an especially popular form.	Any intense physical manipulation of the body, especially of the spine, can be very dangerous, especially if a practitioner lacks training.	When administered correctly, chiropractic medicine has been shown to be effective for joint and bone pain, such as low back pain.[7]
Energy therapies	These forms of treatment focus on fields of energy originating within the body (biofields) or from external sources (electromagnetic fields). Changing or increasing the flow of the fields of energy, practitioners say, can have a variety of health benefits. Qigong, a movement-based component of traditional Chinese medicine, and magnet therapy are examples of energy treatments.	Energy fields are used for a variety of reasons, including stress reduction, pain relief, and improvement of cardiac health.	Risks appear to be relatively minor.	Most of the research done to date is either preliminary or inconclusive. One large analysis of the efficacy of qigong in reducing high blood pressure, for example, found some encouraging evidence, but cautioned that further study is needed.[8]

References: **1.** "The Status and Future of Acupuncture Clinical Research," by J. Park, K. Linde, E. Manheimer, A. Molsberger, K. Sherman, C. Smith, J. Sung, A. Vickers, R. Schnyer. *The Journal of Complementary and Alternative Medicine, 14*(7), pp. 871–881. **2.** "Are the Clinical Effects of Homeopathy Placebo Effects? Comparative Study of Placebo-Controlled Trials of Homoeopathy and Allopathy," by A. Shang, K. Huwiler-Müntener, L. Nartey, P. Juni, S. Dörig, J. Sterne, D. Pewsner, M. Egger, *Lancet, 366,* pp. 726–732. **3.** *Backgrounder: An Introduction to Naturopathy* by the National Center for Complementary and Alternative Medicine, retrieved from http://nccam.nih.gov/health/naturopathy, May 2009. **4.** *Backgrounder: Ayurvedic Medicine: An Introduction* by the National Center for Complementary and Alternative Medicine, retrieved from http://nccam.nih.gov/health/ayurveda/introduction.htm, May 2009. **5.** *Backgrounder: Herbs at a Glance* by the National Center for Complementary and Alternative Medicine, retrieved from http://nccam.nih.gov/health/herbsataglance.htm, May 2009. **6.** "Systematic Review of the Efficacy of Meditation Techniques as Treatments for Mental Illness" by A. Arias, K. Steinberg, A. Banga & R. Trestman. 2006, *The Journal of Alternative and Complementary Medicine, 12*(8), pp. 817–832. **7.** "Diagnosis and Treatment of Low Back Pain: A Joint Clinical Practice Guideline from the American College of Physicians and the American Pain Society" by R. Chou, A. Qaseem, V. Snow, D. Casey, J. Cross, P. Shekelle, D. Owens, and for the Clinical Efficacy Assessment Subcommittee of the American College of Physicians and the American College of Physicians/American Pain Society Low Back Pain Guidelines Panel 2007, *Annals of Internal Medicine, 147,* pp. 478–491. **8.** "Qigong for Hypertension: A Systematic Review of Randomized Clinical Trials" by M. Lee, R. Pittler, M. Guo, & E. Ernst. 2007, *Journal of Hypertension, 25*(8). pp. 1525–1532.

you are on one to begin with), you'll likely find that **health insurance** options that were available to your parents are less likely for you. A growing number of employers don't offer health insurance, provide very limited plans, or make employees pick up a hefty share of the tab. If you work for yourself as a freelancer or contractor, or find yourself between jobs, you'll have to find your own health insurance or pay for your health care yourself. Many insurance companies now offer individual insurance plans targeted to younger customers, but these plans might not cover all the services you'd expect. As the cost of health care continues to rise, most people in the U.S. find they are having to cover more of it out of their own pockets.

We'll start with an overview of the ways that people commonly pay for health care, and then look at some options for getting the best care you can afford, both now and when you graduate.

Discount Programs

Does your student health center cover the cost of your prescriptions? If not, does it offer a program with nearby pharmacies that lets you fill your prescriptions at a reduced price? If so, you are taking part in a **health discount program.** These programs are increasingly offered by employers and large institutions that want to provide some level of assistance with medical costs but don't want to pay for full insurance. Discount programs typically offer prices anywhere from 5 to 25% lower than average, although some programs for students may provide deeper discounts. Some large employers with high numbers of low-paid workers offer little traditional health insurance, instead presenting these employees with a series of discount programs at local retail clinics and pharmacies.

Health Insurance

At its essence, health insurance is your shield against medical costs. You may think you don't need such a safeguard—especially if you are young and currently healthy. But even if you don't get sick often, a sudden illness or an accident could leave you visiting the hospital and facing thousands of dollars in medical bills. Having a basic understanding of health insurance options can save you stress and money down the road.

A health insurance policy is a contract between an insurance company and an individual or group, in which the insurer agrees to cover a defined set of medical costs if the insured party pays a defined price, or *premium*. Insurers either pay your health-care providers directly, or reimburse you for covered health-care expenses. Some experts joke that health insurance is more accurately referred to as "halfway-health insurance," because almost all plans limit the types of care covered. While many plans cover primary

---

health insurance A contract between an insurance company and a group or individual who pays a fee to have some or all health costs covered by the insurer.

health discount program A system of health discounts given to members of groups, such as employees of a particular company or students attending a particular college.

pre-existing condition A health issue that existed prior to application to or enrollment in an insurance plan, which insurers sometimes use to restrict care or set the price paid for insurance.

managed-care plan A type of health insurance in which the insurer contracts with a defined group of health providers, which the consumer must use or face higher out-of-pocket costs.

health maintenance organization (HMO) A type of managed care in which most health care is funneled through and must be approved by the primary care doctor.

preferred provider organization (PPO) A type of managed care in which the consumer is encouraged to stay within an approved network of providers but has more choice over whom is seen when.

point-of-service (POS) plan A type of managed care that lets HMO consumers see a broader list of providers for an additional fee.

mini-med plan A type of managed-care plan, sold individually to younger people, which carries lower costs but does not cover many services.

---

care, for example, they may offer little or no coverage for services such as mental health services, substance abuse programs, or physical therapy. Alternative medicine is rarely covered. Many plans also restrict which doctors you can see and may place rules on seeing specialists. A few plans may refuse or limit your coverage if you already have an illness, or a **pre-existing condition** (although children with pre-existing medical issues now have greater protections against insurance discrimination, some plans still limit coverage of pre-existing conditions for adults).

Insurance plans come in many forms. Some are created for groups, such as collections of people who work at the same company. Others are created for individuals who buy their insurance straight from an insurance company. Common types of policies available to individuals and groups include *managed-care plans, public programs*, and *fee-for-service plans*.

Managed-Care Plans

Managed-care plans offer you lower costs, but also less choice. In a managed-care plan, insurers have contracts with particular doctors, hospitals, and other health-care providers, and you must often limit your visits to these caregivers or face additional expense. Most people with employer-based insurance are in one of three types of managed-care plans. **HMOs, or health maintenance organizations,** restrict choice the most but also usually cost the consumer the least, requiring that all care be funneled through and managed by the primary care doctor. **PPOs, or preferred provider organizations,** offer more choice by letting the consumer see a wider range of providers without a referral, but also usually carry a higher cost to the consumer. **POSs, or point-of-service plans,** offer some HMO members greater flexibility by letting them see outside physicians for an additional fee.

Managed-care plans can also be purchased on the individual insurance market. But this coverage can be expensive, sometimes costing thousands of dollars a year. To reduce monthly premiums, some consumers opt for *high-deductible* or *catastrophic* plans, which carry lower fees up front but only provide coverage after a person has paid for a certain amount of medical expenses out-of-pocket. In addition, many insurers have started offering a special version to younger people who may be out of college and find themselves without health insurance. These so-called **mini-med plans** often come at a more affordable monthly price than other types of individual coverage and pay for some health basics, such as primary care and trips to the emergency room. But they often don't cover other types of care, such as prenatal care and childbirth. If you are considering a mini-med plan, make sure you understand what the plan doesn't cover and see whether its limits fit your life for the next few years before you buy.

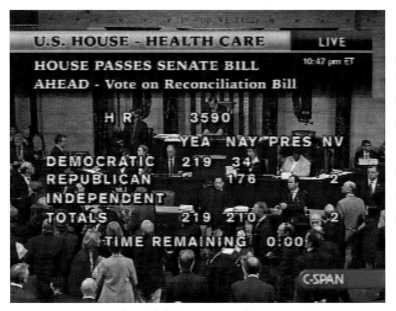

The passage of **health-care reform** in 2010 was a historical and controversial event.

Public Programs

Public programs provide government-sponsored insurance for individuals and families who could otherwise not afford health coverage. These plans usually operate in a way similar to managed care, funneling services through primary care clinics whenever possible. Common types of public insurance include **Medicaid,** usually offered to low-income individuals and families through joint state-federal sponsorship; **Medicare,** a federal program that covers many health costs for all Americans who have certain disabilities or are 65 or older; and state and local children's health programs.

Fee-for-Service Plans

Fee-for-service plans allow you to use any medical provider you choose, and then submit a bill to your insurance company, which pays part of it, leaving you to cover the rest. These plans, once more common, have become less popular as health-care costs have climbed.

Under the federal health insurance reforms passed in 2010, people who are ill and can not find insurance will be able to purchase coverage through a national "high risk pool," a program designed to provide coverage for those who are difficult to insure. Beginning in 2014, states will also create "health exchanges," in which people who don't have insurance can shop for policies at competitive rates. See the special feature, **What Health-Care Reform Means for You.**

Health Savings Accounts and Flexible Spending Accounts

Employers sometimes offer the option to create special savings accounts to help you maximize your health dollars. Two of the most common are **health savings accounts, or HSAs,** and medical **flexible spending accounts, or FSAs.**

HSAs come attached to a health insurance plan, and that plan carries a high **deductible,** or an amount that you must pay out of your HSA before your insurer will cover most health costs. HSA funds can be used to cover medical expenses that are approved by the federal government, such as medical visits and prescriptions costs. By law, HSA deductibles must be at least $1,150 for an individual or $2,300 for a family. In some cases, employers help cover some or all of the deductible. In others, they do not, and a person makes pre-tax contributions to the HSA to save the money necessary to cover the deductible (pre-tax contributions, taken from a person's paycheck before taxes are deducted, help consumers reduce their costs). An estimated 4.5 million people in the U.S. use this form of savings-related health coverage.[16] While backers of this approach say it gives consumers more control and could help lower health-care costs, critics counter that the high deductibles make this option an unaffordable choice for many in this country.[17] One study found that participants in such high-deductible plans were more likely to forego medical care to save money—a decision that may lower health-care costs in the short-term but drive them up later when a person's health suffers.[18]

FSAs, also offered through employers, allow employees to save pre-tax dollars to cover certain medical and health expenses. Unlike an HSA, FSAs do not come attached to an insurance plan. To withdraw money from your FSA to pay for health-related expenses, you must show receipts to prove that you spent the funds for allowed medical or health purposes.

Students and Health Insurance

Most college students have some form of health insurance. But the ways students are insured varies widely. Meanwhile, a significant percentage—about 20%, or 1.7 million students—remain uninsured, according to a federal analysis.[15] The same analysis reveals that:

- About 67% of students have insurance through a family member's employer. This means that someone in the family, most likely a parent, has insurance through work and includes the student in that coverage. While this type of coverage is common, it can also have drawbacks. If your policy requires that you use health providers in your home town, you may be without some types of care if your school is located elsewhere (although your student health center can fill in some of the gaps).

  Under health insurance reforms passed in 2010, a young person can stay on a parent's insurance policy until age 26. This change is likely to benefit many students. In the past, many policies stopped covering dependents when they reached their early 20s, at which age many students became uninsured.

- About 7% of students have insurance through another type of commercial policy, such as a student insurance plan offered by a college or

Medicaid A joint federal-state public insurance program that covers low-income individuals and families.

Medicare A federal public insurance program that covers people with long-term disabilities and anyone 65 or older.

fee-for-service plan A type of health insurance in which you choose your providers, and you and your insurer divide the costs of care.

health savings account (HSA) A consumer-controlled account that comes attached to a high-deductible health insurance plan and covers the costs of the deductible and other health-related expense approved by the federal government.

flexible spending account (FSA) A consumer-controlled account, usually offered through employers, that uses pre-tax dollars to cover approved health-related purchases.

deductible An amount of money that you must pay yourself before your insurer begins to cover the costs of your medical care.

What Health-Care Reform Means for You

In 2010, health insurance made big headlines as national lawmakers passed broad new laws designed to increase health-care access for millions of Americans. Many of the reforms don't take effect until 2014, but some are already in place, and can make a real difference to students and young people. Here are five highlights:

- **Better protections for children with pre-existing conditions.** Children insured through private insurance plans, such as those offered through an employer, can not be denied coverage because of pre-existing conditions.

- **Get sick, stay insured.** Health plans can not cut off coverage if a person becomes sick, a practice known as *rescission*.

- **No lifetime limits.** Insurers can no longer place a lifetime cap on the insurance benefits you receive.

- **For young people, the magic number is 26.** You can now stay on a parent's insurance plan until your 26th birthday, if your parent so chooses.

- **New options for those with health concerns.** People who have had trouble getting insurance because of a pre-existing condition can join a new national "high risk pool," a group that will be provided immediate options for purchasing coverage.

In 2014, even broader reforms take effect, including the creation of new "health exchanges" where people who can not obtain insurance through work can purchase coverage. Adults will also be protected from discrimination based on pre-existing conditions, and women will be shielded from having to pay more for insurance than men.

Source: Affordable Health Care for America: Key Provisions That Take Effect Immediately from the Office of Speaker Nancy Pelosi, May 3, 2010, retrieved from http://docs.house.gov/energycommerce/IMMEDIATE_PROVISIONS.pdf.

university. More than half of all colleges now offer student health plans, with four-year schools far more likely to offer them than two-year schools. Some colleges now require that you enroll in their insurance if you can not provide proof of other coverage. Costs for this coverage vary widely, ranging anywhere from $30 to $2,400 a year, with most plans costing less than $1,000 a year. Many of these plans make use of the campus health center — some don't cover primary care, for example, if the student health center already provides this care.

- About 6% of students are covered by public insurance programs, such as Medicaid, for low-income individuals and families, or Medicare, for students with long-term disabilities. Recipients may also receive some care through their student health centers.

- About 20% of students have no health insurance. Among 18- to 23-year-olds, those aged 22 and older are more likely to be uninsured. Students of color are far more likely to be uninsured than white students, with Latinos more likely to be uninsured than any other group. Students reporting lower family incomes were also more likely to be without coverage. Without other health coverage, a student's only affordable option for services may be the college's student health center. The federal reforms allowing dependents to stay on a parent's insurance policy until they turn 26 are also likely to help.

See **Practical Strategies for Health: Tips for Affordable Health Care** for ideas about how to find health care that won't put you in debt.

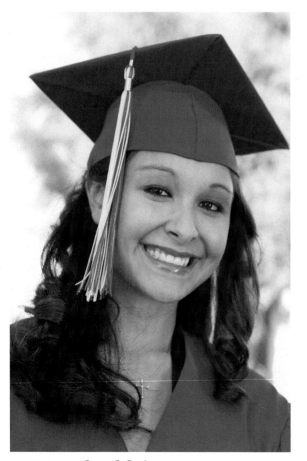

Will you still have **health insurance** when you graduate? If you're not sure, find out.

☺ *Practical Strategies for Health*

Tips for Affordable Health Care

No form of health-care coverage will pay for every penny of your health-care costs. To help ensure you don't wind up with medical bills that you can't afford, keep these strategies in mind:

- If you have your own insurance, make sure you understand the basic limits of the policy. How much do you have to pay in deductibles? What other out-of-pocket payments or "co-payments" are you responsible for? Does your insurance restrict your care geographically? Does it have a separate prescription plan? What services or providers are excluded? Does it stop covering you when you reach a certain age? What are the rules on visiting a hospital in an emergency? Make sure you keep a current copy of your insurance card, which you'll need to show medical providers when you receive care.

- Learn about what services are offered at your college's student health center. If a service isn't provided, ask about discount programs the center may have with other providers. Student health centers may have discount arrangements with local pharmacies, dentists, and other types of health providers.

- If you are uninsured or if your campus doesn't have a health center, ask your health instructor about local resources that provide free or low-cost care. Your campus or community may offer low-cost health coverage. Your campus may also offer health discount programs with local providers. There may be a nonprofit clinic nearby, or a retail clinic available at your local pharmacy.

- If you do need care, avoid heading to the emergency room or calling an ambulance unless you truly require emergency attention. Although emergency rooms are required to treat all patients who enter their doors seeking help (even patients with minor illnesses who don't have insurance), the care they provide is expensive, and you'll be billed directly. For less serious ailments, you can often receive the care you need at a much lower price from a community or retail clinic.

- Take care of your health preventively, which will help reduce the amount and cost of medical care you may need.

What Happens When I Graduate?

When it's time to get your diploma, add one more task to your "to-do" list: Find out what happens to your health insurance. Students going straight to graduate school or a job offering health insurance may have little or no gap in their coverage. But if you will be going without coverage for any length of time, you'll need to take steps to protect yourself.

Waiting for Health Coverage

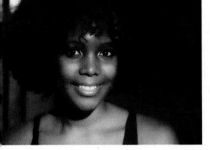

STUDENT STORY

"My name is Anuella.

I don't have health insurance. My mom's insurance only lets her add people once a year. That means I have to wait several months before I can have anything checked out—an ear infection, or if I break a bone—unless I want a really big bill from the hospital coming in the mail. Nobody has the money to pay a $500 bill just to get your ear checked out by a doctor. And even for a prescription, it's like $100. When I had health insurance, it was only about $20 to fill a prescription. Now it costs way more than it should cost for just a couple of little pills."

1: As a college student, what other sources of health coverage may be available to Anuella? What are her options besides waiting to be added to her mother's insurance plan?

2: Assume Anuella gets added to her mother's health insurance plan. What kinds of questions should she ask her insurance provider when she graduates from college?

Do you have a story similar to Anuella's? Share your story at **www.pearsonhighered.com/choosinghealth**.

If you have insurance through your parents, that coverage can continue until you reach the age of 26. If you have health insurance through your school, that coverage often ends around the time of your graduation. In some cases, policies literally stop the day you graduate. In others, you may have a couple of months of coverage before you are no longer eligible. If you are covered through a public program, your insurance is less likely to be tied to your student status, but find out for sure.

When your coverage ends, you'll likely have options to extend it, but at a high price. College and university policies can often be extended, but the cost will likely be at least double the cost of the original premium. For example, if your campus policy cost $1,200 per year, you'd pay at least $2,400 per year for the extension. You may be able to extend your coverage under your family's policy through a program called *COBRA*, but such policies often cost at least $300 or more a month, for a yearly bill of $3,600 or more.

You may also choose to purchase a policy on the individual insurance market. For younger people who are less likely to get sick, these are often more affordable than programs such as COBRA, usually carrying premiums of about $100 to $200 a month. Many of these policies, however, offer the type of "mini-med" coverage described earlier in this chapter. Many types of services probably won't be included. Make sure you understand the limits of your policy, and purchase one that gives you as much flexibility and coverage as possible.

The Genomic Revolution and the Future of Consumer Health

New medical advances against major diseases such as cancer are made each year. In the coming years, however, few advances will have as much potential to fundamentally reshape how you think about your health as personal **genomics**. Defined broadly as the study of the *human genome* (the biological code that "builds" a human being), genomics once seemed largely confined to science fiction. But with the decoding of the human genome completed in 2003, our understanding of this "code of life" has made it possible for us to examine our own genomes and understand some of the information they hold about our health. The goal of this effort is a personalized medicine that is tailored to your individual DNA.

> **genomics** The study of genomes and their effects on health and development.

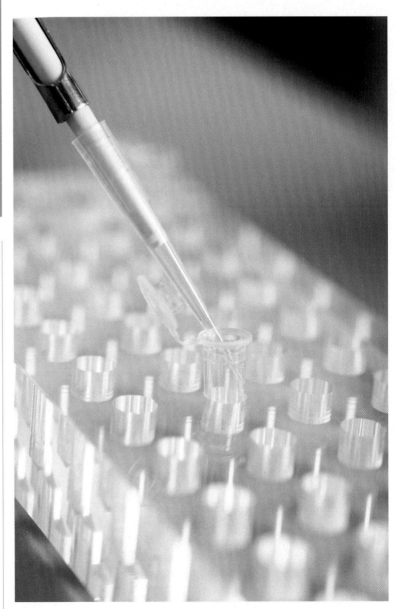

Advances in **genomics** are resulting in high-tech options for personalized health care.

Who Are the Uninsured?

Approximately 46 million people in the United States do not have health insurance.[1] The uninsured are not necessarily unemployed—according to the Kaiser Family Foundation, more than 8 in 10 of the uninsured are members of working families.[2] Many employers, reeling at the rising costs of health care, have scaled back insurance benefits or asked their employees to pick up more of the tab, making affordable health care out of reach for some. Employers also commonly offer health insurance only to full-time employees who work at least 40 hours per week.

Such trends hit blue-collar and young workers especially hard. These workers are less likely to have jobs offering full health benefits, and are also less likely to be able to afford health plans that require a significant financial contribution on their part. They are also more likely to have jobs with variable schedules that don't provide full-time status. Young adults between the ages of 19 and 29 have the highest uninsured rate of any age group—30%—because of low income or variable job status.[2]

Workers who fit this employment profile are also more likely to be members of ethnic minorities. As a result, Latinos, African Americans, Asian Americans, and other communities of color are less likely to have health insurance than Caucasians.[2]

Below are rates of uninsurance by race and ethnicity for the U.S. population as a whole and for college students.

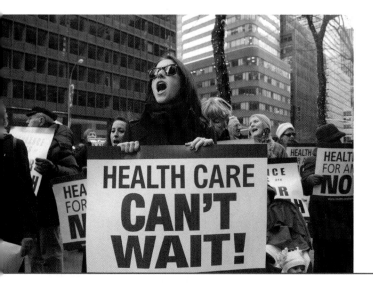

Rates of Uninsurance in Various Communities[2]

	U.S. as a Whole	College Students
Latino	34%	38%
Native American	30%	Data NA
African American	21%	29%
Asian and Asian American	18%	26%
Multiracial	13%	Data NA
Caucasian	12%	15%

References: **1.** "Number Uninsured and Uninsured Rate: 1987 to 2008," in *Current Population Survey, 1988 to 2009 Annual Social and Economic Supplements* by the U.S. Census Bureau, 2008, retrieved from http://www.census.gov/hhes/www/hlthins/data/incpovhlth/2008/fig06.pdf. **2.** *The Uninsured: A Primer - Key Facts About Americans Without Health Insurance* by the Henry J. Kaiser Family Foundation, 2007, retrieved from http://www.kff.org/uninsured/upload/7451-03.pdf.

Genomics sounds complex—and it is—but to get a basic understanding of your own genome, you only need to know a few key concepts:

- **DNA** (deoxyribonucleic acid) is the material that carries the biological instructions that "build" us. These instructions are *genetic*, meaning that they are inherited from our parents and ancestors. For example, your DNA is genetic information because you inherited it from your mother and father, who passed their DNA on to you when you were conceived. If you have a genetic disorder, it means you have a health condition passed on in the DNA you inherited from someone in your family.

- **Genes** are packets of DNA that carry the code for specific building blocks in your body.

- **Chromosomes** are packets of genes and supporting DNA that make up your genome.

- **Your genome** is your entire collection of DNA, coiled in a tight double spiral. Copies of your genome are found in almost every cell in your body. Although all human beings share mostly the same DNA, everyone's genome contains a few unique differences, or *genetic variants.* Your variants make you distinct in many ways, including in some of the ways your health may develop.

- **Your genome is not your destiny.** Though DNA is powerful, it is not the only factor that determines who you are or how healthy you may be. Environment and behavior choices are also powerful forces that can shape your health.

Uses of Genomic Information

As our understanding of the human genome evolves, this information is rapidly transforming health care. In the past, health has often been discussed in terms of "one size fits all" or "one size fits many." But genomic information increasingly enables people, either on their own or through their doctors, to find approaches more likely to work for them on an individual basis. Here are some of the ways genomic understanding is reshaping health.

Family Health Histories

Federal health officials now encourage everyone in the U.S. to create a basic **family health history,** or a record of health conditions that have appeared in a family over time. Health histories used to be reserved for families with rare genetic conditions, such as the blood clotting disorder hemophilia. Now, however, genomic research has revealed that many common health conditions, such as Type 2 diabetes, high cholesterol, and heart disease, have a genetic component. Creating a family health history

genome The genetic material of any living organism.

family health history A detailed record of health issues in one's family that presents a picture of shared health risks.

enables you and your relatives to look for patterns of illness that might indicate genetic risk. If you find that you are at greater risk for a disease, you can then take steps early to minimize your risk by making healthier choices, such as improving your diet or seeking out certain screening tests earlier or more frequently.

> You can find information on creating a family health history at **www.hhs.gov/familyhistory.**

Single-Gene Testing

If you or your doctor think you are at risk for a genetic illness, or that your DNA carries increased risks for certain health conditions, you may opt to have a certain gene or section of a particular chromosome analyzed. Such *single-gene testing* can tell you whether you carry DNA variants known to be linked to particular health conditions. Some women with particular family backgrounds, for example, choose to be tested for breast cancer–related variants in genes called *BRCA1* and *BRCA2*. If they find that they are at increased genetic risk, they may opt for medical treatments that reduce their risk.

These tests are powerful, but they are also expensive and emotionally complex. Most such genetic testing is usually conducted with the help and support of a *genetic counselor*, a medical professional who helps patients understand genetic testing, assess their own feelings and beliefs about such testing, decide whether they want testing, and determine how they will respond to the results. As genomics becomes a larger part of our health system, the number of genetic counselors is growing rapidly.

Whole-Genome Scanning and Sequencing

Other genetic technologies enable you to read your whole genome at once and see what it says about your risk for a variety of health conditions. In some cases, this form of testing only looks at specific points on your genome, a process called **whole-genome scanning.** Scientists can also decode and spell out every point on your genome, a process called **genome sequencing.** Scanning is simpler and cheaper, and is thus more widely available. Full genome sequencing is also available, but it remains far too costly for most people.

Although assessment of your whole genome holds great promise for providing a broad look at what your genome says about your health, this form of testing remains controversial. Proponents say that whole-genome assessment is now ready for widespread use. Critics counter that our understanding of health-related genetic risks is still too limited for the information to be of much practical medical use, and that related ethical considerations can be complicated. If you find yourself thinking about any form of DNA testing, consider speaking with a genetic counselor first to help you find options that are right for you.

DNA Tests and Medical Choices

In addition to providing information about risks for certain illnesses, DNA information can sometimes help us decide how to treat them. Each of us, for example, carries DNA variants that affect how our

whole-genome scanning A form of genetic testing that looks for variants throughout a person's genome.

genome sequencing The full decoding and readout of an entire genome.

pharmacogenomics The use of DNA information to choose medications and make prescribing decisions.

bodies process certain medications. The study of this DNA-drug interaction, called **pharmacogenomics,** has already changed the way doctors prescribe certain blood thinners and other medications. In the case of some cancers, doctors can now analyze the DNA of tumors to determine which treatments might best stop them.

Ethical, Social, and Legal Implications of Genomic Advances

Genomic advances can enable you to take a more personal approach to your health. But for many, it also raises doubts and fears. What about privacy? Will others use your genetic information to discriminate against you? Will DNA differences that you carry appear in medical records that can be used to justify higher insurance premiums?

These questions are already shaping new laws designed to help build a lifetime of better health in the genomic era. In 2008, after more than a decade of debate, U.S. lawmakers enacted the *Genetic Information Nondiscrimination Act*, or *GINA*. This law strengthens the privacy of personal DNA information and prohibits genetic discrimination in health insurance and employment.

Still, other questions remain. Should genetic discrimination also be barred in other types of insurance, such as disability insurance? How widely should personal DNA information be shared? Will DNA knowledge make people feel more empowered about their health, or more hopeless? These and other important questions will continue to spur discussion and regulation as the genomic revolution unfolds.

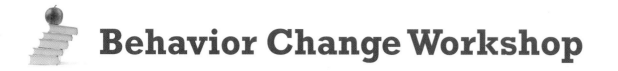

Behavior Change Workshop

To complete this workshop online, visit **www.pearsonhighered.com/choosinghealth**.

Becoming Proactive About Preventive Care

It's easy to be passive about health care, and to not worry about preventive care or having health insurance until you get sick or injured. But a little planning and action in advance can greatly pay off down the line by reducing the risks you will develop an illness and by offering you protection if or when you do need medical care.

Use this worksheet to start becoming more proactive about your health. Begin by taking the Self-Assessment on page 321. Then, fill out the grid below.

	Past Behavior	Future Behavior
Physical exam	When was the last time you had a physical exam?	When will you schedule your next exam?
Gynecological exam with Pap smear (for females)	When was the last time you had a gynecological exam?	When will you schedule your next exam?
Dental care	When was the last time you visited a dentist?	When will you schedule your next exam?
Vision care	When was the last time you had a general vision exam?	When will you schedule your next exam?
Tetanus/diphtheria booster shot	When was the last time you received a tetanus/diphtheria booster shot?	If it's been over 10 years since your last booster, when will you schedule your next vaccination?
Protection from influenza	When was the last time you received an influenza vaccination?	If it's been over a year since your last vaccination, when will you schedule your next one?
Health insurance	Do you have health insurance?	If you do not have health insurance, when will you investigate the options available to you?

Chapter Summary

- Our health system is increasingly one in which individuals have an abundance of choices, but also the responsibility of researching information, critically evaluating it, and making educated decisions.

- *Self-care* includes maintaining basic wellness habits, evaluating health information critically, using over-the-counter medications properly, exercising caution when taking dietary supplements, using home health tests properly, and knowing when it is time to see a doctor.

- Preventive care, such as periodic screenings and checkups, can help prevent health problems or catch them early when they are often easier to treat.

- *Conventional medicine* is characterized by a focus on the physical aspects and treatment of disease; the presence of discernable, defined symptoms; the maintenance of public health; and the use of scientific evidence and the scientific method.

- Conventional care is now available from a wide variety of facilities and providers, ranging from hospitals to student health centers to retail clinics.

- When choosing a doctor, find out whether he or she is covered by your insurance plan, and ask friends and family for recommendations. When you meet a doctor in person, make sure he or she listens to you, answers your questions completely, and treats you with respect. Be vocal and honest with your doctor about all aspects of your health.

- *Complementary and alternative medicine* (CAM) encompasses therapies and practices outside those of conventional medicine. CAM practices often look beyond the physical aspects of disease to issues that connect mind, body, and spirit.

- Examples of CAM include traditional Chinese medicine, biologically based practices such as the use of herbs and botanicals, mind-body therapies, manipulative therapies, and energy therapies.

- CAM is popular, but many CAM practices have not been proven safe or effective. Research any CAM therapy or provider before starting care, and make sure both your CAM and conventional practitioners know the full range of care you are receiving as well as your health history and habits to make sure you are being treated safely.

- Options for paying for health care include discount health programs, health insurance, health savings accounts, and flexible spending accounts.

- Health insurance policies come in many forms, including managed-care plans, fee-for-service plans, and public plans.

- *Genomics* is the study of the human genome. Genomic research is spurring the development of personalized health care based on an individual's DNA.

  Examples of genomic applications in health care include prenatal testing, single-gene testing, whole-genome scanning, and genome sequencing.

Test Your Knowledge

1. In today's health-care system, who needs to be the primary advocate for taking care of your health?
   a. a doctor
   b. a hospital
   c. the government
   d. you

2. What are the typical characteristics of credible health-related research?
   a. publication in a peer-reviewed journal
   b. a large pool of study participants
   c. results that have been replicated by other scientists
   d. all of the above

3. Which of the following is true about dietary supplements?
   a. There is scientific consensus about their health benefits.
   b. They are extensively evaluated by government agencies.
   c. They may not be appropriate for certain populations.
   d. There are regulations for the general marketing claims they can make.

4. Which of the following is not considered a practitioner of conventional medicine?
   a. medical doctors
   b. acupuncturists
   c. nurse practitioners
   d. dentists

5. Being a smart patient includes
   a. being honest and vocal with your doctor.
   b. asking questions when you don't understand something.
   c. following the instructions you receive from your doctor.
   d. all of the above

6. What is chiropractic an example of?
   a. alternative medicine
   b. conventional medicine
   c. energy therapy
   d. naturopathy

7. Which of the following is characteristic of managed-care health insurance plans?
   a. The more flexibility you want in selecting a health-care provider, the more the insurance will cost.
   b. They don't cover medication.
   c. There are no out-of-pocket fees associated with them.
   d. They offer no flexibility for medical care outside of the plan's approved providers.

8. Under the federal health-care reforms passed in 2010, children can stay on their parents' insurance plans until what maximum age?
   a. 18
   b. 21
   c. 26
   d. 30

9. Analyzing a certain gene to assess the risk of developing a genetic disease is an example of
   a. whole-genome sequencing.
   b. single-gene testing.
   c. genomics.
   d. genetic variation.

10. The study of DNA-drug interaction is called
    a. pharmacogenomics
    b. single-gene testing
    c. alternative medicine
    d. carrier testing

Get Critical

What happened:

When a novel infectious disease—a new strain of influenza virus, H1N1, popularly called "swine flu"—caught the world by surprise in 2009, health officials scrambled to try to stop a possible pandemic. One of their responses included quick work on a vaccine protecting against the H1N1 virus. But the race to develop the vaccine triggered intense debate. Some people welcomed such speedy vaccine development, especially in poorer countries most threatened by a large influenza outbreak. Others questioned the safety and efficacy of any vaccine developed so rapidly, saying more needed to be learned about H1N1 before taking steps such as injecting large numbers of people with a new vaccine.

What do you think?

- Have you ever received a seasonal or one-time flu vaccine?
- Do you think the public debate over vaccines is helpful or harmful?
- If given the chance to use a newly developed vaccine, such as one developed quickly for a new strain of flu, what would you do? Would you feel safe? Or would you have concerns?
- For your vaccine questions, where would you look for information, and which sources would you trust?

Get Connected

Health Online Visit the following websites for further information about topics in this chapter:

- The Medical Library Association's Top 100 List: Health Websites You Can Trust
  http://caphis.mlanet.org/consumer/index.html

- Evaluating Health Information on the Internet (from the National Cancer Institute, part of the National Institutes for Health)
  www.cancer.gov/cancertopics/factsheet/Information/internet

- Agency for Healthcare Research and Quality (AHRQ)
  www.ahrq.gov

- National Center for Complementary and Alternative Medicine
  http://nccam.nih.gov

- The Human Genome Project
  www.ornl.gov/sci/techresources/Human_Genome/home.shtml

Website links are subject to change. To access updated web links, please visit **www.pearsonhighered.com/choosinghealth**.

References

i. Pew Internet & American Life Project. (2009). *Generational differences in online activities*. Retrieved from http://www.pewinternet.org/Infographics/Generational-differences-in-online-activities.aspx

ii. Slone Epidemiology Center at Boston University. (2006). *Patterns of medication use in the United States: A report from the Sloane survey*. Retrieved from http://www.bu.edu/slone/SloneSurvey/AnnualRpt/SloneSurveyWebReport2006.pdf.

iii. Stasio, M., Curry, K., Sutton-Skinner, K., & Glassman, D. (2008). Over-the-counter medication and herbal or dietary supplement use in college: Dose frequency and relationship to self-reported distress. *Journal of the American College Health Association,56*(5), 535–547.

iv. U.S. Census Bureau. (2008). Number uninsured and uninsured rate: 1987 to 2008, in *Current population survey, 1988 to 2009. Annual social and economic supplements*. Retrieved from http://www.census.gov/hhes/www/hlthins/data/incpovhlth/2008/fig06.pdf

1. Pew Internet & American Life Project. (2009). *Demographics of Internet users*. Retrieved from http://www.pewinternet.org/Static-Pages/Data-Tools/Download-Data/~/media/Infographics/Trend%20Data/January%202009%20updates/Demographics%20of%20Internet%20Users%201%206%2009.jpg

2. Pew Internet & American Life Project (2009). *Generational differences in online activities*. Retrieved from http://www.pewinternet.org/Infographics/Generational-differences-in-online-activities.aspx

3. Escoffrey, C., Miner, K., Adame, D., Butler, S., McCormick, L., & Mendell, E. (2005). Internet use for health information among college students. *Journal of the American College Health Association, 53*(4), 183–188.

4. Slone Epidemiology Center at Boston University. (2006). *Patterns of medication use in the United States: A report from the Slone survey*. Retrieved from http://www.bu.edu/slone/SloneSurvey/AnnualRpt/SloneSurveyWebReport2006.pdf.

5. U.S. Food and Drug Administration, Center for Drug Evaluation and Research. (2009). *Regulation of nonprescription products*. Retrieved from http://www.fda.gov/cder/Offices/otc/default.htm

6. Stasio, M., Curry, K., Sutton-Skinner, K., & Glassman, D. (2008). Over-the-counter medication and herbal or dietary supplement use in college: Dose frequency and relationship to self-reported distress. *Journal of the American College Health Association, 56*(5), 535–547.

7. Kittinger, P., & Herrick, D. (2005). Patient power: Over-the-counter drugs. *National C*

enter for Policy Analysis, Brief Analysis, 524. Retrieved from http://www.ncpa.org/pub/ba524/.

8. American Academy of Family Physicians. (2010). When Should I Go to the Emergency Department? Retrieved from http://www3.acep.org/patients.aspx?id=26018.

9. Merck & Co., Inc. (2007). *The Merck Manual of Medical Information—Home Edition*. Porter, R. S. (Ed.). Whitehouse Station, NJ. Available at: http://www.merck.com/mmhe.

10. American Academy of Family Physicians. (2009). *Tips for talking to your doctor*; retrieved from http://familydoctor.org/online/famdocen/home/patadvocacy/healthcare/837.html; and *Medical errors: Tips to help prevent them*; retrieved from http://familydoctor.org/online/famdocen/home/healthy/safety/safety/736.html

11. National Center for Complementary and Alternative Medicine. (2007). *CAM basics: What is CAM?* Retrieved from http://nccam.nih.gov/health/whatiscam/overview.htm

12. National Center for Complementary and Alternative Medicine. (2009). *CAM basics: Are you considering complementary and alternative medicine?* Retrieved from http://nccam.nih.gov/health/decisions/consideringcam.htm

13. National Center for Complementary and Alternative Medicine. (2009). *CAM basics: Selecting a complementary and alternative medicine practitioner*. Retrieved from http://nccam.nih.gov/health/decisions/practitioner.htm

14. World Health Organization. (2008). *World health statistics: Global health indicators*. Retrieved from www.who.int/entity/whois/whostat/4.xls

15. U.S. Government Accountability Office. (2008). Health insurance: Most college students are covered through employer-sponsored plans, and some colleges and states are taking steps to increase coverage. Report GAO-08-389. Retrieved from http://www.gao.gov/new.items/d08389.pdf

16. Jost, T. (2008). Access to health care: Is self-help the answer? *The Journal of Legal Medicine, 29,* 23–40.

17. Collins, S. (2008). Consumer-driven health care: Why it won't solve what ails the United States health system. *The Journal of Legal Medicine, 28,* 53–77.

18. Dixon, A., Greene, J., & Hibbard, J. (2008). Do consumer-directed health plans drive change in enrollees' health care behavior? *Health Affairs, 27*(4), 1120–1131.

14

- Approximately 75% of teen and young adult (aged 15–24) deaths are caused by unintentional and intentional injuries.[i]

- Alcohol is a contributing factor in many unintentional injuries and deaths, including those resulting from automobile crashes, falls, fires, drowning, sexual assaults, suicides, and homicides.[ii]

- A person is four times more likely to get in a car crash drinking and driving, and eight times more likely to get in a car crash texting while driving.[iii]

- Of the crimes against students, 93% are committed off-campus.[iv]

Personal Safety and Injury Prevention

IDENTIFY the factors that lead to unintentional injuries and the most common types of unintentional injuries.

UNDERSTAND how you can protect yourself from unintentional injuries.

IDENTIFY the factors that lead to violence and the most common types of intentional injuries and violence.

UNDERSTAND how you can protect yourself from intentional injuries and violence.

UNDERSTAND how unintentional injuries and violence affect college students and develop strategies for staying safe on campus.

LIST ways to prevent violence.

Health Online icons are found throughout the chapter, directing you to web links, videos, podcasts, and other useful online resources.

Personal safety—what does it mean?

Is it wearing a seatbelt? Not getting on your bike without a helmet? Avoiding getting drunk and walking home alone? It means all these things and more. **Personal safety** is the practice of making decisions and taking actions that reduce your risk of injury and death. Injuries come at enormous social and personal cost. According to national estimates, injury-related medical expenses cost the U.S. population billions of dollars each year—in one year alone, about $80 billion in direct medical costs and another $326 billion in productivity losses.[1] And injuries are the number-one killer of people in the U.S. between the ages of 15 and 24.[2] The good news is that in recent years deaths due to injuries have dropped.[2] You can prevent many injuries if you are informed and make good decisions.

Injuries fall into two main categories. **Unintentional injuries,** often called *accidents* by public health officials, are injuries sustained even though no harm was intended. Examples of unintentional injuries are injuries from car accidents, accidental house fires, falls, or accidental drowning. **Intentional injuries,** on the other hand, are purposefully inflicted through violence. Examples of intentional injuries are injuries caused by assault, rape, or murder. Suicide and self-harm are often considered intentional injuries as well.

In this chapter, we will show you how you can avoid injury. We'll start by describing the major types of unintentional injuries, what factors lead to them, and how to avoid each kind. Then we'll discuss injuries due to violence, including murder, assault, and sexual assault. We'll provide you with tips on how to stay safe. And finally, we'll talk about how to prevent violence.

Unintentional Injuries

Unintentional injuries, or those that occur without intent to cause harm, send more than 27 million people to emergency rooms in the U.S. each year.[3] More than 15,000 Americans between the ages of 15 and 24 die from unintentional injuries each year.[2] Many of these tragedies could be prevented by simple decisions. For example, in a national survey of college students, about 5% said they rarely or never wore a seat belt, 69% of bike riders said they rarely or never wore a bike helmet, and about 25% said that in the past month, they'd ridden in a car with a driver who'd been drinking.[4] These situations leave you open to a variety of injuries, and learning to identify and avoid them can reduce your risk.

> The CDC has a number of podcasts on unintentional injuries: www.cdc.gov/ncipc/duip/podcast/index.htm.

Factors That Lead to Unintentional Injuries

Unintentional injuries occur as the result of multiple factors.

- **Risky behaviors.** Often events that cause injury occur because of the behaviors immediately preceding them. For example, heavy alcohol consumption or other substance abuse increases the risk of many types of unintentional injuries. Or, participating in a high-risk activity like drag racing can also lead to injury.
- **Sex.** Males account for almost two-thirds of the deaths attributed to unintentional injuries.[5]

personal safety The practice of making decisions and taking actions that reduce your risk of injury and death.

unintentional injury (accidents) Physical harm that is not deliberately caused.

intentional injury Physical harm that is purposefully inflicted through violence.

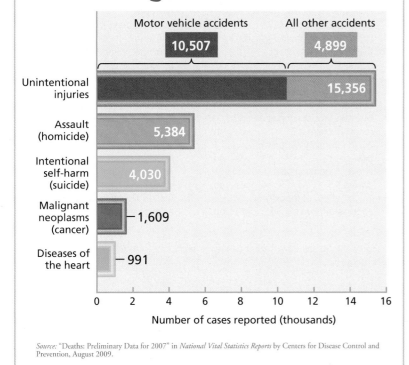

Top Five Causes of Death in the U.S. Among People Aged 15–24

	Motor vehicle accidents	All other accidents
	10,507	4,899

Unintentional injuries: 15,356

Assault (homicide): 5,384

Intentional self-harm (suicide): 4,030

Malignant neoplasms (cancer): 1,609

Diseases of the heart: 991

Number of cases reported (thousands)
0 2 4 6 8 10 12 14 16

Source: "Deaths: Preliminary Data for 2007" in *National Vital Statistics Reports* by Centers for Disease Control and Prevention, August 2009.

safety devices like seatbelts and airbags. Excessive speed is a factor in about 31% of all fatal car accidents, and for men between the ages of 15 and 24 that number climbs to 37%.[6] On average, 1,000 drivers a month are killed in speed-related accidents.[7]

Aggressive driving. Aggressive driving is defined by the National Highway Traffic Safety Administration as the operation of a motor vehicle in a manner that endangers or is likely to endanger people or property. Examples of aggressive driving are driving too quickly for conditions, cutting off other vehicles, tailgating, and abrupt lane changes. Aggressive driving is estimated to be a factor in more than 55% of fatal car crashes.[8] Though drivers can always be pulled over for any laws they break, 14 states now have traffic laws specifically targeting aggressive driving.

Driving while distracted. If you want to dramatically increase your chance of getting into a car accident, distract yourself from the road by talking on your phone, sending a text, or fiddling with your stereo while you drive. The risk of getting into a car accident that causes injury goes up four-fold when a driver is speaking on a cell phone or eight-fold when texting while driving.[9] Studies have found that even if you are speaking on a hands-free cell phone, you are just as distracted as if it was hand held, and one study indicated that you may be just as impaired as a legally intoxicated driver.[10–13] Drivers between the ages of 18 and 21 are especially vulnerable to the dangers of distracted driving because of their relative inexperience behind the wheel.[14] In recent years, multiple deadly transit accidents have occurred in which operators of trains, subway cars, and other large vehicles were using their phones for talking or texting just before or during the crash.

Try the *New York Times* game that tests how distracted you become while trying to text message while driving: www.nytimes.com/interactive/2009/07/19/technology/20090719-driving-game.html.

- **Age.** Compared with other age groups, young people (ages 15 to 29) account for the largest proportion of overall injury-death.
- **Environmental factors.** Factors such as increased traffic volume or poor weather conditions can increase risk of automobile, motorcycle, bicycle, or recreational injury.
- **Divided attention.** Performing any type of potentially dangerous activity without completely focusing on the task at hand increases the risk of injury.

Automobile Injuries

Being on the road is dangerous. More than 3 million people in the U.S. are hurt in motor vehicle accidents each year, and about 40,000 die.[2] About one-quarter of those lives lost are people between the ages of 15 and 24. No other single cause of death claims more young lives than car crashes.

Factors That Lead to Automobile Injuries

Common factors that lead to automobile injuries are:

Speeding. Speeding reduces the amount of time you have to react to conditions in the road in front of you, increases the distance needed to stop in an emergency, and reduces the effectiveness of

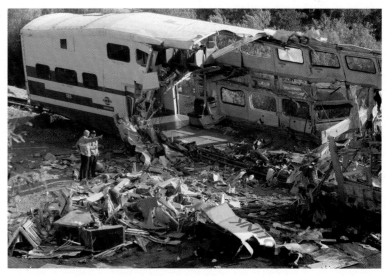

In this 2008 train accident in California **25 people were killed and 135 injured.** The conductor was text messaging just moments before the accident, in violation of transit agency policy.

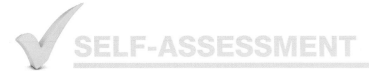

SELF-ASSESSMENT

To complete this self-assessment online, visit **www.pearsonhighered.com/choosinghealth**.

Are You an Aggressive Driver?

Do you have aggressive habits that could threaten your safety or the safety of others on the road? Circle yes or no for each question.

Do you...

1. Overtake other vehicles **only** on the left?   yes   no
2. Avoid blocking passing lanes?   yes   no
3. Yield to faster traffic by moving to the right?   yes   no
4. Keep to the right as much as possible on narrow streets and at intersections?   yes   no
5. Maintain appropriate distance when following other vehicles, bicyclists, or motorcyclists?   yes   no
6. Provide appropriate distance when cutting in after passing a vehicle?   yes   no
7. Use headlights in cloudy, raining, or low light conditions?   yes   no
8. Yield to pedestrians?   yes   no
9. Come to a complete stop at stop signs or before right turn on red?   yes   no
10. Stop for red traffic lights?   yes   no
11. Approach intersections and pedestrians at slow speeds to show your intention and ability to stop?   yes   no
12. Follow right-of-way rules at four-way stops?   yes   no
13. Drive below posted speed limits when conditions warrant?   yes   no
14. Drive at slower speeds in construction zones?   yes   no
15. Maintain speeds appropriate for conditions?   yes   no
16. Use turn signals for turns and lane changes?   yes   no
17. Make eye contact and signal intentions where needed?   yes   no
18. Acknowledge intentions of others?   yes   no
19. Use your horn sparingly around pedestrians, at night, around hospitals, and at other times?   yes   no
20. Avoid unnecessary use of high beam headlights?   yes   no
21. Yield and move to the right for emergency vehicles?   yes   no
22. Refrain from flashing headlights to signal a desire to pass?   yes   no
23. Drive trucks at posted speeds, in the proper lanes, using nonaggressive lane changing?   yes   no
24. Make slow, deliberate U-turns?   yes   no
25. Maintain proper speeds around roadway crashes?   yes   no
26. Avoid returning inappropriate gestures?   yes   no
27. Avoid challenging other drivers?   yes   no
28. Try to get out of the way of aggressive drivers?   yes   no
29. Refrain from momentarily using High Occupancy Vehicle (HOV) lanes to pass vehicles?   yes   no
30. Focus on driving and avoid distracting activities (e.g., smoking, use of a cell phone, reading, shaving)?   yes   no
31. Avoid driving when drowsy?   yes   no
32. Avoid blocking the right-hand turn lane?   yes   no
33. Avoid taking more than one parking space?   yes   no
34. Avoid parking in a disabled space (if you are not disabled)?   yes   no
35. Avoid letting your door hit the car parked next to you?   yes   no
36. Avoid using the cell phone while driving?   yes   no
37. Avoid stopping in the road to talk with a pedestrian or other driver?   yes   no
38. Avoid inflicting loud music on neighboring cars?   yes   no

HOW TO INTERPRET YOUR SCORE

0–3 "No" answers: Excellent
4–7 "No" answers: Good
8–11 "No" answers: Fair
12–38 "No" answers: Poor

Source: Adapted from *Are You an Aggressive Driver or a Smooth Operator?* by the New Jersey Office of the Attorney General, Division of Highway Traffic Safety, retrieved from http://www.state.nj.us/lps/hts/SO_Quiz.pdf.

Drunk or impaired driving. Driving after you've been drinking or using drugs is extremely dangerous, and driving with a blood alcohol concentration of 0.08% or higher is illegal in all 50 states. Drinking alcohol, even a small amount, impairs your vision, lessens motor control and coordination, impedes your ability to do two things at the same time, and reduces judgment and alertness—all necessary skills for driving. Almost 40% of all car crash–related deaths are linked to a driver who's been drinking.[15] Drugs other than alcohol, such as marijuana or cocaine, are a factor in about 18% of all vehicle-related deaths, often in conjunction with alcohol.[16]

Fatigue. Research studies have consistently found that sleepiness and fatigue are a factor in about 20% of crash or near-crash incidents.[17] Fatigue slows your reaction time and reduces your attention level, ability to process information, and the accuracy of your short-term memory, all of which impair your driving and your ability to avoid an accident. Fatigue isn't just brought on by lack of sleep, it can also be due to long work hours or medications that induce drowsiness.

Skipping seatbelts. Almost all states require that drivers and passengers use seatbelts and, if they are young children, child safety seats. Yet about 17% of vehicle occupants don't use these proven lifesavers.[18] Seatbelt use is lowest among people between the ages of 16 and 24. But the benefits of seatbelts are unrivaled. They are the single most effective prevention against injury or death in a car crash.[19] Between 2004 and 2008, seatbelts saved 75,000 lives. One benefit of seatbelts is that they prevent you from being thrown from the car—an event that is five times more deadly than if you remain in the car during an accident.[20] Seatbelts are also essential companions to other safety restraints such as airbags.

Safe Driving

Your first line of defense lies in making smart driving decisions. The following safe driving practices can help you avoid accidents.

- **Allow plenty of time for your trip.** Don't try to rush somewhere once you get in your car.
- **Stay within speed limits.** Driving fast reduces your ability to adjust to driving conditions and avoid accidents.
- **Slow down when the weather is bad.** Poor weather conditions mean it may take longer to stop the car on a wet surface, vision could be reduced, or roads could be icy.
- **Don't tailgate.** Tailgating, or following too closely to the car in front of you, increases your chances of an accident by reducing the amount of time and distance you have to react to events in front of you. Use the 3-second rule when following: Make sure you

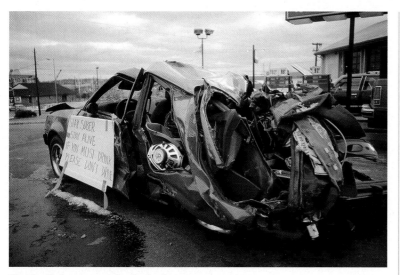

Drinking and driving can kill you or others.

are following at such a distance that it takes at least 3 seconds for your car to cross a fixed reference point after the car in front of you crosses it. When driving at higher speeds, on slippery roads, or when you are being followed by a tailgater, increase your distance even more.

- **Follow the rules of the road.** Signal before turning or changing lanes, look both ways before entering an intersection, check your blind spot, make a full stop at all stop signs, and obey traffic signals.
- **Don't text or otherwise distract yourself.** Put your phone out of reach before you get in the car. If you must talk or text, pull over to the side of the road. Set up your music before you start driving. Don't try to eat, shave, or put on make-up, even if you are stopped in traffic or at a stoplight.
- **Don't drink and drive.** Pick a designated driver, take a cab, or ask a sober friend to take you home. Don't ride with a driver who has been drinking, and if possible, take away the keys of someone who has been drinking and wants to get behind the wheel. One bad decision can kill you or others. It's not worth it.
- **Don't drive when you are sleepy.** If you are drowsy, don't start to drive, or pull over and rest. On long drives, take a break every 2 hours or 100 miles to get out of the car, stretch, and check your level of fatigue.
- **Buckle up.** It only takes a second. And in most states, it's the law.

Automobile Safety Technology

You can also keep yourself safer on the road by keeping your car in good condition and choosing and using additional safety features whenever possible. When you are looking at a new car, consider some of the following safety features.

Airbags. Airbags are safety devices that inflate in a fraction of a second after an accident, protecting you from impact against the car's interior or outside objects. As soon as a crash begins, sensors determine the severity of the crash, and deploy the airbags if it's serious enough. Driver and passenger airbags are required by law for all new passenger cars, SUVs, and light trucks. Some cars also offer optional side-impact airbags, which provide added protection during a sideways collision.

Advancements in airbag technology have led to new "smarter" airbags that not only further reduce the risk of injury in a car crash, but also reduce some of the risks of airbags themselves. In 2007, "advanced" airbags became standard in all light vehicles, which reduce the force at which airbags are deployed in low-speed collisions or shuts off the airbag entirely, reducing risk of injury to smaller occupants. Nonetheless, children under 12 and infants in child safety seats should not be placed in the front seat where a frontal airbag could injure them in a car accident.

Although airbags provide some protection during an accident, they are designed to be used with seatbelts, and adults and children should always wear seatbelts whenever they are in a car.

View just how quickly an airbag deploys at www.iihs.org/video.aspx/info/static_airbag.

Child safety seats. Car crashes are the leading cause of death for children in the U.S.[21] Proper use of child safety seats reduces the risk of death in infants by 71%, and in children 1–4 years old by 54%.[21] Parents should use rear-facing car seats for infants until they reach the height or weight limit for the seat, at least until the child is 1 year old or 20 pounds. After that, forward-facing child safety seats will keep a child safe until he or she is 4 years old or 40 pounds.

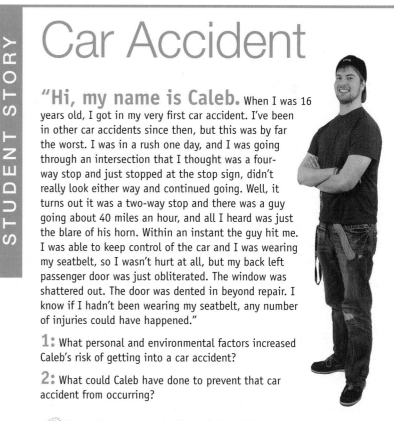

Once children outgrow safety seats parents should use booster seats to ensure that seatbelts are positioned properly against the child—lap belt against the upper thighs and shoulder belt crossing the chest. Once a child is 4 feet, 9 inches tall, seat belts will normally fit them and the booster seat can be removed.

Electronic stability control. New developments in safety technology mean there are more safety options than ever on the market. One new technology that greatly reduces the risk of accidents is electronic stability control (ESC). ESC uses sensors and computers in the car to recognize what the driver is doing. If the driver suddenly turns the steering wheel, a move that can lead to a spin out or a rollover, ESC will make automatic shifts in speed or direction to reduce the risk of loss of control. Studies show that ESC can reduce fatal single-car accidents by 51% and fatal multi-car accidents by 19%, a safety benefit so dramatic that beginning with 2012 models, all cars, SUVs, pickups, and minivans will be required to be equipped with standard ESC.[22]

Motorcycle and Bicycle Injuries

Riding a motorcycle or a bicycle can be dangerous. One of the more common forms of injury that befall motorcycle and bicycle riders is **traumatic brain injury (TBI).** TBI is caused when the head is jolted or hit, or when an object pierces the skull, resulting in a sudden injury that damages the brain. While many TBI patients recover quickly, a significant number face a lifetime of disability, and some die. Among teens, TBIs account for more than 240,000 emergency room visits each year, about 36,000 hospitalizations, and more than 5,700 deaths.[23] Even if it is not legally required in your area, wearing a proper helmet while on a bike or motorcycle is essential for reducing the risk of TBIs.

Motorcycle Injuries

In recent years, our roads have gotten less hazardous—unless you are on a motorcycle. Overall, the number of accident-related vehicle injuries, while still significant, continues to fall, except among motorcycle riders. The rate of motorcyclists injured in crashes almost doubled from 1998 to 2008.[24] In 2008 about 96,000 motorcycle riders and passengers were injured, and of those, more than 5,300 died.[24]

Over half the motorcyclists injured in crashes are involved in "single-vehicle crashes," meaning that no other motorcycle or car was a factor. According to traffic safety statistics, motorcyclists are about 6 times more likely than those riding in a car to die in a motor vehicle traffic crash.[24] Even though motorcycles are known to be more dangerous than cars, only 63% of motorcycle riders wear helmets.[25] Fewer than half of all states require that adults wear a helmet when riding a motorcycle, a factor that contributes to injuries and deaths.

Bicycle Injuries

Bikes may not pack the force or speed of a car or motorcycle, but riding one still carries risks. According to national statistics, about 500,000 people—mostly boys and younger men—wind up in emergency rooms because of bike crash injuries each year in the United States, and more than 700 die.[3, 26]

Although cars need to make room on the road for bikes, bike riders are responsible for road safety as well. In one study of bike crashes, cyclists were found to be at fault about half the time, mostly due to unsafe riding habits such as riding against traffic and running stop signs.[27] As with motorcycles, varying helmet laws contribute to the injury statistics. Though many states have laws requiring bike helmets for teens and children who ride, more than a dozen do not, and in most states, helmets are optional for adults. Experts estimate that only about 25% of riders use a helmet.[26]

How to Avoid Motorcycle and Bicycle Injuries

The likelihood of being in a motorcycle or bicycle accident can be reduced if you follow these simple guidelines.

- **Follow the rules of the road.** Motorcycles and bikes may be more nimble than cars, but avoid the temptation to cut through lanes of traffic, run lights, or blow through stop signs. And always ride with the flow of traffic. You are sharing the road with vehicles far larger and heavier than yours, and you are far less protected.
- **Wear a helmet.** Even if laws in your state don't require one, wear a helmet every time you ride. If all motorcyclists wore helmets, an additional 800 lives could be saved each year.[24] For bicyclists, 70% of bike accident deaths are from head injuries and bike helmets are more than 85% effective at mitigating or preventing these head injuries.[26] For more information on choosing the right bike helmet, see the **Consumer Corner** on the next page.
- **Stay visible.** Don't assume that drivers can see you. Avoid riding in a car's blind spot or passing quickly. Wear at least one piece of brightly colored clothing on your upper body, and if riding at night, make sure your clothes, helmet, and bike are outfitted with reflectors.
- **Don't drink and ride.** About a quarter of bicyclists killed in bike accidents are found to have blood alcohol concentrations at or above legal limits.[27] You face the same increased risks of an accident as an impaired driver of a car.

Home and Recreational Injuries

A surprising number of accidents and injuries occur at home or at play. Whether you live in a house, an apartment, or a dorm, a few basic precautions will help keep you safe.

Falls

Falls are the most common types of home injuries. About 8 million people in the U.S. are injured in falls each year; about 21,000 die. Most victims of falls are adults aged 65 or older, and among older adults, falls are the most common causes of fatal and nonfatal

---

traumatic brain injury (TBI) An injury that disrupts normal functioning of the brain, caused by a jolt or blow to the brain or a penetrating head wound.

> "*In recent years, our roads have gotten less hazardous—unless you are on a motorcycle.*"

How to Choose a Bike Helmet

You've gone into a sporting goods store to buy a new bike helmet, and find yourself with dozens to choose from, ranging in price from $40 to more than $200. Where to start?

Among bike helmets, a higher price does not necessarily equal greater safety. More expensive helmets may be tailored for specialty riders. If you aren't aspiring to be an expert road racer or mountain biker, you may not want to look at expensive specialty helmets.

Instead, you'll only need to focus on the core elements of a quality helmet—the strap, the foam liner, and the hard plastic outer shell. These make sure the helmet protects you by staying on in a crash, absorbing the shock of an impact, and providing a barrier between your head and a hard surface. Select a few helmets and try them on, paying attention to the following:

- **Size.** You need a fit that is snug, but not so tight that the helmet is uncomfortable or rides up. When strapped on, the helmet shouldn't move more than an inch in any direction, and you shouldn't be able to get it off no matter how you try. If your head shape is hard to fit, ask a salesperson for help with extra padding or straps.
- **Sits straight.** The helmet should sit straight on your head, not tilted back or forward. If you have long hair

that you often wear back, consider a helmet with a "ponytail port" so that your ponytail doesn't push your helmet forward.

- **Straps.** Avoid thin straps. Look instead for a set that fits snugly under your chin, with a "V" on either side that meets under your ears. Make sure the buckle is strong and doesn't pop open easily.
- **Sticker.** Helmets sold in the United States must meet safety standards set by the Consumer Product Safety Commission, and carry a CPSC sticker inside. If a helmet doesn't have one, give it a pass.

If you get in a crash, replace your helmet, even if it looks fine. The accident could have caused structural damage that you can't see but that could cause the helmet to fail in another accident. If something on your helmet breaks, don't try to fix it. Invest in a new one. In a crash, you can't count on those repairs to provide the protection you need.

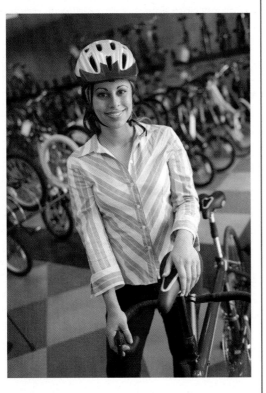

injury.[28] Falls also cause the most nonfatal injuries among children aged 0–19.[29]

Many falls at home are related to slippery or unstable flooring. Mop up spills right away, and use a traction mat in the shower or bath. Keep stairs in good repair and well-lit, and keep carpets and rugs tacked down. If children or older people live with you, use extra safety devices such as gates at the top of stairs, window guards, or handrails in the bathroom.

Poisoning

Every day, about 75 people in the U.S. die from unintentional poisoning and another 2,000 are treated at the hospital.[30] We all know that certain toxic substances, such as cleaning products, solvents, and pesticides are hazardous. But many other common household items, such as medications or even certain houseplants, are poisonous if consumed at high dosages.

Poisoning from overdoses of both legal and illegal drugs has risen steadily in the U.S. since 1970.[31] Prescription painkillers are responsible for the majority of that increase. Common culprits are prescription opioid painkillers such as oxycodone (OxyContin), hydrocodone (Vicodin), and methadone. Because these drugs produce a "high," they are more likely to be abused or used without a prescription, leading to overdose. Another risk is that children can ingest prescription and over-the-counter drugs if they are left within reach. Children are twice as likely to be poisoned by medications as they are by other household products like cleaning supplies.[30]

If you think you or someone you are with has been poisoned, call the National Poison Control Center at 1-800-222-1222. To avoid poisonings, store all potential poisons as directed in their original bottles and keep them out of the reach of children. Follow the directions on medicine labels, and never share or sell your prescriptions. Dispose of any medication you no longer need. For more on dangerous toxics that can be found in the home see Chapter 15.

Fire Injuries

A huge majority, 80%, of all fire deaths occur in the home.[32] In 2008, someone in the U.S. died in a house fire every 158 minutes, and someone was injured every 31 minutes. On college campuses, rates of fires are increasing, mostly due to apathy or ignorance of fire safety and prevention practices.[33] Most of the fires that lead to death are caused by careless smoking, but other common causes of residential fires include candles, cooking, malfunctioning or improperly used heaters, and arson. Alcohol plays a role in about 60% of fatal burn injuries.[34]

Fire safety isn't difficult if you plan ahead. Every home should have a smoke detector on every level and every dorm room should have its own smoke detector. Smoke detectors should be tested monthly, and the batteries replaced twice a year. Several easy tips can protect against fire. If you are using your stove or oven, don't leave it unattended. Don't overload electrical outlets, and make sure extension cords are used properly. If anyone in your home smokes, put out cigarettes in ashtrays, and never smoke in bed. If you use a portable space heater, keep it at least three feet away from anything flammable, and never leave it unattended. Know to dial 911 if you see a fire or smoke, take all fire alarms seriously, make sure you know the escape route for your dorm or create one ahead of time for your home, and participate in practice fire drills. Understanding how to evacuate in advance will help you in the chaos of a real fire.

Prepare for Home Emergencies

Whether you live in a dorm, an apartment, shared housing, or at home with your family, the U.S. Department of Homeland Security recommends taking a few basic safety precautions to prepare yourself for a natural disaster, house fire, or some other type of emergency:

- Be informed about the different types of emergencies that could occur in your area and their appropriate responses.

- Have an emergency plan. If you live on campus, your school has probably developed such plans for student housing. Find out about yours.

- Keep an emergency supply kit on hand.

Here is a list of basic items to stock in your emergency supply kit. Consider adding additional items based on your individual needs.

- Water, one gallon of water per person per day for at least 3 days, for drinking and sanitation

- Food, at least a 3-day supply of nonperishable food

- Battery-powered or hand crank radio and a NOAA (National Oceanic and Atmospheric Administration) Weather Radio with tone alert and extra batteries for both

- Flashlight and extra batteries

- First aid kit

- Whistle to signal for help

- Dust mask, to help filter contaminated air, and plastic sheeting and duct tape to shelter-in-place

- Moist towelettes, garbage bags, and plastic ties for personal sanitation

- Wrench or pliers to turn off utilities

- Can opener for food (if kit contains canned food)

- Local maps

- Cell phone with chargers

Source: *Ready* by the U.S. Department of Homeland Security Ready Campaign, retrieved from http://www .ready.gov.

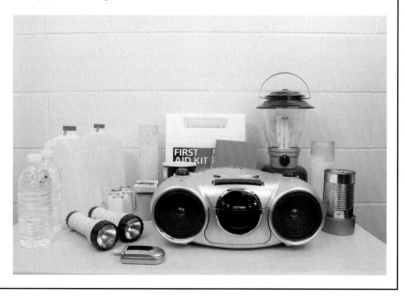

Choking and Suffocation

Small children and older adults are especially vulnerable to choking and suffocation. Make sure foods given to children younger than 3 years old are cut into very small pieces. If someone is choking and can not cough forcefully or speak, the **Heimlich maneuver** can help. To perform the

---

Heimlich maneuver on an adult, stand behind the choking victim and place your arms around him or her; make a fist and grab it with your other hand between the victim's ribcage and belly button. Perform a series of sharp, upward thrusts, until the object is expelled or the victim loses consciousness, at which point you should call 911. You can take a class in the Heimlich maneuver and basic emergency assistance from your local American Red Cross chapter or campus health center.

The Heimlich Institute provides directions on how to perform the Heimlich maneuver on adults, infants, and yourself: www.heimlichinstitute.org.

Accidental Shootings

Some who keep guns at home do so because it makes them feel safer, but having a gun in the home can lead to accidental shootings. In order to prevent accidental injury or death, keep guns and ammunition away from children. Unload your guns before storing them, and treat any gun as though it were loaded, even if you think it isn't. Invest in a gun lock designed specifically for your gun, or buy a gun that comes equipped with such a safety feature. Because 4.3% of college students bring their guns with them to school, consider that accidental shootings can also occur in your home away from home.[35]

Drowning and Water Injuries

Drowning causes an average of 10 deaths a day, not including drownings due to boating accidents.[36] Most children under the age of 4 drown in swimming pools, but pools aren't the only culprits in drowning accidents. Young children also die in bathtubs, buckets, toilets, and hot tubs. For people over 15, most drownings occur in natural water settings like lakes, oceans, or rivers. Alcohol intoxication greatly increases the risk of drowning.

Everyone should swim with a companion, never alone. Do not ever dive or jump into an unknown body of water, and do not ever drink alcohol when you are swimming or operating a boat. To keep children safe in water settings, never leave them alone when they are around water, whether it's in a bathtub, at the beach, or in your backyard pool. Children can drown in less than 5 minutes so you should keep a constant watch on them. And remember to always wear a personal flotation device, or life jacket, when riding in a boat or participating in other water sports like jet skiing or waterskiing.

Work Injuries

Almost 4 million workers in the U.S. are injured on the job each year, and about 5,000 die.[37, 38] Many of those injuries occur in jobs traditionally considered higher risk, such as mining, construction, or trucking and other transit-related industries. But other types of workplaces cause significant numbers of injuries as well, including hospitals, retail stores, and offices. In these sectors, many injuries relate to repetitive motion caused by spending long hours doing computer- or data-related work.

If you work at a job where safety equipment is provided, use it! Safety equipment takes only a few moments to put on and gives invaluable protection. Follow all safety measures required in your workplace, and if you aren't sure what they are, ask. Employers are required to provide nec-

---

Heimlich maneuver A method for helping someone who is choking by dislodging the obstruction through a series of quick upward thrusts below the diaphragm.

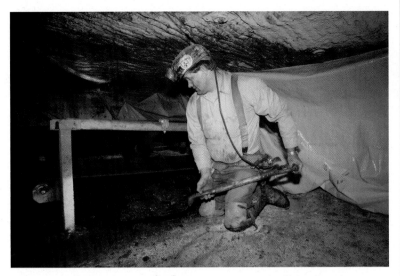

High-risk jobs like **mining** are responsible for the majority of work-related injuries.

essary safety equipment, establish safety procedures, and provide training on both to all employees.

Repetitive Strain Injuries

Performing the same movements over and over, even slight movements with your hands and fingers, can injure and inflame your joints, connective tissues, and nerves. These **repetitive strain injuries, or RSI** (also referred to as *repetitive stress injuries* or *repetitive motion injuries*), can lead to pain, swelling, numbness, loss of motion, and even permanent nerve damage.

One type of RSI, called **carpal tunnel syndrome,** is especially prevalent among those who use any type of computer keyboard or keypad regularly. Symptoms include numbness, tingling, aching, and shooting pain in the hand or wrist. To avoid carpal tunnel, take frequent breaks to give your hands and wrists a rest when you are using a keyboard. See the **Practical Strategies for Health** for more tips on how to work safely at your computer.

Back Injuries

Lifting heavy objects is a leading cause of injury on the job.[39] If you've got a heavy box or other object to pick up and carry, start by making sure your balance is good. Then keep your back straight and crouch down by bending at the knees and hips to pick up the object; do not bend at the waist. Once you've picked up the item, lift by straightening your legs. Keep the object close to your body by holding your elbows close to your body. This helps keep strain off your spine. Don't twist your body while carrying the load; if you need to change directions, change your foot placement. To release the object, lower it down by bending your knees, not your back. If you need to lift something that weighs more than 50 pounds or is an awkward shape, get another person to help you, or use a hand truck or other lifting and carrying device.

repetitive strain injury (RSI) An injury that damages joints, nerves, or connective tissue caused by repeated motions that put strain on one part of the body.

carpal tunnel syndrome A repetitive stress injury of the hand or wrist, often linked to computer keyboard use or other types of repetitive motion.

☺ *Practical Strategies for Health*

Preventing RSI When Working on a Computer

Knowing how to set up your computer for optimal posture can help you avoid RSI.

- Keep your neck in a neutral position by using a laptop stand, monitor risers, books, or packages of paper to raise the top of the screen to about eye level.

- Angle the screen to avoid bending your head forward.

- Use a document holder to position documents you are typing from vertically, rather than bending your head to look at them.

- Allow for good hand and wrist posture by placing your keyboard and mouse on an adjustable keyboard tray that can be moved up or down. Keyboard and mouse should be positioned slightly at or below elbow height. If a laptop is your main computer, set up a work station with a regular-size external keyboard and mouse attached to it.

- When typing, don't bend and twist your hand to reach awkward key combinations. If you need to hit multiple keys at once, use a separate hand for each key, rather than contorting your hand to reach both keys with the same set of fingers.

- Keep your wrists straight. Don't rest your palms on the keyboard so that your hands are angled up from your wrists. Your wrists should be straight and your fingers should reach down slightly to find the keys.

- Use a chair that supports a comfortable upright or slightly reclined posture. Prop your feet up to maintain a comfortable trunk-thigh angle, if needed.

- Position the screen at a right angle to windows to reduce glare. Use a desk lamp or laptop light that plugs into a USB port for extra light, if needed.

- Clean your screen frequently with computer-safe antistatic cleaning material. Dust on the screen can make it difficult to read and increase eyestrain.

- Stop and stretch every 30 to 45 minutes.

- When carrying a laptop, use a wheeled case or a backpack with wide, padded straps, rather than a bag that places all the weight on one shoulder.

Adapted from: Ergonomic Tips for Laptop Users by U.C. Berkeley's Ergonomics Program for Faculty and Staff, 2007, retrieved May 2010 from http://uhs.berkeley.edu/facstaff/pdf/ergonomics/laptop.pdf.

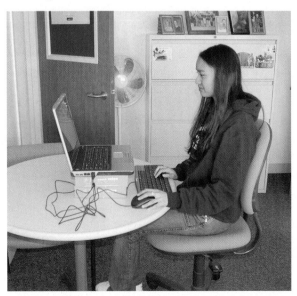

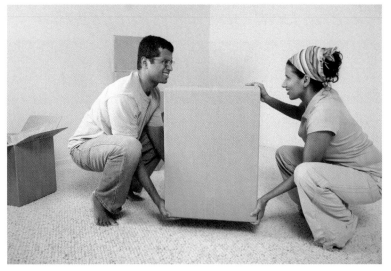

Get help lifting a heavy or awkward object to avoid back injuries.

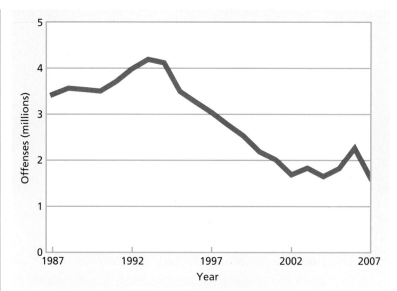

Figure 14.1 **Violent crime rates over the last 20 years.** The serious violent crimes included are rape, robbery, aggravated assault, and homicide. Rates include estimates for crimes not reported to the police.

Source: "Four Measures of Serious Violent Crime" in *Key Facts at a Glance* by the Bureau of Justice Statistics. retrieved from http://bjs.ojp.usdoj.gov/content/glance/cv2.cfm.

Intentional Injuries and Violence

Violence, or the use of physical force—threatened or actual—with the intent of causing harm, is a serious health concern for all of us, especially young people. Intentional injuries—in other words, injuries caused by violence—account for more than 2.4 million emergency room visits each year, and more than a quarter of the victims are young people between the ages of 10 and 24.[3] In 2008, more than 1.4 million violent crimes were committed annually in the United States—about 3,836 a day.[40] Of these attacks:

- About 60% were aggravated assault, or an attack intended to cause serious injury, often involving a weapon.
- About 32% were robberies, or the taking of or attempt to take anything of value from a person by violence and/or by putting the victim in fear.
- About 6% were forcible rapes.
- About 1% were murders.[40]

Although levels of crime in the United States have fluctuated in recent years, the overall amounts of violent crime have dropped in the last two decades **(Figure 14.1)**.[41] By taking some basic precautions to keep yourself safer, and encouraging others to look for nonviolent ways to resolve conflicts, you can help keep yourself from becoming a statistic and build a safer campus and community.

Factors That Lead to Violence

Many attacks have underpinnings in complex webs of personal, family, community, and social factors, including:

- **Sex.** Most violent crime is committed by men. Of the almost 600,000 arrests for murder, rape, robbery, and assault in 2008, 82% of those taken into custody were men. Men are also more often victims—about 78% of all people murdered in the United States in 2008 were male.[42] Crime experts continue to work to pinpoint the links between men and violence.[43] See the **Diversity & Health Box Injuries and Violence:**

Special Concerns for Young Men for more on possible reasons men are at higher risk than women.

- **Age.** Teens and young adults experience the highest rate of violent crime.
- **Guns.** The United States continues to have a high murder rate compared to other industrialized countries, and many experts link this phenomenon to the easy availability of firearms. In 2008, about 67% of the nation's murders, 44% of robberies, and 21% of aggravated assaults were committed with the use of a gun.[5, 44] Almost 85,000 people were killed or injured by gunfire.[40]
- **Poverty.** Regions that are lower in income and status consistently see more crime. Communities that are distressed, with poor housing, high crime rates, high unemployment, and limited community services often have higher rates of violence, especially among young people. Rates of violent crime also tend to be higher among disadvantaged socioeconomic groups. African Americans, who make up about 13% of the U.S. population and are more likely to live in poverty, also comprise about 48% of all murder victims.[42]
- **Interpersonal relationships.** Many crime victims know their attackers. Women are especially vulnerable to criminal acts at the hands of an acquaintance, friend, intimate partner, family member, or spouse.[45]
- **Drugs and alcohol.** Substances that disrupt judgment and impair your ability to control your emotions consistently emerge as a factor in violence. One landmark study of violent crime in the United States found that alcohol was a factor in almost 40% of all cases.[46] In another study that looked at drinking on college campuses over 2 years, more than 600,000 students reported being hit or assaulted by another student who'd been drinking.[47]

violence Use of physical force—threatened or actual—with the intent of causing harm.

Injuries and Violence:
Special Concerns for Young Men

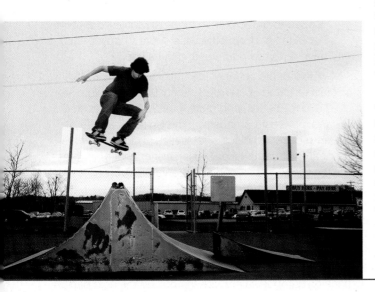

Two of the biggest risk factors for injury and death due to accidents or violence are things none of us can control: age and sex. If you are young, and you are male, your risk for getting hurt or killed in an accident or attack is almost always higher than that of women or any other age group. Sexual assault is one of the few situations where women are in more danger, but for most other types of violence and injuries, young men are at higher risk. In monetary terms, men and boys account for about 70% of the total costs of injuries in the U.S.[1]

The reasons for these higher risks are widely debated among researchers. Some suggest that the influence of the male hormone testosterone leads to more aggression, anger, and risk-taking. Some point to gender roles that encourage men, especially young men, to be tough, aggressive, risk-taking, or confrontational. Others say that a mix of these factors often put young men in harm's way.

Reducing the risk of injury doesn't mean taking all the fun out of your life. Instead, experts suggest, channel your energies in ways less likely to get you hurt or killed. Here are just a few suggestions:

• Your car is no place for an adrenaline rush. Find thrills in sports, video games, or anywhere but behind the wheel.

• Watch how much you drink. As you'll learn throughout this chapter, alcohol is a factor in many accidents and crimes. Whether you are the aggressor or the victim, you don't want to wind up a drinking-related statistic. For more information on alcohol and its effects, see Chapter 8.

• Anger can't help you solve problems. It's natural to get angry, but anger can quickly escalate a conflict into violence. Learning to manage anger and find other ways to resolve problems is one of the manliest things you can do. For more information about reducing stress and anger, see Chapters 2 and 3.

Reference: The Incidence and Economic Burden of Injury in the United States by the Centers for Disease Control and Prevention, 2007, retrieved from http://www.cdc.gov/ncipc/factsheets/costbook/Economic_Burden_of_Injury.htm.

The use of drugs, or their sale, is also a factor in many types of crime.

• **Childhood environment.** Researchers have consistently noted that children raised in violent surroundings are more likely to grow up to be violent adults.[48]

• **Violence in the media.** Between TV shows, movies, video games, and song lyrics, most children and teenagers are exposed to thousands of violent messages each year. Although crime researchers continue to debate the exact level of influence media violence has on personal violence and crime, most agree that violence in the media contributes to some level of aggressive behavior and a perception that violence is normal.

• **Personal and cultural beliefs.** In some cases, personal values or religious beliefs may be interpreted in ways that justify the use of violence. Violence can also be targeted against people of one religious group by those of a different faith.

• **Stress.** Think about the last time you were under a great deal of stress, and how you were quicker to anger than you might have been otherwise. People who are consistently under stress are more likely to react violently, especially if they are prone to anger easily.

aggravated assault An attack intended to cause serious physical harm, often involving a weapon.

murder The act of intentionally and unjustifiably killing another person.

homicide The killing of one human being by another.

Assault

Assault, a physical attack or threat of attack on another person, is one of the leading categories of violent crime. **Aggravated assault** is an assault committed with the intent to cause severe injury, or an assault or threatened attack with a weapon or other means likely to cause death or major injury. More than 834,000 aggravated assaults were committed in 2008.[49] More effective preventions and tougher law enforcement appear to have helped reduce the number of assaults, however. Arrests for assault have dropped dramatically since the late-1990s, especially among teenagers.[50]

Murder

Murder, the act of intentionally and unjustifiably killing another person, is a form of **homicide,** the killing of one person by another, and is second only to unintentional injuries as the leading cause of death in the U.S. among people between the ages of 15 and 24. More than 5,200 15- to 24-year-olds are murdered each year—about 14 lives lost each day.[2] Most murder victims and perpetrators are male, with three times more men than women murdered.[42] In 2008, at least 44% of these crimes were found to have been committed by someone the victim knew.[51] As with assault, prevention and law enforcement efforts appear to be helping, with arrests for murder down since the late-1990s, particularly among teenagers.[50]

Gang Violence

Many violent criminals don't act alone. **Gangs,** or economic and social groups that form to intimidate and control both their members and outsiders through threats and violence, are responsible for many acts of violent crime. According to the FBI, about 1 million gang members belonging to more than 20,000 gangs are criminally active in the United States, and commit as much as 80% of the crime within some communities.[52] They are major factors in the drug trade, and some also participate in armed robbery, assault, auto theft, extortion, fraud, home invasion, weapons dealing, and human trafficking. More and more women are joining gangs, and gangs are also increasing their range, becoming more active in suburban and rural areas.[52] With their sense of inclusion and camaraderie, gangs can seem appealing, especially in distressed neighborhoods where regular jobs are few and families and schools are strained. But once inside, gang members often find themselves caught in a culture of intimidation and crime that is difficult to escape.

School and Campus Violence

When two students went on a murderous rampage at Columbine High School in 1999, it began an era where many equated going to school with some amount of risk. Yet despite several high-profile tragedies, overall trends of crime on elementary, middle, and high school campuses have dropped dramatically since 2004, and a national analysis found that students were 50 times more likely to be seriously hurt or killed off campus than while at school.[53]

What Columbine means to high schools, Virginia Tech has come to mean for colleges and universities. In the horrifying 2007 mass

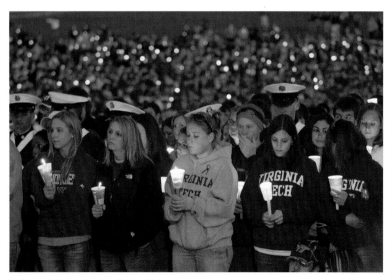

The Virginia Tech shootings in 2007 prompted colleges to reevaluate their safety and alert procedures.

gang An economic or social group that forms to intimidate and control members and outsiders through threats and violence.

hazing Initiation rituals to enter a fraternity or other group that can be humiliating, hazardous, or physically or emotionally abusive, regardless of the person's willingness to participate.

hate crime A crime fueled by bias against another person's or group's race or ethnicity, religion, national origin, sexual orientation, or disability.

shooting, a student killed 32 others and himself. In response to the tragedy, U.S. colleges and universities have reevaluated the effectiveness of their emergency responses and developed new response plans and procedures, upgraded communication systems, and implemented new safety techniques and services.

Few campus crimes are as devastating as the one that took place at Virginia Tech, but any act of violence still affects a campus community. One common problem on college campuses is **hazing,** a set of initiation rituals for fraternities, sports teams, or other groups that can result in injury or death. Hazing is dangerous because peer pressure or other power dynamics induce those being hazed to participate in high-risk activities that they wouldn't perform otherwise. More than one-third, 36%, of students have reported participating in hazing.[54]

Other types of violent crime occur on campus as well. In 2008, law enforcement officials reported 16 murders, almost 2,700 forcible sex offenses, almost 2,000 robberies, and more than 2,700 aggravated assaults on two- and four-year campuses in the United States.[55] All U.S. universities are required to disclose statistics about the crimes reported on and near their campuses. The legislation that mandates this disclosure is the Clery Act, named after Lehigh University student Jeanne Clery, who in 1986 was beaten, raped, and murdered in her dorm room when dormitory security doors were propped open, allowing a perpetrator to enter. Unfortunately, many campus crimes still go unreported, with victims often too embarrassed, ashamed, or afraid to step forward. Reporting a crime is also the first step toward addressing the problem and making a campus safer for everyone. For detailed suggestions on campus safety, see the box on the next page.

Hate Crimes

Certain crimes are fueled by bias against another person's or group's race or ethnicity, religion, national origin, sexual orientation, or disability. Any acts—whether physical assaults or vandalism against property—due to such prejudice have been classified as **hate crimes.** More than 7,500 of these hate crimes are reported each year, with the majority driven by bias against the victim's race. In 2008, 36 hate crimes were reported on college campuses.[55] For the public at large, FBI statistics for 2008 show:

- About 51% of victims were targeted because of their race.
- About 18% of victims were attacked because of their religious beliefs.
- About 18% of victims were targeted because of their sexual orientation.
- About 13% were attacked because of their ethnicity or national origin.
- About 1% were targeted because of a disability.[56]

Hate crimes tend to reflect prevalent social and cultural biases. Hate crimes against Muslims in the U.S., for example, jumped after the terrorist attacks of September 11, 2001. In recent years, hate crimes fueled by ethnicity or national origin bias have been committed against Hispanics in increasing numbers, a phenomenon experts pin to the ongoing debate over immigration.[57]

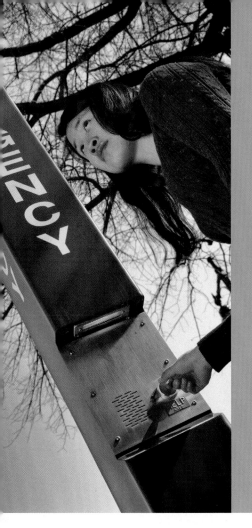

10 Tips for CAMPUS SAFETY

1. Program numbers for campus safety services into your cell phone, since most 911 calls from cell phones go to highway safety dispatchers, not local police. Also program in the direct line for the local police department.

2. If you live in a dorm, keep your room locked, and don't loan out your keys.

3. If you live in a dorm, group house, or apartment building, don't prop open access doors or let strangers in. If someone has arrived to visit another occupant, they can get the person they are visiting to let them in.

4. Whether you live in a dorm, group house, or apartment, know where the smoke detectors are and make sure they are working. Know where the emergency exits are and what your fire escape plan is.

5. Drink in moderation, if at all. Alcohol is a factor in many assaults, date rapes, and other campus crimes.

6. If you make purchases online using your credit card, don't use a shared computer.

7. Don't travel alone after dark. Take a shuttle, go with a friend, or use the security escorts available on many campuses.

8. Give friends or family your schedule of classes, work, and other activities.

9. Keep your valuables hidden. That's not always easy to do in a small dorm room, but it should still be possible to keep money, ATM cards, jewelry, and other valuables out of plain sight.

10. Know your surroundings and trust your instincts. If something doesn't seem right, get help by calling campus security.

Source: Adapted from information provided by: **1.** Security on Campus, Inc. (2008). *Seven tips for campus safety,* retrieved from http://www.securityoncampus.org/index.php?option=com_content&view=article&id=1563. **2.** Livesecure.org. (2009). *College student safety tips,* retrieved from http://www.livesecure.org/college-student-safety-tips/. **3.** Collegesafe.com (2003). *College safety tips—campus safety tips,* retrieved from http://www.collegesafe.com/campus_safety_tips.htm.

Terrorism

Terrorism is premeditated, politically motivated violence against noncombatant individuals, usually in an effort to influence a larger audience. The year 2001 saw more terrorism on U.S. soil than had ever been seen before. The dangerous bacteria that causes anthrax was deliberately dispatched through the U.S. postal system and more than 3,000 people died in the September 11 attacks. Since that point, the numbers of deaths and injuries due to terrorism in the U.S. have dropped greatly, but the effects remain. Terrorism is a crime that operates on many levels: It can maim or kill, but it also alters everyday life through the threat of unexpected violence, making people afraid.

As a result, fighting terrorism requires both physical force and psychological finesse. In response to the terrorist attacks in 2001, the U.S. government created the Department of Homeland Security, a government agency tasked with defending the nation against terrorism and other threats. Other agencies, such as the FBI, CIA, the U.S. military, and state and local law enforcement also guard against terrorism. Ongoing efforts work not just to disarm, catch, or kill terrorists, but to discredit their tactics, diminish the perception of threats, and reduce their abilities to win public support and new recruits. These efforts matter both on U.S. soil and abroad—in 2008, at least 54,000 civilians worldwide were killed, kidnapped, or injured by terrorists, with children being disproportionately affected by terrorism.[58]

Domestic and Intimate Partner Violence

Being close ideally means being supportive and affectionate, but unfortunately, that isn't always the case. In some households, family members may verbally, emotionally, physically, or sexually abuse others, a phenomenon known as **family violence** or **domestic violence.** Such abuse may also occur in relationships where people are intimate but don't share a household, a phenomenon known as **intimate partner violence.** Victims of domestic or intimate partner violence can be married or not married, heterosexual, gay or lesbian, living together, separated, or dating. Some experts believe that moving away from home to college can increase a teen's vulnerability to intimate partner violence, due in part to the decrease in parental monitoring and support and the desire to fit in, which can change behaviors toward others.[59]

Many cases of domestic and intimate partner violence go unreported, so the exact scope of this problem is hard to pin down. But reported cases make it clear that this type of abuse is widespread—each year, about 4.8 million

terrorism Premeditated, politically motivated violence against noncombatant individuals, usually as a means of coercion.

domestic (family) violence An abusive situation in which family members may verbally, emotionally, sexually, or physically abuse others.

intimate partner violence An abusive situation in which one member of a couple or intimate relationship may verbally, emotionally, sexually, or physically abuse the other.

women and 2.9 million men are the victims of violence at the hands of an intimate partner. In 2005, intimate partner violence resulted in 1,510 deaths, of which 78% were women and 22% were men.[60] Although domestic violence is often considered a problem of men abusing women, these statistics show that men can also be the victims of abuse, either by women or homosexual partners. Overall, however, women experience more intimate partner abuse than men.[61]

Physical and Emotional Abuse

At its core, abuse in a family or intimate relationship arises from the abuser's need for control. That effort at control may take the form of abusing others emotionally and psychologically, through comments and actions that try to erode the other person's confidence, independence, and sense of self-worth. Withholding money, keeping a partner from contacting family or friends, stopping a partner from getting or keeping a job, and constant putdowns are all characteristics of emotional abuse. Physical forms of abuse include any type of physical assault or use of physical restraint. In most cases, emotional abuse and controlling behaviors accompany physical abuse when it is present in a relationship.

Some people who find themselves the victim of an episode of abuse end the relationship and leave immediately. But other abuse victims, especially women, stay, and may find themselves subject to further and more severe abuse. Most such domestic and intimate partner abuse captures the victim in a situation that is difficult to escape, described as *the cycle of violence*:

- **Tension building.** A phase in which relatively minor abuse occurs, and the victim responds by trying to please the abuser and avoid provoking another attack.
- **Acute battering.** A phase in which the abuser lashes out more forcefully, no matter how accommodating or conciliatory the victim has been.
- **Remorse.** A phase in which the abuser may feel shock and denial over the abuse and swear it will never happen again. Over time, however, the tensions and need for control that started the cycle resurface, and abuse starts anew, often more seriously than before.

Victims stay in abusive relationships for a variety of reasons. Some are financially dependent on their partners, or have children and don't want to break up their family. Some come from belief systems or cultures that forbid family separation or divorce. Some may still love their abusers. Others may lack the self-confidence to confront their abuser by leaving, or don't know where to go. A variety of organizations provide counseling and shelter to such victims of abuse. One annual survey of domestic violence groups found that on a given day, more than 65,000 adults and children received shelter, housing, legal counseling, emotional counseling, or other types of support related to family and intimate violence.[62] More than 9,000 others seeking such help had to be turned away for lack of adequate services.

Domestic abuse persists, in part, because of a broader lack of understanding of how and why it occurs. In one survey of college students, more than half agreed with myths about domestic vio-

Abusive Relationship

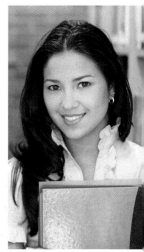

"Hi, I'm Jenny. I was dating a guy for a few months who I really liked and everything seemed great at first, but he slowly started to get more and more controlling. First he didn't want to go out with my friends, then after a while he didn't want *me* to go out with my friends. He got really jealous any time he saw me talking to another guy and he started making me check in with him every day to let him know my schedule. He even checked my cell phone to see who I was talking to. One day we got into a fight about it and he grabbed me and pushed me into a wall. I got really scared and left immediately. I broke up with him by text and I've avoided him ever since."

1: What could have happened if Jenny had stayed with her abusive boyfriend?

2: What else could Jenny have done in response to her boyfriend's behavior along with breaking up with him?

3: Was Jenny right to break up with him with a text or should she have met up with him to explain?

Do you have a story similar to Jenny's? Share your story at www.pearsonhighered.com/choosinghealth.

lence, such as the idea that some such violence is caused by women picking physical fights with their partners, or the idea that most women can get out of an abusive relationship if they really want to.[63] College men taking the survey were more likely to agree with these myths than college women.

Stalking

Intimate partner abuse is closely linked to **stalking,** defined as harassment directed at a specific person that is intended to cause intimidation and fear. According to a national study, about 3 million people over the age of 18 are stalked each year in the U.S.[64] Women were about three times as likely to be stalked as men, and men make up the majority of stalkers. In one survey of college women, about 20% reported having been stalked while in college, and the overwhelming majority of their stalkers were men the victim knew, including acquaintances, classmates, and boyfriends or ex-boyfriends.[65]

stalking A pattern of harassment directed at a specific person that is intended to cause intimidation and fear, often through repeated, unwanted contact.

Common stalking behaviors include:

- Making unwanted phone calls
- Sending unwanted letters or emails
- Following or spying
- Showing up at places where the victim would be, with no legitimate reason

- Waiting for the victim, with no legitimate reason
- Leaving unwanted items or presents for the victim
- Posting information or spreading rumors about the victim online, in a public place, or by word of mouth

Stalking may take the form of direct personal contact, or contact through digital and online communications, a phenomenon called *cyberstalking*. However, fewer than 30% of stalking cases involve elements of cyberstalking.[64]

If you are being stalked, don't try to reason with your stalker. Stalking is not rational behavior. Instead, start by letting the stalker know that the attention is unwelcome. If possible, have someone else deliver this message for you—this thwarts the stalker's goal of trying to force contact with you. If the stalker persists, keep a record of all contacts, and get help from your resident advisor, campus health center, campus security, or law enforcement.

Child Abuse

Unfortunately, children are not immune from family violence. In 2007, child protective services agents reported almost 800,000 cases of child maltreatment or abuse. Almost 60% of these cases involved child neglect, such as failure to provide basic food, shelter, medical care, or education. The remainder of cases were physical, sexual, and emotional in nature. More than 1,700 of these children died, the vast majority of them less than 4 years old.[66] The rates of abuse are highest for children from birth to age 3.[67]

Factors that lead to child abuse are psychological issues in the adult caregiver such as low self-esteem, feelings of being out of control, poor impulse control, depression, anxiety, and antisocial behavior.[67] Substance abuse, single parenthood, poverty, the presence of other domestic violence in the home, negative attitudes about childhood behavior or child development, and teen parenthood also increase the risk of child abuse. In addition, children who are physically, cognitively, or emotionally disabled are almost twice as likely to experience abuse.[67] About a third of children who are abused will go on to abuse their own children.

Elder Abuse

Elder abuse is the physical, emotional, psychological, financial, sexual, or verbal abuse, neglect, or exploitation of someone over the age of 60. Elder abuse can occur in the home, in a nursing home, hospital, or elsewhere. It is believed that more than 500,000 older adults suffer from elder abuse each year.[68] However, it is a largely hidden crime; experts estimate that only one in six cases is reported.[69] Elder abuse occurs across socioeconomic classes, cultures, and races. Women, elders at more advanced ages, those with dementia or mental health issues, and elders who are physically or socially isolated are at higher risk.

Addressing Family and Intimate Partner Violence

Stopping domestic violence begins with recognizing when a situation is abusive. If you have questions or concerns about your own relationship, or are frightened by something you see in the relationship of someone you know, contact your stu-

dent health center or the National Domestic Violence Hotline at 1-800-799-SAFE (7233) or at TTY ("text telephone" for the hearing impaired) 1-800-787-3224, or visit www.thehotline.org.

If you have children or plan to some day, and were abused yourself as a child, you are at risk of continuing that cycle of abuse. Health and child wellness centers around the country offer classes and counseling in positive parenting skills that help prevent child abuse and maltreatment. If you suspect that a child you know is being neglected or abused, seek help. Contact the National Child Abuse Hotline at 1-800-4-A-CHILD (1-800-422-4453).

Sexual Violence

Unwanted sexual advances are a serious, pervasive problem on college campuses and in the world beyond. Sexual violence can take several forms, including attempted but uncompleted sex acts without the victim's consent, unwanted touching, completed sex acts without the victim's consent, and noncontact sexual abuse, such as voyeurism or verbal harassment.

Factors That Lead to Sexual Violence

Influences that can lead to sexual violence include:

- **Negative attitudes about women.** Men who report hostility toward women or who hold low opinions of women are more likely to show higher levels of sexual aggression and to believe in myths like "When she says 'no,' she really means 'yes.'"
- **Rape-tolerant attitudes.** Several studies of college students have confirmed that college men are more likely to hold attitudes that are tolerant of rape, such as "Some women asked to be raped" or "It's all right to get a woman drunk just to have sex with her."[70]
- **Gender role stereotypes.** Outdated social perceptions hold that men should always insist on sex, and that women who decline are just playing "hard to get."
- **Alcohol and drugs.** People who have consumed alcohol to excess, either voluntarily or involuntarily, or used or been given a drug are more vulnerable to sexual assault. Many college women reporting an assault said they were incapacitated at the time, often by alcohol.[71] In one study, about 15% of men reported having used some form of alcohol-related coercion, and 20% admitted having friends who'd gotten a woman drunk or high to have sex with her.[70]
- **"No" isn't always heard as "No."** Studies have found that some young men have problems understanding a young woman's sexual refusals. Less direct refusals, such as body language that displays a lack of interest, or attempts at polite rejection such as "I don't think it's a good idea," were misinterpreted by some young men as agreeing to sex.[72]

Sexual Harassment

Unwanted contact of a sexual nature that arises in the context of school or workplace settings is considered **sexual harassment** when it explicitly or implicitly affects a person's job or academic situation, work or school performance, or creates an intimidating, hostile, or offensive environment. Sexual harassment is a form of discrimination that violates federal civil rights law.

sexual harassment Unwelcome sexual advances that explicitly or implicitly affect academic or employment situations, unreasonably interfere with work or school performance, or create an intimidating, hostile, or offensive work or school environment.

According to legal guidelines, sexual harassment can occur in a variety of circumstances, including but not limited to the following possibilities. In all cases the harasser's conduct must be unwelcome.

- The victim and the harasser may be a woman or man, and the two parties do not have to be of the opposite sex.
- The harasser can be the victim's supervisor (or teacher), an agent of the employer (or school), a coworker (or fellow student), or a nonemployee (nonstudent).
- The victim does not have to be the person harassed, but can be anyone affected by the offensive conduct.
- Harassment may occur even if the victim suffers no economic injury or stays on the job or at school.[73]

On campus, sexual harassment can take the form of everything from one student making the school environment uncomfortable for another to a professor demanding sexual favors from a student in exchange for a better grade. In one survey of college students, about 60% of all students (male and female) reported having been sexually harassed while enrolled in school. About 80% of those harassed said their harasser was a fellow student. About 50% of college men admitted to having harassed someone, and about 22% said they had done so more than once. Only 10% of those harassed said they had reported the incident to a campus official.[74]

If you are being harassed, stop this abuse by first confronting your harasser. State clearly, in person or in writing, that the actions are unwelcome. Be direct: Tell the harasser to stop, and state that you consider these actions to be sexual harassment. If direct communication has no effect, keep a record of all harassing contacts and behavior, and report the problem to campus or workplace supervisors. They are required by law to take your report seriously and investigate.

Rape and Sexual Assault

Any form of coerced sexual activity that relies on the threat of force, the use of force, or takes advantages of circumstances that make a person incapable of consenting to sex is forcible **rape** or **sexual assault.** Any sexual activity with a person younger than the legally defined "age of consent" is also considered a form of rape called **statutory rape,** regardless of whether any coercion or force was involved.

Although rape can happen to both men and women, most rape victims are women, and most rapists are men. In 2008, national crime records

> ## "In one survey of college students, about 60% of all students (male and female) reported having been sexually harassed while enrolled in school."

rape Nonconsensual oral, anal, or vaginal penetration by body parts or objects, using force, threats of bodily harm, or taking advantage of circumstances that make a person incapable of consenting to sex.

sexual assault Any form of coerced sexual activity up to but not including penetration, using force, threats of bodily harm, or taking advantage of circumstances that make a person incapable of consenting to sex.

statutory rape Any sexual activity with a person younger than the legally defined "age of consent," regardless of whether any coercion or force was involved.

date (acquaintance) rape Coerced, forceful, or threatening sexual activity in which the victim knows the attacker.

date rape drugs Drugs used to assist in a sexual assault, often given to the victim without his or her knowledge or consent.

showed that about 89,000 women in the U.S. were raped.[75] Given how many of these crimes go unreported, experts believe the actual number to be much higher. One large-scale national survey found that almost 18 million women and 3 million men in the U.S. had been raped at some point in their lives.[61] For women victims, at least half those assaults occurred before she turned 18; and for men, 71% of rapes occurred before age 18. Nearly two-thirds of women who reported being raped or physically assaulted said their assailant was a spouse, boyfriend, or date. In one survey of college women, almost 20% said they'd been sexually assaulted during their undergraduate years.[71]

Date rape. Of those rapes documented among college students, many took the form of **date (acquaintance) rape.** This form of coerced sexual activity, in which the victim knows the attacker, is a common problem on campus. Just because a victim knows the perpetrator doesn't lessen the emotional impact of the rape. In fact, sometimes the long-term emotional impact is even more severe because a date rape victim is attacked by someone who was trusted. Date rape is sometimes preceded by intimate partner violence that escalates to sexual abuse. As with other types of sexual assault, many cases of date rape go unreported. Drinking and drug use are factors in many cases of date rape, and in some instances the victim is unknowingly given a drug to facilitate rape, called a date rape drug.

Date rape drugs. Drugs used to assist in a sexual assault, or **date rape drugs,** are powerful, dangerous, and difficult to detect once they've been slipped into a drink. They can make you weak or confused, or cause you to pass out—all conditions that leave you unable to refuse sex or fend off an assault. These drugs can also make it difficult to remember what happened while you were drugged. The drugs can be used on both men and women. The most common date rape drugs can come in pill, liquid, or powder form and include flunitrazepam (Rohypnol), Ketamine, or GHB (gamma-hydroxybutyric acid).

Under federal law, any convicted rapists who use a date rape drug to incapacitate a victim will have 20 years added to their sentences.

The following precautions can help you avoid accidentally consuming a date rape drug.

- Don't accept drinks from other people, including nonalcoholic ones.
- Open drink containers yourself.

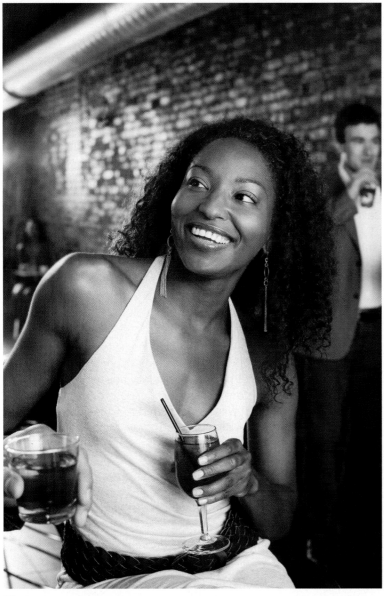

Date rape drugs can be difficult to detect once added to drinks.

- Keep your drink with you at all times. If you've left it unattended, pour it out.
- Don't share drinks, or drink from punch bowls or other open, shared containers.
- If someone offers to get you a drink, go with the person to the bar, and carry it back yourself.
- If you feel drunk and haven't had any alcohol, or have been drinking but feel like the effects are much stronger than usual, get help from a friend or other person nearby right away.

Reducing the risk of date rape. Preventing date rape requires effort from both men and women.

For women:

- When dating someone you don't know well, stay in public or go out on group dates. Arrange for your own transportation; don't rely on your date for transport.

- Watch out for coercive behavior on a date. If your date tries to pressure you into activities such as drinking heavily or any other action you'd rather avoid, you may face similar pressures for sex as well.
- Tell others about what is happening to you. If you are being pressured to drink or have sex by someone aggressive at a party, let your friends know and get out of there.
- Keep in mind that drinking and drugs make it harder for you to communicate clearly and set limits about sex.
- Be assertive and direct. If you are being pressured for sex and don't want to participate, it's no time to be polite. Say "No" clearly and firmly. If the pressure persists or worsens, tell the other person that he or she is committing rape, and that you are calling the police.

For men:

- "No" means "No." Even if you think her outfit means "Yes," or her flirtatious manner means "Yes," pay attention to her reactions and words. When in doubt, back off.
- When a woman is too incapacitated to give consent, that does not mean she has agreed to sex.
- Drinking and drugs make it harder for you to communicate clearly and set limits about sex too.
- Remember what being out on a date means—and what it doesn't. Dating means a chance to get to know someone better in a social setting. It is not an automatic ticket to sex. Your date has the right to set limits and refuse any level of sexual activity.

If you are raped or sexually assaulted. If you are raped or sexually assaulted, remember that you are not to blame. Sexual violence occurs because the attacker is sexually aggressive, not because of something you've said, done, or worn. If you know your attacker and he or she is not armed, you may be successful at fending off the attack by yelling, screaming, hitting, kicking, or running away. If your attacker is a stranger or is armed, however, you may put yourself in more danger by fighting. Every situation is different, so use your best judgment. If you choose not to resist, it does not equal consent.

After an assault, go to a place where you feel safe, and call someone you trust. Write down as many facts about the attack as you can remember. Try not to change your clothes or clean up; you'll destroy physical evidence that may be helpful if you report the attack to the police. Instead, go to a hospital to be treated for any injuries you've received and screened for sexually transmitted infections. If female, you can be checked for pregnancy and possibly given emergency contraception. Physical evidence can be collected at that time while you decide whether to report the attack. When you seek medical care, ask for referrals to a counselor who can help you deal with the many emotional and psychological challenges that can arise after a sexual assault.

The decision to report a rape or sexual assault can be difficult. You may be reluctant to talk about the attack publicly. Top barriers to reporting a sexual assault include shame, guilt, and embarrassment; concerns about confidentiality; and concerns about not being believed.[76] Reporting the crime, however, may give you a renewed sense of power and control. Sexual assailants also tend to repeat their behavior. By reporting a sexual assault, you may prevent your attacker from raping someone else in the future.

Violent Crime and Abusive Relationships on Campus

Students reported experiencing the following within the last 12 months

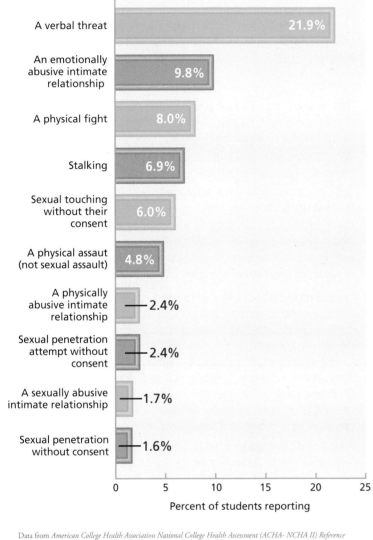

A verbal threat	21.9%
An emotionally abusive intimate relationship	9.8%
A physical fight	8.0%
Stalking	6.9%
Sexual touching without their consent	6.0%
A physical assaut (not sexual assault)	4.8%
A physically abusive intimate relationship	2.4%
Sexual penetration attempt without consent	2.4%
A sexually abusive intimate relationship	1.7%
Sexual penetration without consent	1.6%

Percent of students reporting

Data from *American College Health Association National College Health Assessment (ACHA- NCHA II) Reference Group Executive Summary, Fall 2009* by the American College Health Association, 2009, retrieved from http://www.acha-ncha.org/reports_ACHA-NCHAII.html

Sexual Abuse of Children

Of the 800,000 cases of child abuse documented in 2007, about 64,000 took the form of sexual abuse.[67] This form of assault covers any type of sexual contact, regardless of the apparent willingness of the child, between an adult and a child below the legal age of con-

sent. It is also a hidden crime that often goes unreported, with actual cases estimated at about three times the level of those documented in police files.[77]

This type of abuse takes many forms, including inappropriate touching, exposure of genitalia to a child, and using a child as a pornography subject. Most abusers are men who know the children they abuse, and about one-third of abusers are related to their victims.[78]

For sexually abused children, the long-term emotional and psychological effects are often devastating. If you think a child you know is being sexually abused, get help immediately.

Effects of Sexual Violence

Sexual violence has immediate and long-term consequences on psychological and social health. People who experience sexual violence often experience depression, increased risk of suicide, substance abuse, sleep disorders, sexual dysfunction, and post-traumatic stress disorder. They may also have decreased capacity to form intimate bonds with partners, strained relationships with loved ones, and, in some groups, sexual abuse can lead to rejection of the victim by partners or family.

Children who are sexually abused often come to suffer from low self-esteem, feelings of worthlessness, and abnormal or distorted views of sex. Among other problems, sexually abused children may also develop distrust of adults, difficulty relating to others except on sexual terms, depression, withdrawal from loved ones, secretiveness, delinquency, and feelings of being "dirty" or "damaged."

How to Help Prevent Violence

Violent crimes and abusive relationships unfortunately do occur on college campuses. See the **Student Stats** box for recent statistics. Violent crime is frightening, but it can also be confronted. While in college, you can help by:

- **Knowing your campus safety rules and resources.** Especially since the Virginia Tech shootings, most U.S. college campuses have revised and improved their campus safety rules and resources. Learn what they are and how you can take advantage of them to protect your personal safety.

- **Watching how much you drink.** As you've learned in this chapter, alcohol use is closely tied to many types of violent crime.

- **Steering clear of social pressures that encourage violence.** You may encounter acquaintances or groups that encourage domination of others, hostility to outsiders, binge drinking, or sexual aggression. Don't play along.

- **Making sure any guns in your home are handled safely.** Keep them unloaded, out of sight, and securely away from kids. Invest in a lock-and-load indicator, and use it.

- **Reporting crime.** If you see or hear about a crime, let campus security or police know.

Watch videos of real students discussing personal safety at www.pearsonhighered.com/choosinghealth.

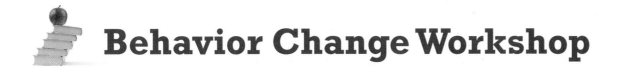

Behavior Change Workshop

To complete this workshop online, visit www.pearsonhighered.com/choosinghealth.

Reducing the risk of injury and violence involves reducing risky behaviors. Think about things you do, perhaps without even thinking about them, that may increase your risk of injury. What can you do to reduce your risk?

Part I. Assessing Your Personal Risk

1. List all the behaviors you do that might increase the risk of injuries. Why do you participate in these risky behaviors? What could be the consequences of them?

Risky behavior	Why do you do it?	Possible consequences
_____	_____	_____
_____	_____	_____
_____	_____	_____
_____	_____	_____
_____	_____	_____

2. Pick one of the behaviors above that you want to target. Ask yourself honestly: How ready am I to commit to a behavior change that will help me reduce that behavior? What stage of behavior change am I in?

Target behavior: _____

_____

Current stage of behavior change: _____

_____

3. Keeping your current stage of behavior change in mind, describe what might be a "next step" to reduce or eliminate the risk of injury due to the risky behavior. Also list your timeline for making your next step.

Next step: _____

_____

_____

Timeline for next step: _____

_____

Part II. Make Your Car a No Phone Zone

According to neuroscientists, the human brain is not capable of fully concentrating on two tasks simultaneously. And yet, millions of drivers in the U.S. attempt to divide their attention between texting or talking on the phone and the complex and dangerous task of driving a car. What about you? Do you risk becoming a casualty of distracted driving? Are you ready to take the pledge to stop this dangerous behavior?

1. While driving, do you:
(place a check next to each behavior you engage in)

_____ talk on your cell phone?

_____ dial numbers on your cell phone?

_____ read text messages (or other mobile email messages)?

_____ type text messages?

Describe your current cell phone use while driving:

_____

_____

_____

2. What are some strategies for avoiding talking on your phone or texting while driving?

_____

_____

_____

3. If you don't think you will stop texting or talking on the phone while you drive, what are the reasons?

_____

_____

_____

Now, list three things that you can do to address these reasons.

_____

_____

_____

The following website provides information about the dangers of being on your phone while driving, true stories of accidents caused by texting and talking on the phone, and a pledge form to stop using the phone while driving: **www.nophonezone.com.**

Chapter Summary

- Unintentional injuries, especially car crashes, are a leading cause of death and injury in the United States, especially among young people.
- Distracted driving, aggressive driving, drunk driving, and poor use of safety features such as seat belts and bike helmets are the top factors behind automobile, bike, and motorcycle accidents and injuries.
- Falls, caused by slippery or unstable flooring, stairs, or ladders, are the top cause of injury at home.
- Careless handling of lit cigarettes or candles, along with improperly used or maintained cooking and heating equipment, are the causes of most home fires. Participate in fire drills. Regularly check smoke detectors and have an emergency plan ready in case of fire, including escape routes.
- If there are guns in your home, keep them unloaded, put away, and away from children. Use a safety lock-and-load indicator, and always treat a gun as if it were loaded, even if you think it isn't.
- Violence is also a leading cause of death and injury among young people, especially young men.

- Violent crimes include murder, forcible rape, robbery, and assault.
- Most violent crimes are committed by men. Men are more likely to be murdered than women, and women are more likely to be raped. Women are also more likely to be victimized by domestic and intimate partner violence.
- Sexual violence can take many forms, including unwanted uncompleted sexual acts, unwanted touching, unwanted completed sexual acts, and noncontact violations such as voyeurism or sexual harassment. Many women who are sexually assaulted know their attackers.
- Date rape is a common problem on college campuses. Drinking and drug use is a factor in many cases of date rape, and the problem persists, in part, because of rape-tolerant attitudes and misconceptions about women held by some college men.
- Declining rates of violent crime show that prevention works, including personal steps such as knowing campus safety rules and resources, drinking moderately, encouraging a culture of safety and respect, handling guns safely, and reporting crime.

Test Your Knowledge

1. What cause of injury most often kills people in the U.S. between the ages of 15 and 24?
   a. car crashes
   b. violence, such as a fight or a gunshot
   c. drowning
   d. bike accidents

2. Which of the following activities is especially dangerous when you are driving?
   a. changing the song on your MP3 player
   b. texting
   c. talking on your phone
   d. all of the above

3. Carpal tunnel syndrome
   a. is due to repetitive motions.
   b. isn't an issue if you mostly use a keypad on a mobile phone or PDA.
   c. isn't an issue for people who use laptops.
   d. does not have long-term consequences.

4. What is the leading cause of unintentional injuries at home?
   a. drowning
   b. fire
   c. gunshots
   d. falls

5. About what percentage of murders are known to have been committed by someone the victim knew?
   a. 14%
   b. 44%
   c. 54%
   d. 84%

Get Critical

What happened:

At an off-campus party thrown in 2007 by members of the De Anza College baseball team in Cupertino, California, three members of the school's women's soccer team were about to head home when someone stopped them, whispering that in a side room, a very drunk teenage girl was alone with a group of guys.

The three friends tried to open the door to the room. When a young man inside held the door closed, the young women forced their way in. The friends described a scene that shocked them—a teenage girl was lying on a mattress unconscious, vomit clinging to the side of her face, while two young men performed sex acts on her and others stood by cheering.[79] The three women then dragged the girl out of the room and took her to a local hospital.

Since that night, the friends have traveled to campuses around the country to tell their story, and have inspired a campaign called "No Woman Left Behind" that urges students to help others in a moment of need.[80]

What do you think?

- If you heard a rumor about a drunk girl in a room with several guys, what would you do? Do you think the soccer players were right to intervene?
- Do young women who get drunk at parties want or deserve extra sexual attention or to be forced to perform sexual acts?
- Where is the line between consensual sex and rape in cases such as these?
- If you were to step in and intervene, how could you do so safely and effectively?

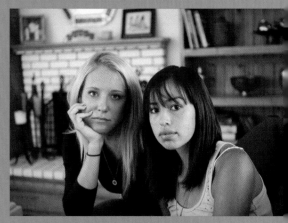

De Anza College students April Groelle and Lauren Chief Elk, who along with another friend rescued a drunk teen from an alleged sexual assault.

6. Are students more or less likely to be victims of violent crime at school than off campus?
   a. more likely to be victims of violent crime at school than off campus
   b. slightly less likely to be victims of violent crime at school than off campus
   c. much less likely to be victims of violent crime at school than off campus
   d. none of the above

7. What are the two most common types of violent crime reported on college campuses?
   a. robbery and sexual assault
   b. robbery and murder
   c. robbery and aggravated assault
   d. sexual assault and aggravated assault

8. What is a hate crime?
   a. a crime driven by dislike of someone personally
   b. a crime driven by bias against a person's or group's race, ethnicity or national origin, sexual orientation, or religious beliefs

   c. a violent crime against anyone
   d. none of the above

9. Sexual harassment
   a. occurs in both schools and workplaces.
   b. isn't a problem for men in college.
   c. only affects young women.
   d. only applies to the two people involved, not anyone else around them.

10. Date rape
   a. is more likely if one or both people on a date have been drinking.
   b. doesn't carry the same legal penalties as other types of rape.
   c. only affects women.
   d. all of the above

Get Connected

Health Online Visit the following websites for further information about the topics in this chapter:

- National Center for Injury Prevention & Control
  www.cdc.gov/injury/index.html
- National Safety Council
  www.nsc.org
- Home Safety Council
  http://homesafetycouncil.org
- American Association of Poison Control Centers
  www.aapcc.org
- Injury Prevention Web
  www.injuryprevention.org
- Motorcycle Safety Foundation
  www.msf-usa.org

- National Domestic Violence Hotline
  www.thehotline.org
- Childhelp National Child Abuse Hotline
  www.childhelp.org
- Rape, Abuse, & Incest National Network (RAINN)
  www.rainn.org
- No Woman Left Behind
  www.facebook.com/No-Woman-Left-Behind_Campaign/ 131828857122#/pages/No-Woman-Left-Behind-Campaign/ 131828857122

Website links are subject to change. To access updated web links, please visit **www.pearsonhighered.com/choosinghealth**.

References

i. Xu, J., Kochanek, K. D., Murphy, S., & Tejada-Vera, B. (2010). Deaths: Final data for 2007. *National Vital Statistics Reports, 58,* (19). Retrieved from http://www.cdc.gov/ NCHS/data/nvsr58/nvsr58_19.pdf

ii. National Institute on Alcohol Abuse and Alcoholism. (2010). *Rethinking drinking: Alcohol and your health.* Retrieved from http://rethinkingdrinking.niaaa.nih.gov/ WhatsTheHarm/WhatAreTheRisks.asp

iii. Austin, M. (2009, June). Texting while driving: How dangerous is it? *Car and Driver.* Retrieved from www.caranddriver.com/ features/09q2/texting_while_driving_how_ dangerous_is_it_-feature

iv. Carr, J. (2005). *Campus violence white paper.* Baltimore, MD: American College Health Association.

1. Centers for Disease Control and Prevention. (2007). *The incidence and economic burden of injury in the United States.* Retrieved from http://www.cdc.gov/ncipc/ factsheets/costbook/Economic_Burden_ of_Injury.htm

2. Xu, J., Kochanek, K. D., Murphy, S., & Tejada-Vera, B. (2010). Deaths: Final data for 2007. *National Vital Statistics Reports, 58,* (19). Retrieved from http://www.cdc.gov/ NCHS/data/nvsr58/nvsr58_19.pdf

3. Centers for Disease Control and Prevention. (2008). National hospital ambulatory medical care summary: 2006 emergency department summary. *National Health Statistics Reports, 7,* 1–38.

4. American College Health Association. (2009). *American College Health Association*

National College Health Assessment (ACHA-NCHA II) reference group executive summary, Spring 2009. Retrieved from http:// www.acha-ncha.org/docs/ACHA-NCHA_ Reference_Group_ExecutiveSummary_ Spring2009.pdf

5. Centers for Disease Control and Prevention. (2008-2009). CDC *WISQARS (Web-based Injury Statistics Query and Reporting System) Fatal injury data.* Retrieved from http://www.cdc.gov/injury/ wisqars/fatal.html

6. National Highway Traffic Safety Administration, National Center for Statistics and Analysis. (2009). Speeding. In *Traffic safety facts: 2008 data.* Retrieved from http:// www-nrd.nhtsa.dot.gov/Pubs/811162 .pdf

7. National Highway Traffic Safety Administration. (n.d.). *Think fast...* Retrieved from http://www.nhtsa.gov/DOT/NHTSA/ Traffic%20Injury%20Control/Articles/ Associated%20Files/think.pdf

8. American Automobile Association, Foundation for Traffic Safety. (2009). *Aggressive driving: Research update,* p. 2. Retrieved from http://www.aaafoundation .org/pdf/AggressiveDrivingResearch Update2009.pdf

9. Austin, M. (2009, June). Texting while driving: How dangerous is it? *Car and Driver.* Retrieved from www.caranddriver.com/ features/09q2/texting_while_driving_how_ dangerous_is_it_-feature

10. Patten, C. J. D., Kircher, A., Ostlund, J., & Nilsson, L. (2004). Using mobile tele-

phones: Cognitive workload and attention resource allocation. *Accident Analysis and Prevention, 36,* 341–350.

11. Redelmeier, D. A., & Tibshirani, R. J. (1997). Association between cellular-telephone calls and motor vehicle collisions. *New England Journal of Medicine, 336,* 453–458.

12. Strayer, D. L., & Johnston, W. A. (2001). Driven to distraction: Dual task studies of simulated driving and conversing on a cellular phone. *Psychological Science, 12,* 462–466.

13. Strayer, D. L., Drews, F. A., & Crouch, D. J. (2006). A comparison of the cell phone driver and the drunk driver. *Human Factors, 48,* 381–391.

14. Hosking, S., Young, K., & Regan, M. (2006). *The effects of text messaging on young novice driver performance* (Report No. 246). Monash University Accident Research Centre. Retrieved from http://www.monash.edu.au/muarc/reports/muarc246.pdf

15. National Highway Traffic Safety Administration, National Center for Statistics and Analysis. (2008). Persons killed, by highest driver blood alcohol concentration (BAC) in the crash, 1994 - 2008 - State : USA. *Fatality Analysis Reporting System Encyclopedia.* Retrieved from http://www-fars.nhtsa.dot.gov/Trends/TrendsAlcohol.aspx

16. Jones, R. K., Shinar, D., & Walsh, J. M. (2003). *State of knowledge of drug-impaired driving* (Report DOT HS 809 642). National Highway Traffic Safety Administration.

17. Wiegand, D., Hanowski, R., Olson, R., & Melvin, W. (2008). *Fatigue analyses: From 16 months of naturalistic commercial motor vehicle driving data.* The National Surface Transportation Safety Center for Excellence. Retrieved from http://scholar.lib.vt.edu/VTTI/reports/FatigueAnalyses_061208.pdf

18. National Highway Traffic Safety Administration. (2009, August). Seat belt use in 2008—Demographic results. *Traffic safety facts: Research note* (Report DOT HS 811 183). Retrieved from http://www-nrd.nhtsa.dot.gov/Pubs/811183.PDF

19. National Highway Traffic Safety Administration. (2010). *The top 5 things you should know about buckling up* (Report DOT HS 811 257). Retrieved from http://trafficsafetymarketing.gov/bua/brochures/general/links/SeatBeltTop5Flyer.pdf

20. California Department of Motor Vehicles. (2010). Seat belts: Mistaken beliefs about seat belts. In *California driver handbook* (p. 19). Retrieved from http://www.dmv.ca.gov/pubs/

21. Centers for Disease Control and Prevention. (2010). *Child passenger safety: Fact-sheet.* Retrieved from http://www.cdc.gov/ncipc/factsheets/childpas.htm

22. Insurance Institute for Highway Safety, Highway Loss Data Institute. (2010). *Q&As: Electronic stability control.* Retrieved from http://www.iihs.org/research/qanda/esc.html

23. Centers for Disease Control and Prevention, National Center for Injury Prevention and Control. (2006). *CDC injury fact book.* Retrieved from http://www.cdc.gov/Injury/Publications/FactBook/

24. National Highway Traffic Safety Administration. (2009). Motorcycles. *Traffic Safety Facts: 2008 Data* (Report DOT HS 811 159). Retrieved from http://www-nrd.nhtsa.dot.gov/pubs/811159.pdf

25. National Highway Traffic Safety Administration. (2009, July). Motorcyclists injured in motor vehicle traffic crashes. *Traffic Safety Facts: Research Note* (Report DOT HS 811 149). Retrieved from http://www-nrd.nhtsa.dot.gov/Pubs/811149.PDF

26. National Highway Traffic Safety Administration. (2008). Bicycle helmet use laws. *Traffic Safety Facts: Laws* (Report DOT HS 810 886W).

27. Federal Highway Administration, Turner-Fairbank Highway Research Center. (2006). *Lesson 3: Pedestrian and bicycle safety.* Federal Highway Administration university course on bicycle and pedestrian transportation. Retrieved from http://www.tfhrc.gov/safety/pedbike/pubs/05085/chapt3.cfm

28. Centers for Disease Control and Prevention. (2009). *Falls among older adults: An overview.* Retrieved from http://www.cdc.gov/HomeandRecreationalSafety/Falls/adultfalls.html

29. Centers for Disease Control and Prevention. (2009). *Falls: The reality.* Retrieved from http://www.cdc.gov/SafeChild/Falls

30. Centers for Disease Control and Prevention. (2010). *Poisoning in the United States: Fact sheet.* Retrieved from http://www.cdc.gov/HomeandRecreationalSafety/Poisoning/poisoning-factsheet.htm

31. Centers for Disease Control and Prevention. (2010). *Unintentional drug poisoning in the United States.* Retrieved from http://www.cdc.gov/HomeandRecreationalSafety/pdf/poison-issue-brief.pdf

32. Centers for Disease Control and Prevention. (2009). *Fire deaths and injuries: Fact sheet.* Retrieved from http://www.cdc.gov/HomeandRecreationalSafety/Fire-Prevention/fires-factsheet.html

33. U.S. Fire Administration. (2006). *Fire safety 101.* Retrieved from http://www.usfa.dhs.gov/citizens/college/101.shtm

34. National Institute on Alcohol Abuse and Alcoholism. (2010). What are the risks? *Rethinking drinking: Alcohol and your health.* Retrieved from http://rethinkingdrinking.niaaa.nih.gov/WhatsTheHarm/WhatAreTheRisks.asp

35. Miller, M., Hemenway, D., & Wechsler, H. (2002). Guns and gun threats at college. *Journal of American College Health, 51*(2), 57–65.

36. Centers for Disease Control and Prevention. (2010). *Unintentional drowning: Fact sheet.* Retrieved from http://www.cdc.gov/HomeandRecreationalSafety/Water-Safety/waterinjuries-factsheet.html

37. Bureau of Labor Statistics. (2009, October 29). *Workplace injuries and illnesses—2008* (USDL-09-1302) [News release]. Retrieved from http://www.bls.gov/news.release/pdf/osh.pdf

38. Bureau of Labor Statistics. (2009). Table A-1: Fatal occupational injuries by industry and event or exposure, all United States, 2008. *Census of fatal occupational injuries.* Retrieved from http://www.bls.gov/iif/oshwc/cfoi/cftb0232.pdf

39. Bureau of Labor Statistics. (2009, November 24). *Nonfatal occupational injuries and illnesses requiring days away from work, 2008* (USDL-09-1454) [News release]. Retrieved from http://www.bls.gov/iif/oshwc/osh/case/osnr0033.pdf

40. Federal Bureau of Investigation, Criminal Justice Information Services Division. (2009). Violent crime. *Uniform crime report: Crime in the United States, 2008.* Retrieved from http://www.fbi.gov/ucr/cius2008/offenses/violent_crime/index.html

41. Federal Bureau of Investigation, Criminal Justice Information Services Division. (2009). Table 1: Crime in the United States by volume and rate per 100,000 inhabitants, 1989–2008. *Uniform crime report: Crime in the United States, 2008.* Retrieved from http://www.fbi.gov/ucr/cius2008/data/table_01.html

42. Federal Bureau of Investigation, Criminal Justice Information Services Division. (2008). Expanded homicide data table 1. *Uniform crime report: Crime in the United States, 2008.* Retrieved from http://www.fbi.gov/ucr/cius2008/offenses/expanded_information/data/shrtable_01.html

43. Feder, J., & Levant, R. (2007). Boys and violence: A gender-informed analysis. *Professional Psychology: Research and Practice, 38*(4), 385–391.

44. Centers for Disease Control and Prevention. (2008-2009). CDC W*ISQARS (Web-based Injury Statistics Query and Reporting System) Non-fatal injury data.* Retrieved from http://www.cdc.gov/injury/wisqars/nonfatal.html

45. Rand, M. (2009, September 2). *Criminal victimization, 2008* (Report NCJ 227777). U.S. Department of Justice, Bureau of Justice Statistics. Retrieved from http://bjs.ojp.usdoj.gov/index.cfm?ty=pbdetail&iid=1975

46. U.S. Department of Justice, Bureau of Justice Statistics. (1998, April 1). *Alcohol and crime.* (Report NCJ 168632). Retrieved from http://bjs.ojp.usdoj.gov/index.cfm?ty=pbdetail&iid=385

47. Hingson, R., Heeren, T., Winter, M., & Wechsler, H. (2005). Magnitude of alcohol-related mortality and morbidity among U.S. college students ages 18–24: Changes from 1998 to 2001. *Annual Review of Public Health, 26,* 259–279. Retrieved from http://arjournals.annualreviews.org/eprint/vcvaePUAKVDCcRnieMGH/full/10.1146/annurev.publhealth.26.021304.144652

48. Krug, E. G., Dahlberg, L. L., Mercy, J. A., Zwi, A. B., & Lozano, R. (Eds.). (2010, June). *World report on violence and health.* Geneva, World Health Organization. Retrieved from http://whqlibdoc.who.int/publications/2002/9241545615_eng.pdf

49. Federal Bureau of Investigation, Criminal Justice Information Services Division. (2009). Aggravated assault. *Uniform crime report: Crime in the United States, 2008.* Retrieved from http://www.fbi.gov/ucr/cius2008/offenses/violent_crime/aggravated_assault.html

50. Federal Bureau of Investigation, Criminal Justice Information Services Division. (2009). Table 32: Ten-ear arrest trends, Totals 1999–2008. *Uniform crime report: Crime in the United States, 2008.* Retrieved from http://www.fbi.gov/ucr/cius2008/data/table_32.html

51. Federal Bureau of Investigation, Criminal Justice Information Services Division. (2009). Expanded homicide data table 10. *Uniform crime report: Crime in the United States, 2008.* Retrieved from http://www.fbi.gov/ucr/cius2008/offenses/expanded_information/data/shrtable_10.html

52. Federal Bureau of Investigation, National Drug Intelligence Center. (2009). *National gang threat assessment 2009.* Retrieved from http://www.usdoj.gov/ndic/pubs32/32146/index.htm#National

53. Bureau of Justice Statistics & National Center for Education Statistics. (2008). *Indicators of school crime and safety: 2007.* Retrieved from http://nces.ed.gov/pubsearch/pubsinfo.asp?pubid=2008021

54. Campo, S., Poulos, G., & Sipple, J. (2005). Prevalence and profiling: Hazing among college students and points of intervention. *American Journal of Health Behaviors, 29*(2), 137–149.

55. U.S. Department of Education, Office of Postsecondary Education. (2008). *The campus security data analysis cutting tool.* Retrieved from http://www.ope.ed.gov/security

56. Federal Bureau of Investigation, Criminal Justice Information Services Division. (2009). Incidents and offenses. *Hate crime statistics, 2008.* Retrieved from http://www.fbi.gov/ucr/hc2008/incidents.html

57. Federal Bureau of Investigation, Criminal Justice Information Services Division. (2008). *Hate crime statistics year 2008.* Retrieved from http://www.fbi.gov/ucr/ucr.htm#hate

58. National Counterterrorism Center. (2009). *2008 report on terrorism.* Retrieved from http://wits-classic.nctc.gov/ReportPDF.do?f=crt2008nctcannexfinal.pdf

59. Forke, C. M., Myers, R. K., Catallozzi, M., & Schwarz, D. F. (2008). Relationship violence among female and male college undergraduate students. *Archives of Pediatrics & Adolescent Medicine, 162*(7), 634–641.

60. Centers for Disease Control and Prevention. (2009). *Understanding intimate partner violence: Fact sheet 2009.* Retrieved from http://www.cdc.gov/violenceprevention/pdf/IPV_factsheet-a.pdf

61. Tjaden, P., & Thoennes, N. (2006). *Extent, nature, and consequences of rape victimization: Findings from the National Violence Against Women Survey.* National Institute of Justice. Retrieved from http://www.ncjrs.gov/pdffiles1/nij/210346.pdf

62. National Network to End Domestic Violence. (2010). *Domestic violence counts 2009: A 24-hour census of domestic violence shelters and services.* Retrieved from http://nnedv.org/resources/census/2009-census-report.html

63. Nabors, E., Dietz, T., & Jasinski, J. (2006). Domestic violence beliefs and perceptions among college students. *Violence and Victims, 21*(6), 779–795.

64. Baum, K., Catalano, S., Rand, M., & Rose, K. (2009). *Stalking victimizations in the United States*. Bureau of Justice Statistics Special Report, National Crime Victimizations Survey. Retrieved August 2009 from http://bjs.ojp.usdoj.gov/index.cfm?ty=pbdetail&iid=1211

65. Buhi, E., Clayton, H., & Surrency, H. (2008). Stalking victimization among college women and subsequent help-seeking behaviors. *Journal of American College Health, 57*(4), 419–425.

66. Centers for Disease Control and Prevention, National Center for Injury Prevention and Control. (2009). *Child maltreatment: Facts at a glance*. Retrieved August 2009 from http://www.cdc.gov/ViolencePrevention/pdf/CM-DataSheet-a.pdf

67. Child Welfare Information Gateway. (2010). *Factors that contribute to child abuse and neglect*. Retrieved from http://www.childwelfare.gov/can/factors/contribute.cfm

68. Centers for Disease Control and Prevention. (2009). *Elder maltreatment prevention*. Retrieved from http://www.cdc.gov/Features/ElderAbuse

69. National Center on Elder Abuse. (2010). *Why should I care about elder abuse?* Retrieved May 2010 from http://www.ncea.aoa.gov/Ncearoot/Main_Site/pdf/publication/NCEA_WhatIsAbuse-2010.pdf

70. Carr, J., & VanDeusen, K. (2004). Risk factors for male sexual aggression on college campuses. *Journal of Family Violence, 19*(5), 279–289.

71. Krebs, C., Lindquist, C., Warner, T., Fisher, B., & Martin, S. (2009). College women's experiences with physically forced, alcohol- or other drug-enabled, and drug-facilitated sexual assault before and since entering college. *Journal of American College Health, 57*(6), 639–647.

72. O'Byrne, R., Hansen, S., & Rapley, M. (2007). "If a girl doesn't say 'no'...: Young men, rape, and claims of 'insufficient knowledge.' *Journal of Community and Applied Social Psychology, 18,* 168–193.

73. U.S. Equal Employment Opportunity Commission. (2009). *Sexual harassment*. Retrieved from http://www.eeoc.gov/laws/types/sexual_harassment.cfm

74. Hill, C., & Silva, E. (2005). *Drawing the line: Sexual harassment on campus*. American Association of University Women Educational Foundation. Retrieved from http://www.aauw.org/learn/research/upload/DTLFinal.pdf

75. Federal Bureau of Investigation, Criminal Justice Information Services Division. (2009). Forcible rape. *Uniform crime report: Crime in the United States, 2008*. Retrieved from http://www.fbi.gov/ucr/cius2008/offenses/violent_crime/forcible_rape.html

76. Sable, M., Danis, F., Mauzy, D., & Gallagher, S. (2006). Barriers to reporting sexual assault for women and men: Perspectives of college students. *American Journal of College Health, 55*(3), 157–162.

77. American Academy of Child and Adolescent Psychiatry. (2008). *Facts for families: Child sexual abuse*. Retrieved from http://aacap.org/page.ww?name=Child+Sexual+Abuse&section=Facts+for+Families

78. National Institutes of Health, National Library of Medicine. (2009). *MedlinePlus health topics: Child sexual abuse*. Retrieved from http://www.nlm.nih.gov/medlineplus/childsexualabuse.html

79. KTVU-TV. (2007, May 24). *Witnesses to alleged De Anza rape speak out*. Retrieved from http://www.ktvu.com/news/13370961/detail.html

80. ABC News. (2009, June 5). *Alleged gang rape ends with no criminal charges but civil suit pending*. Retrieved from http://abcnews.go.com/2020/story?id=7757324&page=1

15

Almost **7 billion people** share this planet.[i]

Since 1979, more than **20%** of the polar ice cap has **melted away**.[ii]

Every day, every person in the United States creates about **4.5 pounds** of **trash**.[iii]

Exposure to **radon gas** is the second most common cause of **lung cancer**.[iv]

Your Environment, Your Health

EXPLAIN why environmental health is a global issue.

DISCUSS how the world's expanding population stresses the environment.

DESCRIBE the effects of air pollution on personal and public health and the global environment.

IDENTIFY the most common routes by which contaminants enter a community's water supply.

COMPARE and contrast municipal and hazardous waste and discuss efforts to manage each.

ANALYZE your home environment for potential sources of inhaled and ingested pollutants.

EXPLAIN the roles of amplitude and duration of noise in promoting hearing loss.

DISTINGUISH between ionizing and non-ionizing radiation and identify several potential sources of harmful levels of radiation.

DISCUSS a variety of strategies to improve your own environmental health and that of your community.

Health Online icons are found throughout the chapter, directing you to web links, videos, podcasts, and other useful online resources.

As a society and individually, the increasing interest in protecting our

environment touches much of what we do, from what we eat to how we get to class to where we live. The importance of this environmental awareness is often framed in terms of "saving our planet." But is that what's really going on?

Studies of planetary history tell us that the Earth has kept on spinning whether it was covered with steamy jungles or with ice. Earth has survived meteor impacts, methane explosions, and volcanic eruptions that have thrown massive amounts of debris into the air, land, and water. So the likelihood that Earth will survive well into the future is not in doubt. The question is, will it remain inhabitable for us?

You might like to think of yourself as an independent agent, but the truth is, we all live in an **ecosystem,** a dynamic collection of organisms and their nonliving surroundings that function as a unit. Consider, for instance, the animals, plants, microbes, soils, and water in a small pond. Although most days your own "pond" probably doesn't feel much bigger than your college campus, we all ultimately live within one giant ecosystem—planet Earth. We depend on it to survive. Yet in recent decades, people have begun to examine how the global ecosystem is maintained, and to question how effectively humans are taking care of it.

As you study this chapter, you'll encounter examples of the consequences on human health when the ecosystem is damaged—increased rates of cancer, respiratory disease, and other health problems. The impact of the environment on personal health, public health, and species survival is the domain of a relatively new field of study known as environmental health. It's also the subject of this chapter.

Overview of Environmental Health

Environmental health is a discipline that addresses all the physical, chemical, and biological factors external to individual human beings, especially those that influence health. Its primary goal is the creation of health-supportive environments.[1] According to the World Health Organization, about 25% of all disease worldwide is linked to environmental hazards, and about 13 million deaths each year could be prevented by making our environments healthier.[2]

Human-made environmental contamination, or **pollution,** is a critical focus of environmental health. That's because pollutants can lead to acute health problems. A dramatic example occurred in Minamata, Japan, between 1932 and 1968; during that period a chemical manufacturer released methyl mercury into a nearby bay and thousands who consumed contaminated seafood suffered paralysis or death. Pollutants can linger in trace amounts in the environment for

ecosystem A dynamic collection of organisms and their nonliving surroundings that function as a unit.

environmental health The discipline that addresses all the physical, chemical, and biological factors external to individual human beings, especially those that influence human health.

pollution Contamination of the natural environment as a result of human activities.

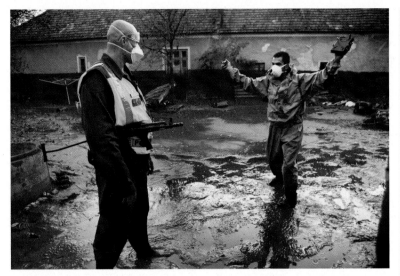

A flood of toxic sludge accidentally released from an alumina refinery in Hungary in 2010 caused environmental devastation, killed nine people, and injured almost 150 more.

we may think that, if our own immediate ecosystem is protected, then we must be as well.

But our local ecosystem is inextricably tied to that of our planet. As a result, no one community or nation can provide an environmental "island of safety." For instance, almost all of us watch for the lowest prices when we shop, and in recent decades, that often means buying goods made in China. This consumer demand has led to an enormous surge in manufacturing in China, a country where environmental enforcement is not as strong as it is in North America and Western Europe. The factories that make the goods we buy, and the coal-burning power plants that fuel them, release large quantities of mercury and other airborne pollutants. These pollutants have profound health effects in China, where air pollution is a leading cause of death.[4] But the damage doesn't end at China's borders. Scooped up by powerful winds, these contaminants blow across the Pacific Ocean and fall upon North America, where scientists have detected them in the air over Los Angeles and in snowfall in Colorado's Rocky Mountains.[5] The affordable flat-screen TVs and digital cameras that we buy here may seem like a bargain, but their affect on the global ecosystem is, in fact, very costly.

centuries, causing chronic health problems. Some are so potent that they change cellular DNA. These DNA changes, or mutations, can lead to birth defects, cancer, and other health problems.

Defining Your Environment

Your environment includes, of course, the features of the natural world that surround you, such as air, water, and soil. It also includes the human-made, or "built," environment, which encompasses physical structures such as schools and homes; manufactured products; components of transportation networks such as streets, sidewalks, subway systems, and airports; waste management systems; and human alterations to the natural world, such as dams or irrigation systems. Your environment also includes social aspects, including your socioeconomic status and factors in your community such as the level of crime. All of these influence human health. For example, a neighborhood where residents can easily walk to a market selling organic produce is likely to promote better health than a neighborhood with no sidewalks and a convenience store selling only sodas, snack foods, and cigarettes.

We said earlier that, although we all live in a local ecosystem, all humans share one global environment. This means that we're affected both by local conditions and by conditions many miles away. The fact that we all share one global ecosystem makes environmental health a global issue.

Environmental Health Is a Global Issue

In the United States, it can be easy to think that environmental health relates only to conditions close to home. The U.S. Environmental Protection Agency (EPA) exists to protect human health and to safeguard the natural environment—air, water, and land—upon which life depends.[3] We enjoy environmental policies that curb pollution, provide safe drinking water, and protect open spaces for relaxation and exercise. We also issue public health warnings if air quality is poor, or the water at a public beach becomes polluted. So

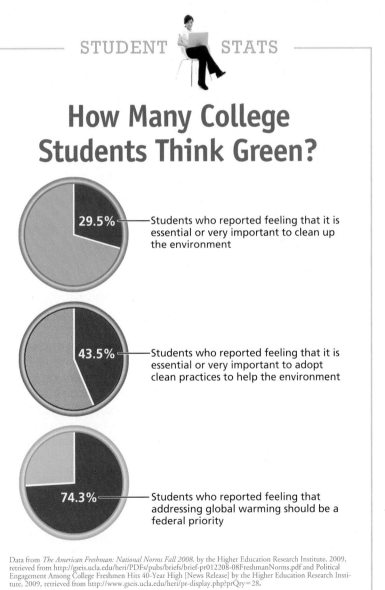

STUDENT STATS

How Many College Students Think Green?

29.5% — Students who reported feeling that it is essential or very important to clean up the environment

43.5% — Students who reported feeling that it is essential or very important to adopt clean practices to help the environment

74.3% — Students who reported feeling that addressing global warming should be a federal priority

Data from *The American Freshman: National Norms Fall 2008,* by the Higher Education Research Institute, 2009, retrieved from http://gseis.ucla.edu/heri/PDFs/pubs/briefs/brief-pr012208-08FreshmanNorms.pdf and Political Engagement Among College Freshmen Hits 40-Year High [News Release] by the Higher Education Research Institute, 2009, retrieved from http://www.gseis.ucla.edu/heri/pr-display.php?prQry=28.

The Evolution of Environmental Health

The environmental health movement got its start over a century ago, when advances in microbiology led to broad acceptance of the germ theory of disease. Public health experts came to understand that the diseases responsible for most illness and death were infectious; that is, that they were caused by harmful microbes in people's drinking water, food, and even in the air they breathed. Public health organizations began to develop policies for safe food-handling practices, the management of trash and sewage, and maintenance of a pure public water supply. These efforts paved the way for the broader developments in environmental health that emerged after Word War II.

The improved standard of living in the United States in the postwar years led to an unprecedented population boom. That meant more mouths to feed, which translated into a need for increased agricultural production. U.S. industry complied by providing a variety of new synthetic fertilizers and pesticides, most notoriously an insecticide called DDT, which began poisoning not just insects, but fish and birds, from the time it was first released for agricultural use in 1945. Then, in 1962, marine biologist Rachel Carson published *Silent Spring,* a book that was to galvanize the environmental movement. In it, Carson warned about the harmful effects of indiscriminate use of DDT and other synthetic pesticides—for example, she asked her readers to consider the effect of pesticides on songbird species, whose extinction might someday lead to a "silent spring."

Skeptics accused Carson of shallow science, but scientists found her research convincing and readers flocked to her cause. In the years that followed, as people in the U.S. learned about the effects of the defoliation tactics used in jungles during the Vietnam War, they became even more concerned about air, water, and soil pollution. The establishment of the EPA in 1970 was significantly influenced by these pivotal events.[6]

Today, environmental health still encompasses efforts to improve sanitation and reduce the use of harmful pesticides and other pollutants. But since the establishment of the Intergovernmental Panel on Climate Change (IPCC) in 1988, it is increasingly focused on studying the health effects of global climate change. An issue as broad as climate change may not seem to have immediate connections to personal health, but a glance at ongoing research shows just how intricately these two issues are related. For example, studies have found that even a slightly warmer planet can lead to more dangerous extreme weather events such as hurricanes, more outbreaks of infectious disease, and more food shortages due to altered growing seasons and crop failures.[7] Other potential health effects include increased air pollution and more cases of illnesses carried by insects and rodents.[8] Melting of polar ice means a rise in sea level that threatens coastal communities and could submerge entire islands. According to the World Health Organization, global warming already claims more than 150,000 lives worldwide every year.[9] It's clear, then, why global climate change has become the primary focus of environmental health. We'll look a little more closely at the mechanics of global warming and its effects later in this chapter.

sustainability The ability to meet society's current needs without compromising future generations' abilities to meet their own needs; includes policies for ensuring that certain components of the environment are not depleted or destroyed.

Toward Sustainability

In the last few decades, environmentalists, environmental health experts, and millions of people around the world have taken steps to reverse the effects of environmental damage or prevent further destruction. The concept of **sustainability** is a key aspect of this new movement toward improved environmental awareness and efforts.

Sustainability, in very general terms, is the ability to meet society's current needs without compromising future generations' abilities to meet their own needs; it includes policies for ensuring that various aspects of our environment do not become overtaxed, depleted, or destroyed. For example, many programs now exist that allow each of us *to offset,* or counterbalance, the global warming emissions we create. For instance, you may opt to take a long plane flight, and then offset the carbon emissions generated during the flight by contributing a few dollars to a program that sustains forests that absorb and recycle such harmful emissions.

Many college campuses have instituted measures to improve sustainability. How sustainable is life on *your* campus? Find out by reading the **Get Critical** at the end of the chapter.

Overpopulation and Globalization

We share the ecosystem that is Earth with countless other organisms—and none has a greater environmental impact than we do. The demands we place on the environment have skyrocketed in the last two centuries, driven largely by an explosion in the number of people living on our planet. Around the time of the founding of the United States, the world's population stood at just over 1 billion people.[10] In 2011, it reached almost 7 billion, and that number is estimated to exceed 9 billion by 2050.[11] Almost 99% of this population growth takes place in less developed countries, especially parts of South America and Asia. India, for example, is projected to add another 400 million people by

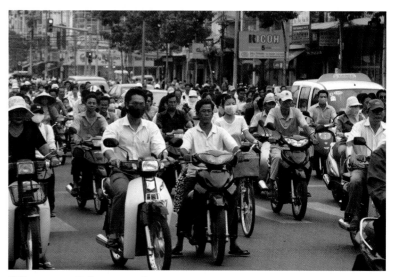

The world population is growing more rapidly than ever, especially in developing countries like Vietnam.

the year 2050, and Brazil another 240 million. The United States is projected to add about another 90 million.[12]

Along with this growth in sheer numbers of people comes a surge in human demands on the environment. Wealthier, more developed countries such as the United States, enjoy a lifestyle that consumes more energy, generates more waste, and uses more natural resources than that of less developed countries. For example, the United States has about 5% of the world's people but uses about 22% of its energy.[13] Overall, industrialized nations, which account for less than 20% of the world's population, contribute roughly 40% of global carbon emissions.[14] In short, industrialized nations have a larger **ecological footprint.** But as more and more nations transition out of poverty, and their citizens strive to achieve a higher standard of living, their ecological footprint grows. This phenomenon is one aspect of **globalization**—the interaction and integration of regional phenomena such as diets, technologies, arts and entertainment, economies, and other factors, on a global scale. Many of the forces behind globalization have positive aims. But they also carry enormous environmental demands. For example, if more of the world's population drives a gasoline-powered car on a regular basis, the effect is more drilling for oil, more pollution-emitting oil refineries, more tailpipe emissions, and more smog. It also means that fewer people walk, ride a bicycle, or take public transportation, leading to a more sedentary lifestyle and the accompanying health risks that you learned about in Chapters 5 and 6.

Global population control is one potential solution to this problem. Japan and more than a dozen countries in Europe have now achieved either *zero population growth*—in which a country's number of live births and immigrations simply replaces the number of deaths and emigrations—or *negative population growth*—in which a country's population actually declines. These achievements have come about less as a result of governmental mandates than of increased access to contraception, higher education, and professional opportunities for women.[15] But population control is only part of the solution, environmental experts say. Industrialized nations must also develop "greener" technologies and services, and share these with the developing world, so that globalization can have a more positive effect on our local and global environments.[16]

Developing these greener technologies and services requires an understanding of some key elements in our environment. First, we'll look at the air we breathe.

Air Pollution

Close to our planet's surface, air provides the oxygen and carbon dioxide that support human, animal, and plant life. Higher up, in the region of our atmosphere called the stratosphere, a natural layer of gas called *ozone* shields us from excessive sunlight. In between, a mixture of water vapor and other naturally occurring gases, called *greenhouse gases,* occurs. This layer allows solar heat to reach our planet, and retains some of this heat close to Earth's surface. This phenomenon helps keep our planet warm enough to sustain life (Figure 15.2 on page 356 illustrates this process).

Want to find out what the world population stands at today? Go to the World Population Clock: www.census.gov/main/www/popclock.html.

ecological footprint The collective impact of an entity on its resources, ecosystems, and other key environmental features.

globalization The interaction and integration of regional phenomena globally.

It's a delicately balanced system, and over the past 200 years, we've disrupted it, largely through the burning of *fossil fuels,* or fuels derived from decayed organic matter buried underground. In the United States, about 83% of the energy we use is derived from burning fossil fuels.[17]

Common Air Pollutants

Many different pollutants dirty our air, from gases that contribute to global warming to tiny particles of soot and other irritants that damage our lungs. In the United States, environmental regulators have identified almost 200 air pollutants that can harm human health and the environment.[18] Of these, seven pollutants receive closest ongoing scrutiny from regulators, health-care researchers, and scientists.[19] These include:

- **Carbon dioxide (CO_2),** a gas naturally found in Earth's atmosphere and, at normal levels, an essential part of life. Carbon dioxide is also a prime ingredient in emissions from the burning of fossil fuels, whether in the boiler room of a factory or the combustion engine of a car. Excessive CO_2 in our atmosphere not only pollutes the air, but serves as a greenhouse gas, trapping heat and contributing heavily to global warming. We'll look more closely at global warming shortly.

- **Carbon monoxide (CO),** also a gas that originates from the burning of fossil fuels. Poisonous to humans, it inhibits the blood's ability to carry oxygen, and excessive exposure can lead to sickness or death. Carbon monoxide can also be a dangerous indoor air pollutant, a facet we'll further address later in this chapter.

- **Sulfur dioxide (SO_2),** a gas that forms when fossil fuels are burned or processed or during metal processing. It is linked to numerous health problems, especially respiratory diseases. SO_2 can also dissolve in water to form acid, and is a primary culprit in the phenomenon of acid rain, discussed shortly.

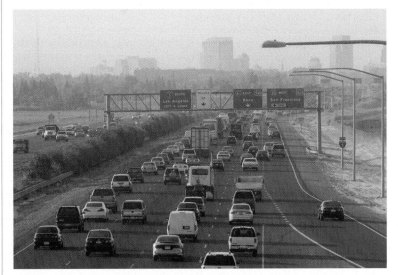

Cars produce many of the emissions that pollute our air.

- **Nitrogen dioxide (NO₂),** a gas also emitted during the burning of fossil fuel. Lower levels can contribute to respiratory illness, and higher levels can be fatal.

- **Ozone (O₃),** a gas composed of three atoms of oxygen, ozone is described by the EPA as "good up high, bad nearby."[20] That is, whereas ozone in the stratosphere is protective, ground-level ozone, which is produced when certain pollutants mix with sunlight, is a harmful component of smog (discussed shortly). Not only is ground-level ozone a potent respiratory irritant, it also damages crops, trees, and other plant life.

- **Hydrocarbons,** gaseous combinations of hydrogen and carbon that form during the burning of fossil fuels. Hydrocarbons are a precursor to ground-level ozone.

- **Particulates,** minute solid pollutants such as soot that form during the burning of fossil fuels, industrial processes, or the production of almost any kind of smoke, including tobacco smoke. Particulates can lodge in the lungs and trigger or worsen respiratory conditions.

In the United States, environmental health officials have established air quality standards for levels of these pollutants to protect public health. National and local air quality officials regularly monitor the air for these pollutants, and issue health advisories as needed through a tool called the **Air Quality Index (AQI).** When you hear of an air pollution–related health alert on your local radio station, for example, the announcement is usually triggered by a potentially hazardous local score on the Air Quality Index. For a guide to this index, see **Figure 15.1.**

Table 15.1 identifies some of the most common types of outdoor air pollution, their sources, composition, and health effects. Next, we'll take a look at how these pollutants accumulate into some broader environmental phenomena.

When the AQI is in this range:	...air quality conditions are	...as symbolized by this color:
0 to 50	Good	Green
51 to 100	Moderate	Yellow
101 to 150	Unhealthy for sensitive groups	Orange
151 to 200	Unhealthy	Red
201 to 300	Very unhealthy	Purple
301 to 500	Hazardous	Maroon

Figure 15.1 Air Quality Index (AQI).

Source: Air Quality Index (AQI) – A Guide to Air Quality and Your Health, by AIRNow, 2010, retrieved from http://www.airnow.gov/index.cfm?action=aqibasics.aqi.

Air Quality Index (AQI) An index for measuring daily air quality according to a list of federal air criteria, published by city or region.

Table 15.1: **Common Types of Outdoor Air Pollution**

Pollutant	Source	Description	Health Effects	Who's Most at Risk
Vehicle exhaust	All motorized vehicles and tools powered by fossil fuels, including cars, trucks, lawnmowers, tanker ships, and airplanes. One gallon of gasoline is estimated to produce about 19 pounds of CO_2, as well as many other air pollutants.[1]	A wide range of pollutants and toxins, including CO_2, CO, SO_2, O_3, and hydrocarbons. Particulate matter is also of high concern, especially from older vehicles and engines and locations where vehicle emissions concentrate, such as near freeways.	Breathing difficulties; increased rates of asthma and other lung diseases, cardiovascular disease, and cancer; increased risk of premature death.[2] Particulate matter in the lungs appear to trigger inflammation and can increase a person's risk of death from cardiovascular causes.[3]	People with chronic heart and lung diseases, older adults, those who live near busy freeways and roadways, and children. Levels of ozone and particulate matter are high enough in many parts of the United States to threaten children's health.[4]
Fossil fuel emissions	Power plants, which burn fossil fuels, including coal and natural gas, to generate electricity; office buildings and manufacturing facilities that burn fossil fuels.	A wide range of pollutants and toxins, including CO_2, CO, SO_2, O_3, and hydrocarbons. Particulate matter and mercury are also of concern, especially from power plants and factories that burn coal. Some factory emissions may also contain toxic metals such as lead, cadmium, or copper.	Cardiovascular and respiratory disease; cancer. At coal-burning plants, the health effects of mercury, a powerful neurotoxin, are also of concern. Emissions of toxic metals can cause developmental damage, lung damage, and certain cancers.	People with chronic heart and lung diseases and children may be especially vulnerable.
Smoke	By-product of burning both fossil fuels and plant matter, such as wood or tobacco. Can arise from large events like forest fires or small daily sources, such as a home fireplace or even a cigarette being smoked nearby.	Gases from wood smoke include toxins such as benzene. Pollutants include soot and fine particulate matter, which can settle in eyes and lungs.[5] Tobacco smoke releases approximately 4,000 chemicals, including 60 carcinogens.	*Mild:* burning eyes, runny nose, bronchitis. *Severe:* aggravation of chronic heart and lung diseases; increased risk of cancer.[6]	Wood smoke: people with chronic heart or lung diseases, including asthma; older adults; children. Tobacco smoke: both smokers and those who breathe secondhand smoke.
Deforestation and dust	Deforestation leads to soil dehydration and damage and excessive airborne dust. Because trees and plants recycle CO_2, deforestation also increases the levels of CO_2 in our atmosphere.	Fine particulate matter from a variety of sources (soil, vegetation, surface pollutants) in the form of dust; excessive CO_2 in the atmosphere contributes to global warming.	On an individual level, breathing difficulties and reduced lung function; on a public health level, increased risk of certain diseases and dangerous weather events due to global warming.	Given global wind and weather patterns, deforestation and dust affect both those who live near deforested or dust-producing areas and people half a world away.

References: 1. *Emission Facts: Greenhouse Gas Emissions from a Typical Passenger Vehicle,* by the Environmental Protection Agency, 2005, retrieved from http://www.epa.gov/oms/climate/420f05004.htm. 2. "Health Effects Associated with Exposure to Ambient Air Pollution," by J. Samet, & D. Krewski. 2007, *Journal of Toxicology and Environmental Health, Part A, 70,* 227–242. 3. "Mortality Effects of Longer Term Exposures to Fine Particulate Air Pollution: Review of Recent Epidemiological Evidence," by C. Pope, 2007, *Inhalation Toxicology, 19*(1), 33–38. 4. "Ambient Air Pollution: Health Hazards to Children," by the American Academy of Pediatrics Committee on Environmental Health, 2004, *Pediatrics, 114*(6), 1699–1707. 5. "Woodsmoke Health Effects: A Review," by L. Naeher, M. Brauer, M. Lipsett, J. Zelikoff, C. Simpson, J. Koenig, & K. Smith, 2007, *Inhalation Toxicology, (19),* 67–106. 6. "How Smoke from Fires Can Affect Your Health," in *AIRNOW: Quality of Air Means Quality of Life,* by AIRNow, n.d., retrieved from http://www.airnow.gov/index.cfm?action=smoke.index.

Environmental Phenomena Associated with Air Pollution

Air pollution increases the risk of asthma and other diseases in humans, and is harmful to animal and plant life. In addition, air pollution causes several broad environmental phenomena, including smog, global warming, thinning of the stratospheric ozone layer, and acid rain.

Production of Smog

A term originally coined from the words "smoke" and "fog," smog describes a brown, murky, ozone-laden mixture of pollutants that arises from motor vehicle exhaust, coal burning, and the manufacturing and use of paints, solvents, pesticides, and several other compounds. Weather and geography usually play a hand in creating this brew. In valleys where air is trapped by surrounding mountains, a weather phenomenon called a *temperature inversion* can maintain a cooler layer of air under a layer of warmer air. Sunlight then triggers chemical changes in the pollutants suspended in that air, forming ozone-rich smog that lingers until winds blow it away. Smog is most likely to develop during the summer months, when temperature inversions are more likely, and in warmer climates. According to the American Lung Association, almost 60% of the U.S. population lives in areas with unhealthful levels of ozone-rich smog.[21]

global warming A sustained increase in the Earth's temperature due to an increase in the greenhouse effect resulting from pollution.

Global Warming

As discussed earlier in this chapter, Earth supports life, in part, because layers of gases in our atmosphere provide a *greenhouse effect,* allowing the sun's energy to enter and then trapping some of it close to the surface of the planet. At the right levels, the greenhouse effect is necessary to our survival. But human-made air pollution has increased it **(Figure 15.2).** The result is **global warming,** or a type of global climate change that results in sustained rise in the planet's atmospheric temperature across geographic regions. Earlier in the chapter, we identified a range of health effects of global warming, from increases in infectious disease to loss of entire communities.

What's the evidence for global warming? Here are some sobering statistics:

- The global temperature record shows an average warming of about 1.3°F (0.74°C) over the past century.
- Seven of the eight warmest years on record have occurred since 2001.
- Within the past 30 years, the rate of warming across the globe has been approximately three times greater than the rate over the last 100 years.
- Past climate information suggests the warmth of the last half-century is unusual in at least the previous 1,300 years in the Northern Hemisphere.[22]

In light of this data, the Intergovernmental Panel on Climate Change (IPCC) has concluded that warming of the Earth's climate system is now "unequivocal."[22] The IPCC bases this conclusion on observations of increases in average air and ocean temperatures, melting of snow and ice, and average sea level across the globe.

What's the relationship between air pollution and global warming? Many of the gases that produce the greenhouse effect, such as carbon dioxide, methane, and hydrocarbons, are the same as those emitted in vehicle exhaust and other human activities that burn fossil fuels **(Figure 15.3).** The United States is currently the global leader in producing greenhouse gases, responsible for about 21% of all emissions.[23] But while the industrialized world has long led the way in producing greenhouse gases, the developing world is catching up. U.S. environmental regulators estimate that by 2015, emissions produced by developing nations will equal, and then surpass, those produced by more developed countries.[24]

But fossil fuel emissions are not solely responsible for global warming. Two additional, interrelated factors include deforestation and worldwide meat consumption. As you may remember from a discussion of photosynthesis in your high school biology class, plants use energy from sunlight to convert CO_2 and hydrogen into carbohydrates. In the process, they release oxygen as a by-product. The clearing of huge forests—typically rainforests—for residential, agricultural, and industrial use thus deprives us of a natural mechanism for the removal of CO_2 from our atmosphere. The importance of maintaining forested lands is acknowledged

Car vs. Campus Shuttle

"Hi, I'm Toby. Don't get me wrong, I feel like I'm a pretty 'green' person. I recycle and I've even started buying notebooks that are made out of recycled paper. But I grew up in LA where everyone drives, and I'm very attached to my car. There's a free campus shuttle that goes from my apartment complex to school, and all my friends try to get me to take it, but I don't. I like the freedom that driving gives me—I don't have to wait for the shuttle, I can put my music on the stereo, and I can leave stuff in my car if I want to. It's only a 15 minute drive; I don't think it's really that bad to take my car."

1: What do you think about Toby's decision to drive instead of take the campus shuttle? Would you take the shuttle or drive if you were in his shoes?

2: Toby lists some of the benefits of driving over taking the shuttle, what might be some of the benefits of taking the shuttle?

3: If Toby continues to drive, what could he do to help protect the environment as a driver?

Do you have a story similar to Toby's? Share your story at **www.pearsonhighered.com/choosinghealth.**

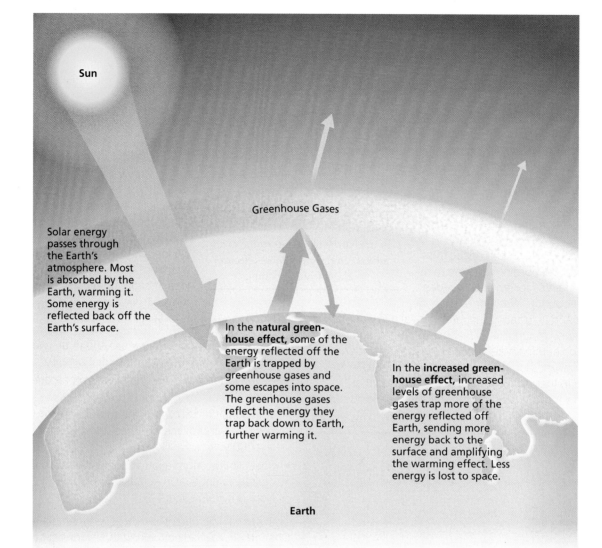

Sun

Greenhouse Gases

Solar energy passes through the Earth's atmosphere. Most is absorbed by the Earth, warming it. Some energy is reflected back off the Earth's surface.

In the **natural greenhouse effect,** some of the energy reflected off the Earth is trapped by greenhouse gases and some escapes into space. The greenhouse gases reflect the energy they trap back down to Earth, further warming it.

In the **increased greenhouse effect,** increased levels of greenhouse gases trap more of the energy reflected off Earth, sending more energy back to the surface and amplifying the warming effect. Less energy is lost to space.

Earth

Figure 15.2 The greenhouse effect.

internationally; nevertheless, the Nature Conservancy reports that every second of every day, a rainforest area the size of a football field is destroyed.[25]

Often, forests are cut down to clear land for the grazing of cattle and other ruminant animals raised for meat. Moreover, meat production is directly harmful because the digestive tracts of these animals produce methane, a potent greenhouse gas. Cows and other ruminant animals exhale methane with every breath, and excrete it in their wastes. A molecule of methane produces more than 20 times the warming of a molecule of CO_2 and remains in the atmosphere for up to 15 years.[26] Still, a blanket recommendation to choose vegetarian meals to help the environment may be overly simplistic, since highly processed soy products require significant energy to produce. Thus, the content of vegetarian meals matters, with locally grown whole foods a superior choice to packaged vegetarian meals.

In addition to choosing three times a day what to eat, you make choices each day about

> Want to take a trip through the Amazon rainforest? Log onto www.nature.org/rainforests/explore/video.html.

> What's your carbon footprint? Find carbon footprint calculators at www.nature.org/initiatives/climatechange/calculator and www.climatecrisis.net/take_action/become_carbon_neutral.php.

how to get from home to school to work, how to light, heat, and cool your home, whether or not to reuse, recycle, and compost, and what products to buy and avoid. Since each of these choices influences the generation of greenhouse gases, each contributes in a small way to your individual *carbon footprint*—the total greenhouse gas emissions for which you are personally responsible.

Thinning of the Ozone Layer

As you learned earlier in this chapter, the layer of ozone many miles up in the stratosphere is protective, shielding us from excessive solar radiation.

Certain industrial chemicals called *chlorofluorocarbons (CFCs)* can drift into the stratosphere and eat away at this blanket of planetary protection. Although this term may not be familiar, CFCs are actually a part of everyday life. Your refrigerator and air conditioner most likely rely on them, as CFCs are used in coolants. CFCs are also used as foaming agents in some rigid foam products, such as foam-based coffee

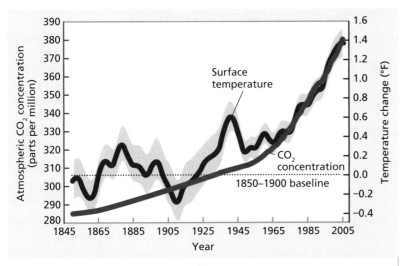

Figure 15.3 Increase in global surface temperature and in atmospheric CO₂ levels, 1850–2005. The increase in atmospheric CO₂ levels is mainly due to the burning of fossil fuels. The shaded gray area represents the 95% uncertainty range.

Source: Observed Temperature & Greenhouse Gas Trends: 2B. Atmospheric GHG Concentrations & Global Surface Temperature Trends, the Last 150 Years. by the Pew Center on Global Climate Change, 2006, retrieved from http://www.pewclimate.org/global-warming-basics/facts_and_figures/temp_ghg_trends/co2_and_temp.cfm. Used by permission.

cups or takeout containers. You can also find them in some spray propellants, some types of fire extinguishers, and some industrial solvents.

Over the last 30 years, CFCs have led to significant **ozone depletion,** a gradual thinning of the ozone layer worldwide, and a more dramatic loss of ozone—referred to as the development of "ozone holes"—over some parts of the world. Ozone depletion poses serious problems because it allows more UV radiation to reach the Earth. This increases your risk for sunburn, skin cancer, and cataracts (cloudy regions that develop over the lens of the eyes).[27] It also disrupts plant reproduction and threatens the survival of microscopic aquatic plant life—called *phytoplankton*—that is the foundation of the marine food chain. Scientists once thought that only regions closest to the poles, especially Antarctica, Australia, and parts of South America, were seriously affected. But research has revealed seasonal ozone thinning over other regions as well, including North America, where ozone levels declined by as much as 10% over the last three decades.[18]

Many countries, recognizing the dangers of CFCs and ozone depletion, have been phasing out their use of these chemicals. As a result, the ozone layer has started to recover. But because CFCs can persist in the atmosphere for decades, the ozone layer likely will only be fully restored decades after these chemicals are no longer released.

Production of Acid Rain
Some air pollutants do more than burn your eyes or form clouds of smog. They can also dissolve in water, turning the precipitation that nourishes our ecosystem into a hazardous deluge.

ozone depletion Destruction of the stratospheric ozone layer, which shields the Earth from harmful levels of ultraviolet radiation, resulting from pollution.

acid rain A phenomenon in which airborne pollutants are transformed by chemical processes into acidic compounds, then mix with rain, snow, or fog and are deposited on Earth.

groundwater The supply of fresh water beneath the Earth's surface, which is a major source of drinking water.

When sulfur dioxide and nitrogen oxide are released into the air from the burning of fossil fuels, they can react with other airborne matter to form acidic compounds. These acids then dissolve in rain, snow, or fog, falling to Earth and making waterways and soil more acidic. This phenomenon, commonly called **acid rain,** can harm fish, birds, animals, vegetation, and even damage human-made structures such as buildings and monuments.

In the United States, the regions that have been most affected by acid rain include industrial sections of the Northeast, upper Midwest, and Great Lakes area. Although environmental measurements show a reduction in acid deposits in these areas over the last 20 years, many affected waterways still show significant levels of acid, and scientists are working to study the long-term health and environmental effects of this type of pollution.[18]

What Can You Do to Reduce Air Pollution?

To reduce air pollution, reduce your carbon footprint, and improve the quality of the air you breathe, one way to begin is to reduce your energy consumption. For example, vehicle exhaust accounts for about one-half of all air-polluting emissions in the United States.[28] And every time you flick a switch, you increase your local power plant's use of fossil fuels. To find out how to curb your energy appetite, see **Practical Strategies for Change: Reducing Your Energy Consumption** on page 358.

Water Pollution

Water covers about 75% of the Earth's surface and supports almost all aspects of life on our planet. We derive our drinking water from two sources: surface-level fresh water, and more than 1 million cubic miles of **groundwater** found beneath our feet.[18]

Although water may seem like an endlessly available and renewable resource, only about 1% of the planet's entire water supply is accessible. As populations grow and global warming alters weather patterns, water shortages loom. By the year 2025, about 800 million people are likely to face water scarcity on a regular basis.[29] In addition to overpopulation and climate change, contamination reduces the amount of usable water.

> *By the year 2025, about 800 million people are likely to face water scarcity on a regular basis.*

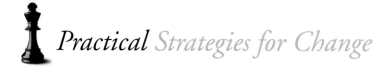
Reducing Your Energy Consumption

One way to reduce global warming and the other effects of air pollution is to reduce your consumption of electricity and fossil fuels. The following personal steps can make a real difference:

- **Drive less.** Few choices you make matter more than this when it comes to outdoor air pollution. Walk, cycle, take public transit, or ride-share. You'll get yourself in better shape, and you'll also save money.

- **Take care of your car.** When you do drive, fill your gas tank with cleaner fuels, keep your tires properly inflated, and keep your car tuned up. A better-functioning vehicle releases fewer pollutants and emissions.

- **Don't idle.** If your car is stopped while you wait to pick someone up, turn off the engine and cut your emissions.

- **Limit your use of other gasoline engines.** Do you really need that gas-powered lawn mower or snow blower when a push mower or shovel could do the trick? Many local air quality protection agencies offer incentives to get these polluting devices out of our communities, so find out what options are available to you.

- **Use less electricity.** Every time you turn on an appliance, you increase demand on your local power plant, which then has to burn more fuel. Turn off lights, electronics, and appliances when not in use. Watch out for "energy vampires"—devices such as computers that can stay on indefinitely and drive up energy use and your utility bills. Use power strips with a single on-off switch that let you turn connected electronics (such as your computer, scanner, and printer or TV, stereo, and DVD player) on and off all at once. And finally, replace incandescent light bulbs with energy-saving compact fluorescent bulbs.

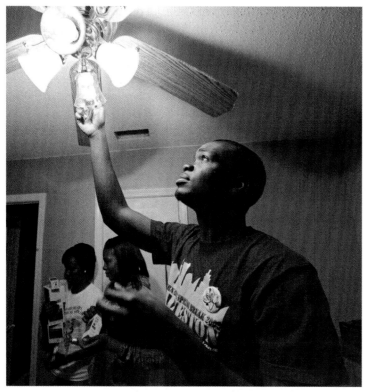

Compact fluorescent lightbulbs use about 75% less energy than traditional bulbs.

Types of Pollutants Found in Water

Many of the pollutants released into our environment can enter our water supplies, reducing water quality and creating significant health risks. One form of this pollution is infectious microorganisms spread by a lack of basic sanitation. According to the World Health Organization, about 1.5 million children worldwide die from illnesses related to contaminated water. About 2.5 million people lack access to improved sanitation, and more than 880 million people lack access to safe drinking water.[30]

In the developed world, too, water supplies can be contaminated by harmful microbes. However, a more common source of contamination is a variety of chemical and industrial pollutants. These include:

- **Petroleum products,** such as gasoline and motor oil. Petroleum products contain a wide variety of toxins, such as benzene, which is linked to cancer.

- **Polychlorinated biphenyls (PCBs),** which were used as insulating materials in electrical equipment and in paints, motor oils, floor finishes, and many other products until they were banned in the U.S. in 1979. They are highly stable and persist for many years in the environment.[31] PCBs have been linked to birth defects and cancer.

- **Dioxins,** chemicals found in herbicides and pesticides and also created during industrial combustion, such as when a power plant burns coal to generate electricity. Dioxins linger in the environment—and in the human body—for years, are extremely toxic, and have been linked to a wide variety of health problems, including immune disorders, liver damage, and cancer. Because dioxins accumulate in the fatty tissues of animals, more than 95% of dioxin exposure in humans is thought to occur through dietary intake of meat, dairy, and seafood.[32]

- **Chemicals used in agriculture,** such as pesticides and herbicides. According to the Environmental Protection Agency, more than 1,055 active ingredients are registered in the United States as pesticides, used everywhere from the fields that grow our food to our own backyards.[33] Pesticides have been linked to a wide variety of health concerns, including birth defects and nervous system disorders.

Some common sources of water pollution are identified in **Table 15.2.** Many of us try to protect ourselves from such pollutants by reaching for bottled water. Before you reach for your next bottle, however, it's worth looking at how healthful bottled water really is.

Is Bottled Water Worth It?

In the developed world, most of us have access to a ready supply of clean water. According to national estimates, about 85% of the U.S. population gets its drinking water from a community water system, and the rest from private wells.[34] Still, over the last decade, many of us have also reached for another source of water—from bottles. In 2008, bottled water represented the second-largest category of all beverage sales, pulling in more than $11 billion. People in the United States now drink about 28 gallons of bottled water per person each year, an increase of about 15 gallons in a decade.[35]

Many of us opt for bottled water because we assume it is more healthful or more pure. But those assumptions aren't necessarily true. Contrary to what many people believe, bottled water is not required to exceed most health and safety standards set for drinking water

Table 15.2: **Common Types of Water Pollution**

Pollutant	Source	Health Risks
Bacteria	Inadequate sanitation. According to the World Health Organization, about 2.6 million people lack access to adequate sanitation.[1]	A wide variety of waterborne diseases, such as cholera and trachoma.
Lead	Older plumbing that uses leaded pipes. About 15–20% of lead exposure in the U.S. comes from drinking water affected by leaded pipes.[2]	A variety of health problems. This heavy metal poses an especially serious risk of developmental delay and brain damage in young children.
Petroleum products	Leaking underground gasoline storage tanks. In 2009, more than 100,000 underground storage tanks awaited cleanup.[3] Used motor oil poured down storm drains.	Contain a number of toxins, such as benzene, which is linked to cancer.
Chemical contaminants	Industrial and home use of chemicals and improper disposal into waterways. Leaky underground storage containers. Worldwide, the extent of industrial water pollution is too vast to tally accurately. In the U.S., the Great Lakes region alone has 43 polluted zones officially deemed "areas of concern."[4]	A wide variety of health problems, including cancers, thyroid disorders, and developmental disorders.
Pesticides and fertilizers	Crop production and horticulture that cause irrigation runoff or use aerial spraying. More than 1,000 pesticides are registered in the U.S. Since 1960, the use of fertilizers in the U.S. has increased sharply, with combined use of three common fertilizers climbing from 46 pounds per acre in 1960 to 138 pounds per acre in 2005.[5]	A wide variety of health problems, including nervous system disorders and cancers. Fertilizers flow into runoff and contaminate waterways, stripping water of oxygen and leading to hazardous algae blooms and death of aquatic life.
Raw animal sewage; antibiotics and hormones given to livestock	Industrial meat production facilities and feed lots, where animals and their wastes are kept in confined areas. The U.S. has about 450,000 feedlot operations.[6] Leaky or inadequate storage facilities for waste or improper waste disposal spread this waste into the water supply.	Infectious disease; development of strains of microbes resistant to conventional antibiotics; exposure to hormones. One study found that standard livestock waste management practices do not adequately protect nearby water resources.[7]
Pharmaceuticals	Discarding medications and health and beauty products improperly, such as pouring them down the drain or flushing them down the toilet; wastewater treatment doesn't yet address these substances. Traces of more than 100 different pharmaceuticals have been detected in drinking water in the U.S. and Europe.[8]	Studies of health effects are still underway. Concerns have prompted increased regulation to keep these substances out of water supplies.

References: **1.** World Health Organization. (2010). Climate change and human health: Water services for health. Retrieved from http://www.who.int/globalchange/ecosystems/water/en/index.html. **2.** "Reducing Lead Exposure from Drinking Water: Recent History and Current Events," by R. Mass, S. Patch, D. Morgan, & T. Pandolo, 2005, *Public Health Reports, 120*(3), 316–321. **3.** *American Recovery and Reinvestment Act of 2009 – Environmental Protection Agency Recovery Act Program Plan: Underground Storage Tanks Program,* by the Environmental Protection Agency, May 15, 2009, retrieved from http://www.epa.gov/recovery/plans/oust.pdf. **4.** *Great Lakes,* by the Environmental Protection Agency, 2009, retrieved from http://www.epa.gov/greatlakes/index.html. **5.** *EPA's 2008 Report on the Environment: Highlights of National Trends,* by the Environmental Protection Agency, 2008, pp. 1–37, retrieved from http://oaspub.epa.gov/hd/downloads. **6.** *Animal Feeding Operations Unified Strategy,* by the Environmental Protection Agency, National Pollutant Discharge Elimination System, 2002, retrieved from http://cfpub.epa.gov/npdes/afo/ustrategy.cfm. **7.** "Impacts of Waste from Concentrated Animal Feeding Operations on Water Quality," by Burkholder, J., Libra, B., Weyer, P., Heathcote, S., Kolpin, D., Thorne, P., Wichman, M., 2007, *Environmental Health Perspectives, 2,* 308–312. **8.** "Damming the Flow of Drugs into Drinking Water," by Pat Hemminger, 2005, *Environmental Health Perspectives, 113*(10), retrieved from http://www.ehponline.org/members/2005/113-10/spheres.html.

from the tap. Federal environmental and health regulators do not certify bottled water, and do not require that bottled water come from a particular source. Some brands are actually made from tap water.

Don't assume that bottled water is always free from contaminants. In one study of bottled water sold in the Houston, Texas, area, 4 of the 35 brands analyzed were found to be contaminated with bacteria.[36] A federal study found that safety and consumer protections for bottled water are often less stringent than those applied to tap water.[37]

Federal rules, however, do require that bottlers use certain terms and definitions when labeling their water, including:

- **Artesian, ground, spring, or well water.** Water from an underground source, which may or may not be treated.
- **Distilled water.** Water that has been boiled and recondensed, a process that kills microbes and removes natural minerals.
- **Drinking water.** Water intended for human consumption and sealed in containers with no additional ingredients except for disinfectants.
- **Mineral water.** Groundwater containing certain levels of dissolved mineral solids.
- **Purified water.** Water from any source that has been treated to be essentially free of chemicals, and possibly microbes.
- **Sterile water.** Water from any source that has been sterilized to remove microbes.[38]

The convenience of bottled water also presents its own environmental challenges. Every year, people in the U.S. throw away millions of empty plastic water bottles. These bottles can be difficult and costly to recycle, and often wind up in landfills. In the next section, we'll look more closely at this and other forms of pollution that affect the land.

What Can You Do to Reduce Water Pollution?

The choices you make each day have a direct effect on your ability to enjoy access to clean water. To reduce water pollution, take the following actions:

- Dispose of motor oil and similar products properly. Yes, it's a little more inconvenient to save used oil and take it to a disposal site, but it's worth the effort.
- Throw old soaps, lotions, and cosmetics away in the trash. Don't pour them down the drain or flush them down the toilet.
- Bring outdated medications to a medication or hazardous waste drop-off site, the location of which can be found by using the search tool at http://earth911.com. If such a program is not available in your community, ask your health-care provider for tips for proper disposal. And don't forget to recycle the plastic container!
- Limit the use of pesticides, herbicides, and fertilizers around your home.
- Choose environmentally friendly soaps and cleaning products that are biodegradable and don't contain chemicals called phosphates.
- Take your dirty car to the local car wash rather than cleaning it yourself. Most car washes are better equipped to treat such wastewater properly.

What's in That Bottle?

Since one brand of bottled water can be very different from the one next to it on the store shelf, it pays to take a look at the label before you buy. Reading the label may help you understand where the water came from, how it was processed, what health benefits it claims to offer, and how those claims are backed up. You may also find that the label doesn't provide direct answers—if so, switch brands or contact the company for more information.

Before taking a bottle of water to the register, ask yourself the following questions:

- What is the source of this water? Does it say artesian, ground, spring, or well water? Or does the label contain the abbreviation "P.W.S.," indicating that the water comes from a public (tap) water source?

- Even once you know the source, purity isn't guaranteed. Is the water labeled as purified? What processing, if any, has the water undergone? Two effective methods for removing microbes are *micron filtration* and *reverse osmosis* (also called ultrafiltration).

- Are there added sugars, as in the case of "vitamin" waters or energy waters? It is best to avoid waters with added sugars, which provide empty calories.

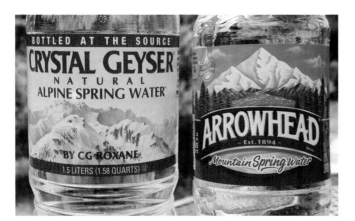

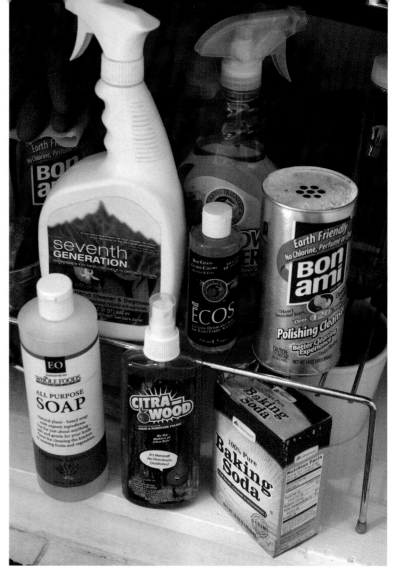

Environmentally friendly cleaners can help reduce water pollution.

tics. People in the U.S. throw out more than 250 million tons of this garbage each year.[18]

Garbage may be made up of items we no longer want, but it still requires a great deal of handling—and that handling is often far more complex than simply hauling it to a landfill or burning it in an incinerator. As landfill space becomes less available, more U.S. communities are encouraging residents to reduce, reuse, and recycle:

- *Reduction* is the altering of manufacturing and consumption processes to reduce the amount and toxicity of trash. For example, many food manufacturers are designing packaging that uses less plastic. For their part, consumers can choose to buy these products rather than versions with more plastic packaging. And there are other ways to reduce your trash as well. Switch to online bill payment wherever it's offered. And stop using a tray in the dining hall! More and more campuses are going "trayless," asking students to only choose food and drink they can carry to their tables without a tray. The move substantially cuts food packaging, uneaten food waste, and other garbage, encourages eating smaller meals, and reduces the use of water for washing.[39]

- When making choices at the grocery store or farmer's market, whenever possible opt for locally grown produce that is organic or grown without pesticides, and choose meats from animals raised by smaller, local, or organic producers.

Land Pollution

Every day, the average person in the United States creates about 4.5 pounds of trash.[18] Two types of trash are of concern: municipal waste and hazardous waste.

Municipal Waste and Its Management

Formally referred to as **municipal solid waste (MSW),** this refuse typically consists of discarded food, packaging, yard clippings, paper, and plas-

> **municipal solid waste (MSW)**
> Nonhazardous garbage or trash generated by industries, businesses, institutions, and homes.

- *Reuse* means switching from single-use items to versions that last. For instance, canvas shopping bags, cloth napkins, porcelain travel mugs, stainless steel water bottles, and rechargeable batteries.

- *Recycling* is the processing of discarded paper, glass, metal, and plastics to turn it back into usable goods. Your role in recycling is twofold: First, stop and think each time you're tempted to throw an item into the trash. Can it be recycled? If you're not sure, contact your local recycling center and find out. Second, purchase goods made from recycled materials whenever possible: notebooks, tote bags, jewelry, wallets, door mats, lawn chairs . . . you name it, a recycled version is probably available.

- A related action is *composting,* the conversion of organic waste such as food scraps and yard trimmings into a natural fertilizer. Composting is now done in both residential backyards and on a large scale to provide soil boosters for organic farming. According to national estimates, about 33% of municipal solid waste is now composted or recycled.[18]

See the **Behavior Change Workshop** on page 370 for more ideas about how to reduce, reuse, and recycle. If practiced consistently, these actions can make significant reductions in the amount of trash trucked to landfills. In 2003, for example, the city of San Francisco set aggressive goals of diverting 75% of the city's waste from landfills by 2010, and 100% by 2020.[40] Through the use of waste reduction measures, including a city-wide composting program, the city reported in early 2010 that 72% of all waste was being diverted from landfills.[41]

To find recycling centers in your neighborhood, go to **http://earth911.com.**

STUDENT STORY

Recycling Cell Phones

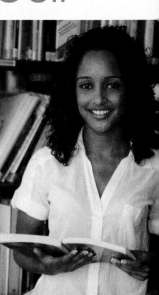

"Hi, I'm Camille. Like most of my fellow students, I feel like I'm pretty into the environment. But I recently got a new cell phone and when my boyfriend saw me throwing out my old one he told me that I should recycle it. Well, I didn't even know you could or should recycle cell phones and I didn't know how or where I could take it. We looked up cell phone recycling and found a center, but it's all the way on the other side of town. I don't know if I want to travel that far just for a tiny little cell phone."

1: Have you ever recycled a cell phone or other electronic device? Where did you take it?

2: What's in a cell phone that would make you want to recycle it?

3: If you think about the fact that some cell phone plans let you get a new cell phone every two years, why might it seem more important to start recycling them?

Do you have a story similar to Camille's? Share your story at **www.pearsonhighered.com/choosinghealth.**

Hazardous Waste and Its Management

Some waste is too toxic to be processed alongside regular trash. **Hazardous waste,** defined as refuse with characteristics or properties capable of harming human health or the environment, must be handled separately. This type of waste often consists of industrial chemicals or products containing heavy metals, which are difficult to treat or reuse safely.

Many of us equate hazardous waste with barrels of residue from factories. But we all share in the generation of hazardous waste. Many household products, such as paint, cleaners, garden products, and batteries, are too hazardous to simply throw in the trash. Many of the digital communication devices we use every day also generate toxic waste. Old computers, for example, can contain toxins and heavy metals. These machines, part of a phenomenon called **e-waste,** often end up dumped in developing countries, where people try to eke out a living by salvaging wires and other reusable parts amid the mountains of hazardous high-tech refuse.

Where does e-waste end up? These videos show where some of our e-waste ends up: **www.youtube.com/watch?v=OJZey9GJQPO, www.youtube.com/watch?v=ZHTWRYXy2gE&feature=related.**

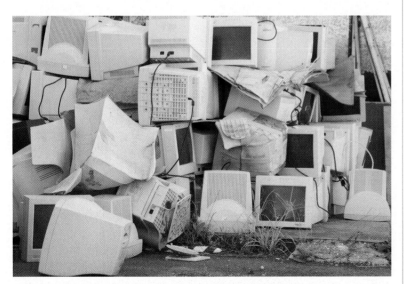

A new category of hazardous waste is "e-waste," items such as old cell phones and computers, which contain toxins and heavy metals.

The nature of hazardous waste means that handlers are typically inclined to dispose of it as quickly as possible, even if that disposal isn't always safe. Then, when toxic components leak or spill at a site, handlers may simply let the problem sit, unsure of how to clean it up—or

hazardous waste Garbage or byproducts that can pose a hazard to human health or the environment when improperly managed.

e-waste Hazardous waste generated by the production or disposal or electronic or digital devices.

Working for
Environmental Justice

Although we all feel the effects of environmental damage, its burden falls more heavily on some. In study after study, environmental regulators and researchers have noted that low-income and minority communities typically face increased health risks from the environment. Here are just a few recent examples documented by environmental scientists:

- Minority and low-income populations are more likely to live near high-priority

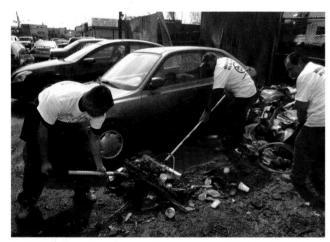

Volunteers from Queens, NY, help clean up garbage in their neighborhood.

Superfund sites, but are less likely to benefit from Superfund cleanup efforts, even after federal efforts to make the Superfund more equitable.[1]

- In North Carolina, schools with higher numbers of minority and low-income students were more likely to be located near large swine feedlots, which emit pollution that can affect air quality, water quality, and increase the prevalence of asthma symptoms.[2]

- Despite advances in the medical treatment of asthma, the condition continues to cause more sickness and death among African American and Hispanic children than Caucasian children, especially among those living in low-income urban areas.[3]

The reasons for these disparities are complex, but a few key factors stand out. Members of minority and low-income communities are more likely to live near businesses and industries that emit large amounts of pollutants, often because of zoning laws and tax incentives that make such businesses more likely to locate in these areas.[4] Members of these communities are also more likely to live in poor-quality housing, which may increase exposure to environmental hazards such as inadequate ventilation or mold.

These disparities have given rise to the movement for *environmental justice*, a two-part process that works to ensure that everyone:

- Enjoys the same degree of protection from environmental and health hazards.

- Has equal access to decision-making processes that influence the regional environment.

Environmental justice can be very global in its focus, or extremely local. Some community groups, for example, work to help give people half a world away access to clean drinking water. Others work in their own neighborhoods on issues such as trash pickup, tree planting, or the reduction of industrial emissions. If you are interested in helping to promote environmental justice, you can start by checking with your health instructor or environmental studies department on campus. These resources are likely to know of or be involved in efforts or research related to environmental equity.

References: **1.** "Superfund: Evaluating the Impact of Executive Order 12898," by S. O'Neal, 2007, *Environmental Health Perspectives, 115*(7), pp. 1087–1093. **2.** "Race, Poverty, and Potential Exposure of Middle-School Students to Air Emissions from Confined Swine Feeding Operations," by M. Mirabelli, S. Wing, S. Marshall, & T. Wilcosky, 2006, *Environmental Health Perspectives, 114*(4), pp. 591–596. **3.** "Asthma Disparities in Urban Environments," by T. Bryant-Stephens, 2009. *Journal of Allergy and Clinical Immunology, 123*(6), pp. 1199–1206. **4.** "Which Came First? Toxic Facilities, Minority Move-In, and Environmental Justice," by M. Pastor, J. Sadd, & J. Hipp, 2001, *Journal of Urban Affairs, 23*(1), pp. 1–21.

---

unwilling to bear the financial burden of doing so. As a result, the United States, along with many other countries, is dotted with hazardous waste "hot spots." U.S. environmental regulators started a concerted campaign to address hazardous waste sites in 1980 by passing the Comprehensive Environmental Response and Liability Act, commonly referred to as the **Superfund.** This fund, financed largely by taxes on the chemical and petroleum industries, pays for ongoing hazardous waste cleanup of land, surface water, and groundwater. Although more than 32,000 potentially hazardous sites have been identified under the Superfund, and almost 1,500 have been listed as high priority, only a fraction of these have been fully cleaned up. The program has managed, however, to contain or control serious health risks emanating from most of these sites. According to federal statistics, human exposure to contaminants is under control at about 82% of high-priority Superfund sites; the

Superfund A federal program that funds and carries out emergency and long-term identification, analysis, removal, and cleanup of toxic sites.

rest either show no documented health exposure or remain unclassified.[18] Most states also keep track of hazardous waste sites, conduct or supervise cleanups, and monitor any possible environmental hazards.

What Can You Do to Manage Household Hazardous Waste?

People in the U.S. generate 1.6 million tons of household hazardous waste (HHW) each year.[42] HHW includes products that contain corrosive, ignitable, toxic, or reactive ingredients. Any such product requires special care during disposal.

What can you do to reduce your contribution to HHW and clean up the HHW in your home and community? Try these ideas:

- First, don't purchase products with hazardous ingredients unless you have no alternative. For instance, skip the pesticides, switch to rechargeable batteries, and use common ingredients in your kitchen—such as baking soda and white vinegar—as cleaning solutions. See the **Get Connected** links at the end of this chapter for tips on how to make your own natural cleaning products.

- Think before you toss. Recognize hazardous household waste and dispose of it properly. Don't throw batteries, paint, or other chemicals in the trash. Instead, take these products to the collection site on your campus or in your community.

- As suggested earlier, don't allow motor oil to flow into open drains. Collect it and take it to your local collection site. Alternatively, some local garages will accept used motor oil.

- Take your e-waste to an approved disposal center in your community. If your community waste-management facility doesn't accept e-waste, ask a staff member to identify the nearest collection site. Some local businesses have special drop-off days, and some campuses schedule e-waste collection days.

- Even empty containers of HHW can pose hazards because of residual chemicals that might remain. Keep the lid or cap on containers and take them to your campus or community collection site.[42]

- Get involved! Identify the scope of the problem, the impact on the environment, the items that qualify as HHW, and the collection sites in your area. If you live in a dorm, for example, help organize a collection drive or collection center where students can turn in dead batteries, old florescent light bulbs, and other common HHW.

Pollution at Home

At home, you encounter pollutants in the foods and beverages you ingest and the indoor air you breathe. Let's take a closer look at how this occurs, as well as some changes you can make to reduce your exposure.

Pollutants in Foods and Beverages

When you eat an apple and drink a glass of milk, any pollutants present in your snack will enter your bloodstream and circulate through your body. Depending on their chemical makeup, some of these will then be quickly excreted. Others, however, are *fat-soluble,* which means that they will be transported into your body's fat cells, where they can be stored for long periods of time, building up gradually in a process called **bioaccumulation.** The role of human beings at the top of the food chain exacerbates this process, because we also ingest contaminants that have built up in the fats found in the animal products we eat, including meats and dairy foods. In a process called **biomagnification,** these pollutants have become more and more concentrated as they've traveled up the food chain **(Figure 15.4)**.

If you're concerned about the buildup of pollutants in the foods you eat, a few simple steps can reduce your exposure. If you eat meat, choose lean cuts and trim off all visible fat. Drink skim milk, and buy lower-fat cheeses whenever possible. Choose organic for both animal-based foods and produce. If you're concerned about the higher cost of organic foods, check out the **Consumer Corner** on page 84 of Chapter 4 for information on which foods retain the most pesticide residues and pick organic for those.

bioaccumulation The process by which substances increase in concentration in the fat tissues of living organisms as the organisms take in contaminated air, water, or food.

biomagnification The process by which certain contaminants become more concentrated in animal tissue as they move up the food chain.

Mercury is a toxin that commonly bioaccumulates in fish (and in your own body if you eat contaminated seafood). Use this mercury calculator to see if you're consuming too much mercury: www.gotmercury.org.

We also ingest pollutants that were not originally present in the food itself, but have leached into it from the product packaging, or from plastic containers in which we've stored it. For example, a pollutant called bisphenol A, or BPA, is found in baby bottles, plastic dinnerware, plastic beverage and food storage containers, food can linings, and other products. Although the health effects of this chemical are still being researched, it's a form of synthetic estrogen, and scientists have linked it to breast cancer in both males and females, prostate cancer, miscarriage, reduced sperm count, genital abnormalities, heart disease, and diabetes.

In October 2010, the Canadian government declared BPA a toxic substance, and earlier that year the U.S. FDA announced that it had "raised its level of concern" about BPA and was supporting industry efforts to replace it.[43] The FDA advises that, in the meantime, you avoid carrying, storing, or microwave-heating foods or liquids in containers with the recycling code 3 or 7. Although number 2, 4, 5, and 6 plastics are generally considered to be BPA-free and safe for carrying or storing food, water, and other beverages, always use glass or ceramics to microwave foods and fluids.

Pollutants in Indoor Air

Aspects of your home environment that you encounter every day—including paints, insulation materials, flooring, and furniture—may release toxic fumes or other contaminants into the indoor air. Other aspects of home life, such as exposure to smoke from a woodstove or fireplace, tobacco smoke, mold spores, lead dust, rodent droppings, dust mites, or pet dander can also build up in indoor air, especially in the winter when the windows are closed. When these pollutants are inhaled, they enter the bloodstream, travel throughout the body, and can be stored in fat tissues.

One indoor air pollutant of significant concern is radon. A radioactive gas released from uranium present naturally in rocks and soil, radon can leach into indoor air through a home's foundation. It can also enter groundwater and be released into the air as the water flows from faucets. The radioactive particles in radon are highly damaging to cells in the lungs. In fact, the National Cancer Institute lists radon exposure as second only to cigarette smoking as a cause of lung cancer.[44]

Another deadly indoor toxin is carbon monoxide (CO), which we mentioned earlier is a gas that impairs the ability of your bloodstream to carry oxygen. It is produced whenever any fuel such as gas, oil, wood, or charcoal is burned. If, for example, a wood-burning stove is not installed or maintained properly, dangerous levels of CO can be released. Unfortunately, CO is invisible and produces no odor, so its presence typically goes undetected. Low to moderate levels can produce headaches, nausea, confusion, and other symptoms, but can be fatal if allowed to persist. High levels can be fatal in minutes.[45]

Volatile organic compounds (VOCs) are a group of gases emitted from more than a thousand products, including paints, paint strippers, cleaning supplies, building materials, furnishings, glues, permanent markers, and office

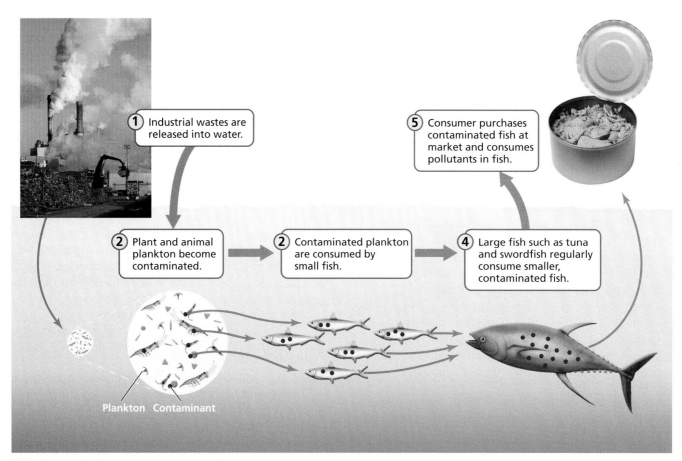

Figure 15.4 Biomagnification. In biomagnification, the concentration of contaminants increases as animals higher and higher in the food chain consume contaminated animal tissue. Biomagnification can increase the concentration of pollutants like mercury in fish that we commonly eat, like tuna.

In the figure:
1. Industrial wastes are released into water.
2. Plant and animal plankton become contaminated.
2. Contaminated plankton are consumed by small fish.
4. Large fish such as tuna and swordfish regularly consume smaller, contaminated fish.
5. Consumer purchases contaminated fish at market and consumes pollutants in fish.

Plankton Contaminant

equipment. In addition to irritating the eyes, nose, throat, and skin, they can cause headaches, difficulty breathing, dizziness, nausea, and other symptoms, and some are known to cause cancer.[46]

For a closer look at sources of pollution at home, see **Table 15.3.**

Health Effects of Pollutants at Home

Of course, we don't only eat or breathe indoor air when we're at home! The pollutants we encounter at school, work, shopping, or eating out can also influence our health. In fact, in parts of the world with a modern infrastructure, people spend more than 90% of their time indoors, giving indoor air quality significant potential to affect your well-being.[47] Some of the effects of foodborne and indoor air pollutants have been researched for decades and are well understood:

- Some substances, such as certain pesticides found in fruits and vegetables, radon gas, some VOCs, and toxins found in wood and tobacco smoke, are known carcinogens, meaning that they are capable of causing cancer.

- Some substances, such as BPA and other compounds found in plastics or agricultural chemi-

cals, are **endocrine disruptors,** meaning that they interfere with the body's hormones and endocrine system.

- Some substances, such as certain pesticides, mercury, and lead, are nervous system disruptors or **neurotoxins,** meaning that they have the potential to harm the brain or nervous system or interfere with childhood development.

- Some substances, such as sulfites used as food preservatives, cigarette smoke, pet dander, dust mites, and rodent droppings, are *allergens*, substances capable of causing allergies and asthma. For example, many studies have implicated "mouse allergen" as a significant cause of asthma in inner-city children.[48]

In other cases, the health effects of contaminants are not yet well understood. Just because a chemical is present in your body does not mean that it is harmful. Most contaminants must be present at a certain level before exerting any clear health effects. Scientists and medical experts are working to better define those thresholds. They are also trying to understand the cumulative effects of contaminants when they combine or are present together in a person's body.

Body burden is a person's cumulative exposure to and storage of chemicals and other pollu-

endocrine disruptor A substance that stops the production or blocks the use of hormones in the body and that can have harmful effects on health or development.

neurotoxin A substance that interferes with or harms the functioning of the brain and nervous system.

body burden The amount of a chemical stored in the body at a given time, especially a potential toxin in the body as the result of environmental exposure.

Table 15.3: **Common Types of Pollution at Home**

Pollutant	Source	Pathway into Body	Health Effects
Pesticides and herbicides	Fruits, vegetables, meat, milk, and other foods. In annual surveys conducted since 1994, up to 71% of food samples have shown detectable amounts of pesticide residue.[1]	Consumed in the diet, either directly or as stored in the tissues of animal products. Public health officials are currently tracking the presence of more than 35 agricultural chemicals in the bodies of people in the U.S.[2]	Varied. Some pesticides and herbicides are neurotoxins, while others are endocrine disruptors or have been linked to cancer.
Asbestos	Construction materials used before the 1970s and designed to resist fire, including insulation, roofing, flooring, cement, and surface coatings, also natural sources.[3]	Inhalation—asbestos fibers are light and small.	Asbestosis (scarring of lung tissue), lung and other cancers.
Lead	Old paint, gasoline, and pesticides containing lead. Lead paint was commonly used in the United States until 1978; lead-based pesticides were used even earlier but can remain in soil.	Inhalation or ingestion. Lead can be inhaled in dust or ingested through the mouth, especially by small children. Old lead paint flecks and chips can fall off surfaces and mix with soil outside homes or dust inside homes. Old lead-based pesticides can remain in soil for decades or longer.	Developmental delays and brain damage in children; reproductive problems and a variety of brain and nervous system disorders in adults.[4]
Mercury	Fish; emissions from combustion.	Inhalation or ingestion. Mercury, a heavy metal once commonly used in industry, bioaccumulates in tissues, including the tissues of fish, and is ingested when contaminated fish are eaten. It can also be inhaled from combustion emissions.	Varied. Mercury is a powerful neurotoxin, and at high levels, exposure is fatal. Large fish that are higher up in the food chain, such as tuna, Chilean sea bass, mackerel, and shark, carry more mercury than others.
Formaldehyde	Furniture made from plywood, particle board, or compressed wood; carpeting; some upholstery	Inhalation. Formaldehyde, a chemical found in glues and bonding agents, is released into the air and can be inhaled, especially in indoor spaces.	Coughing; eye, nose, and throat irritation; skin rashes; headaches; dizziness. Some people appear to be more sensitive to formaldehyde than others.[5]
Carbon monoxide (CO)	Indoor combustion units, including gas heaters, fireplaces, and gas stoves.	Inhalation. Because it is colorless and odorless, people are often unaware of the presence of this gas.	Dizziness, headaches, confusion, and even death resulting from interference with the blood's ability to carry oxygen. About 500 people in the U.S. die each year from unintentional CO poisioning.[6]
Radon	Decay of uranium in rocks and soil beneath or surrounding a home.	Inhalation of radioactive particles leached into indoor air or into well water. The particles become airborne when the water is used and are then inhaled.	Increased risk of lung cancer.
Mold (fungus) and other biological pollutants	Damp spaces, including basements, bathrooms, ventilation systems, and spaces within walls; dander from cats and dogs; allergens from dust mites in bedding and furniture.	Inhalation of airborne spores from mold, pet dander, or dust mite allergens.	Allergies and other respiratory problems. Although it isn't possible to remove all traces of mold, dander, or dust mites from a home, regular cleaning and moisture control can usually keep it contained.[7] Regular bathing of pets and housecleaning can help reduce pet dander in the air.
Phthalates, bisphenol A (BPA), and other chemicals found in packaging	Plastic products, including drinking cups, baby bottles, food containers, and water bottles; cans lined with plastic.	Ingested when food or drink that has touched plastic is consumed. In one study, people who used plastic bottles containing BPA showed a two-thirds increase in the level of the chemical in their urine after one week.[8]	Still being studied. However, a growing body of evidence indicates that these compounds may be endocrine disruptors, and BPA has also been linked to heart disease and diabetes.[9]
Volatile organic compounds (VOCs)	Cleaning products, paints, adhesives, solvents such as paint thinner and paint stripper, petroleum-based fuels.	Inhalation. VOCs readily evaporate at room temperature and are inhaled, often as fumes that have a distinct chemical odor. Outdoors, they are a precursor to ground-level ozone.	Varied. Known immediate effects of some VOCs include eye and respiratory tract irritation, headaches, dizziness, visual disorders, and memory impairment. Many VOCs are known to cause cancer in animals. Some are suspected of causing, or are known to cause, cancer in humans.[10]

References: 1. *EPA's 2008 Report on the Environment: Highlights of National Trends,* by the Environmental Protection Agency, 2008, pp. 1–37, retrieved from http://oaspub.epa.gov/hd/downloads. 2. *Third National Report on Human Exposure to Environmental Chemicals,* by the Centers for Disease Control and Prevention, 2005, retrieved from http://www.cdc.gov/exposurereport/report.htm. 3. *Understanding Asbestosis,* by the American Lung Association, 2010, retrieved from http://www.lungusa.org/lung-disease/asbestosis/understanding-asbestosis.html. 4. *Lead in Paint, Dust, and Soil: Basic Information,* by the Environmental Protection Agency, 2009, retrieved from http://www.epa.gov/lead/pubs/leadinfo.htm. 5. *An Introduction to Indoor Air Quality: Formaldehyde,* by the Environmental Protection Agency, 2009, retrieved from http://www.epa.gov/iaq/formalde.html. 6. "Carbon Monoxide—Related Deaths: United States, 1999–2004," by M. King & C. Bailey, National Center for Environmental Health, 2007. *Morbidity and Mortality Weekly Report, 56*(50), 1309–1312, retrieved from http://www.cdc.gov/mmwr/preview/mmwrhtml/mm5650a1.htm?s_cid=mm5650a1_e. 7. *Mold and Moisture,* by the Environmental Protection Agency, 2008, retrieved from http://www.epa.gov/mold/index.html. 8. "Polycarbonate Bottle Use and Urinary Bisphenol A Concentrations," by Jenny Carwile, Henry Luu, Laura Bassett, Daniel Driscoll, Caterina Yuan, Jennifer Chang, . . . & Karin Michels, 2009, *Environmental Health Perspectives, 117*(9), retrieved from http://www.ehponline.org/members/2009/0900604/0900604.pdf. 9. "Association of Urinary Bisphenol A Concentration with Medical Disorders and Laboratory Abnormalities in Adults," by I. Lang, T. Galloway, A. Scarlett, W. Henley, M. Depledge, & R. Wallace, 2008, *Journal of the American Medical Association, 300*(5), 1303–1310. 10. *An Introduction to Indoor Air Quality: Volatile Organic Compounds (VOCs),* by the Environmental Protection Agency, 2009, retrieved from http://www.epa.gov/iaq/voc.html.

tants. Scientists and health experts are assessing the effects of body burden through a process called **biomonitoring,** in which individuals' levels of certain contaminants are measured over time and then monitored to see what health effects develop. In the United States, biomonitoring is

biomonitoring Analysis of blood, urine, tissues, and so forth to measure chemical exposure in humans.

now a part of an ongoing national health survey, and some state and local governments have similar programs. Key findings from the most recent national biomonitoring survey include the following:

- Levels of lead in children's blood continue to decline, a positive sign that improved awareness and lead containment efforts are working.

Reducing Pollution at Home

When you eat:

- Choose organic when available and affordable.

- If you can't buy organic produce, scrub your fruits and vegetables with a dilute solution of dish detergent and room-temperature water. Remove the outer leaves of lettuce heads. For the inner leaves and other soft or small produce, swirl in the detergent solution for several seconds, then rinse.

- Reduce the amount of meat and animal-based products in your diet.

- Opt for fresh, whole foods over processed foods. Read food labels—the more ingredients you don't recognize or can't pronounce, the more processed the item is.

- Limit your use of plastic containers and utensils. Be especially careful to avoid microwave-heating food in plastic containers or plastic wrap.

- Choose the fish you eat carefully. The EPA recommends avoiding a few types of fish high in mercury, including swordfish, king mackerel, and shark, and limiting consumption of some types of tuna. To download a wallet card with specific recommendations, see the **Get Connected** links at the end of this chapter.

Where you live:

- Test your home for radon. To find out how, visit www.epa.gov/radon/radontest.html

- Install a carbon monoxide detector.

- Learn whether or not your home has surfaces covered with lead paint, and repaint, remove, or contain them. If you do repaint, opt for zero- or low-VOC paint.

- Help prevent mold by making sure bathrooms, kitchens, and basements have good air circulation and are cleaned often.

- When purchasing new furniture, mattresses, rugs, or carpeting, look for low-VOC options and keep it outdoors (or in a room with the windows open) for a few days before using or installing it.

- Vacuum thoroughly and frequently to remove dust mites, pet hair and dander, and other potential allergens.

- If you smoke, take it outside. If a roommate smokes, insist that he or she do the same.

- A majority of states in the U.S. have banned smoking in all enclosed public spaces. If your state is in the minority, avoid bars and restaurants where you'll be exposed to secondhand smoke.

- In all indoor spaces, good ventilation is key to air quality. If you suspect a ventilation problem in a dorm or classroom building on campus, let the building supervisor know.

- Get involved in green efforts on your campus that encourage administrators to make changes such as using low-VOC paint, carpet, and other products.

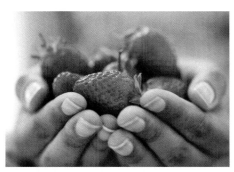

Choosing fresh, whole foods that have not been sprayed by pesticides can reduce your wastes and exposure to pollutants.

- Levels of cotinine, a by-product of the nicotine found in tobacco smoke, have dropped in the blood of nonsmokers over the past decade, a sign that efforts to ban smoking in indoor and outdoor spaces is working. But about 5% of U.S. adults have potentially risky levels of cadmium, with smoking the likely source, indicating that further research and smoking cessation efforts are needed.

- African-American adults carry higher levels of potentially risky mercury than Caucasians or Mexican Americans. At elevated levels, mercury is a powerful neurotoxin that can affect adults, children, and developing babies.

- Many other chemicals were found in the blood of U.S. adults and children, including phthalates (plasticizers that make plastic materials flexible), PCBs, insecticides, herbicides, and heavy metals. However, it's important to note that health effects of these exposures remains unclear in many cases.[49]

Now that you understand the potential health effects of pollutants that might be lurking in your home, you're probably wondering what you can do about them. Check out the **Practical Strategies for Change: Reducing Pollution at Home.**

Noise Pollution

What did you say? Something about noise pollution? Hold on—I need to take out my earbuds first.

Noise is a fact of contemporary life, in the streets, on campus, and in our homes. But noise pollution takes a toll on our hearing: According to national estimates, about 30 million people in the U.S. are exposed to daily noise levels that are likely to lead to early hearing loss.[50] Of the 28 million individuals with impaired hearing, about half have hearing loss at least partly related to damage from noise. Noise pollution can also trigger other health effects, including elevated blood pressure, headaches, irritability, sleep disturbances, and increased heart rate.

The loudness—or amplitude—of sound is measured in **decibels,** and in many aspects of our lives, those decibels are

decibel The unit of measurement used to express sound intensity.

high. Prolonged exposure to any sound over 85 decibels—the noise level of heavy city traffic—can damage the delicate hair cells of the inner ear and lead to gradual hearing loss. Sustained exposure to louder sounds can result in hearing loss more quickly. In fact, the surge in popularity of personal music devices such as MP3 players has resulted in a corresponding increase in hearing loss among people in their twenties.[51] If you turn the volume on your MP3 player all the way up, you'll be exposed to 120 decibels. Not only the volume, but the duration of exposure is important, too. More than 30 minutes of exposure to high-decibel noise—such as during a rock concert, or with an MP3 player set at more than three-quarters of maximum volume—can impair hearing. For a look at the decibel levels of some common sounds, see **Figure 15.5.**

> MedlinePlus illustrates how we hear: www.nlm.nih.gov/medlineplus/ency/anatomyvideos/000063.htm.

> Dangerous Decibels is an organization that provides information on hearing loss and protecting your ears: www.dangerousdecibels.org.

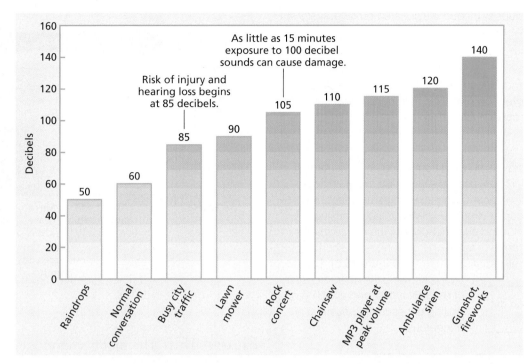

Figure 15.5 Decibel levels for common noises. Noise-related hearing damage can be caused not only by high decibel levels but also by prolonged exposure to noises above 85 decibels.

Source: Adapted from *Reduce Your Chance of Noise-Induced Hearing Loss,* by Emergency Medical Products, March 26, 2009, retrieved from http://www.buyempblog.com/2009/03/reduce-your-chance-of-noise-induced-hearing-loss/111, and *How Loud Is Too Loud? Bookmark,* by the National Institute on Deafness and Other Communication Disorders, 2009, retrieved from http://www.nidcd.nih.gov/health/hearing/ruler.asp.

What can you do to limit your exposure to noise pollution and protect your hearing? Try the following:

- Give your ears a break from your earbuds. Switch to over-the-ear headphones, which block outside noise and provide fewer decibels at the same volume setting. And follow the 60/60 rule: Don't go past about 60% of the device's volume, and don't listen for more than 60 minutes a day.
- When you go to concerts, stay away from the speakers, and wear ear plugs. The music is usually so loud (about 105 decibels) that you'll still be able to hear through them just fine.

> *The surge in popularity of personal music devices such as MP3 players has resulted in a corresponding increase in hearing loss among people in their twenties.*"

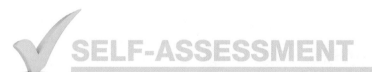

SELF-ASSESSMENT

Is Loud Music Damaging Your Hearing?

Is your hearing at risk because of loud music? Answer these questions to find out.

1. Do you hear a ringing or buzzing in your ear (tinnitus) immediately after exposure to music?   yes   no
2. Do you experience slight muffling of sounds after exposure, making it difficult to understand people when you leave the area with loud music?   yes   no
3. While listening to music, do you experience difficulty understanding speech; that is, you can hear all the words, but you can't understand all of them?   yes   no
4. Do people who are only three feet away have to shout to be heard while you are listening to music?   yes   no

HOW TO INTERPRET YOUR SCORE

A "yes" on any item means the music may be too loud and pose a risk to your hearing. Wear earplugs at clubs or concerts, and turn the music down on your MP3 player. If you think you may have hearing loss, make an appointment with an audiologist (a hearing professional who can measure hearing loss).

Adapted from information available at Center for Hearing and Communication. (2010). Noise & music fact sheet, retrieved from http://www.chchearing.org/noise-center-home/facts-noise/noise-music.

To complete this self-assessment online, visit **www.pearsonhighered.com/choosinghealth**.

- If you go to bars and clubs with loud music, step outside every so often to give your ears a break.
- If you work around noise, use protective headphones. Most workplaces supply them.
- Loud music, movies, and TV can be fun. But pace yourself. By keeping the volume lower now, you'll be helping to make sure you can enjoy those same sounds later in life too.

Radiation

Radiation, or energy that travels outward from a source in the form of invisible rays, waves, or particles, usually sounds like the stuff of warfare or science fiction. That's because radiation, in some cases, has the power to alter the molecular structure of living things, causing changes that can be harmful and even deadly. But the *electromagnetic spectrum*—the complete range of radiation from longest to shortest waves—is broad, and not all radiation is harmful **(Figure 15.6).** The trick is knowing the characteristics of different types, and avoiding or limiting exposure to those that are dangerous.

radiation Energy that travels in the form of rays, waves, or particles.

Types of Radiation and Their Health Effects

As you can see in Figure 15.6, radiation can be quite low in energy, like radio waves, which we typically don't even think of as a form of radiation. This is called non-ionizing radiation. In contrast,

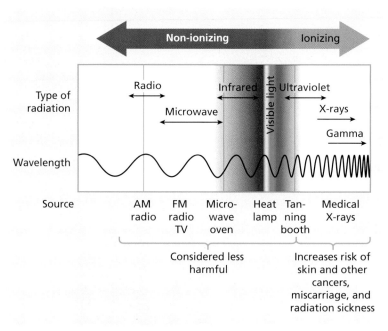

Figure 15.6 **The electromagnetic spectrum and sources of radiation.** Non-ionizing radiation is considered less harmful than ionizing radiation.

Source: Adapted from *Radiation Protection: Ionizing & Non-Ionizing Radiation*, by the Environmental Protection Agency, 2009, retrieved from http://www.epa.gov/radiation/understand/ionize_nonionize.html.

MYTH OR FACT?

Does Using a Cell Phone Fry Your Brain?

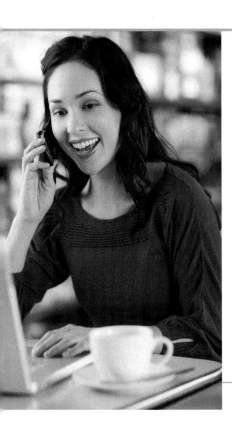

For most of us, cell phones are indispensable. But every time you use it, your cell phone emits radiation in the form of high-frequency electromagnetic waves. That fact has fueled a long-running controversy over whether this

radiation exposure can damage your brain or lead to brain cancer, especially when you talk with your phone held close to your ear.

Numerous scientific studies have tackled this question, but so far, the jury is still out. While some evidence points to a correlation between cell phone use and an increased risk of brain cancer,

scientists still aren't sure how significant this risk is. To find out, they'll need to track the health of cell phone users over long periods of time.[1] Only time will tell whether cell phones pose any real danger. In the meantime, you can play it safe by using a headset. Or put your cell on speaker and set it down. And remember that while

the risk of brain cancer and cell phone use isn't yet clear, another risk is—driving while distracted. Going hands-free with your cell phone is not the solution. If your phone rings while you're driving, pull over before taking the call.

Reference: **1.** "Review: The Controversy About a Possible Relationship Between Mobile Phone Use and Cancer," by M. Kundi, 2009. *Environmental Health Perspectives, 117*(3), pp. 316–324.

> *Not all radiation is harmful. The trick is knowing the characteristics of different types, and avoiding or limiting exposure to those that are dangerous.*

high-energy radiation, like medical and dental X-rays, is ionizing. The difference between the two has implications for your health:

- *Non-ionizing radiation* travels in the form of relatively long, shallow electromagnetic waves. It can cause molecules in matter to move, but can't alter them. Everyday examples include microwaves, radio waves, and visible light. In general, this form of radiation is considered less harmful, although questions have arisen about some electronic devices that rely on radio frequency (RF) waves, such as cell phones. For a closer look at this issue, see the **Myth or Fact?** box.

- *Ionizing radiation* carries enough energy to cause changes in molecules of matter, and exposure is considered more harmful, especially at higher or sustained levels. Ultraviolent (UV) rays

from the sun or tanning beds, X-rays from medical diagnostic devices, radon, and the fuel found in nuclear weapons and nuclear power plants are common forms of ionizing radiation. Radiation exposure is measured in units called *radiation absorbed doses,* or *rads,* and can cause damage at relatively low levels. Health risks include cancer, such as skin cancer arising from prolonged exposure to UV sunlight, and miscarriages. At higher levels of exposure, radiation can lead to *radiation sickness,* a multisymptom condition that can cause nausea, fatigue, and hair loss. At very high levels, radiation destroys the body's ability to make white blood cells and is fatal.

What Can You Do to Reduce Your Exposure to Radiation?

You can reduce your exposure—and your health risks, with a few simple steps:

- Watch your sun exposure. Protect yourself with sunscreen, sunglasses, and a hat.
- Skip the tanning salon. That bronze glow is actually a sign of radiation-induced skin damage.
- Use a headset when talking on your cell phone, or put it on speaker and set it down.
- Work with your doctor and dentist to limit your exposure to X-rays and other imaging devices that use radiation.
- Test your home for radon. To find out how, visit www.epa.gov/radon/radontest.html.

Curious about how much radiation you're exposed to in an average year? Let the EPA help you calculate your annual radiation dose at **www.epa.gov/radiation/understand/calculate.html.**

Watch videos of real students discussing environmental health at **www.pearsonhighered.com/choosinghealth.**

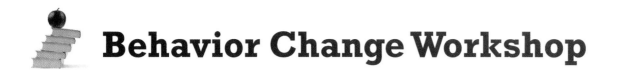

Behavior Change Workshop

To complete this workshop online, visit **www.pearsonhighered.com/choosinghealth**.

As you've learned from this chapter, many of your everyday actions can have an impact on the environment. While you may feel that you are just one person and nothing you do personally can make much difference in improving the environment, all the little things you do to "REDUCE, REUSE, RECYCLE" do add up.

Part I. Assess Your Behaviors

1. Consider the following list of little things you can do to Reduce, Reuse, or Recycle. Place a checkmark next to the items that you already do.

Reduce

❑ Raise (in the summer) or lower (in the winter) your thermostat 2 degrees.

❑ Cancel all junk mail. (Go to www.dmachoice .org/dma/member/regist.action to stop direct mail advertising and to www.optoutprescreen.com to stop credit card solicitations.)

❑ Switch to online bill payment.

❑ Turn off all TVs, computers, lights, printers etc. when you aren't using them.

❑ Turn off the faucet when brushing your teeth.

❑ Commit to walking to one place you normally drive to.

❑ Replace incandescent light bulbs with compact fluorescent bulbs.

❑ Don't buy products with lots of packaging.

❑ Go "trayless" in the dining hall.

Reuse

❑ Bring your own reusable bags to stores.

❑ Use cloth napkins or dishtowels rather than disposable napkins or paper towels.

❑ Use a reusable bottle rather than buying bottled water or other drinks.

❑ Don't throw away items (clothing, furniture, appliances) that you don't want anymore. Take them to a center that collects donations or give them to your friends.

❑ Take your own cup to the coffee shop.

❑ Buy rechargeable batteries instead of using disposable ones.

Recycle

❑ Check with your local recycling company to find out what items can be easily recycled near you.

❑ Always put paper and other recyclable trash in an appropriate container.

❑ Buy products that contain recycled materials.

❑ Take any e-wastes (old computers, cell phone, MP3 players, or other electronics) to certified e-waste recyclers.

❑ Purchase goods made from recycled materials whenever you can.

2. Target one behavior that you currently don't do. Ask yourself honestly: How ready am I to commit to a behavior change for each? What stage of behavior change am I in?

Target behavior: _____

Current stage of behavior change: _____

_____

Part II. Take Action

1. Describe what next step you will take to make this change.

Example: *I will purchase an insulated water bottle to take to class with me instead of buying bottled water at the campus snack bar.*

_____

_____

_____

2. Describe what obstacles might get in your way and how you will address them.

Obstacle   **How to Overcome**

_____   _____

_____   _____

_____   _____

_____   _____

● Chapter Summary

- Your environment has a direct effect on your health, and the choices you and others make help shape your environment and determine its quality. Environmental health is global—decisions made in one part of the world have the potential to affect all of us.

- Environmental health issues have changed over time, expanding from issues of hygiene and clean water to food production, industrial pollution, and global warming.

- Human population growth stresses our environment and can have effects that harm our health.

- Air pollution is primarily caused by the burning of fossil fuels. Some air pollutants cause smog or acid rain. Others lead to global warming or damage the Earth's protective ozone layer.

- Water pollution can arise from biological contaminants, such as disease-causing microbes, or chemical contaminants, such as industrial compounds or pesticides and fertilizers.

- Although many of us reach for bottled water as a safer, more healthful choice, there is no guarantee that bottled water is any purer than tap water.

- Land pollution is a result of our disposable society. The average person in the U.S. throws away about 4.5 pounds of solid waste each day. Some of this waste can be recycled or composted; some of it, however, contains toxins that make it too hazardous to dispose of without special containment or treatment.

- At home, we're exposed to pollution from the foods and beverages we ingest and the air we inhale. Some contaminants found in food can build up in our bodies' tissues over long periods of time, a process called bioaccumulation.

- Noise pollution damages hearing and causes other adverse health effects, including headaches, tension, and irritability. Exposure to about 85 decibels or lower is considered safe.

- We are all exposed to radiation on a regular basis, but only some forms are harmful, including UV radiation from the sun and ionizing radiation released by X-ray machines and other medical imaging devices.

- Through the personal decisions you make, you can improve both your own environmental health and that of those around you. Drive less. Carry reusable bags when you go shopping. Buy organic produce. Carry your own stainless steel water bottle and porcelain coffee mug, rather than getting a new disposable container every time you need a drink of water or buy a latte. These small choices add up to a healthier planet—and healthier people.

Test Your Knowledge

1. Which of the following statements about population is true?
   a. No countries of the world have yet achieved negative population growth.
   b. By 2050, the United States will have achieved zero population growth.
   c. Population growth typically slows as women become better educated.
   d. The world's population will probably peak at about 8 billion around the year 2050.

2. Which of these statements accurately characterizes global warming?
   a. Global warming harms wildlife, but hasn't hurt people yet.
   b. Global warming is a climate problem, not a health problem.
   c. Global warming is due to radon and stratospheric ozone.
   d. Global warming already has negatively affected human health.

3. Why is deforestation a problem?
   a. because it reduces the Earth's ability to remove CO_2 from the atmosphere
   b. because it reduces the Earth's ability to remove ozone from the atmosphere
   c. because it releases too much oxygen into the atmosphere all at once
   d. all of the above

4. Which of these statements about bottled water is true?
   a. Bottled water is not necessarily more healthful than tap water.
   b. Bottled water has less environmental impact than tap water.
   c. Bottled water is cheaper than tap water.
   d. all of the above

5. Why should you consider going trayless the next time you visit the dining hall?
   a. because you'll probably generate less trash
   b. because you'll probably waste less food
   c. because you'll probably eat less
   d. all of the above

6. Which common but potentially fatal indoor pollutant is released from the burning of fuels such as gas, oil, wood, or charcoal?
   a. carbon monoxide
   b. carbon dioxide
   c. radon
   d. mold spores

7. In modern societies, people spend about what percentage of their time indoors?
   a. 90%
   b. 75%
   c. 50%
   d. 40%

8. Which of these statements about endocrine disruptors is true?
   a. Endocrine disruptors are one way to clean up industrial air pollution.
   b. Endocrine disruptors haven't been linked to plastics.
   c. Endocrine disruptors only affect animals.
   d. Endocrine disruptors harm the functioning of the body's hormones.

9. What does biomonitoring refer to?
   a. ongoing studies that measure the levels of certain chemicals in people
   b. ongoing studies that measure the health of our biosphere
   c. ongoing studies that measure the amount of biofuels we burn
   d. none of the above

10. Which of these statements about cell phone use is true?
    a. Cell phone use can result in some exposure to radiation.
    b. Cell phone use has been clearly linked to brain cancer.
    c. Cell phone use has been clearly linked to cancer of the mouth, nose, and throat.
    d. all of the above

Get Critical

What happened:

Thousands of college campuses are "going green" with initiatives like offering low-emission shuttles to and from campus to cut down on driving, designing new buildings to be "green" or retrofitting older ones to be energy efficient, using energy-efficient appliances and light bulbs in residence halls, recycling paper in classrooms and offices, and composting food wastes in dining halls. Some schools have taken small steps, while others have set ambitious goals to become environmentally friendly fast.

How green is your campus? The nonprofit Sustainable Endowments Institute publishes report cards on at least 300 public and private campuses. You can find out if your school is included, see its ranking, and compare schools at www.greenreportcard.org.

What do you think?

- How important is it to you that your campus be "green"? Should student tuition money be used to develop and implement environmental initiatives at your school?

- What could be done on your campus to make it greener? How could the student body help to promote green initiatives?

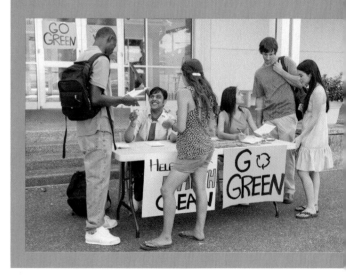

Health Online Visit the following websites for further information about the topics in this chapter:

- National Center for Environmental Health (NCEH)
  www.cdc.gov/nceh
- Environmental Protection Agency
  www.epa.gov
- Natural Resources Defense Council, Mercury in Fish wallet card
  www.nrdc.org/health/effects/mercury/walletcard.PDF
- Centers for Disease Control and Prevention National Biomonitoring Program
  www.cdc.gov/biomonitoring

- Environmental Working Group Shopper's Guide to Pesticides
  www.foodnews.org/fulllist.php
- Eartheasy Non-Toxic Home Cleaning
  http://eartheasy.com/live_nontoxic_solutions.htm
- College Sustainability Report Card
  www.greenreportcard.org
- Bottled Water Everywhere: Keeping it Safe
  www.fda.gov/ForConsumers/ConsumerUpdates/ucm203620.htm

Website links are subject to change. To access updated web links, please visit **www.pearsonhighered.com/choosinghealth.**

i. Census Bureau, International Data Base. (2010). *World population summary.* Retrieved from http://www.census.gov/ipc/www/idb/worldpopinfo.php

ii. Pew Center on Global Climate Change. (2010). Summer Arctic Sea ice decline. In *Global warming basics: Facts and figures.* Retrieved from http://www.pewclimate.org/global-warming-basics/facts_and_figures/impacts/seaice.cfm

iii. Environmental Protection Agency. (2008). *U.S EPA's 2008 report on the environment: Highlights of national trends*, pp. 1–37. Retrieved from http://cfpub.epa.gov/ncea/cfm/recordisplay.cfm?deid=190806

iv. National Cancer Institute. (2004). *Radon and cancer: Questions and answers.* Retrieved from http://www.cancer.gov/cancertopics/factsheet/Risk/radon

1. World Health Organization. (2010). *Environmental health.* Retrieved from http://www.who.int/topics/environmental_health/en

2. World Health Organization. (2008). *10 facts on preventing disease through healthy environments.* Retrieved from http://www.who.int/features/factfiles/environmental_health/en/index.html

3. Environmental Protection Agency. (2010). *About EPA: EPA's mission.* Retrieved from http://www.epa.gov/aboutepa/index.html

4. World Health Organization. (2009). *Country profile of environmental burden of disease: China.* Retrieved from http://www.who.int/quantifying_ehimpacts/national/countryprofile/china.pdf

5. Obrist, D., Hallar, A., McCubbin, I., Stephens, B., & Rahn, T. (2008). Measurements of atmospheric mercury at Storm Peak Laboratory in the Rocky Mountains: Evidence for long-range transport from Asia, boundary layer contributions, and plant mercury uptake. *Atmospheric Environment, 42*(33), 7579–7589.

6. Lewis, J. (1985, November). The birth of EPA. *EPA Journal.* Retrieved from http://www.epa.gov/history/topics/epa/15c.htm

7. McMichael, A., Woodruff, R., & Hales, S. (2006). Climate change and human health: Present and future risks. *The Lancet, 367*(5), 859–869.

8. Ebi, K., Mills, D., Smith, J., & Grambach, A. (2006). Climate change and human health impacts in the United States: An update on the results of the U.S. national assessment. *Environmental Health Perspectives, 114*(9), 1318–1324.

9. Patz, J., Campbell-Lendrum, D., Holloway, T., & Foley, J., (2005). Impact of regional climate change on human health. *Nature, 438*(17), 310–317.

10. U.S. Census Bureau. (n.d.). *International programs: Historical estimates of world population.* Retrieved from http://www.census.gov/ipc/www/worldhis.html

11. U.S. Census Bureau, International Data Base. (2010). *World population summary.* Retrieved from http://www.census.gov/ipc/www/idb/worldpopinfo.php

12. United Nations Population Division. (2009). *World population prospects: The 2008 revision population database.* Retrieved from http://esa.un.org/unpp/.

13. Energy Information Administration. (2006). *Energy kids.* Retrieved from http://www.eia.doe.gov/kids/classactivities/CrunchTheNumbers.pdf

14. Worldwatch Institute. (2008). *State of the world 2008.* Retrieved from http://www.worldwatch.org/node/5568

15. Population Reference Bureau. (2010). *Human population.* Retrieved from http://www.prb.org/Educators/TeachersGuides/HumanPopulation.aspx

16. Kjellstrom, T., Hakansta, C., & Hogstedt, C. (2007). Globalisation and public health: Overview and a Swedish perspective.

Scandinavian Journal of Public Health, 70(35), 2–68.

17. Energy Information Administration, Independent Statistics and Analysis. (2010). *Renewable energy consumption and electricity preliminary statistics 2009.* Retrieved from http://www.eia.doe.gov/cneaf/alternate/page/renew_energy_consump/rea_prereport.html

18. Environmental Protection Agency. (2008). *U.S. EPA's 2008 report on the environment: Highlights of national trends*, pp. 1–37. Retrieved from http://cfpub.epa.gov/ncea/cfm/recordisplay.cfm?deid=190806

19. AIRNow. (2003). *AIRNOW Air Quality Index: A guide to air quality and your health.* Retrieved from http://www.airnow.gov/index.cfm?action=aqibasics.aqi

20. Environmental Protection Agency. (2009). *Bad nearby.* Retrieved from http://www.epa.gov/oar/oaqps/gooduphigh/bad.html

21. American Lung Association. (2009). *State of the air 2009.* Retrieved from http://www.lungusa2.org/sota/2009/SOTA-2009-Full-Print.pdf

22. Environmental Protection Agency. (2009). *Recent climate change: Temperature changes.* Retrieved from http://www.epa.gov/climatechange/science/recenttc.html

23. Energy Information Administration. (2008). *Emissions of greenhouse gases report.* Retrieved from http://www.eia.doe.gov/oiaf/1605/ggrpt

24. Environmental Protection Agency. (2009). *Climate change – Greenhouse gas emissions: U.S. greenhouse gas inventory.* Retrieved from http://www.epa.gov/climatechange/emissions/usginventory.html

25. Nature Conservancy. (2009). *Rainforests at risk.* Retrieved from http://www.nature.org/rainforests/explore/threats.html

26. Environmental Protection Agency. (2010). *Methane.* Retrieved from http://www.epa.gov/methane

27. Environmental Protection Agency. (2010). *Health and environmental effects of ozone layer depletion.* Retrieved from http://www.epa.gov/ozone/science/effects

28. Environmental Protection Agency. (2008). *Key elements of the Clean Air Act: Cars, trucks, buses, and "nonroad" equipment.* Retrieved from http://www.epa.gov/air/caa/peg/carstrucks.html

29. United Nations. (2006). *UN-Water thematic initiatives: Coping with water scarcity.* Retrieved from ftp://ftp.fao.org/agl/aglw/docs/waterscarcity.pdf

30. World Health Organization / UNICEF Joint Monitoring Programme for Water Supply and Sanitation. (2009). *Millennium development goal assessment report.* Retrieved from http://mdgs.un.org/unsd/mdg/Resources/Static/Products/Progress2009/MDG_Report_2009_En.pdf

31. Environmental Protection Agency. (2009). *Polychlorinated biphenyls (PCBs).* Retrieved from http://www.epa.gov/osw/hazard/tsd/pcbs/pubs/about.htm

32. Food and Drug Administration. (2009). *Questions and answers about dioxins.* Retrieved from http://www.fda.gov/Food/FoodSafety/FoodContaminantsAdulteration/ChemicalContaminants/DioxinsPCBs/ucm077524.htm

33. Environmental Protection Agency. (2007). *Assessing health risks from pesticides.* Retrieved from http://www.epa.gov/opp00001/factsheets/riskassess.htm

34. Environmental Protection Agency. (2009). *Factoids: Drinking water and ground water statistics for 2009.* Retrieved from http://www

.epa.gov/ogwdw000/databases/pdfs/
data_factoids_2009.pdf

35. Rodwan, J. (2009). *Confronting challenges: U.S. and international bottled water developments and statistics for 2008.* Retrieved from http://www.bottledwater.org/public/2008%20Market%20Report%20Findings%20reported%20in%20April%202009.pdf

36. Saleha, M., Abdel-Rahmanb, F., Woodarda, B., Clarka, S., Wallacea, C., Aboabaa, A., . . . Nancea, J. (2008). Chemical, microbial, and physical evaluation of commercial bottled waters in the greater Houston area of Texas. *Journal of Environmental Science and Health, 43,* 335–347.

37. Government Accountability Office. (2009). *Bottled water: FDA safety and consumer protections are often less stringent than comparable EPA protections for tap water.* Retrieved from http://www.gao.gov/new.items/d09610.pdf

38. Environmental Protection Agency. (2006). *Water health series: Bottled water ba-*sics. Retrieved from http://www.epa.gov/safewater/faq/pdfs/fs_healthseries_bottlewater.pdf

39. Foderaro, L. (2009, April 28). Without cafeteria trays, colleges find savings. *New York Times.* Retrieved from http://www.nytimes.com/2009/04/29/nyregion/29tray.html?_r=2

40. San Francisco Department of the Environment. (2003). *Resolution setting zero waste date.* Retrieved from http://www.sfenvironment.org/downloads/library/resolutionzerowastedate.pdf

41. San Francisco Planning and Urban Research Association. (2010, February). Toward zero waste. *Urbanist.* Retrieved from http://www.spur.org/publications/library/article/toward_zero_waste

42. Environmental Protection Agency. (2008). *Household hazardous waste.* Retrieved from http://www.epa.gov/osw/conserve/materials/hhw.htm

43. Food and Drug Administration. (2010). *Bisphenol A (BPA).* Retrieved from http://www.fda.gov/NewsEvents/PublicHealthFocus/ucm064437.htm

44. National Cancer Institute. (2004). *Radon and cancer: Questions and answers.* Retrieved from http://www.cancer.gov/cancertopics/factsheet/Risk/radon

45. Environmental Protection Agency. (2010). *Protect your family and yourself from carbon monoxide poisoning.* Retrieved from http://www.epa.gov/iaq/pubs/coftsht.html

46. Environmental Protection Agency. (2010). *Volatile organic compounds (VOCs).* Retrieved from http://www.epa.gov/iaq/voc.html

47. Wu, F., Jacobs, D., Mitchell, C., Miller, D., & Karol, M. (2007). Improving indoor environmental quality for public health: Impediments and policy recommendations. *Environmental Health Perspectives, (115)*6, 953–957.

48. Matsui, E. C., Eggleston, P. A., Buckley, T. J., Krishnan, J. A., Breysse, P. N., Rand, C. S., & Diette, G. B. (2006, October). Household mouse allergen exposure and asthma morbidity in inner-city preschool children. *Annals of Allergy, Asthma & Immunology, 97*(4), 514–520.

Pongracic, J. A., Visness, C. M., Gruchella, R. S., Evans, R., & Mitchell, H. E. (2008, July). Effect of mouse allergen and rodent environmental intervention on asthma in inner-city children. *Annals of Allergy, Asthma & Immunology, 101*(1), 35–41.

49. Centers for Disease Control and Prevention. (2010). *Fourth national report on human exposure to environmental chemicals.* Retrieved from http://www.cdc.gov/exposurereport/

50. Daniel, E. (2007). Noise and hearing loss: A review. *Journal of School Health, 77*(5), 225–231.

51. American Speech-Language-Hearing Association. (2010). *Unsafe usage of portable music players may damage your hearing.* Retrieved from http://www.asha.org/about/news/atitbtot/mp3players.htm

- More than 1 in 8 people in the United States is over age 65.[i]

- Almost 40% of noninstitutionalized older people in the U.S. rate their health as very good or excellent.[i]

- The 55-and-older crowd is the fastest-growing age group on Facebook.[ii]

DISCUSS the changes in life expectancy and longevity in the United States that have occurred in the past several decades.

DESCRIBE the physical and psychosocial changes that typically accompany aging.

IDENTIFY at least five key strategies for aging successfully.

EXPLAIN how people develop a concept of death.

IDENTIFY six qualities of a good death.

COMPARE and contrast the available options when planning for end-of-life care.

IDENTIFY the five stages of grief.

DEVELOP strategies to create personal health and wellness throughout your lifetime, and face end-of-life issues with maturity and grace.

Health Online icons are found throughout the chapter, directing you to web links, videos, podcasts, and other useful online resources.

College life is a whirlwind of shifting possibilities.

Does a week ever go by that you don't think about changing your classes, projects, career goals, relationships, housing, diet, how you spend your free time . . . ? But in the midst of all the changes of your college years, one constant remains—every day, you are getting a little older.

Aging brings many gifts: a stronger sense of who you are and what you'd like out of life; greater power to make your way in the world; a broader range of experiences that, in turn, expands your appreciation of the people and situations around you and deepens your compassion. But aging also bring challenges. Your body starts to show the wear and tear of time. You experience the loss of loved ones, and face the task of defining for yourself what is a good life, and a good death.

This chapter can help deepen your appreciation of the gifts of aging, and help you meet its challenges. Although you might find yourself arguing that you're too young to "connect" with these goals, they're relevant for everyone simply because aging and dying are part of the human experience. What's more, the healthy choices you make today will help you to age with vitality and grace. And finally, understanding end-of-life issues can help you cope with the death of loved ones, and clarify your values, beliefs, and feelings about your own passing.

As with other key aspects of health, aging is as social as it is personal. We'll start by looking at how America, as a whole, is growing older.

Aging in the U.S.

Stand in front of a typical magazine rack and you'll see one headline after another that promises new strategies for how to stop feeling older, looking older, and growing older. These stories seem to suggest that, as a culture, we're afraid of growing old. The truth, however, is quite different. Rather than fearing aging, we're transforming it.

The United States is gearing up for a longevity revolution.[1] Already, about 12.5% of the U.S. population are over the age of 65. By the year 2050, according to federal government estimates, more than 88 million people in the U.S. will fall within this age category— about 20% of the population **(Figure 16.1).** Older people, in another significant shift from the past, are becoming more racially and ethnically diverse. In 2003, about 83% of older adults in the United States were Caucasians. By 2030, that figure will fall to about 72%, with Hispanics, African Americans, and Asian Americans representing growing segments of the older population.

Trends in Health and Health Care

At the same time that the number of older people in the U.S. is growing, key aspects of aging—health and wellness—are also changing:

- More older people are giving a positive report on their overall health. The number of people older than 65 rating their own health as only fair or poor has fallen steadily since 1993, with about 25% choosing such ratings in 2008.[2] Older African Americans, Native Americans, and Hispanics are less likely to rate their own health as excellent or good than Asian Americans or Caucasians.[3]

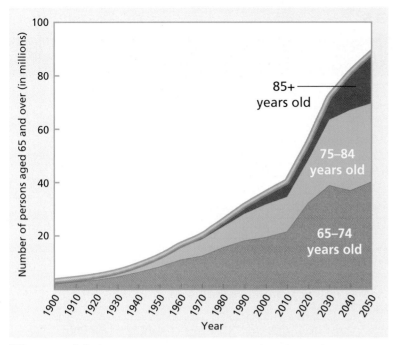

Figure 16.1 **Number of older people in the U.S. population, 1900–2050.**

Data from *Projected Future Growth of the Older Population – By Age: 1900–2050.* Administration on Aging, 2010, retrieved from http://www.aoa.gov/aoaroot/aging_statistics/future_growth/future_growth.aspx.

- At the same time, other key indicators of health, such as the mean number of physically or mentally unhealthy days a person experiences each month, have not improved. Older adults report having about 5 physically unhealthy days each month, and about 2 days per month when they experience significant mental distress.[4, 5]

- Most older Americans have at least one chronic health condition, such as hypertension, heart disease, cancer, diabetes, or arthritis, and many have multiple chronic conditions.[3] But major contributors to poor health among older people are also preventable or reversible. About 74% of older Americans report no leisure time physical activity and about 27% are obese.[6]

- The cost of providing health care for an older person in this country is about three to five times higher than the cost for someone younger than 65. So without overall improvements in the health of older people, our increasingly older population means that the nation's health-care spending will only continue to increase.[7]

The keys to better health as you age—a balanced diet, regular exercise, and avoidance of tobacco and alcohol abuse—lie within the reach of most people. As we'll see next, these choices affect not only how well, but also how long you can expect to live.

Life Expectancy

While you can't know for certain how long you'll live, your personal choices greatly influence the answer. **Life expectancy** in the U.S. has climbed steadily over the last century, due in large part to the growing availability of preventive health measures, such as vaccines, and public health campaigns, such as those that discourage smoking. Life ex-

life expectancy The length of time a person can expect to live, usually measured in years.

pectancy for a person born in the United States in 2010 is now projected at 78.3 years, with all races and ethnicities seeing gains over previous years.[8] There also appears to be ample room for further improvement. Some of the leading causes of death, such as heart disease, stroke, and type 2 diabetes, can be prevented or moderated through more healthful lifestyle choices. In fact, some researchers are concerned that the high rate of obesity in this country could reduce our life expectancy in coming years.[9]

Even with these gains, noteworthy gaps remain. One research study described the United States as a country of "eight Americas" in terms of longevity, distinguishing between these eight groups using a variety of racial, ethnic, economic, and geographic factors. According to this analysis, Asian Americans can expect to live the longest—almost 85 years. On the other end of the spectrum, African Americans living in the rural South or high-risk urban areas can expect to live about 71 years.[10] For an overview of the study's findings, see **Table 16.1.**

> While nothing can predict how long you'll live, you can calculate your life expectancy based on your health, habits, and lifestyle: **http://longevitycalculator.aarp.org.**

Gender and Longevity

Men, in general, cannot expect to live as long as women. Life expectancy for U.S. men now stands at about 75.3 years, almost 5 years less than women, who have a life expectancy of about 80.4 years.[7] This gender-based longevity gap is not unique to the United States. Throughout the developed world, women tend to live several years longer than men.[11]

As with aging itself, the factors at work in the gender longevity gap are complex and still under study. But researchers have pinpointed a few critical reasons behind women's longer lives, including:

- **Delayed cardiovascular risks.** Women tend to develop conditions such as heart disease or stroke in their 70s and 80s, about 20 years later than men.

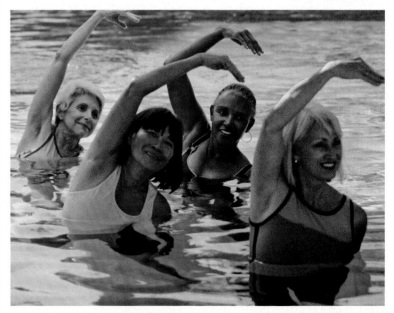

Women in the U.S. have a life expectancy almost 5 years longer than men.

Table 16.1: **Longevity Gap in "8 Americas"**

America Number	General Description	Definition	Average Life Expectancy (years)
1	Asian American	Asians living in counties where Pacific Islanders make up less than 40% of the total Asian population	84.9
2	North Central, low-income, rural Caucasians	Caucasians living in Northern Plains and Dakotas with 1990 county-level per capita income below $11,775 and population density less than 100 persons per square kilometer	79.0
3	Caucasian Middle America	All other Caucasians not included in Americas 2 and 4, Asians not included in America 1, and Native Americans not included in America 5	77.9
4	Low-income Caucasians in Appalachia and the Mississippi Valley	Caucasians in Appalachia and the Mississippi Valley with 1990 county-level per capita income below $11,775	75.0
5	Western Native American	Native American populations in the mountain and plains areas, predominantly on reservations	72.7
6	African American Middle America	All other African American populations not included in counties in Americas 7 and 8	72.9
7	Southern, low-income, rural African Americans	African Americans living in counties in the Mississippi Valley and the Deep South with population density below 100 persons per square kilometer, 1990 county-level per capita income below $7,500, and total population size above 1,000 persons	71.2
8	High-risk urban African American	Urban populations of more than 150,000 African Americans living in counties with cumulative probability of homicide death between 15 and 74 years old greater than 1%	71.1

Source: Adapted from "Eight Americas: Investigating Mortality Disparities Across Races, Counties, and Race-Counties in the United States," by C. J. L. Murray, S. C. Kulkarni, C. Michaud, N. Tomijima, M. T. Bulzacchelli, T. J. Iandiorio, & M. Ezzati, 2006, *PloS Medicine, 3*(9), Table 1, retrieved from http://www.plosmedicine.org/article/slideshow.action?uri=info:doi/10.1371/journal.pmed.0030260&imageURI=info:doi/10.1371/journal.pmed.0030260.t001.

- **Sex chromosomes.** Human beings have one pair of sex chromosomes, which determine—along with many other traits—whether you are male or female. Women have two X chromosomes. Men have one X chromosome and one Y. The X chromosome is larger than the Y chromosome and holds many more genes, some of which perform important functions. Because they have two X chromosomes, women basically have a back-up set of these genes, allowing their genomes to choose the best of the pair.

- **Fewer risk-taking behaviors.** As you learned in Chapter 14, men are much more likely than women to die from unintentional injuries such as car crashes, or intentional injuries caused by violence.

- **Emotional health and stress management.** As you learned in Chapter 2, women are less likely to internalize stress, loneliness, or anger than men. These emotions can have powerful health effects, especially over time.[12]

Being a man or a woman, however, is just one factor influencing how long you'll live.

What Happens As You Age?

When they hear the term *aging*, most people think of *biological aging*—the normal, ongoing, irreversible changes to the body that start at birth and continue until death. But like health and wellness, aging is much more than a physical phenomenon. *Psychological aging* encompasses changes to the brain and to mental health—including cognition, memory, and mood—that can come with advancing years. And *social aging* involves changes in relationships, career, and income. Not all of these changes happen to everyone, and if they do, the age at which they first occur varies widely from person to person. Moreover, they're interrelated: physical limitations can affect mood and so-cial life, and a reduction in work and income can influence physical and mental health.

If you find yourself feeling discouraged when reading the following discussion of age-related changes, bear in mind that the healthful behaviors you engage in right now can help to delay or reduce them. We discuss strategies for successful aging later in this chapter.

Physical Changes

While you can avert or reduce much of the toll that age takes on your body, you can't avoid physical aging completely. We don't yet completely understand why, but certain systems in the body change the way they work over time. The results range from changes in appearance, such as gray hair at the temples, to diminished function in one or more of the body's key organ systems **(Figure 16.2).**

Hearing Loss

Losing the ability to hear clearly is a common sign of aging, but that doesn't make the change any easier to accept. The reasons for age-related hearing loss, called **presbycusis,** vary from person to person, but the condition usually arises from damage to microscopic hair cells in the inner ear. Loss of the ability to hear conversation can cause the person to feel confused and frustrated and to withdraw from social contact. This in turn can lead to isolation.

Any hearing loss should be tested and treated. A variety of devices, such as hearing aids or phone amplifiers, may help. In severe cases, surgery may restore some hearing. When you are still young, do all you can to protect your hearing. For a refresher on basic hearing safety, see Chapter 15.

presbycusis Age-related hearing loss, which usually develops gradually, often due to damage to or changes in the inner ear.

Vision Loss

Vision usually declines with age. By their mid-40s, many people have developed **presbyopia,** a gradual decline in the ability to focus on objects up close, especially in low light. This vision disorder

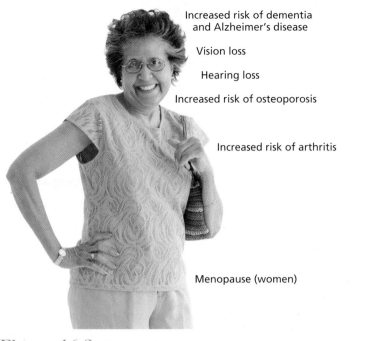

Increased risk of dementia
and Alzheimer's disease

Vision loss

Hearing loss

Increased risk of osteoporosis

Increased risk of arthritis

Menopause (women)

Figure 16.2 Physical changes due to aging.

can be addressed by wearing reading glasses when looking at objects at close range.

Some older adults develop **cataracts,** a clouding of the lens of the eye that dims vision **(Figure 16.3a).** This condition usually arises in a person's 60s, and can be treated through surgery.

Glaucoma arises when fluid builds up in one or both eyes, increasing internal pressure and damaging the optic nerve **(Figure 16.3b).** If untreated, glaucoma can result in a loss of peripheral vision or even total blindness. The condition can be detected through an eye exam, and is treated through medication, laser therapy, or surgery.

Age-related macular degeneration (AMD) impairs the center of a person's vision rather than peripheral eyesight **(Figure 16.3c).** The condition arises when the *macula,* a region of tissue at the center of the retina, deteriorates. The condition can be detected through an eye exam, but is difficult to treat. Surgery or light therapy may help some patients. A study from the National Eye Institute indicates that taking a specific formulation of antioxidants and zinc may be able to slow the progression of the disease.[13]

Menopause

Menopause, or the permanent cessation of a woman's menstrual cycle and fertile years, is a normal, natural process, not an illness. But the hormonal changes

presbyopia Age-related decline in the ability to focus on objects up close, especially in low light.

cataracts An age-related vision disorder marked by clouding of the lens of the eye.

glaucoma An age-related vision disorder arising from an increase in internal eye pressure that damages the optic nerve and reduces peripheral vision.

age-related macular degeneration (AMD) An age-related vision disorder caused by deterioration of the macula that reduces central vision.

menopause The permanent end of a woman's menstrual cycle and reproductive capacity.

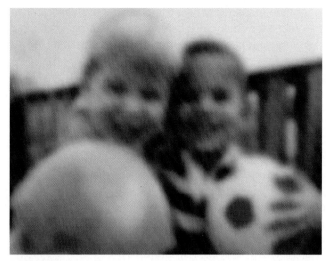

(a) Cataract

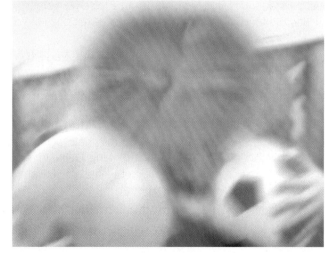

(b) Glaucoma

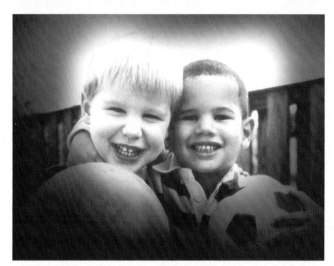

(c) Age-related macular degeneration

Figure 16.3 Vision problems common to aging.

that trigger menopause may cause temporary physical discomfort, as well as increase a woman's risk for cardiovascular disease and osteoporosis. For these reasons, some women turn to health remedies to address the effects of menopause.

Menopause officially begins one year after a woman's last menstrual period. In the United States, that usually occurs in a woman's early fifties, but menopause-related changes often begin several years earlier. In *perimenopause,* women may notice changes in their periods, find they are more likely to build up stores of abdominal fat, have trouble sleeping, or start experiencing some of the classic symptoms of menopause, such as mood swings, vaginal dryness, bursts of perspiration known as hot flashes, and night sweats. These symptoms usually arise from the natural decline of reproductive hormones. Once a woman is 12 months past her last period, her ovaries produce much less estrogen and no progesterone, and no longer release eggs. The years that follow menopause are referred to as *postmenopause.*

After decades of the monthly hassles that having a period brings, some women welcome menopause. This is especially true if a woman experiences relatively few symptoms and side effects. For others, the process brings more mixed feelings. Some women may mourn the loss of their fertility, feel less feminine, or equate menopause with old age. Some may experience extremely uncomfortable or even debilitating physical or psychological symptoms. In these cases, treatments may include:

- **Psychotherapy to help combat fears surrounding menopause.** For instance, the end of menstruation doesn't mean that a woman is facing death: the average woman lives about 30 years after menopause.
- **Hormone replacement therapy (HRT).** Estrogen therapy remains the most effective treatment for hot flashes and other menopausal symptoms. Combination HRT, a mix of estrogen and progestin (synthetic progesterone), was once routinely prescribed for many years before and after menopause, but a large study about 10 years ago linked long-term combination HRT to an elevated risk of breast cancer and cardiovascular disease in some women.[14] Now, doctors tend to prescribe HRT at the lowest possible dose for a shorter period of time.
- **Vaginal estrogen.** This topical medication relieves vaginal dryness and discomfort.
- **Bone-building medications.** These nonhormonal drugs, such as Fosamax or Boniva, help prevent or treat postmenopausal bone loss and reduce the risk of osteoporosis in older women.
- **Antidepressants.** Some antidepressants may help with hot flashes or the mood swings surrounding menopause. In more severe cases, women may find that a combination of HRT and antidepressants provides the greatest benefit.

Many women also have success with home remedies, including:

- **Avoiding hot flash triggers.** Some women find that certain factors, such as spicy food, hot beverages, or sleeping quarters that are too warm, worsen the number and intensity of hot flashes.
- **Quitting cigarettes.** Smoking increases hot flashes and brings on earlier menopause.
- **Exercising regularly.** Exercise not only reduces the risk of postmenopausal health concerns such as osteoporosis and heart disease, but helps control weight and promotes healthful sleep.

CONSUMER CORNER

Alternative Medications for Menopause?

Since a 2002 study linked pharmaceutical HRT to an increased risk of breast cancer and other health problems, interest has surged in alternative therapies to treat menopause symptoms. Some women have switched to a form of treatment called bioidentical hormones, which are chemically identical to ovarian hormones, but are derived from plants. Others have tried herbs such as black cohosh or dong quai.

But so far, evidence of any benefit is mixed at best. One large scientific analysis found that many alternatives to HRT hadn't been studied at all, a few offered mixed results, and some showed no benefit.[1] In addition, many questions of safety remain unanswered. For example, bioidentical hormones are said to be superior to pharmaceutical HRT because the prescription is precisely mixed to meet each woman's hormone needs, based on a test of her saliva. Unfortunately, the hormone levels in saliva don't correspond to those in the bloodstream, nor does a measurement of hormone levels correspond in any way to the menopause symptoms a woman experiences.[2] Moreover, the pharmacies used to produce these preparations are not subject to the same rigorous safety standards as conventional pharmaceutical manufacturers. In addition, neither black cohosh nor dong quai has been shown to be more effective than a placebo in reducing menopause symptoms, and in rare instances the use of black cohosh has been associated with liver failure.[3]

If you are considering an alternative treatment for menopause symptoms, research the therapy carefully, and talk to your doctor.

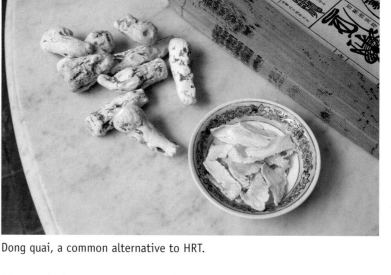

Dong quai, a common alternative to HRT.

References: **1.** "Complementary and Alternative Therapies for the Management of Menopause-Related Symptoms: A Systematic Evidence Review," by A. Nedrow, J. Miller, M. Walker, P. Nygren, L. Huffman, & H. Nelson, 2007, *Archives of Internal Medicine. 166*(14), pp. 1453–1465. **2.** "Bioidentical Hormones: Are They Safer?" by Mary Gallenberg, 2009, retrieved from http://www.mayoclinic.com/health/bioidentical-hormones/AN01133. **3.** *Menopausal Symptoms and CAM* (NCCAM Publication No. D406), by the National Center for Complementary and Alternative Medicine, 2008, retrieved from http://nccam.nih.gov/health/menopause/menopausesymptoms.htm.

Some women also turn to alternative remedies to try to address menopausal symptoms or promote their health after menopause. For a closer look at these alternatives, see the **Consumer Corner.**

Sexuality

An active sex life is usually associated with the young, but older people are far from out of the game. As people age, sexual desire and activity may ebb and flow, but sexuality remains an important aspect of life. If older people remain healthy and have a receptive partner, a substantial number remain sexually active. Several studies have found that while sexual activity may decrease with age, sexual desire does not. An active sex life, as a reflection of social and emotional connections to others, may also help increase longevity. Sexual desire, valuing sexuality, and high sexual self-esteem are important to a woman's sexual activity; for men, high sexual self-esteem, good health, and active sexual history make the most difference for sexual activity later in life.[15]

Chronic Diseases

Aging increases your risk of many chronic diseases. Rates of cardiovascular disease, type 2 diabetes, and some cancers all rise significantly after age 65. For a review of these major chronic diseases and how to address them, see Chapter 12. Next we discuss two chronic diseases especially associated with aging: arthritis and osteoporosis.

Arthritis. More than 46 million people in the U.S.—almost one in seven—has some form of **arthritis.**[16] The condition is characterized by inflammation of one or more joints, resulting in pain, stiffness, warmth in the joint, and loss of motion. The condition usually arises from a breakdown of *cartilage,* protective tissue that lines the joints.

Although there are more than 100 forms of arthritis, affecting people of all ages, the most common form is *osteoarthritis,* a type that often arises with age. In people with osteoarthritis, cartilage wears away in the hands and weight-bearing joints of the body, such as the knees, hips, and ankles. Osteoarthritis often arises from a mix of genetic factors and damaging force, such as injury, repetitive motion, or excessive body weight.

There is no cure for osteoarthritis. But rest, physical therapy, and medication can all prevent further joint damage, reduce pain and swelling, and help restore daily activities. Low-impact exercises, such as swimming, walking, gentler forms of yoga, and tai chi are all good options for staying physically active even when diagnosed with osteoarthritis.

Osteoporosis. As we noted in Chapter 4, **osteoporosis** is a disease characterized by thin, brittle bones that break more easily than normal **(Figure 16.4).** Osteoporosis arises when bone density decreases with age, and it is one of the leading disabling conditions among older people in the United States. According to the National Institutes of Health, about 10 million people already have osteoporosis and another 34 million are at increased risk because of low bone mass.[17]

---

arthritis Inflammation of one or more joints in the body, resulting in pain, swelling, and limited movement.

osteoporosis A disease characterized by low bone mass and deterioration of bone tissue, leading to fragile bones and an increased risk of fractures.

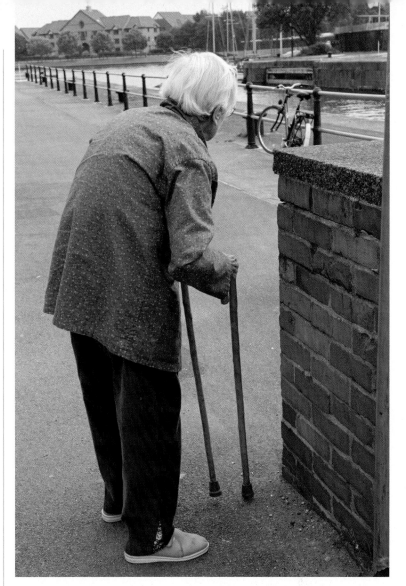

A hunched spine is a characteristic effect of osteoporosis.

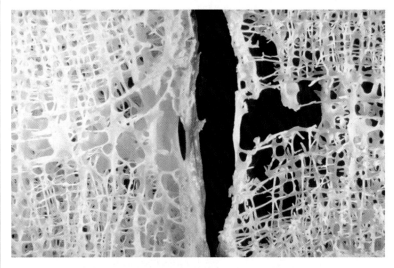

Figure 16.4 **Effects of osteoporosis on the vertebrae of the spine.** The vertebrae of a person with osteoporosis (right), and the vertebrae of a healthy person (left).

Although men are also at risk, osteoporosis is about twice as common in women for several reasons. The female hormone estrogen helps maintain bone mass, and after menopause, the resulting drop in estrogen accelerates bone loss. Moreover, women who strive for a slender body weight throughout their lives deprive their bones of the weight-bearing stress necessary to prompt bone-building. Finally, women live an average of five years longer than men, and since bone loss increases with age, osteoporosis is more likely to show up in women.

About 1.5 million fractures each year are due to osteoporosis. The bones of the wrist, spine, and hip are most at risk.[17] Hip fractures are especially debilitating—up to 20% of all people who suffer a hip fracture die within a year of the injury.

Some risk factors for osteoporosis, such as sex, age, and family history, can't be changed. Body size and ethnicity also matter—small, thin-boned women, as well as women of European and Asian descent, are at higher risk. But other risk factors are within your control. Smoking, excessive alcohol consumption, a sedentary lifestyle, underweight, and a diet low in calcium and vitamin D all increase the risk of developing osteoporosis. Both males and females 14–18 years of age need 1,300 milligrams of calcium each day. Beginning at age 19, adults should consume 1,000 milligrams of calcium each day, and after age 50, that number goes up to 1,200 milligrams a day. The current vitamin D recommendation is 200 IU through age 50, 400 IU through age 70, and 600 IU thereafter; however, these recommendations are under study and may be revised upward.[18]

Changes Affecting Cognition and Memory

Issues once thought to be a routine part of aging, such as forgetfulness and confusion, are no longer considered inevitable. Instead, like the rest of the body, the brain appears to age quite well. Though brain mass does decrease slightly, especially in areas related to complex memory and problem-solving, this change does not have to be debilitating.[19] In fact, many people become wiser with age, as their decades of accumulated experiences help them solve new problems and give them a broad, balanced perspective on life.

Normal age-related changes include more difficulty in multitasking, remembering names of people and places, and learning new information quickly. Many of these skills, however, can be boosted through "brain fitness" activities, which are discussed later in this chapter. It's also important to recognize that poor physical health overall appears to be a greater predictor of cognitive impairment in older adults than is age.[20]

Some older adults, however, do experience true neurological disorders. These include various forms of dementia, the most severe form of which is Alzheimer's disease.

Dementia. In some older adults, memory loss may be severe, and brain function may be so impaired that performing everyday tasks such as preparing food or getting dressed becomes difficult. **Dementia,** a broad term for a group of mental and psychological disorders related to memory and everyday tasks, is used to describe the condition of someone with two or more such impairments. De-

dementia A group of cognitive impairments and other disorders that affect the brain and the ability to perform basic everyday tasks.

Alzheimer's disease (AD) A progressive, fatal form of age-related dementia.

mentia may arise at any point in life, but is much more common in people over the age of 80.

Dementia appears to arise from many causes, only some of which are well understood. Genetics may play a role. People who suffer multiple brain-damaging strokes may also develop a form of dementia.

Although there is no guaranteed path to preventing dementia, healthful behaviors may make a difference. Researchers are currently investigating the role of body weight, diet, exercise, and participation in socially and intellectually stimulating activities in preventing all forms of age-related dementia, including the most common form—Alzheimer's disease.[21]

Alzheimer's Disease. Few age-related illnesses are more feared than this progressive, fatal brain disorder. In **Alzheimer's disease (AD),** nerve cells in the brain stop functioning and disconnect from one another **(Figure 16.5).** Thus, their ability to transmit messages is lost. Eventually, the affected nerve cells die. As they do, affected regions of brain tissue atrophy (shrink), and brain mass is lost. Affected nerve cells are found to be filled with abnormal collections of twisted protein threads called *tangles,* and deposits of apparently toxic protein fragments called *amyloid-beta plaque*s, but it is still unclear whether these tangles and plaques cause the condition or are merely a symptom.[22]

The damage is typically slow but progressive, and may begin as many as 10 to 20 years before any problems become evident. Eventually, however, the disease steals memory and the ability to concentrate, and the ability to perform most daily tasks. In normal age-related memory loss, the person typically forgets only certain details of an event. In contrast, in AD, all memory of an event is typically lost. Recent memory is severely affected: for example, a person may watch a favorite television program, and a few minutes after it ends ask when

To view a video showing what happens to the brain in AD, go to www.nia.nih.gov/Alzheimers/ADvideo.

the program is going to begin. Gradually, AD also affects mood and personality, leaving the person depressed, highly anxious, irritable, combative, and even paranoid and subject to delusions.

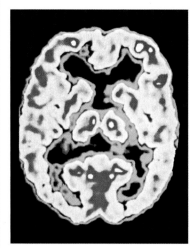

(a) Healthy brain

(b) Brain with Alzheimer's disease

Figure 16.5 Brain activity and Alzheimer's disease. Reds and yellows indicate high activity in tissues; blues and greens represent lower activity in tissues.

Almost 5 million people in the U.S. are living with Alzheimer's disease. This number is expected to quadruple in the next 50 years as more people live longer.[23] Alzheimer's is now the sixth leading cause of death in the United States. Despite the common nature of the disease, however, understanding its causes and finding a cure have so far remained out of reach. Leading risk factors include:

- **Age.** Most cases of Alzheimer's disease occur in people older than 60, and risk jumps dramatically after the age of 80. This version of the condition, known as *late-onset Alzheimer's,* is the most common. A rarer form of the disease, known as *early-onset Alzheimer's,* has a strong genetic component and often begins in a person's 30s or 40s.

- **Genetics and family history.** If Alzheimer's runs in your family, you are at increased risk for developing the disease yourself. With the help of affected families, researchers are zeroing in on genetic factors linked to Alzheimer's risk. One such factor is related to a gene called *apolipoprotein E,* or *ApoE,* which helps the body regulate cholesterol. People with a particular variant of this gene have a substantially increased risk of Alzheimer's disease. Other genetic factors are now also the focus of intense scientific scrutiny.

- **Poor cardiovascular health.** A growing body of research indicates that the factors that harm the cardiovascular system, such as a high-fat diet, high cholesterol, and a sedentary lifestyle, also increase Alzheimer's risk. Interestingly, the ApoE gene linked to Alzheimer's affects how the body processes cholesterol, another indication that vascular health and the body's ability to move blood through the brain plays a role in the disease.

There are currently no cures or long-term treatments for Alzheimer's disease, although several prescription medications may ease some of the cognitive symptoms, such as memory loss, for a relatively short period of time. There are also no proven prevention strategies. However, maintaining a healthful body weight, keeping physically, socially, and intellectually active, and eating a healthful diet might reduce your risk, especially if Alzheimer's disease runs in your family. Following a diet rich in fruits, vegetables, whole grains, and healthy plant oils may be particularly beneficial, especially when combined with regular physical activity.[24] For an overview of good nutrition, see Chapter 4.

> The Alzheimer's Society provides information for people affected by Alzheimer's disease and their families and caregivers: www.alzheimer.ca/english/disease/intro.htm

Psychosocial Changes

If you are a student of typical college age, you are probably experiencing some powerful psychosocial changes. You may recently have moved out of your parents' home to live with others of your own age, or on your own. You'll soon be moving from the world of education—an environment you've known since you were a small child—to the world of work. You may even be thinking of marriage and starting a family of your own. If you think about the challenges that such shifts represent for you, you can begin to imagine how challenging similar changes can be in the lives of older adults.

Family Changes

Your move to college doesn't just affect you. It also affects your parents or guardians. After spending decades raising you, day in and

day out, they may welcome their newfound freedom, yet struggle with feelings of emptiness and loss. This so-called "Empty Nest Syndrome" challenges older adults to rethink not only their day-to-day responsibilities, but also how they define their identities.

The Empty Nest Syndrome also challenges couples. Older people who've raised children together will suddenly find themselves spending more time alone than they have in years, and will probably need to get to know each other again as individuals. Some couples, once their children have left home, find that the bonds that connected them as individuals have frayed, and they may separate. Others find that their connection is stronger than ever, and enjoy the extra time they have together. Some find new happiness by moving to communities for older adults, where social activities and physical environments are arranged to promote fun and well-being for people in older age brackets.

At the same time that they are adjusting to their own aging, many older adults begin taking on significant care-giving tasks for very elderly parents. They may purchase a larger home that can accommodate a parent who can no longer live independently, or they may move into the parent's home. Even when living arrangements stay the same, older adults may find themselves spending many hours each week "parenting" their elderly parents, taking them to medical appointments, shopping for them, and making a variety of arrangements for their care. This change in family dynamics can be highly stressful, but it can also give older adults and their elderly parents precious opportunities to share memories and feelings, resolve conflicts, and affirm their love and caring.

Changes in Employment

Most older adults have been working for decades, deriving a strong sense of identity and self-worth from their careers. Although retirement is meant to bring freedom from work, some seniors may find themselves unsure of who they are if they aren't attached to a profession. Having diverse interests outside of work earlier in life can help. Many seniors find that using their professional skills to volunteer or work part-time provides an easier transition from the professional world to retirement.

Economic Changes

Retirement may bring more free time—but it also means less money. Reduced work translates into reduced income. Many seniors find themselves living on fixed incomes from federal programs such as Social Security or private programs such as employer pensions, and

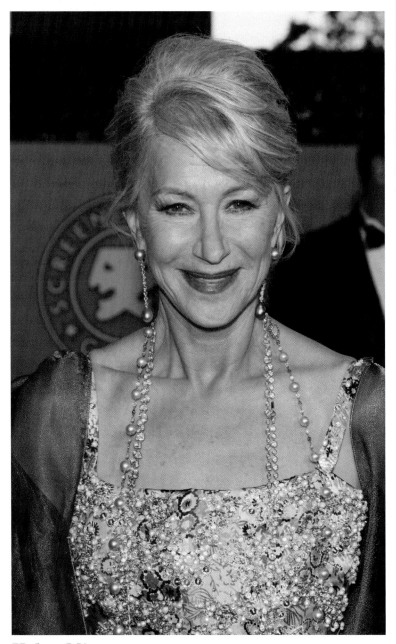

Helen Mirren, at age 65, is at a high point in her career.

need to reduce their spending as a result, even as some costs, such as medical expenses, rise. Personal savings are also often critical—but people in the U.S. are notoriously poor at funding their retirement savings accounts. In a survey of the most common type of employer-based retirement account, the 401(k), most workers were contributing less than half of the federally allowed limit each year, which means they'll have less money to live on after they retire.[25] Many 401(k) accounts are also invested in the stock market, which can fluctuate and, in some cases, substantially diminish the value of a person's retirement savings just as they are getting ready to leave the workforce.

As a result of these factors, the traditional view of retirement as a time of leisure has changed. Increased life expectancy means that people will need an income longer. Some U.S. workers are retiring later, working at full-time jobs well into their 70s. Others find themselves coming out of retirement and taking part-time jobs or starting small businesses to boost their income.

Mood Changes

Changing roles, such as leaving the workforce or having children move away, leave some men and women feeling unnecessary, even irrelevant. Vision and hearing losses, chronic pain, and functional limitations can further narrow an older adult's world. As friends and loved ones, including spouses, fall ill or die, older adults may feel increasingly isolated in their grief.

As a result, rates of depression and suicide are relatively high among older adults. Whereas the suicide rate is about 11 per 100,000 in the general population, about 14 of every 100,000 people age 65 and older die by suicide. Caucasian men age 85 and older are most likely to take their own lives, with a rate of nearly 50 suicides per 100,000 persons in that age group.[26]

If an older relative or friend talks about feeling sad or hopeless, listen carefully and offer to help him or her find care. Many hospitals and senior centers offer support groups and mental health services designed for older adults. Above all, spend time with your loved one. Showing older adults that they are important to you can help them reject feelings of abandonment.

How Can I Age Successfully?

If you are the age of a traditional college student, in your late teens or early 20s, the idea of being a senior citizen probably sounds like something from another planet. But though you won't face the concerns of being an older adult yourself for decades, you are probably already seeing the effects of age on your parents and grandparents. Someday, perhaps sooner than you think, you may be called upon to help them. And eventually, you'll find yourself in their shoes. By establishing healthful habits now, you can help set yourself on a path to successful aging.

But what, exactly, does successful aging look like? Experts agree that it includes the following characteristics:

- An ability to maintain autonomy and independence.
- The capability to function physically, cognitively, and socially.
- A personal view of aging that is self-defined, individualistic, and reflects who you truly are.
- An ability to continuously adapt to the changes that life brings.
- A desire to live life fully and embrace all of its stages.[27]

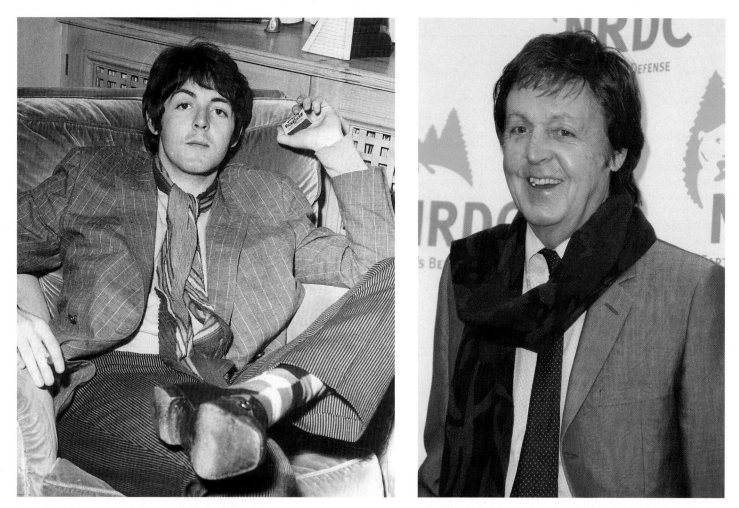

Aging happens to everyone. Beatle Paul McCartney in his 20s, and today at 68.

Sounds good, right? So how do you get there? Genetic factors do appear to play some role in how long and how well a person lives. However, about 70% of life expectancy appears to be due to lifestyle, income, and other nongenetic influences.[28] So instead of waiting to respond to health crises in old age, it makes sense to do all you can to preserve your health along the way. Through consistent efforts at **health preservation,** you can help yourself grow older successfully. Let's start with a habit you've learned about throughout this book—exercise.

Stay (or Become) Physically Active

As you age, you may not be able to run as fast as you could when you were 12, but that's no reason to stop moving. Regular physical activity is one of the most beneficial things you can do for your health, at any point in life. As you've learned in Chapters 5 and 12, consistent exercise greatly reduces a person's risk of dying from cardiovascular diseases and decreases risks for type 2 diabetes, hypertension, and several types of cancer. Physical activity also slows many of the physical aspects of aging, such as a loss of bone density and muscle mass and increased body fat, helps relieve the pain of joint conditions such as arthritis, and eases mental health concerns such as anxiety and depression.

health preservation Performing activities that seek to maintain health, rather than simply responding to health crises as they occur.

It's never too late to enjoy the benefits of exercise. For people who are 65 years of age or older, are generally fit, and have no limiting health conditions, public health experts recommend at least:

- Two hours and 30 minutes of moderate-intensity aerobic activity, such as brisk walking, each week AND muscle-strengthening activities that work all major muscle groups at least 2 days a week, OR

- One hour and 15 minutes of vigorous-intensity aerobic activity, such as jogging, every week AND muscle-strengthening activities that work all major muscle groups at least 2 days a week, OR

- An equivalent mix of moderate- and vigorous-intensity aerobic activity AND muscle-strengthening activities that work all major muscle groups at least 2 days a week.[29]

For a refresher on physical activity, including aerobic exercise, muscle-strengthening fitness, and overall types and intensities of exercise, see Chapter 5.

Eat for the Long Term

No matter your age, good nutrition is vital to maintaining good health. This means a varied diet that is low in saturated fats, *trans* fats, and added sugar, and high in fruits, vegetables, and whole

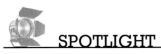
Exercise: The Life Preserver

Want to live longer? Work out more.

Numerous studies show that fitness, especially higher levels of cardiorespiratory fitness, is among the best predictors of longevity. One set of research findings revealed that people with higher levels of cardiorespiratory fitness faced a lower risk of death even if they were overweight or carried a few extra pounds around their midsection.[1] Another study found that people between the ages of 70 and 88 were more likely to live longer if they either continued an existing exercise program or started a new one.[2]

Cardiorespiratory activities, such as brisk walking, biking, or running, matter most. But so do strength training and flexibility. At any age, we all need a regular mix of these types of activities. For an overview of fitness and exercise options, see Chapter 5.

References: 1. "Cardiorespiratory Fitness and Adiposity as Mortality Predictors in Older Adults," by X. Sui, M. J. LaMonte, J. N. Laditka, J. W. Hardin, N. Chase, S. P. Hooker, & S. N. Blair. , 2007, *Journal of the American Medical Association. 298*(21), pp. 2507–2516. 2. "Physical Activity, Function, and Longevity Among the Very Old," by J. Stessman, R. Hammerman-Rozenberg, A. Cohen, E. Ein-Mor, & J. Jacobs, 2009, *Archives of Internal Medicine, 169*(16), pp. 1476–1483.

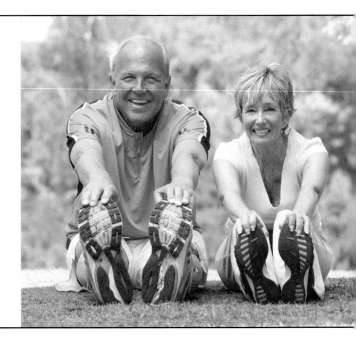

grains. A healthful diet can extend your productive years and reduce your risk of chronic conditions such as cardiovascular disease, stroke, some types of cancer, diabetes, and osteoporosis.

In addition to the essentials of good nutrition you learned in Chapter 4, nutritional guidelines for older adults recommend that you:

- Get enough calcium and vitamins D and B$_{12}$ from foods and/or supplements.
- Limit sodium intake to 1,500 milligrams per day and get at least 4,700 milligrams of potassium per day to help control blood pressure.
- Choose high-fiber fruits, vegetables, and whole grains and drink plenty of water to help prevent constipation.[30]

For a special version of the food pyramid created for older adults, see **Figure 16.6.**

Maintain a Healthful Weight

As we mentioned earlier in this chapter, about 20% of older adults are obese, and that percentage is expected to grow. As you learned in Chapter 6, being overweight or obese isn't simply a matter of appearance. The real risks come from the cascade of health conditions and complications that can follow, including increased risks for cardiovascular disease, type 2 diabetes, cancer, and arthritis. Being overweight or obese—usually the result of a high-calorie diet, lack of physical activity, and stress—is also increasingly linked to a greater risk of Alzheimer's disease or other cognitive impairments as a person ages.

The good news is, if you establish health habits that enable you to manage your weight now, you'll find it easier to maintain those habits—and your healthful weight—as you age. For a review of how to maintain a healthful weight, see Chapter 6.

Limit Drinking and Dependence on Medications

When feeling sad, stressed, or unwell, resist the temptation to reach for a bottle or a pill. Dependence on alcohol, medications, and other

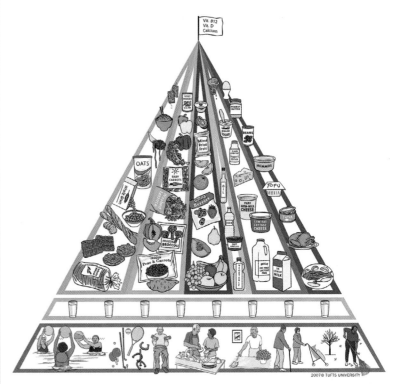

Figure 16.6 **Modified MyPyramid for Older Adults.** Nutrition guidelines for adults aged 70 and older. The base of the pyramid emphasizes the importance of physical activity and proper hydration. The body of the pyramid suggests healthful foods that seniors can eat to meet their nutrition recommendations.

Source: Modified MyPyramid for Older Adults: Tufts Researchers Update Their Food Guide Pyramid for Older Adults [News Release], 2007, Tufts University, retrieved from: http://nutrition.tufts.edu/1197972031385/Nutrition-Page-nl2w_1198058402614.html.

Old Age, Okinawa Style

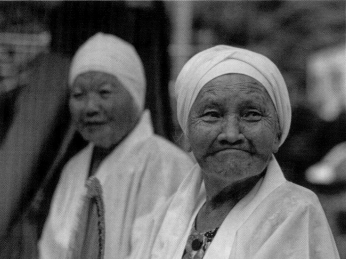

Okinawa, an island that is part of Japan, is at the center of current research on aging. More Okinawans live to see 100 than just about any other large population group in the world. And Okinawa's seniors age in remarkably good health, with clean arteries, low cholesterol levels, relatively few cases of cancer or serious osteoporosis, and low rates of dementia. Many remain active throughout their later years.

Part of the secret appears to lie in the traditional Okinawan diet, which centers around vegetables such as soybeans, leafy greens, and native gourds. This vegan diet provides protein and is high in protective nutrients such as folate and flavonoids. Older Okinawans also get a lot of physical activity each day. Genetics may also play some role.

As younger Okinawans are influenced by contemporary global lifestyles and adopt a less healthful, more Westernized diet and become more sedentary, researchers will see how life expectancy on the island changes.

You can follow this ongoing research yourself, by visiting the Okinawa Centenarian Study at www.okicent.org/study.html.

controlled substances is harmful for seniors, and harmful to you as you age.

You learned about the effects of excessive alcohol in Chapter 8. These effects actually increase with age. That's because, as you get older, your ability to metabolize alcohol diminishes. This means that alcohol stays in your body at higher levels longer, increasing your risk of impaired judgment or physical injury while under its influence.

Many seniors who drink alcohol also take one or more medications, which may interact in a way that is harmful. One recent study found that about 81% of seniors were using at least one prescription medication, about 42% were taking an over-the-counter medication, and about 49% were taking a dietary supplement. About 29% of older adults were taking five or more prescription medications concurrently. Many older adults combine medications, supplements, and/or alcohol without informing their primary care provider, and without researching their potential combined effects.[31]

If you or an older person you know is taking multiple medications and supplements, with or without alcohol, make an appointment to discuss this issue with your physician immediately. Bring to your appointment a complete list of all substances you use. Make sure to discuss not only their safety as individual products, but their potential for harmful interactions. Also discuss the potential for limiting your dependence on these substances by making more healthful choices—a balanced diet, regular exercise, and techniques for managing stress.[32]

Don't Smoke

Few choices shave more years off your life, and reduce the quality of the years you have, than lighting up. Someone who smokes one pack a day can expect to die about 10 years earlier than

someone who has never smoked. Moreover, a person who smokes has a reduced quality of life: smoking 20 or more cigarettes a day ages you by about 10 years, limiting your cardiovascular functions and your ability to perform everyday tasks and enjoy your life.[33] Smoking has also been linked to premature balding, wrinkles, and osteoporosis. For an overview of the health problems linked to smoking, and suggestions on how to quit, see Chapter 8.

Challenge Your Mind

No matter how long you live, there will always be something new to learn or an old skill to hone. Just as exercise can maintain or restore your physical fitness, a daily "brain workout" can contribute to a state known as **brain fitness.** One study found that brain-engaging activities such as completing crossword puzzles, reading books, playing a musical instrument, or playing cards not only helped prevent cognitive decline overall, but slowed memory loss among those who had already developed dementia.[34] Religious or spiritual involvement, such as religious studies or involvement in religious or spiritual services and practices, may also have a positive effect on brain function.[35]

The key to beneficial activities lies in their interactivity. Any pastime that makes you think and requires that you connect with an object or another person—be it a musical instrument, an iPad, a grandchild, or a religious advisor—engages your brain and helps preserve thought and function. Staying connected through email, social networking sites, blogs, and Skype can also help. Conversely, activities that let you tune out and diminish your interactions with the world, such as watching television for extended periods of time on a regular basis, may have the opposite effect on brain fitness. So as you age, keep engaged!

brain fitness A person's ability to meet the cognitive requirements and demands of daily life, such as problem solving and memory recall.

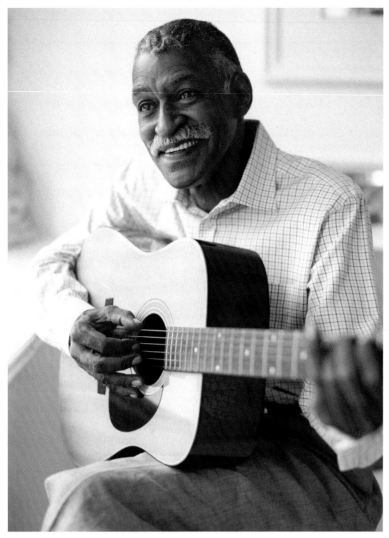

Playing a musical instrument is one way to keep your mind sharp as you age.

Want to see how fast you can match squeaks, squawks, and croaking sounds to the animals that make them? Or decipher encrypted quotations? Have fun playing the American Association of Retired Persons' Brain Games at **http://games.aarp.org**.

Recognize and Reduce Stress

You might think that, when you are older, you'll be retired, without any work obligations or a care in the world. You'll be able to spend your time however you'd like—what could be less stressful?

Tell that to an older adult, and watch them smile. While being older brings many benefits, it's hardly a stress-free time of life. Along with health concerns, there are also many practical changes to juggle. If you've worked all your life, the challenge of building a new identity after retirement can be stressful. Children may be grown and living on their own, but you're still concerned about them—and any grandchildren. As noted earlier, you might also be coping with parents in failing health. And except for the very few independently wealthy among us, the financial pressures of living on a reduced or fixed income can take a heavy toll.

So beginning today, challenge yourself to recognize signs of excessive stress in your life, and address them. Be sure to get enough sleep on a regular basis. Limit your consumption of alcohol, eat right, and exercise. Maintain a healthy network of personal relationships and friends who can serve as a sounding board and help you find your way through life's challenges. For a refresher on stress and stress management techniques, see Chapter 3.

Understanding Death

About 2.4 million people die each year in the United States—about 6,575 a day.[7] Yet many of us rarely even think of death. It's only when we lose someone we love that we pay attention. Yet, as with other essential stages of health and life, death merits consideration—even contemplation. Let's begin by defining death.

What Is Death?

Historically, a person was pronounced dead if he or she had stopped breathing and had no heartbeat. But because of advances in **life support systems,** medical technologies that artificially sustain physiological functions, clinicians now recognize several different definitions of death.

- **Brain death** is the cessation of brain activity as indicated by various medical devices and diagnostic criteria.
- **Functional death** is the end of all vital physiological functions, including heartbeat, breathing, and blood flow.
- **Cellular death** is the end of all vital functions at the cellular level, such as cellular respiration and other metabolic processes.

life support systems Medical technologies that artificially sustain one or more vital functions.

brain death The cessation of brain activity as indicated by various medical devices and diagnostic criteria.

functional death The end of all vital physiological functions, including heartbeat, breathing, and blood flow.

cellular death The end of all vital functions at the cellular level, such as cellular respiration and other metabolic processes.

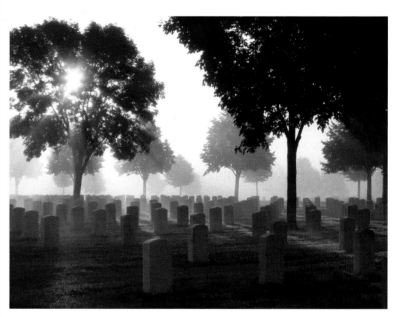

Death is an inevitable part of life.

Are You Comfortable with Death?

In order to comfort others, to grieve authentically, and to live life fully, it is important to accept death as an inevitable and natural stage of life. To assess your ability to do so, consider the following questions.

1. Do you avoid discussing death with your loved ones? yes no
2. Are you unable to listen or be supportive of a friend or family member's "plans" about death such as wills, organ donation, advanced directives, etc.? yes no
3. Do you avoid people who are grieving? yes no
4. Do you try to change the subject if someone wants to talk about the death of a loved one because you believe they will feel better if not reminded of it? yes no
5. Do you typically substitute other words for "death" such as "passed," "gone to a better place," "with the angels," etc.? yes no

HOW TO INTERPRET YOUR SCORE

The more times you answer "yes", the less comfortable you are with death. Consider making an appointment at your school's counseling center to discuss your feelings about death, or explore a spiritual or philosophical study of death.

Sources: Information adapted from Hospice Foundation of America, www.hospicefoundation.org, and BeyondIndigo.com, www.beyondindigo.com.

To complete this self-assessment online, visit www.pearsonhighered.com/ choosinghealth.

> *A rational, mature understanding of death often takes a lifetime to process and personally accept.*

- **Clinical death** is a medical determination that life has ceased, and is often defined by medical criteria that focus on a combination of functional and neurological factors.

These physiologic definitions of death give us a shared standard for determining death of the body. However, your larger ideas about death are influenced by your age, life experiences, and the values and beliefs you cherish.

clinical death A medical determination that life has ceased according to medical criteria that often combine aspects of functional and neurological factors.

Developing a Concept of Death

Most young children are unaware of death's permanence. They may realize that some absence occurs with death, but consider it just a passing phase. In kids' cartoons, characters get knocked off cliffs, hit by anvils, and run over by speeding cars. Yet they always bounce back. This resiliency echoes children's beliefs about the temporary nature of death.

Yet over time, personal experiences teach us that death is irreversible and permanent. A family pet dies, and its bed and toys sit idle for weeks, until a parent tucks them away out of sight. Perhaps a beloved grandparent passes on, and with each family celebration they don't attend, we realize that they really aren't coming back. Or we may even know a child who is terminally ill, and be comforted and inspired as we witness them embrace the life they have before their passing. Slowly, we come to understand that death of the physical body is universal—a physiological process that will come to everyone. Yet this rational, mature understanding of death often takes a lifetime to process and personally accept.

Just as we accept only slowly the reality that others will die, we develop only slowly the understanding that our own lifetime will end. Most of us, not only as children, but even through adolescence and young adulthood, haven't fully acknowledged to ourselves that we will someday die. Although such denial of death may feel life-affirming, it can actually be life-threatening if it causes you to skip the seatbelt or bring alcohol on a boating trip. While it's true of course that most people who die are older, death strikes every age group, with unintentional injuries representing the single largest cause of death for people from age 1 to 44. (For a review of the leading causes of death, for the population as a whole and for younger people, see Chapter 1 and Chapter 14.) As we witness or hear about the deaths of people our own age, we begin to confront our own mortality.

Moreover, youth doesn't always mean perfect health. A younger adult who gets surprised by a high blood pressure or high blood sugar reading at a routine checkup often realizes that his body doesn't work the way it once did, and that these changes will continue to present challenges as the years add up. Most people are eventually presented with ample reminders that their body is aging and that, some day, death will come.

The beliefs and values with which we were raised, or which we adopt as adults, significantly

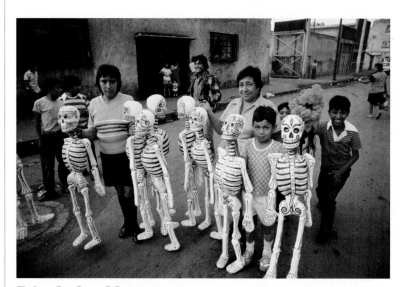

Día de los Muertos, a holiday begun in Mexico, helps those who celebrate it remember friends and family members who have died.

influence our concept of death. Many adults turn to philosophical, religious, or spiritual teachings to help further their understanding of death. Many strive more earnestly to live their values, dedicating themselves to social causes or environmental stewardship as they contemplate the legacy they would like to leave behind. For many, developing a realistic concept of death involves making the most of each day, and connecting more deeply with those around us. This perspective can help us provide genuine support to friends and loved ones at one of the most difficult times imaginable—when they are confronting their own end-of-life issues.

End of Life: Personal and Practical Considerations

Although it may seem odd to "plan ahead" for death, doing so will make the transition smoother, both for loved ones and for yourself. When death is gradual, the dying person needs and deserves support. When it is sudden and unexpected, important decisions must sometimes be made under emotional duress. Preparation makes these steps, though never easy, less distressing.

Supporting a Dying Person

A **terminal illness** is an irreversible condition that will result in death in the near future. If someone you love is diagnosed with a terminal illness, you may have several weeks or months to support the person as he or she prepares for the end of life. When called on to support someone who is dying, you may welcome the opportunity to comfort and help, yet not know exactly how. Fortunately, the dying person will probably share with you quite candidly what he or she would find most helpful.

Many terminally ill people seek a "good death," or an exit handled on their own terms as much as possible. While everyone's definition of a good death may be a little different, researchers have identified six factors of high importance to the dying, their loved ones, and caregivers:

- **Pain and symptom management.** Most people are understandably anxious about spending the end of life in pain.
- **Clear decision making.** It's essential to know the dying person's preferences on medical, spiritual, financial, and other issues as much as possible. We'll look at some options for clarifying these preferences later in this chapter.
- **Preparation for death.** The dying are more at ease when they've had an opportunity to take steps such as prepare a will or help plan for a memorial service after their passing. They and their families also want to know what physical and medical changes might occur as death approaches.
- **Completion.** People who are dying do not want to leave unfinished business behind. They prefer to resolve outstanding disputes, spend time with loved ones, and say good-byes. Many also seek counsel and conversation with a spiritual advisor.
- **Contributing to others.** The dying wish to interact with those around them, not just receive care. They want their caregivers to respect their wishes and listen to their suggestions, and they want to share their memories, insights, and life lessons with loved ones.
- **Affirmation of the whole person.** People who are dying want to be affirmed as the complex, well-rounded human beings they have always been. They do not want to be perceived as merely a collection of illnesses and symptoms.[36]

If you want to support someone who is dying, ask him or her these questions:

- Would you prefer to die at home, in a hospice, or in a hospital? (These care options are discussed shortly.)
- Would you like to have spiritual counseling? If so, what type? Do you have someone in mind?
- Whom do you wish to see before your passing?
- Are there any practical matters you'd like to resolve?

Helping the person think through such questions, and then working to make the answers a reality before the person's passing, is an invaluable gift.

If in doubt, just be there. As one hospital chaplain says, "Never underestimate the power of your presence. Just being present, even when feeling helpless or powerless, can be an important source of strength and comfort for your loved one and for you."[37]

Completing Advance Directives

Advance directives are legal documents allowing a person to specify personal treatment preferences in case of a medical crisis. Without these documents, it can be difficult for loved ones and care providers to make important decisions on a person's behalf, and actions may be taken that the person would not have agreed with. Several types of advance directives are in common use, although some vary from state to state.

Health-Care Proxy

A *health-care proxy* gives someone else the power to make health decisions on your behalf, should you become unable to do so. Also called a *durable power of attorney for health care*, this document usually authorizes a person to have access to medical records and make a wide range of decisions, including:

- Refusing or agreeing to treatments.
- Changing health-care providers, hospitals, or care facilities.
- Deciding on organ donation.
- Deciding about starting or continuing life support.
- Deciding whether a dying person will end life at home or in a care facility.

Many people typically name a relative or trusted friend as their proxy. It's important that all health-care providers know the name and contact information of a patient's health-care proxy. State laws govern the authorities given to health-care proxies, so find out what your state will allow. Although you can find state-specific forms online (see the **Get Connected** section at the end of this chapter), and a lawyer's help isn't required to create a health-care proxy, a legal review of any forms can help ensure that they'll be binding later.

terminal illness An irreversible condition that will result in death in the near future.

advance directive Formal documents that state a person's preferences regarding medical treatment and medical crisis management.

Living Will

A *living will*, or *health-care directive*, states a person's wishes for medical treatment near the end of life. This document may:

- Specify the extent of life-sustaining treatment and major medical interventions the person wants.
- Protect a doctor or hospital from legal liability for following the person's instructions.
- Detail how much discretion the person specifically gives his or her proxy about end-of-life issues.

As with health-care proxies, living wills are governed by state law. You can find state-specific forms online (see the **Get Connected** section at the end of this chapter). Some doctors and hospitals now help patients draft living wills.

The Five Wishes

A less formal type of advance directive, a document called "Five Wishes," includes key aspects of a health-care proxy and a living will. In addition, it helps people express preferences about their level of comfort, relationships, and legacy. The Five Wishes are as follows:

1. The person I want to make health-care decisions for me when I can't make them for myself.
2. My wish for the kind of medical treatment I want or don't want.
3. My wish for how comfortable I want to be.
4. My wish for how I want people to treat me.
5. My wish for what I want my loved ones to know.[38]

The Five Wishes document was created by a patient advocacy group with help from national legal experts, and supporters state that it meets the legal requirements of about 40 states. Some legal experts, however, warn that some of the language in the Five Wishes may be legally ambiguous and create confusion, and recommend that a person using the Five Wishes also complete a standard health-care proxy and living will.[39]

Do Not Resuscitate (DNR) Order

A *Do Not Resuscitate (DNR) order* instructs health-care providers, including doctors, nurses, and paramedics, not to try to restart a person's heart or lungs if heartbeat or breathing stops. Most DNR orders are used in hospitals, and must be signed by a doctor and placed in a person's medical chart. Some states, however, also allow DNR orders to be used at home, should paramedics receive a call about a medical emergency at the home of a terminally ill person.

Writing a Will

If you were to die, what would you want to have happen to your money? Your possessions? If you have them, your children, or even your pets? You probably have preferences, but without a will, it may be difficult to have them carried out.

A **will,** a legally binding document expressing your intention of what should be done with your property after death, is the best way to plan for the distribution of your **estate,** or money, property, and other possessions. During your life, your will can be changed or replaced at any time. You may opt

will A legally binding document stating what should be done with a person's property after death.

estate A person's personal holdings, including money, property, and other possessions.

intestate Dying without leaving a legal will.

palliative care Type of care that focuses on reducing pain and suffering and caring for the whole person, rather than prolonging life or curing disease.

to create a *trust,* another legal document that conveys your property to those you designate, instead. If you die **intestate,** or without a will or similar document, your state's laws will determine who receives your property. Those guidelines may or may not match your personal wishes.

Wills allow you to:

- Name a person as your estate's *executor,* or the individual who makes sure your wishes are carried out.
- List your possessions in detail and specify what individuals or organizations should inherit them.
- Select a guardian for any children you have and specify how they should be cared for.
- Detail any funeral arrangements you would like.

Despite the clarity that wills provide, most people in the United States don't have one. About 55% of U.S. adults have not drafted one. Among ethnic and racial minorities, the percentages are even lower, with only 32% of African American adults and 26% of Hispanic adults having wills.[40]

Software programs and online services are available for creating a will, and many states accept handwritten wills as legally binding. Still, wills vary greatly in complexity, and creating one often requires legal assistance. You can hire a private estate attorney, or inquire about will assistance programs from your local legal aid society or state bar association.

Options for End-of-Life Care

If you or someone in your family were diagnosed with a terminal illness, what would be the best setting for providing care? Answering that question often requires consideration of a mix of personal preferences, family concerns, and medical needs. Three common settings for end-of-life care include the dying person's home, a hospital or nursing home, or a hospice facility. In any of these settings, the type of care most often given to people with a terminal illness is **palliative care.** The goal of palliative care is to relieve pain and suffering, rather than to prolong life or cure the disease. Although it is often given along with treatment-based care—for instance, the administration of pain medication to a person recovering from heart surgery would be classified as palliative care—for people at the end of life, it seeks to provide as much comfort as possible, rather than to prolong life.[41]

Home Care

When surveyed, most older Americans say they would prefer to die at home, yet less than a quarter actually do.[42] This duality reflects the difficulties of providing end-of-life care. Home is familiar and comforting, with loved ones nearby. But it's not always possible to provide intensive medical care in a home setting. Professional caregivers may be needed to provide intravenous pain medications, nutrition, or fluids, for example, or to perform any number of other types of highly skilled tasks. Caring for a terminally ill person can also be an around-the-clock job, which may prove difficult for family members. If the quality of a person's

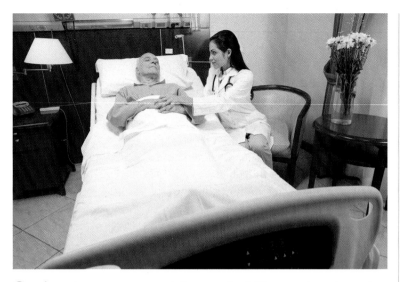

Caring for someone at the end of life can be done in a home, hospital, or hospice.

final days is being eroded by a lack of access to care, it may be best to consider a move to a professional care facility.

Hospital-Based Care

More than half of older Americans die in hospitals or nursing homes.[42] Although these facilities have traditionally focused on treating and curing illness and sustaining life, they are increasingly offering the dying hospital-based palliative care. Some hospitals and nursing homes have separate palliative care units, whereas others are trying to integrate this approach into wider aspects of the care they provide.

Hospice Care

Hospice care seeks to strike a balance between the comforting environment of home and the health-care expertise of a professional care setting. Hospice care focuses on providing the best possible quality of life for the dying and their families, usually within the last six months of a person's life, and does not concentrate on curing or treating disease. Instead, pain management, physical comfort, emotional and spiritual counseling, and similar services form the core of hospice care. Loved ones also receive additional support and counseling, both before and after the person dies. Some train to become hospice volunteers, providing support for patients and family members by visiting, reading aloud, accompanying the patient on walks, and the like.

Whereas people with complex palliative care needs are cared for in hospice facilities, in most cases, hospice services are provided at home.[43] Along with regular home visits from a hospice nurse, chaplain (if desired), and other professional staff, home care also includes volunteers who provide assistance with household tasks, child care, pet care, errands, and so forth. More than 1.4 million Americans receive hospice care each year, with most major insurance companies covering these services.[44]

Ethical Considerations

Hospice care can provide much-needed comfort, counseling, and caregiving to the dying and their families. But choosing hospice care

hospice A home-care program or facility that focuses exclusively on the dying and their loved ones, with a goal of providing comfort rather than facilitating a cure.

requires taking an important step—acknowledging that death is imminent, and that no further medical interventions will be sought to stop it. What if a person decided he was ready to take that step—but his family wasn't? Or what if health-care providers and family members understand that death is imminent, but the dying person wants to "keep fighting"? These complicated decisions often arise at the end of life, requiring complex ethical deliberations. Here are just some of the ethical issues that frequently arise at end of life:

- **When should life support be used or continued?** Medical technology can keep the body alive, even if the heart, lungs, or brain no longer functions independently and the person has no reasonable chance of recovering these functions. Some people fall into a *persistent vegetative state,* in which they are deeply unconscious, would not survive without life support, and have no reasonable hope of improvement. If the person hasn't stated life-support preferences beforehand, the decision whether to start or continue life support can be wrenching for their loved ones. (For a real-life example of this dilemma, see the **Get Critical** section at the end of this chapter.)

- **When should treatment be stopped or withheld?** Doctors can turn to numerous medical remedies to try to help severely ill people, but many of these may have limited effect and be exhausting or painful. What if your grandmother had terminal cancer, and decided to refuse any further chemotherapy or radiation, saying she wanted to live out her remaining days without nausea, exhaustion, or other side effects? What if your grandfather, whose congestive heart failure has drained his bank account, decides against pursuing more expensive therapies, opting instead for hospice? Law and medical practice acknowledge the right of patients to refuse treatment. But the dying and their loved ones may sometimes disagree on the right moment to take that step.

- **Should doctors help someone die?** Some people, facing the prospect of great suffering, may seek their care providers' help in providing a relatively quick, painless passage. These actions could take a more passive form, such as withholding oxygen to a person who is unconscious, or a more active form, such as administering a lethal dose of drugs. Such *physician-assisted suicide* remains deeply controversial. Some professional groups, such as the American Medical Association, take the position that doctors should never help hasten or enable the end of life. Some patient advocacy groups, however, argue that providing a comfortable death should be a core medical responsibility. One state, Oregon, has legalized physician-assisted suicide for terminally ill people who retain the judgment to make such a decision.

These dilemmas are painful to contemplate while you are young and healthy, and even more wrenching when they arise during a crisis. Advance directives offer a helpful way to think through some of these issues for family members and yourself, and express preferences before emergencies arise.

Giving the Gift of Life

If you are at least 18 years old, you can choose to become an organ donor. If you formally agree, either by filling out a donor card or enrolling while signing up for your driver's license, some of your organs, such as your heart, liver, kidneys, or the corneas of your eyes may be donated to a person awaiting an organ transplant. About half of all U.S. adults say they have registered as an organ donor. But in a critical gap, only about half of those who had registered said they had told their family.[45] Informing relatives of your decision is key. Without being aware of your preference, your loved ones may resist having your organs donated after your death.

At any given time, more than 100,000 people in the United States are typically waiting to receive an organ transplant. About 77 people receive a transplant each day—but another 19 die waiting for one.[46]

After a Death

When a loved one dies, the living face many immediate demands. Legal documents, such as a certificate of death, must be signed. Relatives, friends, and colleagues must be notified. Arrangements must be made for burial or cremation, and usually for some form of memorial service. An obituary is typically submitted to the press. Final bills must be paid. And amid all this work, overwhelming feelings of grief may leave survivors unable to focus on the tasks at hand, instead in need of support themselves. Here, we discuss the major tasks that immediately follow death, and the grief that typically accompanies them.

Taking Care of the Body

In decades past, family members typically bathed and dressed the body of the dead in a final act of love and respect before a simple burial. Although many families now relinquish these tasks to professional funeral homes, others still choose to maintain such care within the family. In fact, many religions encourage care of the body as an essential spiritual practice. By law, bodies can be buried or cremated. *Burial* in a cemetery plot can cost a few hundred to a few thousand dollars. Expenses can be even higher if families opt for a traditional coffin—or *casket*—and embalming of the body, in which tissues are preserved with chemicals. Many families forego embalming, and some are choosing a plain wooden or plywood box instead of a casket. An emerging trend is the choice of a "green burial," in which a body is simply wrapped in cloth and placed in the ground. In many states, laws allow for burying a body on the family's property as long as it is outside the village, town, or city limits.[47] *Cremation,* incineration of the body, uses extremely high heat to reduce the corpse to fragments of bone, which are then pulverized. The resulting 4 to 6 pounds of bone "ash" can then be scattered, buried, or preserved in a memorial urn or box. There is no environmental or health risk from cremated remains.

Planning a Service

After death, our loved ones leave behind not only material remains but also the legacy of their lifetime. To comfort the survivors, many choose to hold one or more formal services such as the following:

- **Wake.** The traditional *wake* was a period of hours to days during which loved ones gathered in the home of the deceased to clean, dress, and watch over the body, pray, and support the bereaved. Today, a wake may be held in a funeral home, church, or chapel, and may include a brief religious service, opportunities for individual prayer, and time for offering condolences. Food may be served.
- **Funeral.** To accompany the burial or cremation rites, some families choose to hold a funeral, usually a traditional religious service

in which prayers are said for the deceased and the person's life is remembered by loved ones and friends. Music, poems, and a formal eulogy may be offered. The burial of the body or scattering of the ashes may be held immediately after the service.

- **Memorial service.** Although memorial services often include prayers and music of a spiritual nature, they are typically less formal, involving less religious ritual than a funeral. Others take a more secular approach. Over time, the concept of a memorial service has evolved from a somber remembrance to a joyful celebration of the person's life, full of personal reminiscences, poems, songs, photos, and often a slide show or video. Food is typically a part of such services, and some even include dancing.

Experiencing Grief

Every one of the more than 2.4 million deaths in the United States each year touches the lives of the living. That experience brings a wide mix of feelings and responses, including sadness, anger, guilt, loss, loneliness, financial anxiety, and stress. These feelings can last for months or even years, reflecting the depth of the relationship and shifting as the reality of the death takes hold.

Stages of Grief

Grieving the loss of a loved one is a deeply personal experience that is different for everyone. Still, caregivers have noted that many who grieve experience one or more of the following stages:

- Disbelief, especially if a death is sudden or unexpected.
- Yearning, reflecting the desire to have the person back in your life in a vibrant, vital way.
- Anger, directed at everything from the death itself to the events surrounding the person's passing.

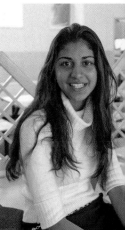

STUDENT STORY

Grieving

"Hi, I'm Michelle. When I was in high school, my uncle was killed in a car accident. It was a big shock to my family because he was still young and we weren't expecting it. I felt like a big part of what I had to do after it happened was support my mom and aunt, both of whom were really upset. Everyone felt so sad because we never had a chance to say good-bye. After the funeral, though, we all told stories and shared how he touched our lives. That made me feel a little better, and to this day I still try to talk about him and remember his spirit."

1: What types of things might Michelle have done to support her mom and aunt as they grieved for her uncle?

2: Why do you think telling stories about her uncle made Michelle feel better? What other types of things do people do to remember someone who's passed away?

3: What stage of grief do you think Michelle is in now?

Do you have a story similar to Michelle's? Share your story at **www.pearsonhighered.com/choosinghealth.**

- Depression, a persistent sadness that pervades daily life as the reality of the person's passing sets in.
- Acceptance, blending together the joys of the person's life and the changes following his or her loss into a new perspective that reflects the totality of the experience.[48]

Each person works through these stages in his or her own way, and some experiences of grief can be more complex than others. If a loved one has lived a long life and died after an illness, it may be easier to find peace with the death. If a person dies at a young age, passes violently, commits suicide, or is a victim of a natural disaster or other unexpected, traumatic event, grief may be much more complex, intense, and long-lasting. Such *complicated grief* may benefit from the assistance of a grief counselor, therapist, or support group attended by several people who have shared such a loss.

The Effects of Grief on Health

Death of a spouse or close family member is widely acknowledged as one of the top stressors that a human being can experience. (See Chapter 3.) People grieving a death, but especially those experiencing complicated grief, may suffer such severe stress that it becomes a risk to their own health. For example, one study found that loss of a spouse resulted in an immediate 12% reduction in life expectancy.[49]

The effects of grief on health may include any of the following symptoms or conditions:

- External symptoms, such as digestive upset, changes in eating habits, headaches, fatigue, weakness, vague pain, and disturbed sleep.
- Cardiac symptoms, such as higher blood pressure or irregular heartbeat.
- Psychosocial symptoms, such as increased drinking, depression, suicidal thoughts, feelings of guilt, isolation from others, and significant spiritual conflict.

If you or someone you know is grieving, social support is key. A grieving person may need a hug or someone to listen. Or they might want to step away from their grief, and seek company in activities that they find life-affirming. Extended support is also important. If a close family member has died, the first few days afterward require almost constant support of loved ones and friends. But in the weeks and months that follow, social support continues to be important, especially on occasions such as holidays and the one-year anniversary of the person's death. In supporting someone who is grieving a death, you are also doing something that the person who has passed would likely welcome—building bonds that affirm life.

☺ *Practical Strategies for Health*

Coping with Grief

If you or someone you know has lost a loved one, the following suggestions may help cope with the loss:

- **Connect with others.** Draw friends and loved ones close. Talk about your loss, your memories, and your experience of the life and death of your loved one. Don't try to protect your family and friends by not expressing your sadness. Find and talk to others who have also lost a loved one.

- **Expect—and allow yourself to feel—a range of emotions.** Don't tell yourself how to feel or let others tell you how you should feel.

- **Have patience with the process.** Accept that you need to experience your grief and your healing in your own time. Don't judge your emotions or compare yourself to others.

- **Take care of yourself: Eat well, exercise, and get enough sleep.** Physical activity is a good way to release tension. If your

grief hampers your appetite, try having small, healthful meals and snacks throughout the day. Resist the urge to eat only those foods that comfort you.

- **Try to maintain your normal lifestyle.** Avoid major life changes (for example, moving, changing jobs, changing important relationships) within the first year of your loss.

- **Forgive yourself for all the things you said or didn't say or do.** Compassion and forgiveness for yourself and others is important in healing.

- **Avoid quick fixes.** Substances such as drugs, alcohol, or over-the-counter sleep aids can be harmful, slow your recovery, and may actually cause new problems.

- **Be prepared for holidays and anniversaries. At these important times, strong feelings may come back.** Decide whether you want to keep certain traditions or create new ones. Plan in advance how you want to

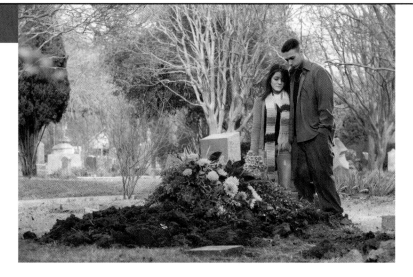

spend your time and with whom. You might be fearful of being overwhelmed by painful memories and emotions, only to find that you work through some of your grief as you cope with the stress of the approaching reminder.

- **When you feel ready, express your feelings by doing something creative.** You could:
  - Write a letter to the person who died to say everything you wish you could say to them.

- Make a scrapbook.
- Plant flowers or trees.
- Involve yourself in a cause or activity that the deceased loved.

Source: Adapted from: **1.** *Coping with the Loss of a Loved One,* by the American Cancer Society, 2009, retrieved from http://www.cancer.org/Treatment/ TreatmentsandSideEffects/EmotionalSideEffects/ GriefandLoss/index. **2.** *End of Life,* by the Mayo Clinic, 2010, retrieved from http://www.mayoclinic.com/health/ grief/MH00036/NSECTIONGROUP=2. **3.** *Grief and Grieving – Home Treatment,* by WebMD, last updated 2009, retrieved from http://www.webmd.com/balance/tc/ grief-and-grieving-home-treatment.

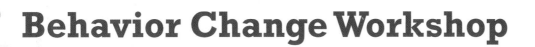

Behavior Change Workshop

To complete this workshop online, visit www.pearsonhighered.com/choosinghealth.

As you've learned in this chapter, many of the health behaviors you choose today affect not only your life expectancy, but also your quality of life as an older adult. A recent study concluded that smoking, alcohol consumption, poor nutrition, and inactivity can age your body up to 12 years![50] The good news, according to the researchers, is that "modest but achievable adjustments to lifestyle behaviors are likely to have a considerable impact." So, healthy behaviors you adopt today will significantly impact your health and quality of life tomorrow!

Part I. Assess Your Behaviors

1. The study found that the following behaviors positively impact health as people age:
- Not smoking
- Eating 3 or more servings of fruits and vegetables each day
- Getting 2 or more hours of "leisure-time physical activity" per week
- Drinking no more that 7 alcoholic drinks per week for women or 10.5 per week for men

Consider these four behaviors. Which are you currently participating in?

_____

_____

_____

Which of the above behaviors are you not participating in?

_____

_____

_____

2. Target one of the above behaviors that needs improvement. Ask yourself honestly, "How ready am I to commit to a behavior change?" What stage of behavior change are you in?

Target behavior: _____

Current stage of behavior change: _____

_____

_____

_____

Part II. Take Action

1. Keeping your current stage of behavior change in mind, describe what you might do differently so that you can adhere to the beneficial behaviors shown in Part I.

Example: I will take salsa dancing lessons at the student recreation center. Because I enjoy dancing, this will be a leisure-time physical activity that I will be motivated to do and that I can do for a lifetime.

Next step: _____

_____

_____

2. What obstacles might get in your way to making long-lasting change? How you will address them?

Obstacle:	How to address:

Chapter Summary

- The United States is heading toward a "longevity revolution," with life expectancy increasing and a growing percentage of the population falling into older age brackets.

- Not everyone, however, can expect a longer life span. Women tend to live at least 5 years longer than men, and life expectancy also correlates closely with a person's racial or ethnic background, income, and region of residence.

- Aging brings changes. Some are physical, such as declines in vision and hearing. Women experience menopause, the loss of reproductive capacity. Chronic diseases, including arthritis and osteoporosis, become more common. Psychosocial changes include shifts in family dynamics, retirement, economic changes, and an increased risk of depression as the aging person is challenged to adapt to the changing circumstances.

- Some older adults experience impairments in cognition and memory. The more mild form of this condition is referred to as age-related dementia. The more severe, progressive, and fatal form is Alzheimer's disease.

- Through lifelong habits that promote health preservation, you can avoid or limit some of the challenges of aging, especially when it comes to reducing your risk of chronic conditions such as cardiovascular disease, type 2 diabetes, and osteoporosis.

- Key steps in healthy aging include engaging in regular physical activity, following a healthy diet, getting enough sleep, avoiding smoking, limiting use of alcohol and medications, challenging your mind, and reducing stress. Put these healthy habits in place when you are young.

- Death is often defined by the cessation of heartbeat, breathing, and other vital functions, but may also be defined by other factors, such as the end of discernable brain-wave activity.

- Our concept of death evolves as we mature from childhood to adulthood, and is influenced by our life experiences as well as our beliefs and values.

- Numerous planning aids can help a person think through end-of-life issues ahead of time, state preferences, and make plans. These include advance directives for health, wills, and registration opportunities for organ donation.

- Options for end-of-life care include home care, hospital-based care, and hospice care, carried out either in a hospice facility or in the person's home. In any setting, palliative care is a key aspect of care for the dying. The goal of palliative care is to decrease pain and suffering rather than to prolong the person's life.

- After a death, a person's body may be buried or cremated, and his or her life remembered and celebrated at a wake, funeral, or memorial service.

- Grieving is a natural part of and reaction to death, and those experiencing grief, especially complicated grief, need the support of friends and loved ones through the long process of coming to terms with their loss.

- In acknowledging death, preparing for it, and coping with its aftermath, you learn much about yourself, including new ways to affirm life.

Test Your Knowledge

1. What percentage of older U.S. adults report getting no leisure time physical activity?
   a. about 12%
   b. about 22%
   c. about 32%
   d. more than 50%

2. What is the life expectancy for someone born in 2010 in the U.S.?
   a. about 68 years
   b. about 78 years
   c. about 88 years
   d. about 98 years

3. Which of the following accurately characterizes arthritis?
   a. Arthritis happens to everyone when they get older.
   b. Arthritis damages your ligaments.
   c. Arthritis is caused by loss of bone density.
   d. Arthritis typically affects the hands and weight-bearing joints.

4. What does Alzheimer's disease affect?
   a. how the brain functions
   b. how the body functions
   c. length of life
   d. all of the above

5. Older adults should limit their sodium intake to what level?
   a. 1,500 milligrams a day
   b. 2,000 milligrams a day
   c. 2,500 milligrams a day
   d. none of the above—sodium isn't a special concern

6. What can people who smoke one pack of cigarettes a day expect?
   a. to experience reduced quality of life as they age
   b. to appear older than others who are the same age but have never smoked
   c. to die about 10 years earlier than those who have never smoked
   d. all of the above

7. What is the Five Wishes an example of?
   a. a health-care proxy
   b. a DNR order
   c. an advance directive
   d. a will

8. What percentage of U.S. adults have drafted a will?
   a. 30%
   b. 45%
   c. 55%
   d. 70%

9. What is the goal of palliative care?
   a. to prolong life
   b. to prevent further deterioration in the patient's condition
   c. to cure disease
   d. to relieve pain and suffering

10. If someone is grieving, what is the best way to help him or her?
    a. talk about something else
    b. be present and offer support, both in the moment and over the long term
    c. distract him or her
    d. talk about others who have died, to show that this particular death was a normal thing

Get Critical

What happened:

In 2005, a 41-year-old woman named Terry Schiavo passed away in a Florida hospice after spending about 15 years in a persistent vegetative state. She had suffered cardiac arrest at her home in 1990, and endured extensive brain damage due to lack of oxygen. Her husband and parents spent several years trying multiple therapies in an attempt to restore consciousness, with no success. Schiavo had left no written advance directives or other formal indications of how she wished to be cared for under such circumstances.

Her husband, however, said that his wife, prior to her collapse, had verbally stated that she would never want to be kept alive by artificial means. After deciding there was no reasonable hope for her recovery, he began petitioning Schiavo's care providers and Florida courts to have her feeding tube removed. Schiavo's parents, however, disagreed, and launched legal proceedings to have her feeding tube kept in place. A lengthy, complicated court battle followed, drawing intense media scrutiny and eventually involving advocacy groups, members of the U.S. Congress, and even former President George W. Bush.

In 2005, a Florida court ultimately issued a ruling agreeing that sufficient evidence of Schiavo's wishes not to continue life support existed, and her feeding tube was removed. Schiavo died several days later.

What do you think?

- If you were on life support, and medical experts agreed that there was no chance of recovery, what would you want your loved ones to do on your behalf?

- How involved should multiple family members be in such decisions? Who should have primary deciding power?

- How might an advance directive have simplified Schiavo's situation?

- Should advocacy groups and politicians get involved in such cases? Or should they remain private family matters?

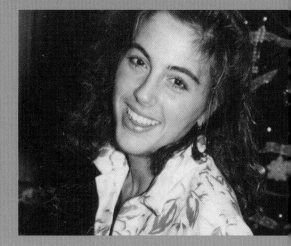

Get Connected

References

i. Administration on Aging. (2009). *Profile of older Americans*. Retrieved from http://www.aoa.gov/AoARoot/Aging_Statistics/Profile/index.aspx

ii. Rocheleau, M. (2010, July 26). Seniors get their tech on. *Christian Science Monitor, 102*/Issue 35, 29.

iii. Centers for Disease Control and Prevention. (2010). *Deaths by 10-year age groups: United States and each state, 2007*. Retrieved from http://www.cdc.gov/nchs/data/dvs/MortFinal2007_Worktable23f.pdf

1. Centers for Disease Control and Prevention and the Merck Company Foundation. (2007). *The state of aging and health in America*. Retrieved from http://www.cdc.gov/aging/pdf/saha_2007.pdf

2. Centers for Disease Control and Prevention. (2009). *Health-related quality of life: National trend – Percentage with fair or poor self-rated health: Age group*. Retrieved from http://apps.nccd.cdc.gov/HRQOL/TrendV.asp?State=1&Measure=1&Category=3&submit1=Go

3. Administration on Aging. (2008). *A profile of older Americans: 2008 – Health and health care*. Retrieved from http://www.aoa.gov/AoARoot/Aging_Statistics/Profile/2008/14.aspx

4. Centers for Disease Control and Prevention. (2008). *Health-related quality of life: National trend – Mean physically unhealthy days: Age group*. Retrieved from http://apps.nccd.cdc.gov/HRQOL/TrendV.asp?State=1&Measure=2&Category=3&submit1=Go

5. Centers for Disease Control and Prevention. (2008). *Health-related quality of life: National trend – Mean mentally unhealthy days: Age group*. Retrieved from http://apps.nccd.cdc.gov/HRQOL/TrendV.asp?State=1&Measure=3&Category=3&submit1=Go

6. U.S. Department of Health and Human Services Administration on Aging. (2009). A Profile of Older Americans: 2009. p. 14. Retrieved from http://www.aoa.gov/AoARoot/Aging_Statistics/Profile/2009/docs/2009profile_508.pdf

7. Xu, J., Kochanek, K. D., & Tejada-Vera, B. (2009, August 19). Deaths: Preliminary data for 2007. *National Vital Statistics Reports, 58*(1). Retrieved from http://www.cdc.gov/nchs/data/nvsr/nvsr58/nvsr58_01.pdf

8. National Center for Health Statistics. (2009, April 17). Expectation of life at birth, 1970 to 2006, and projections 2010 to 2020. Table 102 in Deaths: Final data for 2006. *National Vital Statistics Reports, 57*(14). Retrieved from http://www.census.gov/compendia/statab/2010/tables/10s0102.pdf

9. National Institutes of Health. (2005). *Obesity threatens to cut U.S. life expectancy, new analysis suggests* [News Release]. Retrieved from http://www.nih.gov/news/pr/mar2005/nia-16.htm

10. Murray, C. J. L., Kulkarni, S. C., Michaud, C., Tomijima, N., Bulzacchelli, M. T., Iandiorio, T. J., & Ezzati, M. (2006, September). Eight Americas: Investigating mortality disparities across races, counties, and race-counties in the United States. *PLoS Medicine*. Retrieved from http://www.plosmedicine.org/article/info%3Adoi%2F10.1371%2Fjournal.pmed.0030260

11. Central Intelligence Agency. (2009). Field listing: Life expectancy at birth. In *The World Factbook*. Retrieved from https://www.cia.gov/library/publications/the-world-factbook/fields/2102.html

12. Felder, S. (2006). The gender longevity gap: Explaining the difference between singles and couples. *Journal of Population Economics, 19*(1), 543–557.

13. National Eye Institute. (2010). *Facts about age-related macular degeneration*. Retrieved from http://www.nei.nih.gov/health/maculardegen/armd_facts.asp

14. Writing Group for the Women's Health Initiative Investigators. (2002). Risks and benefits of estrogen plus progestin in healthy postmenopausal women: Principal results from the Women's Health Initiative randomized controlled trial. *Journal of the American Medical Association, 288*(3), 321–333.

15. Kontula, O., & Haavio-Manilla, E. (2009). The impact of aging on human sexual activity and sexual desire. *Journal of Sex Research, 46*(1), 46–56.

16. Centers for Disease Control and Prevention. (2009). *Arthritis: Data and statistics*. Retrieved from http://www.cdc.gov/arthritis/data_statistics.htm

17. National Institutes of Health, Osteoporosis and Related Bone Diseases National Resource Center. (2009). *Osteoporosis*. Retrieved from http://www.niams.nih.gov/Health_Info/Bone/Osteoporosis/default.asp

18. Yetley, E. A., Brulé, B., Cheney, M. C., Davis, C. D., Esslinger, K. A., Fischer, P. W. F. . . . & McMurry, K. Y. (2009). Dietary reference intakes for vitamin D: Justification for a review of the 1997 values. *American Journal of Clinical Nutrition, 89*, 719–727.

19. Gunning-Dixon, F., Brickman, A., Cheng, J., & Alexopoulos, G. (2009). Aging of cerebral white matter: A review of MRI findings. *International Journal of Geriatric Psychiatry, 24*, 109–117.

20. Bergman, I., Blomberg, M., & Almkvist, O. (2007). The importance of impaired physical health and age in normal cognitive aging. *Scandinavian Journal of Psychology, 48*, 115–125.

21. National Institute on Aging. (2010). *The search for AD prevention strategies*. Retrieved from http://www.nia.nih.gov/Alzheimers/Publications/ADPrevented/strategies.htm

22. National Institute on Aging. (2008). *The hallmarks of AD*. Retrieved from http://www.nia.nih.gov/Alzheimers/Publications/Unraveling/Part2/hallmarks.htm

23. Alzheimer's Association. (2009). *2009 Alzheimer's disease facts and figures*. Retrieved from http://www.alz.org/national/documents/report_alzfactsfigures2009.pdf

24. Scarmeas, N., Luchsinger, J. A., Schupf, N., Brickman, A. M., Cosentino, S., Tang, M. X., & Stern, Y. (2009). Physical activity, diet, and risk of Alzheimer's disease. *Journal of the American Medical Association, 302*(6), 627–637.

25. Middleton, T. (2007). Fixing the 5 biggest 401(k) blunders. *MSN Money: Personal Finance*. Retrieved from http://articles.moneycentral.msn.com/Investing/MutualFunds/The5biggest401kBlunders.aspx

26. National Institute of Mental Health. (2009). *Older adults: Depression and suicide facts (fact sheet)*. Retrieved from http://www.nimh.nih.gov/health/publications/older-adults-depression-and-suicide-facts-fact-sheet/index.shtml

27. Hansen-Kyle, L. (2005). A concept analysis of healthy aging. *Nursing Forum, 40*(2), 45–57.

28. Barondess, J. (2008). Toward healthy aging: The preservation of health. *Journal of the American Geriatrics Society, 56*(1), 145–148.

29. Centers for Disease Control and Prevention. (2009). *Physical activity for everyone: How much physical activity do older adults need?* Retrieved from http://www.cdc.gov/physicalactivity/everyone/guidelines/olderadults.html

30. Lichtenstein, A., Rasmussen, H., Yu, W., Epstein, S., & Russell, R. (2008). Modified MyPyramid for older adults. *Journal of Nutrition, 138*, 78–82.

31. Qato, D. M., Alexander, G. C., Conti, R. M., Johnson, M., Schumm, P., & Lindau, S. T. (2008). Use of prescription and over-the-counter medications and dietary supplements among older adults in the United States. *Journal of the American Medical Association, 300*(24), 2867–2878.

32. Dominguez, L., Barbagallo, M., & Morley, J. (2009). Anti-aging medicine: Pitfalls and hopes. *The Aging Male, 12*(1), 13–20.

33. Strandberg, A., Strandberg, T. E., Pitkala, K., Salomaa, V. V., Tilvis, R. S., & Miettinen, T. A. (2008). The effect of smoking in midlife on health-related quality of life in old age. *Archives of Internal Medicine, 168*(18), 1968–1974.

34. Hall, C. B., Lipton, R. B., Sliwinski, M., Katz, M. J., Derby, C. A., & Verghese, J. (2009). Cognitive activities delay onset of

memory decline in persons who develop dementia. *Neurology, 73,* 356–361.

35. Hill, T. (2006). Religion, spirituality, and healthy cognitive aging. *Southern Medical Journal, 99*(10), 1176–1177.

36. Steinhauser, K., Clipp, E., McNeilly, M., Christakis, N., McIntyre, L., & Tulsky, J. (2000). In search of a good death: Observations of patients, families, and providers. *Annals of Internal Medicine, 132*(10), 825–832.

37. Mayo Clinic. (2008). *Terminal illness: Supporting a terminally ill loved one.* Retrieved from http://www.mayoclinic.com/health/grief/CA00041

38. Aging with Dignity. (2009). *Five wishes.* Retrieved from http://www.agingwithdignity.org/forms/5wishes.pdf

39. Koenig, R., & Hyde, M. (2009). Be careful what you wish for: Analyzing the "Five Wishes" advance directive. *Illinois Bar Journal, 97*(5), 242–245.

40. Harris Interactive. (2007). *News: Majority of American adults remain without wills, new lawyers.com survey finds..* Retrieved from http://www.lawyers.com/understand-your-legal-issue/press-room/Majority-of-American-Adults-Remain-Without-Wills.html

41. American Medical Association. (2006, September 20). Palliative care. *Journal of the American Medical Association, 296*(11). Retrieved from http://jama.ama-assn.org/cgi/reprint/296/11/1428.pdf

42. Muramatsu, N., Hoyem, R. L., Yin, H., & Campbell, R. T. (2008). Place of death among older Americans: Does state spending on home- and community-based services promote home death? *Medical Care, 46*(8), 829–838.

43. Hospice Foundation of America. (2010). *Choosing hospice.* Retrieved from http://www.hospicefoundation.org/pages/page.asp?page_id=53053

44. National Hospice and Palliative Care Organization. (2009). *NHPCO facts and figures: Hospice care in America.* Retrieved from http://www.nhpco.org/files/public/Statistics_Research/NHPCO_facts_and_figures.pdf

45. Harris Interactive. (2007). *Most U.S. adults believe in the importance of organ donation but are ambivalent about how to increase the numbers of donors.* Retrieved from http://www.harrisinteractive.com/news/allnewsbydate.asp?NewsID=1226

46. U.S. Department of Health and Human Services, Organdonor.gov. (2009). *Waiting list candidates.* Retrieved from http://www.organdonor.gov

47. Funeral Consumers Alliance. (2007). *Earth burial, tradition in simplicity.* Retrieved from http://www.funerals.org/faq/74-earth-burial-tradition-in-simplicity

48. Maciejewski, P., Zhang, B., Block, S., & Prigerson, H. (2007). An empirical examination of the stage theory of grief. *Journal of the American Medical Association, 297*(7), 716–723.

49. van den Berg, G. J., Lindeboom, M., & Portrait, F. (2006). *Conjugal bereavement effects on health and mortality at advanced ages.* Institute of Labor. IZA DP No. 2358. Retrieved from http://ftp.iza.org/dp2358.pdf

50. Kvaavik, E., Batty, G. D., Ursin, G., Huxley, R., & Gale, C. R. (2010). Influence of individual and combined health behaviors on total and cause-specific mortality in men and women: The United Kingdom health and lifestyle survey. *Archives of Internal Medicine, 170*(8):711–718.

Test Your Knowledge Answers

Chapter 1:
1. c   2. b   3. d   4. a   5. c   6. d   7. c   8. b
9. a   10. d

Chapter 2:
1. d   2. a   3. b   4. b   5. c   6. d   7. a   8. c
9. d   10. c

Chapter 3:
1. a   2. d   3. d   4. c   5. d   6. b   7. b   8. d
9. a   10. a

Chapter 4:
1. a   2. c   3. d   4. c   5. b   6. b   7. c   8. a
9. d   10. d

Chapter 5:
1. d   2. d   3. d   4. c   5. b   6. d   7. b   8. a
9. c   10. a

Chapter 6:
1. c   2. d   3. c   4. b   5. a   6. a   7. b   8. d
9. d   10. b

Chapter 7:
1. d   2. a   3. d   4. c   5. d   6. c   7. d   8. d
9. d   10. c

Chapter 8:
1. a   2. d   3. a   4. b   5. d   6. c   7. b   8. a
9. c   10. c

Chapter 9:
1. d   2. b   3. b   4. d   5. d   6. b   7. c   8. d
9. a   10. b

Chapter 10:
1. c   2. a   3. b   4. a   5. c   6. b   7. d   8. c
9. c   10. d

Chapter 11:
1. b   2. b   3. d   4. a   5. b   6. a   7. a   8. d
9. d   10. c

Chapter 12:
1. d   2. c   3. b   4. b   5. c   6. b   7. d   8. b
9. d   10. a

Chapter 13:
1. d   2. d   3. c   4. b   5. d   6. a   7. a   8. c
9. b   10. a

Chapter 14:
1. a   2. d   3. a   4. d   5. b   6. c   7. d   8. b
9. a   10. a

Chapter 15:
1. c   2. d   3. a   4. a   5. d   6. a   7. a   8. d
9. a   10. a

Chapter 16:
1. c   2. b   3. d   4. a   5. a   6. d   7. c   8. b
9. d   10. b

Behavior Change Workshop Sample Answers

Chapter 6:

There are many things you can do to make this meal lower calorie and more healthful.

Hamburger: Your burger is going to set you back almost 700 calories—you could split it with a friend to cut that amount in half, or you could replace it with a lower calorie option like a grilled chicken sandwich (without sauce) or soup and a salad.

French fries: Your French fries contain around 400 calories; you could replace them with a baked potato and 1/2 T. butter, only 180 calories.

Side salad: The ranch dressing on your salad adds 130 calories to your diet; either switch to a fat-free version and save around 80 calories or consider replacing your salad with steamed broccoli, a 1/2 cup of which only contains around 30 calories!

Coke: You can switch to a diet Cola or water, saving you at least 150 calories.

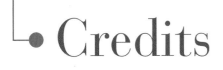

Credits

Photo Credits

p. iv, top: April Lynch; **p. iv, middle:** Barry Elmore; **p. iv, bottom:** Tanya Morgan

Chapter 1 opener: Shannon Fagan/Getty Images; **p. 3:** Daniel Hurst/Newscom; **p. 4:** John Dawson; **p. 5:** Lane Erickson/Dreamstime; **p. 6:** Graham Salter/Alamy; **p. 7, left:** Friedrich Stark/Alamy; **p. 7, right:** Fancy/Alamy; **p. 9:** Nativestock.com/Marilyn Angel Wynn/Getty Images; **p. 10:** Cultura/Alamy; **p. 11:** John Dawson; **p. 12:** Fox Broadcasting Company/Newscom; **p. 13:** alvarez/istockphoto; **p. 17:** Johnny Green/AP Images

Chapter 2 opener: Laura Doss/Corbis; **p. 21:** Newscom; **p. 22:** Jeff Greenberg/Alamy; **p. 23:** Blend Images/Alamy; **p. 24:** Dylan Ellis/Corbis; **p. 25:** Newscom; **p. 26:** Andres Rodriguez/Alamy; **p. 27:** Design Pics Inc./Alamy; **p. 29:** indeed/Getty Images; **p. 30:** Radius Images/Alamy; **p. 31:** catenarymedia/iStockphoto; **p. 32:** MBI/Alamy; **p. 33:** John Bell/iStockphoto; **p. 34:** Jewel Samad/Newscom; **p. 35:** John Dawson; **p. 36:** Ghislain & Marie David de Lossy/Getty Images; **p. 37:** Firefoxfoto/Alamy; **p. 38:** Newscom; **p. 41:** Heather Ainsworth/AP Photo

Chapter 3 opener: Jupiterimages/Getty Images; **p. 46:** Tim McGuire/Getty Images; **p. 47:** Nikolay Suslov/iStockphoto; **p. 48, left:** Steven Le; **p. 48, right:** Stockbyte/Getty Images; **p. 49:** RadiusImages/Alamy; **p. 50:** Maciej Korzekwa/iStockphoto; **p. 51:** Newscom; **p. 52:** Adam Borkowski/iStockphoto; **p. 54:** iStockphoto; **p. 55, left:** Adrian Sherratt/Alamy; **p. 55, right:** Douglas Pulsipher/Alamy; **p. 56:** Justin Horrocks/iStockphoto; **p. 57:** Stockbyte/Getty Images; **p. 58:** Juice Images/Alamy; **p. 60:** AdamGregor/iStockphoto; **p. 63:** Jason DeCrow/AP Images

Chapter 4 opener: Marnie Burkhart/Corbis; **p. 67:** Tom Grill/Corbis; **p. 68:** Feng Yu/Shutterstock; **p. 69, left:** Corbis; **p. 69, right:** Fotocrisis/Shutterstock; **p. 70:** Gustavo Caballero/Getty Images; **p. 71:** Flashon Studio/Shutterstock; **p. 72:** Regien Paassen/Shutterstock; **pp. 72-73, Table 4.1:** all Corbis; **p. 74, Table 4.2, top 4:** Corbis; **bottom:** Shutterstock; **p. 75:** Lana Langlois/Shutterstock; **p. 76, left:** Kati Molin/Shutterstock; **p. 76, right:** Jesse Kunerth/Alamy; **p. 78:** Tetra Images/Corbis; **p. 80:** PLG Learning Studio; **p. 81:** Michael Newman/Photo Edit; **p. 82:** John Dawson; **p. 83, left:** Bramalia/Dreamstime; **p. 83, right:** Shutterstock; **p. 84:** Taylor S. Kennedy/Alamy; **p. 87:** Clive Brunskill/Getty Images

Chapter 5 opener: Dennis Welsh/Getty Images; **p. 92:** Blue Jean Images/Alamy; **p. 94, left:** Newscom; **p. 94, right:** Newscom; **p. 96, Table 5.1, top to bottom:** Richard Smith/Masterfile; Doug Menuez/Photodisc/Getty Images; Stockbyte/Getty Images; **p. 97:** Blue Jean Images/Getty Images; **p. 98, a, b, c:** Elena Dorfman; **d:** Jac Mat; **p. 99, e, f:** Jac Mat; **g:** Rolland A. Renaud; **h, i:** Elena Dorfman; **j:** Rolland A. Renaud; **p. 100:** Image Source/Getty Images; **p. 101:a:** Jac Mat; **b, c, d, e:** Elena Dorfman; **p. 102: f:** Jac Mat; **g:** Denis Gendron; **h:** Rolland A. Renaud; **i:** Elena Dorfman; **j, k:** Jac Mat; **p. 103:** Walter Lockwood/Corbis; **p. 106:** Olivier Blondeau/iStockphoto; **p. 107, left:** RubberBall Selects/Alamy; **p. 107, right:** Newscom; **p. 109:** Newscom; **p. 110, left:** Image Source/Alamy; **p. 110, right:** motorolka/iStockphoto; **p. 113:** Pat Benic/Newscom

Chapter 6 opener: Michael A. Keller/Corbis; **p. 118:** Ace Stock Limited/Alamy; **p. 120:** Newscom; **p. 123:** Frederic J. Brown/Newscom; **p. 125,**

Table 6.1, top to bottom: Sean Aidan/Corbis; David Young-Wolff/PhotoEdit; Life Measurement, Inc; BSIP/SPL/Photo Researchers; **p. 126, top:** George Doyle/Getty Images; **p. 126, bottom:** Newscom; **p. 129:** Creative Digital Creations; **p. 130:** AlexMax/iStockphoto; **p. 132:** Losevsky Pavel/Alamy; **p. 133:** Giulio Marcocchi/Newscom; **p. 134:** Blake Little/Getty Images; **p. 135:** igor kisselev/Alamy; **p. 136:** AFP/Getty Images; **p. 138, top to bottom:** Brand X Pictures/Getty Images; Brand X Pictures/Getty Images; Nikola Bilic/Shutterstock; Corbis

Chapter 7 opener: Chat Roberts/Corbis; **p. 145:** Christopher Hudson/iStockphoto; **p. 147:** Joy Scheller/Newscom; **p. 148, top:** Newscom; **p. 148, bottom:** Newscom; **p. 149:** Jon Schulte/iStockphoto; **p. 150, left:** Radius Images/Alamy; **p. 150, right:** Angela Maynard/Getty Images; **p. 151:** Multnomah County Sheriff/Newscom; **p. 152:** Newscom; **p. 153:** Courtesy of DEA; **p. 155:** Ken Inness/iStockphoto; **p. 155, Table 7.3, top:** nicholas belton/iStockphoto; **bottom:** Courtesy of DEA; **p. 156, Table 7.3, top to bottom:** Joe Bird/Alamy; David Lee/Alamy; Wikipedia; Courtesy of DEA; Courtesy of DEA; **p. 157:** Patrick Kociniak/Alamy; **p. 159:** Tim Pannell/Corbis; **p. 162:** WENN/Newscom

Chapter 8 opener: Robert Lawson/PhotoLibrary; **p. 166:** Jamie Grill/Corbis; **p. 168:** Kristin Piljay; **p. 169:** David Wile/Getty Images; **p. 170:** ZZ/Alamy; **p. 171:** Stockbroker/Alamy; **p. 172:** Paul Piebinga/istockphoto; **p. 173:** Juice Images/Alamy; **p. 174:** Tatiana Popova/Shutterstock; **p. 178:** beti gorse/iStockphoto; **p. 179:** John Dawson; **p. 180:** Philip Hall/Newscom; **p. 181, top:** Image Source/Alamy; **p. 181, bottom:** Mark Goddard/iStockphoto; **p. 182:** Alamogordo Daily News, Ellis Neel/AP Photo; **p. 183:** Milos Luzanin/Shutterstock; **p. 186:** Universal Pictures/Newscom

Chapter 9 opener: www.photo-chick.com/Getty Images; **p. 191:** Tom Chance/Alamy; **p. 192:** Datacraft - Sozaijiten/Alamy; **p. 193:** Randy Faris/Corbis; **p. 194:** John Dawson; **p. 195:** Laurence Mouton/PhotoAlto/Corbis; **p. 196:** John Dawson; **p. 198:** Hill Street Studios/Getty Images; **p. 200:** Amy Sancetta/AP Images; **p. 201:** Ambient Images Inc./Alamy; **p. 202:** Jeff Steinberg/Matt Smith/Newscom; **p. 203:** Newscom; **p. 206:** Peter Sorel/Newscom

Chapter 10 opener: Pierre Bourrier/PhotoLibrary; **p. 213:** Jose Luis Pelaez Inc/Alamy; **p. 214:** John Dawson; **p. 215:** Fancy/Alamy; **p. 218:** Ardelean Andreea/Shutterstock; **p. 219:** ZUMA Press/Newscom; **p. 220:** Rawdon Wyatt/Alamy; **p. 221:** Tammy Hanratty/Alamy; **p. 222:** Adam Nemser/Newscom; **p. 228, left:** Exactostock/SuperStock; **p. 228, right:** IndexStock/SuperStock; **p. 229:** Barbara J. Petrick/Shutterstock; **p. 230:** John Dawson; **p. 233:** Ian Hooton/Alamy; **p. 235, top to bottom:** Lennart Nilsson/Scanpix; Lennart Nilsson/Scanpix; Neil Bromhall/Photo Researchers; Marc Kurschner/Getty Images; **p. 242:** Newscom

Chapter 11 opener: Latin Stock Collection/Corbis; **p. 246:** detwo/Shutterstock; **p. 247:** John Dawson; **p. 249:** Mandel NGAN/Newscom; **p. 251, Table 11.2, top to bottom:** Photo Researchers; Dr. Ray Butler/CDC; Dr. Libero Ajello/CDC; Eye of Science/Photo Researchers; Andrew Syred/Photo Researchers; **p. 252:** Polka Dot/Thinkstock; **p. 254:** Bruno Coignard, M.D.; Jeff Hageman, M.H.S./CDC; **p. 255:** James Gathany/AP Images; **p. 256:** Stringer Shanghai/Reuters/Corbis; **p. 257:** Paul Bradbury/Alamy; **p. 261:** Jose Luis Pelaez Inc/Alamy; **p. 262, left:** Dr. P. Marazzi/

Glossary

12-step programs Addiction recovery self-help programs based on the principles of Alcoholics Anonymous.

A

abortion A medical or surgical procedure used to terminate a pregnancy.

absorption The process by which alcohol passes from the stomach or small intestine into the bloodstream.

abstinence The avoidance of sexual intercourse.

accessory glands Glands (seminal vesicles, prostate gland, and Cowper's gland) which lubricate the reproductive system and nourish sperm.

acid rain A phenomenon in which airborne pollutants are transformed by chemical processes into acidic compounds, then mix with rain, snow, or fog and are deposited on Earth.

acquired immunity The body's ability to quickly identify and attack a pathogen that it recognizes from previous exposure. In some cases acquired immunity leads to life-long protection against the same infection.

acute intoxication (alcohol poisoning) Potentially fatal concentration of alcohol in the blood.

adaptive response Protective physiological adaptations in response to stressors.

addiction A complex, relapsing condition characterized by uncontrollable craving for a substance or behavior despite the harmful consequences.

adrenaline Adrenal gland hormone that is secreted at higher levels during the stress response; also called *epinephrine*.

advance directive Formal documents that state a person's preferences regarding medical treatment and medical crisis management.

aerobic exercise Prolonged physical activity that raises the heart rate and works the large muscle groups.

age-related macular degeneration (AMD) An age-related vision disorder caused by deterioration of the macula that reduces central vision.

aggravated assault An attack intended to cause serious physical harm, often involving a weapon.

Air Quality Index (AQI) An index for measuring daily air quality according to a list of federal air criteria, published by city or region.

alcohol abuse Drinking alcohol to excess, either regularly or on individual occasions, resulting in disruption of work, school, or home life and causing interpersonal, social, or legal problems.

alcohol intoxication The state of physical and/or mental impairment brought on by excessive alcohol consumption (in legal terms, a BAC of 0.08% or greater).

alcohol poisoning Dangerously high level of alcohol consumption, resulting in depression of the central nervous system, slowed breathing and heart rate, and compromised gag reflex.

alcoholism (alcohol dependence) A physical dependence on alcohol to the extent that stopping drinking brings on withdrawal symptoms.

allergies Abnormal immune system reactions to substances that are otherwise harmless.

allostasis The body's process of restoring homeostasis through short-term adaptive mechanisms.

allostatic overload The wear and tear the body experiences as the result of the continuous or repeated demands of allostasis.

altruism The practice of helping and giving to others out of genuine concern for their well-being.

Alzheimer's disease (AD) A progressive, fatal form of age-related dementia.

amenorrhea Cessation of menstrual periods.

amino acids The building blocks of protein; 20 common amino acids are found in food.

amniotic fluid Fluid that surrounds the developing fetus that aids in temperature regulation and allows the baby to move freely.

amphetamines Central nervous system stimulants that are chemically similar to the natural stimulants adrenaline and noradrenalin.

anaerobic exercise Short, intense exercise that causes an oxygen deficit in the muscles.

anal intercourse Intercourse characterized by the insertion of the penis into a partner's anus and rectum.

anaphylactic shock A result of anaphylaxis where the release of histamine and other chemicals into the body leads to a drop in blood pressure, tightening of airways, and possible unconsciousness and even death.

angina pectoris Chest pain due to coronary heart disease.

anorexia nervosa An eating disorder characterized by extremely low body weight, body image distortion, severe calorie restriction, and an obsessive fear of gaining weight.

antibiotic resistance When a bacterium is able to overcome the effects of an antibiotic through a random mutation, or change in the bacterium's genetic code.

antibodies Proteins released by B cells that bind tightly to infectious agents and mark them for destruction.

antigen Tiny regions on the surface of an infectious agent that can be detected by B cells and T cells.

antioxidants Compounds in food that help protect the body from harmful molecules called free radicals.

anxiety disorders A category of mental disorders characterized by persistent feelings of fear, dread, and worry.

Apgar score A measurement of how well a newborn tolerated the stresses of birth, as well as how well he or she is adapting to the new environment.

appetite The psychological response to the sight, smell, thought, or taste of food that prompts or postpones eating.

arrhythmia Any irregularity in the heart's rhythm.

arteries Blood vessels that flow away from the heart, delivering oxygen-rich blood to the body periphery and oxygen-poor blood to the lungs.

arthritis Inflammation of one or more joints in the body, resulting in pain, swelling, and limited movement.

assertiveness The ability to clearly express your needs and wants to others in an appropriate way.

assortative mating The tendency to be attracted to people who are similar to us.

asthma A chronic pulmonary disease in which the air passages become inflamed, making breathing difficult.

asthma Chronic constriction and inflammation of the airways, making breathing difficult and causing shortness of breath, wheezing, coughing, and chest tightness.

atherosclerosis Condition characterized by narrowing of the arteries because of inflammation, scarring, and the buildup of fatty deposits.

atria The two upper chambers of the heart, which receive blood from the body periphery and lungs.

attachment theory The theory that the patterns of attachment in our earliest relationships with others form the template for attachment in later relationships.

attention disorders A category of mental disorders characterized by problems with mental focus.

attention-deficit/hyperactivity disorder (ADHD) A type of attention disorder characterized by inattention, hyperactive behavior, fidgeting, and a tendency toward impulsive behavior.

autonomy The capacity to make informed, un-coerced decisions.

B

bacteria (singular *bacterium*) Single-celled microorganisms that invade a host and reproduce inside. Harmful bacteria release toxic enzymes and chemicals.

ballistic stretching Performing rhythmic bouncing movements in a stretch to increase the intensity of the stretch.

balloon angioplasty An arterial treatment that uses a small balloon to flatten plaque deposits against the arterial wall.

barbiturates A type of central nervous system depressant often prescribed to induce sleep.

bariatric surgery Weight-loss surgery using various procedures to modify the stomach or other sections of the gastrointestinal tract in order to reduce calorie intake or absorption.

basal metabolic rate (BMR) The rate at which the body expends energy for only the basic functioning of vital organs.

behavior change A change in an action or habit that affects health.

behavioral therapy A type of therapy that focuses on a patient's behavior and its relationship to psychological health.

benign tumor A tumor that grows slowly, does not spread, and is not cancerous.

benzodiazepines Medications commonly prescribed to treat anxiety and panic attacks.

binge drinking A pattern of drinking alcohol that results in a blood alcohol concentration of 0.08 or above (about five or more alcoholic drinks within 2 hours for men, or four or more alcoholic drinks within 2 hours for women).

binge eating The rapid consumption of an excessive amount of food.

bioaccumulation The process by which substances increase in concentration in the fat tissues of living organisms as the organisms take in contaminated air, water, or food.

biomagnification The process by which certain contaminants become more concentrated in animal tissue as they move up the food chain.

biomonitoring Analysis of blood, urine, tissues, and so forth to measure chemical exposure in humans.

biopsy A test for cancer in which a small sample of the abnormal growth is removed and studied.

bipolar disorder (manic-depressive disorder) A mental disorder characterized by occurrences of abnormally elevated mood (or mania), often alternating with depressive episodes, with periods of normal mood in between.

birth control pills Pills containing combinations of hormones that prevent pregnancy when taken regularly as directed.

bisexuals People who are attracted to partners of both the same and the opposite sex.

blood alcohol concentration (BAC) The amount of alcohol present in blood, measured in grams of alcohol per deciliter of blood.

blood pressure The force of the blood moving against the arterial walls.

body burden The amount of a chemical stored in the body at a given time, especially a potential toxin in the body as the result of environmental exposure.

body composition The relative proportions of the body's lean tissue and fat tissue.

body image A person's perceptions, feelings, and critiques of his or her own body.

body mass index (BMI) A numerical measurement, calculated from height and weight measurements, that provides an indicator of health risk categories.

bradycardia A slow arrhythmia.

brain death The cessation of brain activity as indicated by various medical devices and diagnostic criteria.

brain fitness A person's ability to meet the cognitive requirements and demands of daily life, such as problem solving and memory recall.

bulimia nervosa An eating disorder characterized by episodes of binge eating followed by a purge behavior such as vomiting, laxative abuse, or extreme exercise.

bypass surgery A procedure to build new pathways for blood to flow around areas of arterial blockage.

C

caffeine A widely used stimulant found in coffee, tea, soft drinks, chocolate, and some medicines.

calorie Also called *kilocalorie*. A unit of measure that indicates the amount of energy that food provides, specifically, the amount of energy required to raise the temperature of one kilogram of water by one degree Celsius.

cancer A group of diseases marked by the uncontrolled multiplication of abnormal cells.

capillaries The smallest blood vessels, delivering blood and nutrients to individual cells and picking up wastes.

carbohydrates A macronutrient that is the body's universal energy source, supplying sugar to all body cells.

carbon monoxide A gas that inhibits the delivery of oxygen to the body's vital organs.

carcinogen A substance known to trigger DNA mutations that can lead to cancer.

carcinogenic Cancer-causing.

carcinoma Cancer of tissues that line or cover the body.

cardiorespiratory fitness The ability of your heart and lungs to effectively deliver oxygen to your muscles during prolonged physical activity.

cardiovascular disease (CVD) Diseases of the heart or blood vessels.

carpal tunnel syndrome A repetitive stress injury of the hand or wrist, often linked to computer keyboard use or other types of repetitive motion.

carrier A person infected with a pathogen who does not show symptoms but who is infectious.

cataracts An age-related vision disorder marked by clouding of the lens of the eye.

cellular death The end of all vital functions at the cellular level, such as cellular respiration and other metabolic processes.

central nervous system cancer Cancer of the brain or spinal cord.

cesarean section (C-section) A surgical procedure involving the incision of a woman's abdominal and uterine walls in order to deliver the baby.

changing self-talk Shifting one's internal dialogue in a more positive, empowering direction.

chronic bronchitis Inflammation of the main airways in the lungs that continues for at least three months.

chronic disease A disease with a gradual onset of symptoms that last a long time or recur.

chronic obstructive pulmonary disease (COPD) A category of diseases that includes emphysema, chronic bronchitis, and asthma.

chronic stress syndrome Collection of symptoms resulting from the long-term effects of prolonged exposure to the body's physiological stress responses.

circumcision The surgical removal of the foreskin.

clinical death A medical determination that life has ceased according to medical criteria that often combine aspects of functional and neurological factors.

clitoris An organ composed of spongy tissue and nerve endings which is very sensitive to sexual stimulation.

club drugs Illicit substances, including MDMA (ecstasy), GHB, and ketamine that are most commonly encountered at nightclubs and raves.

cocaine A potent and addictive stimulant derived from leaves of the coca shrub.

codependency When a friend or family member is part of a pattern that may perpetuate behaviors that sustain addiction.

cognitive therapy A type of therapy that focuses on thoughts and beliefs and how they influence your mood.

cohabitation The state of living together in the same household; usually refers to unmarried couples.

complementary and alternative medicine (CAM) Health practices and traditions not typically part of conventional Western medicine, either used alone (alternative medicine) or in conjunction with conventional medicine (complementary medicine).

complex carbohydrates Contain chains of multiple sugar molecules; commonly called *starches* but also come in two non-starch forms: *glycogen* and *fiber.*

conception The fertilization of a female egg with male sperm.

condom (male condom) A thin sheath typically made of latex, polyurethane, or lambskin that is unrolled over the erect penis prior to vaginal penetration.

conflict avoidance The active avoidance of discussing concerns, annoyances, and conflict with another person.

conflict escalation Increasing conflict to a more confrontational, painful, or otherwise less comfortable level.

conflict resolution Resolving a conflict in a manner that both people can accept and that minimizes future occurrences of the conflict.

congestive heart failure A gradual loss of heart function.

consumer health An umbrella term encompassing topics related to the purchase and consumption of health-related products and services.

continuation rate The percentage of couples who continue to practice a given form of birth control.

contraception Any method used to prevent pregnancy.

contraceptive sponge A flexible foam disk containing spermicide that is inserted in the vagina prior to sex.

conventional medicine Commonly called Western medicine, this system of care is based on the principles of the scientific method; the belief that diseases are caused by identifiable physical factors and have a characteristic set of symptoms; and the treatment of physical causes through drugs, surgery, or other physical interventions.

coronary arteries The blood vessels that feed the heart.

coronary heart disease (coronary artery disease) Atherosclerosis of the arteries that feed the heart.

cortisol Adrenal gland hormone that is secreted at higher levels during the stress response.

cramp An involuntary contracted muscle that does not relax resulting in localized intense pain.

cunnilingus Oral stimulation of the vulva or clitoris.

D

date (acquaintance) rape Coerced, forceful, or threatening sexual activity in which the victim knows the attacker.

date rape drugs Drugs used to assist in a sexual assault, often given to the victim without his or her knowledge or consent.

decibel The unit of measurement used to express sound intensity.

deductible An amount of money that you must pay yourself before your insurer begins to cover the costs of your medical care.

dementia A group of cognitive impairments and other disorders that affect the brain and the ability to perform basic everyday tasks.

dentist A conventional medicine practitioner who specializes in care of the teeth, gums, and mouth.

depressants Substances that depress the activity of the central nervous system including barbiturates, benzodiazepines, and alcohol.

depressive disorder A mental disorder usually characterized by profound, long-term sadness or loss of interest that interferes with daily life and normal functioning.

diabetes mellitus A group of diseases in which the body does not make or use insulin properly, resulting in elevated blood glucose.

diaphragm A flexible silicone cup filled with spermicide and inserted in the vagina prior to sex to prevent pregnancy.

diet The food you regularly consume.

Dietary Reference Intakes (DRIs) A set of energy and nutrient recommendations for supporting good health.

dilation and evacuation (D&E) A multistep method of surgical abortion that may be used in pregnancies that have progressed beyond 12 weeks.

disordered eating A range of unhealthful eating behaviors used to deal with emotional issues that does not warrant a diagnosis of a specific eating disorder.

dissociative drug A medication that distorts perceptions of sight and sound and produces feelings of detachment from the environment and self.

distress Stress resulting from negative stressors.

domestic (family) violence An abusive situation in which family members may verbally, emotionally, sexually, or physically abuse others.

domestic partnership A legal arrangement in which a couple lives together in a long-term committed relationship and receives some, but not all, of the rights of married couples.

dopamine A neurotransmitter that stimulates feelings of pleasure.

drug abuse The use (most often the excessive use) of any legal or illegal drug in a way that is detrimental to your health.

drug misuse The inappropriate use of a legal drug, either for a reason for which it was not medically intended, or by a person without a prescription.

drug A chemical substance that alters the body physically or mentally for a non-nutritional purpose.

dynamic flexibility The ability to move quickly and fluidly through a joint's entire range of motion with little resistance.

dysmenorrhea Pain during menstruation that is severe enough to limit normal activities or require medication.

dysthymic disorder (dysthymia) A milder, chronic type of depressive disorder that lasts two years or more.

E

e-waste Hazardous waste generated by the production or disposal or electronic or digital devices.

eating disorders A group of mental disorders, including anorexia nervosa, bulimia nervosa, and binge-eating disorder, that is characterized by physiological and psychological disturbances in appetite or food intake.

ecological footprint The collective impact of an entity on its resources, ecosystems, and other key environmental features.

ecosystem A dynamic collection of organisms and their nonliving surroundings that function as a unit.

ectopic pregnancy A pregnancy that occurs when a fertilized egg implants within one of the fallopian tubes instead of the uterus; considered a medical emergency.

electrocardiogram A test that measures the heart's electrical activity.

embryo The growing collection of cells that ultimately become a baby.

emergency contraception (EC; "morning after" pill) A pill containing levonorgestrel, a synthetic hormone that is used to prevent pregnancy after unprotected sex.

emotional health The subjective side of psychological health, including your feelings and moods.

emotional intelligence The ability to accurately monitor, assess, and manage your emotions and those of others.

emphysema A chronic disease in which the air sacs in the lung become damaged, making breathing difficult.

enablers People who protect addicts from the negative consequences of their behavior.

enabling factor A skill, asset, or capacity that shapes behavior.

endocrine disruptor A substance that stops the production or blocks the use of hormones in the body and that can have harmful effects on health or development.

endometriosis A condition in which endometrial tissue grows in areas outside of the uterus.

energy balance The state achieved when energy consumed from food is equal to energy expended, maintaining body weight.

environmental health The discipline that addresses all the physical, chemical, and biological factors external to individual human beings, especially those that influence human health.

epididymis A coiled tube on top of each testicle where sperm are held until they mature.

erectile dysfunction (ED) The inability of a male to obtain or maintain an erection.

erection The process of the penis filling up with blood as a result of sexual stimulation.

essential nutrients Nutrients you must obtain from food or supplements because your body either cannot produce them or cannot make them in sufficient quantities to maintain health.

estate A person's personal holdings, including money, property, and other possessions.

ethyl alcohol (ethanol) The intoxicating ingredient in beer, wine, and distilled liquor.

euphoria A feeling of intense pleasure.

eustress Stress resulting from positive stressors.

evidence-based medicine Health-care policies and practices based on systematic, scientific study.

excitement The first phase of the sexual response cycle, marked by erection in men, and lubrication and clitoral swelling in women.

exercise A type of physical activity that is planned and structured.

F

failure rate The percentage of women who typically get pregnant after using a given contraceptive method for one year.

fallopian tubes A pair of tubes that connect the ovaries to the uterus.

family health history A detailed record of health issues in one's family that presents a picture of shared health risks.

fats (lipids) A major source of energy that helps the body absorb fat-soluble vitamins, cushions and insulates organs, and adds flavor and tenderness to foods.

fee-for-service plan A type of health insurance in which you choose your providers, and you and your insurer divide the costs of care.

fellatio Oral stimulation of the penis.

fertility awareness (rhythm or calendar method) The tracking of a woman's monthly menstrual cycle; may be used as a method of preventing pregnancy if the woman tracks carefully and has regular periods, though is not failsafe.

fetal alcohol syndrome A pattern of mental and physical birth defects found in some children of mothers who drank excessively during pregnancy.

fetus The name given to the developing embryo 8 weeks after fertilization.

fiber A non-digestible complex carbohydrate that aids in digestion.

fight-or-flight response A series of physiological reactions to a stressor designed to enable the body to stand and fight or to flee.

FITT Exercise variables that can be modified in order to accomplish progressive overload: frequency, intensity, time, and type.

flexibility The ability of joints to move through their full ranges of motion.

flexible spending account (FSA) A consumer-controlled account, usually offered through employers, that uses pre-tax dollars to cover approved health-related purchases.

food additive A substance added to foods during processing to improve color, texture, flavor, aroma, nutrition content, or shelf life.

food allergy An adverse reaction of the body's immune system to a food or food component.

Food Guide Pyramid (MyPyramid) A graphic representation of the Dietary Guidelines for Americans, which encourage intake of complex carbohydrates and discourage intake of fats and sweets.

foodborne illness (food poisoning) Illness caused by pathogenic microorganisms consumed through food or beverages.

functional death The end of all vital physiological functions, including heartbeat, breathing, and blood flow.

fungi Multicellular or single-celled organisms that obtain their food from organic matter, in some cases human tissue.

G

gang An economic or social group that forms to intimidate and control members and outsiders through threats and violence.

gender roles Behaviors and tasks considered appropriate by society based on whether someone is a man or a woman.

general adaptation syndrome (GAS) An adaptive response consisting of three stages (alarm, resistance, exhaustion) through which the body strives to maintain or restore homeostasis.

generalized anxiety disorder (GAD) An anxiety disorder characterized by chronic worry and pessimism about everyday events that lasts at least six months and may be accompanied by physical symptoms.

genetic modification Altering a plant's or animal's genetic material in order to produce desirable traits such as resistance to pests, poor soil tolerance, or lower fat.

genome sequencing The full decoding and readout of an entire genome.

genome The complete genetic material of any living organism.

genomics The study of genomes and their effects on health and development.

GHB (gamma-hydroxybutyric acid) A central nervous system depressant known as a "date rape drug" because of its use to impair potential victims of sexual assault.

glaucoma An age-related vision disorder arising from an increase in internal eye pressure that damages the optic nerve and reduces peripheral vision.

global warming A sustained increase in the Earth's temperature due to an increase in the greenhouse effect resulting from pollution.

globalization The interaction and integration of regional phenomena globally.

groundwater The supply of fresh water beneath the Earth's surface, which is a major source of drinking water.

H

hallucinogens Drugs that alter perception and are capable of causing auditory and visual hallucinations.

hangover Alcohol withdrawal symptoms, including headache and nausea, caused by an earlier bout of heavy drinking.

hate crime A crime fueled by bias against another person's or group's race or ethnicity, religion, national origin, sexual orientation, or disability.

hazardous waste Garbage or byproducts that can pose a hazard to human health or the environment when improperly managed.

hazing Initiation rituals to enter a fraternity or other group that can be humiliating, hazardous, or physically or emotionally abusive, regardless of the person's willingness to participate.

health belief model A model of behavior change emphasizing personal beliefs in the process of creating effective change.

health discount program A system of health discounts given to members of groups, such as employees of a particular company or students attending a particular college.

health disparities Differences in quality of health among various segments of the population.

health insurance A contract between an insurance company and a group or individual who pays a fee to have some or all health costs covered by the insurer.

health literacy The ability to evaluate and understand health information and to make informed choices for your health care.

health maintenance organization (HMO) A type of managed care in which most health care is funneled through and must be approved by the primary care doctor.

health preservation Performing activities that seek to maintain health, rather than simply responding to health crises as they occur.

health savings account (HSA) A consumer-controlled account that comes attached to a high-deductible health insurance plan and covers the costs of the deductible and other health-related expense approved by the federal government.

health-related fitness The ability to perform activities of daily living with vigor.

health More than merely the absence of illness or injury, a state of well-being that encompasses physical, social, psychological, spiritual, intellectual, environmental, and occupational dimensions.

healthful weight The weight at which health risks are lowest for an individual; usually a weight that will result in a BMI between 18.5 and 24.9.

Healthy Campus An offshoot of the Healthy People initiative, specifically geared toward college students.

Healthy People initiative A federal initiative to facilitate broad, positive health changes in large segments of the U.S. population every 10 years.

heat exhaustion A mild form of heat-related illness that usually occurs as the result of exercising in hot weather without adequate hydration.

heatstroke A life-threatening heat-related illness that occurs when your core temperature rises above 105 degrees Fahrenheit.

Heimlich maneuver A method for helping someone who is choking by dislodging the obstruction through a series of quick upward thrusts below the diaphragm.

hemorrhagic stroke A stroke caused by a ruptured blood vessel.

hepatitis Inflammation of the liver that affects liver function.

herd immunity The condition where greater than 90% of a community is vaccinated against a disease, giving it little ability to spread through the community, providing some protection against the disease to members of the community who are not vaccinated.

heroin The most widely abused of opioids; typically sold as a white or brown powder or as a sticky black substance known as "black tar heroin."

heterosexual A person sexually attracted to someone of the opposite sex.

high-density lipoprotein (HDL) A cholesterol-containing compound that removes excess cholesterol from the bloodstream; often referred to as "good cholesterol."

homeostasis The body's desired state of physiological equilibrium or balance.

homicide The killing of one human being by another.

homophobia The irrational fear of, aversion to, or discrimination against homosexuals or homosexuality.

homosexual A person sexually attracted to someone of the same sex.

hooking up Casual, noncommittal, physical encounters that may range from kissing and "making out" to oral sex and intercourse.

hospice A home-care program or facility that focuses exclusively on the dying and their loved ones, with a goal of providing comfort rather than facilitating a cure.

host A person, plant, or animal in which or on which pathogens live and reproduce.

human sexual response cycle Distinct phases extending from the first moment of sexual desire until the calm after orgasm.

hunger The physiological sensation caused by the lack of food.

hyperglycemia A persistent state of elevated levels of blood glucose.

hypertension (high blood pressure) A persistent state of elevated blood pressure.

hypothermia A potentially fatal condition in which your core body temperature becomes too low.

I

immune system Your body's cellular and chemical defenses against pathogens.

immunization Creating immunity to a pathogen through vaccination or through the injection of antibodies.

implantation The lodging of a fertilized egg in the endometrium of the uterus.

individuality The principle that individuals will respond to fitness training in their own unique ways.

infant mortality rate A calculation of the ratio of babies who die before their first birthday to those who survive until their first birthday.

infection The invasion of body tissues by microorganisms that use the body's environment to multiply and cause disease.

infertility The inability to conceive after trying for at least a year.

inflammatory response A response to damaged body tissues designed to kill any pathogens in the damaged tissue, promote healing, and prevent the spread of infection to other parts of the body.

influenza A group of viruses that cause the flu, a contagious respiratory condition.

inhalants Chemical vapors that, when inhaled, produce mind-altering effects.

insulin A hormone necessary for glucose transport into cells.

intentional injury Physical harm that is purposefully inflicted through violence.

intervention A technique used by family and friends of an addict to encourage the addict to seek help for a drug problem.

intestate Dying without leaving a legal will.

intimacy A sense of closeness with another person formed by being emotionally open and caring.

intimate partner violence An abusive situation in which one member of a couple or intimate relationship may verbally, emotionally, sexually, or physically abuse the other.

intoxicate To cause physical and psychological changes as a result of the consumption of psychoactive substances.

intrauterine device (IUD) A plastic, T-shaped device that is inserted in the uterus for long-term pregnancy prevention.

ischemic stroke A stroke caused by a blocked blood vessel.

isometric exercise Exercise where the muscle contracts but the body does not move.

isotonic exercise Exercise where the muscle contraction causes body movement.

J

jaundice A yellowing of the skin, mucous membranes, and sometimes the whites of the eyes often caused by liver malfunction.

jealousy The response to a threat to a relationship from an actual or imagined rival for a partner's attention.

K

ketamine An anesthetic that can cause hallucinations and a dream-like state; commonly known as "special K."

L

labia Two pairs (majora and minora) of fleshy lips surrounding and protecting the clitoris and the vaginal and urethral openings.

labor The physical processes involved in giving birth.

leukemia Cancer of blood-forming tissue.

leukoplakia White spots on the mucous membranes in the mouth that may become cancerous.

life expectancy The length of time a person can expect to live, usually measured in years.

life support systems Medical technologies that artificially sustain one or more vital functions.

locus of control A person's belief about where the center of power lies in his or her life; can be external or internal.

low birth-weight The term given to birth-weights less than 5 pounds, 8 ounces.

low-density lipoprotein (LDL) A cholesterol-containing compound that, as it degrades, releases its cholesterol load into the bloodstream; often referred to as "bad cholesterol."

LSD (lysergic acid diethylamide) A powerful hallucinogen manufactured from lysergic acid, a substance found in a fungus that grows on rye and other grains.

lymphoma Cancer of the lymph system.

M

mainstream smoke Smoke exhaled from the lungs of smokers.

major depressive disorder (major depression) A type of depressive disorder characterized by experiencing five or more symptoms of depression, including either depressed mood or loss of interest or pleasure, for at least two weeks straight.

malaria A serious disease that causes fever and chills that appear in cycles. In some cases malaria can be life-threatening.

malignant melanoma An especially aggressive form of skin cancer.

malignant tumor A tumor that grows aggressively, invades surrounding tissue, and can spread to other parts of the body; all cancers are malignant.

managed-care plan A type of health insurance in which the insurer contracts with a defined group of health providers, which the consumer must use or face higher out-of-pocket costs.

marijuana The most commonly used illegal drug in the U.S.; derived from the plant *cannabis sativa*.

mast cell A type of cell in the skin and mucous membranes that releases histamine and other chemicals into the bloodstream during an allergic reaction.

masturbation Manipulation of one's own genitals for sexual pleasure.

MDMA (methylenedioxymethamphetamine) A synthetic drug, commonly called "ecstasy," that works as both a stimulant and hallucinogen.

Medicaid A joint federal-state public insurance program that covers low-income individuals and families.

medical doctor A physician trained in conventional medicine, with many years of additional formal education and training and a professional license.

Medicare A federal public insurance program that covers people with long-term disabilities and anyone 65 or older.

menarche The first onset of menstruation.

menopause The permanent end of a woman's menstrual cycle and reproductive capacity.

menstrual cycle A monthly physiological cycle marked by *menstruation*.

menstrual phase Phase of the menstrual cycle characterized by menstrual flow, the release of follicle-stimulating hormone from the pituitary gland to the brain, and the release of estrogen into the bloodstream.

menstruation The cyclical discharge of blood and tissue from the vagina.

mental disorders Significant behavioral and psychological disorders that disrupt thoughts and feelings, impair ability to function, and increase risk of pain, disability, or even death.

mental health The "thinking" component of psychological health that allows you to perceive reality accurately and respond rationally and effectively.

metabolic syndrome A group of obesity-related factors that increase the risk of cardiovascular disease and diabetes, including large waistline, high triglycerides, low HDL cholesterol, high blood pressure, and high fasting blood glucose.

metabolism The breakdown of food and beverages in the body to transform them into energy.

metastasis The process by which a malignant tumor spreads to other body sites.

methamphetamine A highly addictive and dangerous stimulant that is chemically similar to amphetamine, but more potent and harmful.

methicillin-resistant *Staphylococcus aureus* (MRSA) A strain of staph that is resistant to the broad-spectrum antibiotics commonly used to treat staph infections.

minerals Elements, with no energy value of their own, that regulate body processes and provide structure; constituents of all cells.

mini-med plan A type of managed-care plan, sold individually to younger people, which carries lower costs but does not cover many services.

miscarriage A pregnancy that suddenly terminates on its own before the 20th week.

modeling A behavior change technique based on watching and learning from others.

mononucleosis A viral disease that causes fatigue, weakness, sore throat, fever, headaches, swollen lymph nodes and tonsils, and loss of appetite.

mons pubis The fatty, rounded areas of tissue in front of the pubic bone.

moods Prolonged emotional states.

municipal solid waste (MSW) Nonhazardous garbage or trash generated by industries, businesses, institutions, and homes.

murder The act of intentionally and unjustifiably killing another person.

muscular endurance The capacity of muscles to repeatedly exert force, or to maintain a force, over a period of time.

muscular strength The maximum force your muscles can apply in a single maximum effort of lifting, pushing, or pressing.

myeloma Cancer of the bone marrow.

myocardial infarction (heart attack) A cardiac crisis in which a region of heart muscle is damaged or destroyed by reduced blood flow.

myocardium The heart's muscle tissue.

N

neurotoxin A substance that interferes with or harms the functioning of the brain and nervous system.

nicotine An alkaloid derived from the tobacco plant that is responsible for smoking's psychoactive and addictive effects.

nonverbal communication Communication that is conveyed by body language.

nurse practitioner Registered nurses who have undergone additional training and can perform some of the care provided by a medical doctor.

nurse A licensed professional who provides a wide range of health-care services and supports the work of medical doctors.

nutrients Chemical substances in food that you need for energy, growth, and survival.

nutrition The scientific study of food and its physiological functions.

O

obese A weight disorder in which excess accumulations of nonessential body fat result in increased risk of health problems. A weight resulting in a BMI of 30 or above.

obsessive-compulsive disorder (OCD) An anxiety disorder characterized by repeated and unwanted thoughts (obsessions) that lead to rituals (compulsions) in an attempt to control the anxiety.

oncogene A mutated gene that encourages the uncontrolled cell division that results in cancer.

opioids (narcotics) Drugs derived from opium or synthetic drugs that have similar sleep-inducing, pain-reducing effects.

opportunistic diseases Infections and other disorders that take advantage of a weakened immune system.

optimism The psychological tendency to have a positive interpretation of life's events.

optometrist A licensed professional who provides vision care.

oral sex Stimulation of the genitals by the tongue or mouth.

orgasm The peak, or climax, of sexual response, characterized by rhythmic muscle contractions of the genitals and surrounding areas, and ejaculation in men.

osteoporosis A disease characterized by low bone mass and deterioration of bone tissue, leading to fragile bones and an increased risk of fractures.

outercourse Sexual intimacy without penetration of the vagina or anus.

ovaries The two female reproductive organs where ova (eggs) reside.

over-the-counter (OTC) medication A medication available for purchase without a prescription.

overload Increasing the stress placed on your body through exercise, which results in an improved fitness level.

overweight The condition of having a body weight that exceeds what is generally considered healthful for a particular height. A weight resulting in a BMI of 25–29.9.

ovulate Release an egg from the ovary.

ozone depletion Destruction of the stratospheric ozone layer, which shields the Earth from harmful levels of ultraviolet radiation, resulting from pollution.

P

palliative care Type of care that focuses on reducing pain and suffering and caring for the whole person, rather than prolonging life or curing disease.

pancreas An abdominal organ that produces insulin as well as certain compounds helpful in digestion.

pandemic A worldwide epidemic of a disease.

panic attacks Episodes of sudden terror that strike without warning.

panic disorder A mental disorder characterized both by recurring panic attacks and the fear of a panic attack occurring.

parasitic worms (helminths) Multicellular creatures that compete with a host body for nutrients.

passive stretching Stretching performed with a partner who increases the intensity of the stretch by gently applying pressure to your body as it stretches.

pathogen An agent that causes disease.

PCP (phencyclidine) A dangerous synthetic hallucinogen that reduces and distorts sensory input and can unpredictably cause both euphoria and dysphoria.

penis The male sexual and reproductive organ.

percent Daily Value (% DV) Nutrient standards that estimate how much a serving of a given food contributes to the overall intake of nutrients listed on the food label.

personal safety The practice of making decisions and taking actions that reduce your risk of injury and death.

pharmacogenomics The use of DNA information to choose medications and make prescribing decisions.

phobia An extreme, disabling, irrational fear of something that poses little or no actual danger.

physical activity Bodily movement that substantially increases energy expenditure.

physical dependence The physical need for a drug.

physical fitness The ability to perform moderate to vigorous levels of activity and to respond to physical demands without excessive fatigue.

physician assistant (P.A.) A licensed health professional who practices under the supervision of a physician and provides a broad range of care.

phytochemicals Naturally occurring plant substances thought to have disease-preventing qualities and health-promoting properties.

placenta The tissue that connects mother and baby.

plateau The second phase of the sexual response cycle, characterized by intense excitement, rapid heartbeat, genital sensitivity, the secretion of pre-ejaculatory fluid in men, and vaginal swelling in women.

podiatrist A licensed professional who specializes in the care of the feet.

point-of-service (POS) plan A type of managed care that lets HMO consumers see a broader list of providers for an additional fee.

pollution Contamination of the natural environment as a result of human activities.

polyabuser A person who abuses more than one drug.

portion control A method of reducing overconsumption of calories by limiting serving sizes of food.

positive psychology A new field of psychology that focuses on increasing psychological strengths and improving happiness, rather than on psychological problems.

post-traumatic stress disorder (PTSD) An anxiety disorder characterized by recurrent fear, anger, and depression occurring after a traumatic event.

pre-existing condition A health issue that existed prior to application to or enrollment in an insurance plan, which insurers sometimes use to restrict care or set the price paid for insurance.

prediabetes A persistent state of blood glucose levels higher than normal, but not yet high enough to qualify as diabetes.

predisposing factor A physical, mental, emotional, or surrounding influence that shapes behavior.

preeclampsia A serious health condition characterized by high blood pressure in the pregnant woman.

preferred provider organization (PPO) A type of managed care in which the consumer is encouraged to stay within an approved network of providers but has more choice over whom is seen when.

premature ejaculation (PE) A condition in which a male ejaculates earlier than he would like to.

premenstrual dysphoric disorder (PMDD) Severe and debilitating psychological symptoms experienced just prior to menstruation.

premenstrual syndrome (PMS) A collection of emotional and physical symptoms that occur just prior to menstruation.

prenatal care Nutritional counseling and regular medical screenings throughout pregnancy to aid the growth and development of the fetus.

presbycusis Age-related hearing loss, which usually develops gradually, often due to damage to or changes in the inner ear.

presbyopia Age-related decline in the ability to focus on objects up close, especially in low light.

probiotics Living, beneficial microbes that develop naturally in food and that help maintain digestive functions.

progressive overload Gradually overloading the body over time in order to avoid injury.

proliferative phase Phase of the menstrual cycle characterized by a thickening of the lining of the uterus and discharge of cervical mucus. This phase ends when luteinizing hormone triggers the release of a mature egg.

proof value A measurement of alcoholic strength, corresponding to twice the alcohol percentage (13% alcohol equals 26 proof).

prostate gland A walnut-sized gland that produces part of the semen. It is prone to malignancy.

protein A macronutrient that helps build many body parts, including muscle, bone, skin, and blood; key component of enzymes, hormones, transport proteins, and antibodies.

protozoa Single-celled parasites that rely on other living things for food and shelter.

psilocybin A hallucinogenic substance obtained from certain types of mushrooms that are indigenous to tropical regions of South America.

psychoactive A drug that alters feelings, mood, perceptions, or psychological functioning.

psychodynamic therapy A type of therapy that focuses on the unconscious sources for a patient's behavior and psychological state.

psychological dependence A mental attachment to a drug.

psychological health The broad measure of well-being that encompasses the mental, emotional, and spiritual dimensions of health.

psychoneuroimmunology The study of the interactions among psychological processes, the nervous system, hormones, and the immune system.

purging Behaviors, such as vomiting, laxative abuse, or overexercising, intended to reduce the calories absorbed by the body.

R

radiation Energy that travels in the form of rays, waves, or particles.

rape Nonconsensual oral, anal, or vaginal penetration by body parts or objects, using force, threats of bodily harm, or taking advantage of circumstances that make a person incapable of consenting to sex.

realism The ability to perceive life as it really is so that you can rationally respond to its demands.

recovery The period necessary for the body to recover from exercise demands and adapt to higher levels of fitness.

reinforcement A motivational behavior change technique that rewards steps toward positive change.

reinforcing factor An encouragement or a reward that promotes behavior change.

relapse The return to an addictive substance or behavior after a period of conscious abstinence.

relaxation response The physiological opposite response to fight-or-flight that can be activated through relaxation techniques.

repetitions The number of times you perform an exercise repeatedly.

repetitive strain injury (RSI) An injury that damages joints, nerves, or connective tissue caused by repeated motions that put strain on one part of the body.

reservoir The natural environment for any particular pathogen, where it accumulates in large numbers.

residential programs Live-in drug treatment centers.

resolution The stage of the sexual response cycle in which the body returns to normal functioning.

reversibility The principle that fitness levels decline when the demand placed on the body is decreased.

Rohypnol (roofies) A powerful sedative known as a "date rape drug" because of its use to impair potential victims of sexual assault.

S

sarcoma Cancer of muscle or connective tissues.

satiety Physical fullness; the state in which there is no longer the desire to eat.

saturated fats Fats that typically are solid at room temperature; generally found in animal products, dairy products, and tropical oils.

schizophrenia A severe mental disorder characterized by incorrect perceptions of reality, an altered sense of self, and radical changes in emotions, movements, and behaviors.

scrotum The skin sac at the base of the penis that contains the testes.

seasonal affective disorder (SAD) A type of depressive disorder caused by fewer hours of daylight during the winter months.

secondhand smoke (environmental tobacco smoke) The smoke nonsmokers are exposed to when someone has been smoking nearby; a combination of sidestream smoke and mainstream smoke.

secretory phase Phase of the menstrual cycle characterized by the degeneration of the follicle sac, rising levels of progesterone in the bloodstream, and further increase of the endometrial lining.

self-actualization The pinnacle of Maslow's hierarchy of needs pyramid, which indicates truly fulfilling your potential.

self-care Actions you take to keep yourself healthy.

self-disclosure The sharing of honest feelings and personal information about yourself with another person.

self-esteem A sense of positive self-regard, resulting in elevated levels of self-respect, self-worth, self-confidence, and self-satisfaction.

self-medicating Using alcohol or drugs to cope with sadness, grief, pain, or mental health problems.

semen The male ejaculate consisting of sperm and other fluids from the accessory glands.

sets Separate groups of repetitions.

sex The biological and physiological features that differentiate a male from a female.

sexting The use of cell phones or similar electronic devices to send sexually explicit text, photos, or videos.

sexual assault Any form of coerced sexual activity up to but not including penetration, using force, threats of bodily harm, or taking advantage of circumstances that make a person incapable of consenting to sex.

sexual dysfunctions Problems occurring during any stage of the sexual response cycle.

sexual harassment Unwelcome sexual advances that explicitly or implicitly affect academic or employment situations, unreasonably interfere with work or school performance, or create an intimidating, hostile, or offensive work or school environment.

sexual orientation Romantic and physical attraction toward others.

sexuality The biological, physical, emotional, and psychosocial aspects of sexual attraction and expression.

sexually transmitted infections (STIs) Infections transmitted mainly through sexual activity, such as vaginal, anal, or oral sex.

shaping A behavior change technique based on breaking large tasks into more manageable parts.

shyness The feeling of apprehension or intimidation in social situations, especially in reaction to unfamiliar people or new environments.

sidestream smoke Smoke emanating from the burning end of a cigarette or pipe.

simple carbohydrates The most basic unit of carbohydrates, consisting of one or two sugar molecules.

sinus node A group of cells in the right atrium that generate the electricity that keeps the heart beating evenly.

skills-related fitness The capacity to perform specific physical skills related to a sport or other physically demanding activity.

sleep debt A condition occurring when the amount of sleep you attain is less than the amount you need for optimal functioning.

social anxiety disorder (social phobia) An anxiety disorder characterized by an intense fear of being judged by others and of being humiliated by your own actions, which may be accompanied by physical symptoms.

specificity The principle that a fitness component is improved only by exercises that address that specific component.

spermicide A substance containing chemicals that kill or immobilize sperm.

spiritual health A component of psychological health that provides a sense of connection to a larger purpose coupled with a system of core values that provide direction and meaning in life.

spirituality A sense of connection to something larger than yourself.

stalking A pattern of harassment directed at a specific person that is intended to cause intimidation and fear, often through repeated, unwanted contact.

standard drink A drink containing about 14 grams pure alcohol (one 12-oz. can of beer, one 5-oz. glass of wine, or 1.5 oz. of 80-proof liquor).

static flexibility The ability to reach and hold a stretch at one endpoint of a joint's range of motion.

static stretching Gradually lengthening a muscle to an elongated position and sustaining that position.

statins A group of cholesterol-lowering prescription medications.

statutory rape Any sexual activity with a person younger than the legally defined "age of consent," regardless of whether any coercion or force was involved.

stimulants A class of drugs that stimulate the central nervous system causing acceleration of mental and physical processes in the body.

stress response The specific psychobiological changes that occur as the body attempts to cope with a stressor and return to homeostasis.

stress test An analysis of heart function during monitored exercise.

stress The collective psychobiological condition that occurs in reaction to a disruptive, unexpected, or exciting stimulus.

stressor Any physical or psychological condition, event, or factor that causes positive or negative stress.

stroke A medical emergency in which blood flow to or in the brain is impaired.

suction curettage A method of surgical abortion characterized by vacuum aspiration; typically used in the first 6 to 12 weeks of pregnancy.

sudden cardiac arrest A life-threatening cardiac crisis marked by loss of heartbeat and unconsciousness.

sudden infant death syndrome (SIDS) The sudden death of a seemingly healthy infant while sleeping.

Superfund A federal program that funds and carries out emergency and long-term identification, analysis, removal, and cleanup of toxic sites.

supplements Chemical compounds taken for a perceived health benefit.

sustainability The ability to meet society's current needs without compromising future generations' abilities to meet their own needs; includes policies for ensuring that certain components of the environment are not depleted or destroyed.

T

tachycardia A fast arrhythmia.

tar A sticky, thick brown residue that forms when tobacco is burned and its chemical particles condense.

target heart rate range The heart rate range to aim for during exercise. A target heart rate range of 64–91% of your maximum heart rate is recommended.

terminal illness An irreversible condition that will result in death in the near future.

terrorism Premeditated, politically motivated violence against noncombatant individuals, usually as a means of coercion.

testes (testicles) The two reproductive glands that manufacture sperm.

tolerance Reduced sensitivity to a drug so that increased amounts are needed to achieve the usual effect.

toxic shock syndrome (TSS) A rare, serious illness caused by staph bacteria that begins with severe flu symptoms but can quickly progress to a medical emergency.

toxicity The dosage level at which a drug becomes poisonous to the body.

trans **fats** Fats that are produced when liquid fat (oil) is turned into solid fat during food processing.

transgenderism The state in which someone's gender identity or gender expression is different from his or her assigned sex at birth.

transient ischemic attack (TIA) A temporary episode of stroke-like symptoms, indicative of high stroke risk.

transition The final phase of the first stage of labor, characterized by the dilation of the cervix and strong, prolonged contractions.

transsexual A transgendered individual who lives as the gender opposite to their assigned sex.

transtheoretical model of behavior change A model of behavior change that focuses on decision-making steps and abilities. Also called the *Stages of Change* model.

traumatic brain injury (TBI) An injury that disrupts normal functioning of the brain, caused by a jolt or blow to the brain or a penetrating head wound.

tumor An abnormal growth of tissue with no physiological function.

type 1 diabetes A form of diabetes that usually begins early in life and arises when the pancreas produces insufficient insulin.

type 2 diabetes A form of diabetes that usually begins later in life and arises when cells resist the effects of insulin.

U

umbilical cord A vessel linking the bloodstream of the placenta to that of the baby and enabling the exchange of gases, nutrients, and wastes.

underweight A weight resulting in a BMI below 18.5.

unintentional injury (accidents) Physical harm that is not deliberately caused.

unsaturated fats (oils) Fats that typically are liquid at room temperature; generally come from plant sources.

urethra A duct that travels from the bladder through the shaft of the penis, carrying fluids to the outside of the body.

uterus (womb) The pear-shaped organ where a growing fetus is nurtured.

V

vagina The tube that connects a woman's external sex organs with her uterus.

vaginal intercourse Intercourse characterized by the insertion of the penis into the vagina.

values Internal guidelines used to make decisions and evaluate the world around you.

vas deferens A tube ascending from the epididymis that transports sperm.

vector An animal or insect that transports pathogens from one point to another.

vegetarian A person who avoids some or all foods from animal sources: red meat, poultry, seafood, eggs, and dairy products.

veins Blood vessels that flow toward the heart, delivering oxygen-poor blood from the body periphery or oxygen-rich blood from the lungs.

ventricles The two lower chambers of the heart, which pump blood to the body and lungs.

ventricular fibrillation A life-threatening arrhythmia marked by ineffective pumping of the ventricles.

violence Use of physical force—threatened or actual—with the intent of causing harm.

virus A microscopic organism that can not multiply without invading body cells.

vitamins Substances, with no energy value of their own, needed by the body in small amounts for normal growth and function.

vulva All of the female external organs, collectively. Also called *genitals*.

W

water A liquid necessary for life.

wellness The process of actively making choices to achieve optimal health.

whole grains Unrefined grains that contain bran, germ, and endosperm.

whole-genome scanning A form of genetic testing that looks for variants throughout a person's genome.

will A legally binding document stating what should be done with a person's property after death.

withdrawal (drug use) Physical symptoms that develop when a person stops using a drug.

withdrawal (sexual activity) The withdrawal of the penis from the vagina before ejaculation.

Z

zygote A fertilized egg.

Index

Assess How You're Doing in Various Dimensions of Health

Be Smart About Online Health Information

Do Four Things to Live Longer and More Healthfully

Check Out Six Useful Sources of Health Information

Choose To...
Be Smart About Online Health Information

You can find lots of health information online. But is it accurate and credible? Here are some questions to ask:

- Is the sponsor of the site identified? Is it a commercial, nonprofit, academic, or government site?
- What is the purpose of the site? Is it to inform and educate, or is it to sell something?
- Does the site tell you where the information it presents came from? If so, is the content based on scientific evidence?
- Does the site specify when it was last updated?
- Does the site list a reputable professional accreditation?

Choose To...
Assess How You're Doing in Various Dimensions of Health

Health is a multidimensional concept. Ask yourself, "What dimensions of health am I strong in? What dimensions of health do I want to work on?" Remember that the dimensions of health include:

- Physical health
- Intellectual health
- Psychological health
- Social health
- Spiritual health
- Environmental health
- Occupational health

Choose To...
Check Out Six Useful Sources of Health Information

There are many reputable websites that provide useful, credible health-related information. Here are six to begin exploring:

- Centers for Disease Control and Prevention
  www.cdc.gov
- Go Ask Alice
  www.goaskalice.columbia.edu/index.html
- Healthfinder.gov
  http://healthfinder.gov
- Medline Plus
  www.nlm.nih.gov/medlineplus
- Mayo Clinic
  www.mayoclinic.com
- World Health Organization
  www.who.org

Choose To...
Do Four Things to Live Longer and More Healthfully

Just four key behaviors can have a profound influence on your health and life expectancy. They are:

- Eating nutritiously
- Being physically active
- Avoiding smoking
- Avoiding drinking alcohol in excess

What can you do today to engage in at least two of these behaviors?

Step Beyond Shyness

www.pearsonhighered.com/choosinghealth

Beat a Bad Mood

www.pearsonhighered.com/choosinghealth

Build Your Emotional Intelligence

www.pearsonhighered.com/choosinghealth

Help Prevent Suicide

www.pearsonhighered.com/choosinghealth

Choose To...
Beat a Bad Mood

Sometimes a bad mood can't be helped, but it doesn't have to ruin your whole day.

- Talk to a good friend. Even if you are busy, venting for 10 minutes and listening to a friend's input and support can make a big difference.

- Help someone else. Find out about volunteering opportunities in your local community. Focusing on helping others can put your own problems in perspective.

- Spruce up your environment. Clean your room, wash your car, buy some plants, or frame some photos. Improving your surroundings can help you feel better.

- Get outside. Go for a jog in your neighborhood, or take a walk in a local park. Exercise and fresh air can work wonders for a bad mood.

- Do something nice for yourself. Download a couple of songs you love, or treat yourself to a small indulgence.

Choose To...
Step Beyond Shyness

Most of us feel shy at some point. Here are some suggestions to move beyond shyness and meet new groups of friends.

- Start by asking yourself, "What do I enjoy? What am I good at?"

- Find out how your hobbies and talents might help you connect with others. Is there a club you can join? A group you can volunteer with? A class you can take?

- If you feel nervous joining a new group alone, take a friend along to your first gathering.

- When you're in a new group, don't feel like you have to meet every single person. Introducing yourself to just one or two new people is a great start.

- Join the group's email list or social networking page. Stay connected.

- Go to at least three of the group's gatherings. Chances are good you'll make connections with new friends.

Choose To...
Help Prevent Suicide

If someone you know shows any of the following warning signs, get help by calling the National Suicide Prevention Lifeline at 1-800-273-TALK:

- Talking about wanting to hurt or kill him- or herself

- Feeling hopeless

- Acting reckless or engaging in risky activities

- Increasing drinking or drug use

- Seeing no reason for living or purpose in life

- Talking or writing about death or suicide, especially when these actions are out of the ordinary for this person

Choose To...
Build Your Emotional Intelligence

Here are three ways to boost your emotional IQ:

- When you're upset, try to express your feelings honestly rather than put others down. For example, try saying "I feel impatient because you all were late," rather than "My study group is a bunch of rude jerks." It'll help resolve the problem more smoothly.

- In any conflict, imagine yourself in the other person's shoes and try to see his or her perspective. Acknowledging the other person's position can help reduce tensions so that you can resolve the problem.

- Listen before you advise, criticize, or judge. It's easy to make snap judgments about others, but that's rarely accurate or helpful. Listen to others first, without interruption or judgment. What are they really saying? What are they really asking you for?

Reduce Stress Through Wellness Habits

Relax Through Visualization

Get a Good Night's Sleep

Manage Your Time

Choose To...
Relax Through Visualization

1. Get comfortable. Dim the lights, sit or lie down, breathe deeply.
2. Imagine a scene where you feel relaxed, comfortable, and safe. For example, floating on a cloud, lying on the beach, or walking through a meadow. Imagine it with all your senses. Who is with you? What is the temperature like? Do you smell or taste anything? What are you wearing or touching? What do you hear?
3. Or, visualize stress as dark smoke flowing out of your body through your fingers and toes, or of "throwing away" your stress and worries into a garbage can or down a drain.
4. Once you feel relaxed, take a few minutes to breathe slowly and enjoy.
5. As you slowly emerge from the visualization, repeat to yourself that you feel relaxed and refreshed.

Choose To...
Reduce Stress Through Wellness Habits

You can reduce stress by following these basic guidelines. See pages 53–54 for more information.

- Manage your time effectively.
- Get enough sleep.
- Eat well.
- Exercise.
- Strengthen your support network.
- Communicate.
- Take time for hobbies and leisure.
- Keep a journal.

Choose To...
Manage Your Time

- Use a daily planner.
- Mark the due dates of big assignments, tests, and events in your planner.
- Break down big jobs into smaller tasks.
- Hate it? Do it first.
- Leave time for surprises. Don't completely book your schedule.
- Reward yourself.
- Limit time wasters, such as:
    - Facebook, instant messaging, or text messaging
    - Emailing or shopping online
    - Talking on the phone, watching TV, or playing video games

Choose To...
Get a Good Night's Sleep

- Have a regular sleep schedule.
- Avoid caffeine after lunch.
- Avoid alcohol and cigarettes before bedtime.
- Exercise earlier in the day.
- Try not to nap.
- Avoid all-nighters.
- Don't work in bed.
- Give yourself time to wind down.
- Try not to sleep-in on weekends.

Make a High-Fiber Snack

Get More Antioxidants

Get Enough Calcium Today

Know Your Portion Sizes

Get More Antioxidants

Get more color, fun, and nutrients in your diet from some of the foods that the USDA has found to be highest in antioxidants:

- Small red beans
- Blueberries
- Red kidney beans
- Pinto beans
- Cranberries
- Artichokes
- Blackberries
- Prunes
- Raspberries
- Strawberries

Make a High-Fiber Snack

Get more fiber in your diet by making your own great-tasting trail mix. It's high in fiber, but also packs calories, so try having just a half-cup as an afternoon snack.

- Start with two unsweetened dried fruits, such as pineapple, raisins, apricots, cranberries, or bananas.
- Then select two types of nuts, such as walnuts, almonds, cashews, pistachios, or pecans.
- Optional: Choose one additional salty or naturally sweet ingredient, such as pretzel sticks or shredded coconut.
- Measure out one cup of each type of nut and each type of dried fruit, for a total of four cups. If using a salty or sweet ingredient, add as well. Combine in a mixing bowl.
- Store in a sealed plastic bag or airtight container.

Know Your Portion Sizes

- 1 cup = a baseball
- 1/2 cup = a light bulb
- 1 ounce = a golf ball
- 1 teaspoon = a poker chip
- 3 ounces of chicken or meat = a deck of cards
- 3 ounces of fish = a check book
- 1 medium fruit = a baseball
- 1 cup carrots = 12 baby carrots

Get Enough Calcium Today

Young adults need anywhere from 1,000 to 1,200 mg of calcium each day. To get there, reach for:

- Cheddar cheese: About 200 mg per ounce
- Milk or orange juice: About 300 mg per 8-oz. glass
- Soy or rice milk (calcium-fortified): 200 to 300 mg per 8-oz. glass
- Yogurt: About 400 mg per 8-oz. serving
- Cottage cheese: About 800 mg per cup
- Kale, cooked: About 180 mg per cup

Build Up Your Cardiorespiratory Fitness

Know How to Measure Your Heart Rate

Add More Physical Activity to Your Life

Get Enough Exercise Each Week

Choose To...
Know How to Measure Your Heart Rate

Your heart rate is a useful measurement of how hard your heart is working during exercise. To determine your heart rate:

- While you exercise, take your pulse by placing your first two fingers (not your thumb) on the side of your neck next to your windpipe.
- Using a clock or watch, take your pulse for six seconds.
- Multiply that number by 10. The result will be your number of heartbeats per minute, which is your heart rate.

Choose To...
Build Up Your Cardiorespiratory Fitness

Aerobic exercise is a great way to improve your cardiorespiratory fitness. Below are a few fun, easy ways to incorporate more aerobic exercise into your life.

- Swimming
- Hiking
- Cycling
- Jumping rope
- Running or jogging
- Cardio classes, such as step aerobics
- Stair-climbing

Choose To...
Get Enough Exercise Each Week

How much exercise do you need each week? At minimum, try to get:

- At least 30 minutes of moderate-intensity activity 5 days per week.

For greater health benefits, try:

- 5 hours of moderate-intensity activity or 2.5 hours of high-intensity activity AND
- Strength-training 2–3 times per week AND
- Stretching 2–3 times per week.

Choose To...
Add More Physical Activity to Your Life

Here are six easy ways to add more physical activity to your daily life:

- Park your car at the far end of the parking lot to increase the amount of walking you do.
- Walk briskly or ride a bike to class instead of driving.
- Take the stairs instead of the elevator.
- Join a gym that offers classes you are interested in.
- Get a friend to exercise with you. Being social as you exercise will help keep you motivated.
- If you have a dog, walk him/her daily—it will be good for both of you!

Choosing Health Weight Management

Reduce Your Calorie Intake

Choosing Health Weight Management

Get More Exercise

Choosing Health Weight Management

Boost Your Body Image

Choosing Health Weight Management

Make a Low-calorie Snack

Choose To...
Get More Exercise

Slow and steady is the way to use exercise to keep weight off. Studies show that consistent, lower intensity exercise is more helpful than random bursts of intense activity.

- Sign up for a yoga, tennis, or other exercise class. Or, join your campus hiking club and take a hike each weekend.
- Use the stairs each day.
- Park your car at the far end of the lot, so you maximize your chance to walk.
- Take active study breaks: Do 5 minutes of exercise after every 45 minutes of work.
- Relaxing in front of the TV? Make commercial breaks activity breaks. Get up and do some light exercise while the commercials are on.

Choose To...
Reduce Your Calorie Intake

Reduce calories with the following guidelines.

- Practice portion control.
- Drink water instead of sugary drinks.
- Use artificial sweeteners in moderation.
- Choose low-calorie fruits and vegetables rather than high-calorie processed foods like frozen pizza.
- Don't skip meals.
- Share food with others.
- Reach for healthful snacks that are higher in bulk, to make you feel fuller.
- Save high-calorie snacks for special treats.
- Look for emotions—such as stress or happiness—that might make you eat, and think of non-food ways to manage them.

Choose To...
Make a Low-calorie Snack

MEXI-BEAN BAKE

Servings: 6

6–8 corn tortillas, torn
One 15 oz. can of corn or 1.5 cups frozen corn
3 cups canned low-fat chili
1.5 cups shredded low-fat cheddar cheese
Nonstick cooking spray
12 Tbsp. salsa

Spray an 8.5 x 11-inch baking dish with nonstick cooking spray. Cover bottom of dish with 1/3 tortillas, then 1/3 corn, 1/3 chili, and 1/3 cheese. Repeat layers two more times. Bake at 350°F for 25–30 minutes. Serve with 2 Tbsp. salsa per serving.

Calories per serving: approximately 265

Choose To...
Boost Your Body Image

Any of these simple tips can boost your body image.

- Exercise. Anything from swimming to mountain biking will help you love your body.
- Pick your favorite body feature—your nose, your hair, your legs. Look yourself in the mirror and compliment yourself, out loud.
- Stand up straight, square your shoulders, and don't look down. You'll feel more confident and look more confident too.
- Do nice things for your body. Get a massage, buy some nice smelling lotion, or take a nap.
- Don't let your size or shape stop you from doing something you want to do. Participating in activities will make you feel good and show you all that your body can accomplish.

Watch Your Caffeine Intake

Use Prescription Drugs Properly

Know the Signs of Drug Addiction

Seek Natural Highs

Choose To...
Use Prescription Drugs Properly

An estimated half of all prescriptions dispensed in the United States each year aren't taken according to directions. Before taking a prescription drug:

- Be sure you understand exactly how to take the medicine. Read the label on the drug bottle carefully, and talk to your pharmacist or doctor if you have any questions at all.
- Make sure you understand the proper dosage.
- Make sure you understand *when* and *how often* you should take the medication.
- Be sure the medication does not interfere with any other drugs you may be taking. Let your doctor know right away if you are taking any other drugs.
- Find out if there are side effects to the medication.

Choose To...
Watch Your Caffeine Intake

Below is the estimated caffeine content for some common products and beverages.

- Brewed coffee, 8 oz.: 95–200 mg
- NoDoz, maximum strength, 1 tablet: 200 mg
- Rockstar energy drink: 80 mg
- Black tea, 8 oz.: 40–120 mg
- Mountain Dew, 12 oz.: 54 mg
- Coca Cola Classic, 12 oz.: 35 mg
- Decaffeinated brewed coffee, 8 oz.: 2–12 mg
- Hershey's milk chocolate bar, 1.55 oz.: 9 mg

Choose To...
Seek Natural Highs

You don't need to turn to drugs to achieve a "high." Below are some drug-free methods of feeling good.

- **Exercise.** It's true—exercise releases endorphins in the brain, which produces a feeling of euphoria commonly known as "runner's high."
- **Spend time with your loved ones.** Good times spent with family members, a significant other, or a friend can produce an emotional "high" that is more meaningful than a drug-induced chemical "high."
- **Do things you love.** Go to a live sporting event. Attend a rock concert. Travel someplace you've never been. Figure out what excites you, and then make plans to do it.

Choose To...
Know the Signs of Drug Addiction

How can you tell if you or someone you care about has an addiction? Look for the following signs:

- **Compulsion.** Is there an obsession with doing drugs?
- **Loss of control.** Does the person have a pattern of behaving recklessly?
- **Negative consequences.** Does the person have a pattern of destructive behavior?
- **Denial.** Does the person fail to recognize that the addiction is causing problems?

A great resource for helping someone with a drug problem is the Partnership at Drugfree.org website at www.drugfree.org.

Recognize a "Standard" Drink

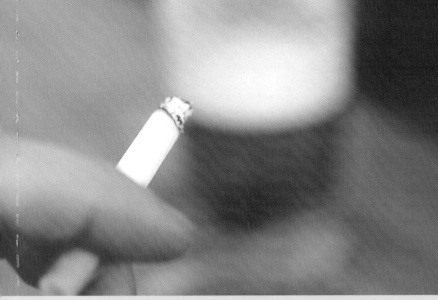

www.pearsonhighered.com/choosinghealth

Be Smart When Dealing with a Hangover

www.pearsonhighered.com/choosinghealth

Avoid Secondhand Smoke

www.pearsonhighered.com/choosinghealth

Kick a Tobacco Habit

www.pearsonhighered.com/choosinghealth

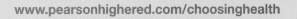

Choose To...
Be Smart When Dealing with a Hangover

A hangover is your body's way of telling you that you have consumed too much alcohol. The only way to prevent a hangover is to avoid drinking to excess. If you do get a hangover:

- **Drink water or a sports drink.** It may not make the headache go away, but it will provide the rehydration your body needs.
- **Do not drink coffee.** The caffeine in it will only make you more dehydrated.
- **Do not drink more alcohol.** Although this may postpone the effects of a hangover, it will not prevent them, and may ultimately make you feel worse.
- **Do not take acetaminophen** (e.g., Tylenol), which is dangerous when mixed with alcohol.

Choose To...
Recognize a "Standard" Drink

It's easy to underestimate how much alcohol a person has consumed. "One drink" can mean anything. Depending on the size of the glass or can, the alcohol content may be one "standard" drink, or much more than that. Technically, one "standard" serving of alcohol is equivalent to:

- A 5-oz. glass of wine
- A 1.5-oz. shot (standard shot glass size) of hard liquor, such as whiskey or vodka
- A 12-oz. can of beer
- About 8 or 9 oz. of malt liquor

Note that each of these servings contains about the same amount of alcohol—14 g, or about 1/2 oz.

Choose To...
Kick a Tobacco Habit

Quitting isn't easy, but it's worth it. Here's how to S.T.A.R.T:

- **S**et a quit date.
- **T**ell others that you plan to quit.
- **A**nticipate and plan for the challenges you'll face while quitting.
- **R**emove cigarettes and other tobacco products from your home, car, and work.
- **T**alk to your doctor about getting help to quit.

In addition, visit these excellent online resources: www.smokefree.gov and www.cancer.gov/help.

Choose To...
Avoid Secondhand Smoke

Millions of Americans are essentially passive smokers, thanks to others' tobacco habits. Here are some ways to avoid secondhand smoke:

- Request smoke-free living situations (dorms, apartments, etc.) whenever possible.
- If you live with a smoker, ask him or her to smoke outside and far away from doors and windows.
- Stick to bars and clubs that are smoke-free. One night in a smoky bar can expose you to hours of hazardous toxins (and leave you smelling like an ashtray).

Relationships and Communication

Be a Good Listener

www.pearsonhighered.com/choosinghealth

Relationships and Communication

Be Smart About Facebook

www.pearsonhighered.com/choosinghealth

Relationships and Communication

Try Online Dating Safely

www.pearsonhighered.com/choosinghealth

Relationships and Communication

Maintain a Strong Relationship

www.pearsonhighered.com/choosinghealth

Be Smart About Facebook

Use Facebook safely and effectively by:

- Limiting your "friends" to people you really care about.

- Avoiding tagging friends in unflattering or problematic photos.

- Using personal messaging instead of posting on a friend's public "wall" when discussing sensitive matters.

- Keeping personal information off your profile—like your birthday and where you live.

- Activating your privacy settings.

- Logging off. Facebook is fun and can help you keep in touch with far-away friends, but don't forget to make time for face-to-face friendships.

Be a Good Listener

Listening is a critical part of good communication. Some strategies for being a good listener:

- Be silent while another person is sharing his or her feelings or concerns. Overcome the urge to interrupt.

- Try to put yourself in the other person's shoes and understand where he or she is coming from.

- Maintain eye contact, keep a relaxed posture, and nod and smile so that the other person knows you are listening.

- Give the speaker your undivided attention. Get rid of any distractions. Close the door and turn off your cell phone.

Maintain a Strong Relationship

The following are a few strategies for maintaining a strong relationship:

- Be honest with each other.

- Trust each other.

- Respect each other.

- Communicate effectively.

- Give your loved one freedom and encouragement.

- Take time for activities and hobbies you both enjoy.

- Be kind to one another

- Show affection for each other.

- Share decision making.

Try Online Dating Safely

Remember that people you meet online are basically strangers. Keep a few precautions in mind:

- Never give out your full name, address, or other personal information until you've met online contacts in person and know them well enough to tell if they are trustworthy.

- Make sure you meet your date the first few times in a public place, and tell a friend where you'll be going.

- Don't have a new date pick you up at home.

- If something doesn't seem right on the date, don't be afraid to cut it short and move on.

Choosing Health Sexuality, Contraception, and Reproductive Choices

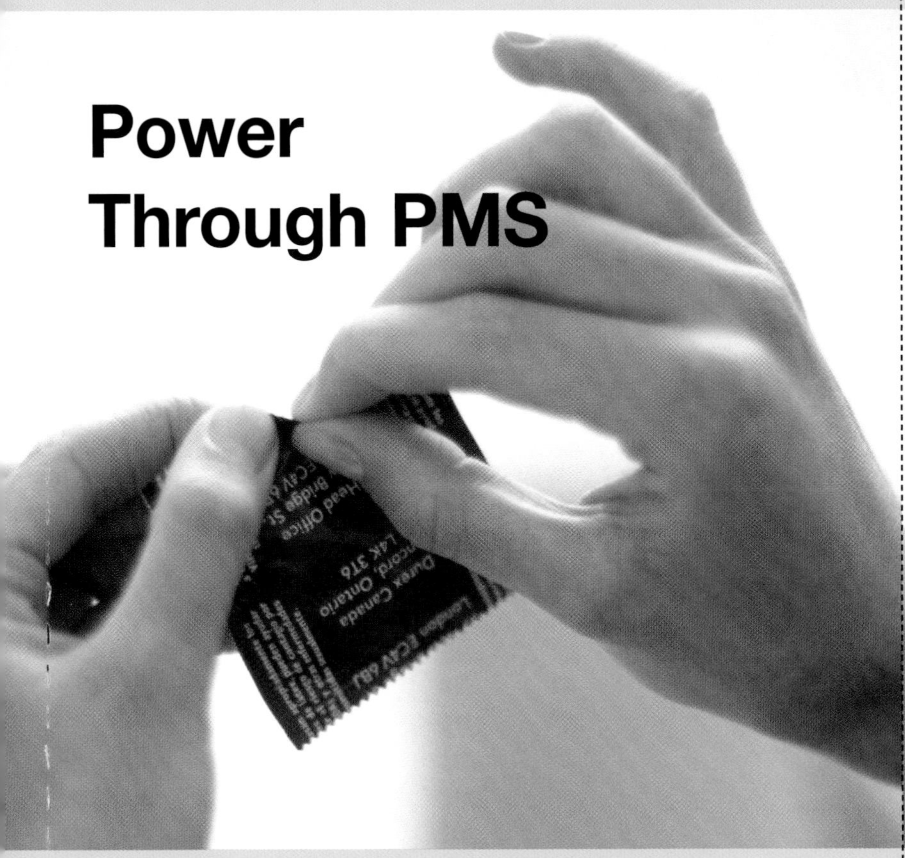

www.pearsonhighered.com/choosinghealth

Choosing Health Sexuality, Contraception, and Reproductive Choices

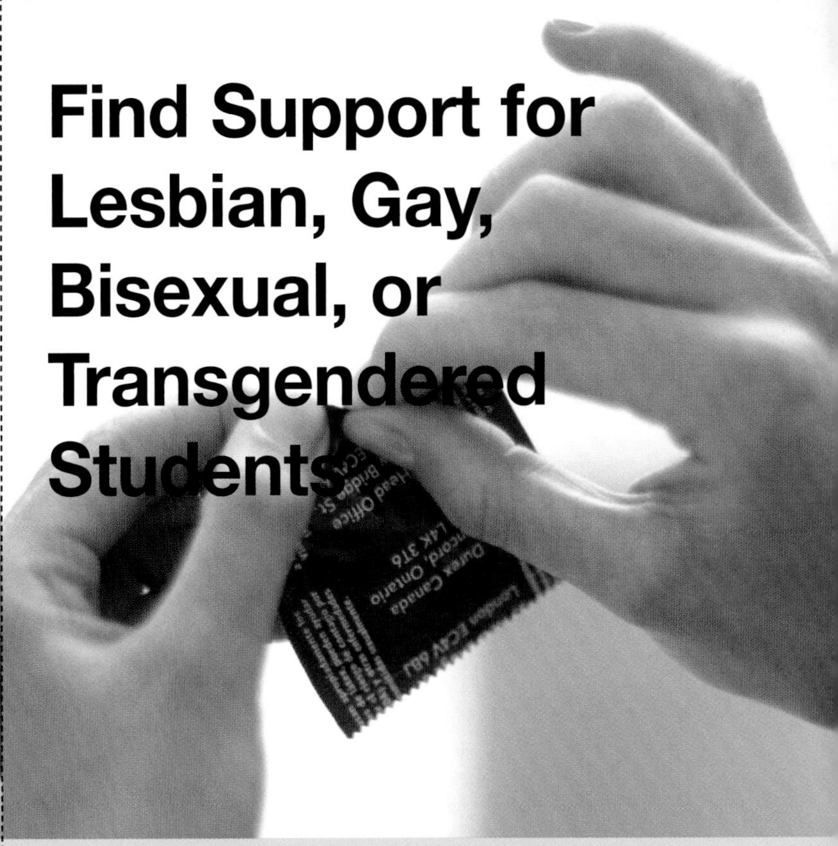

www.pearsonhighered.com/choosinghealth

Choosing Health Sexuality, Contraception, and Reproductive Choices

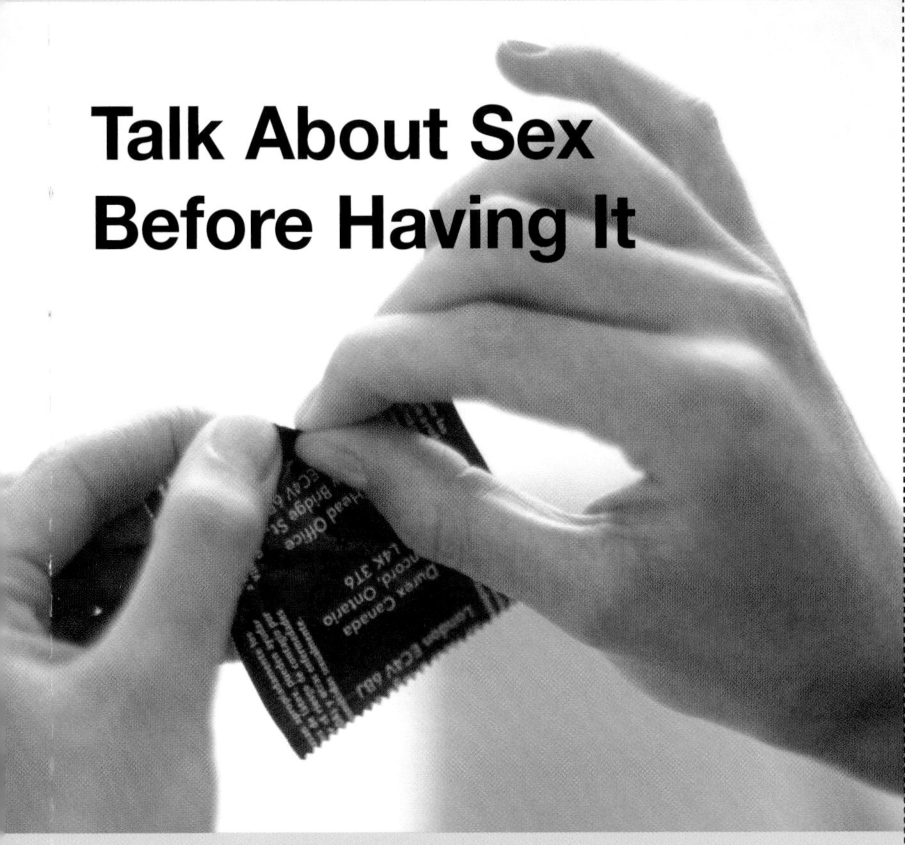

www.pearsonhighered.com/choosinghealth

Choosing Health Sexuality, Contraception, and Reproductive Choices

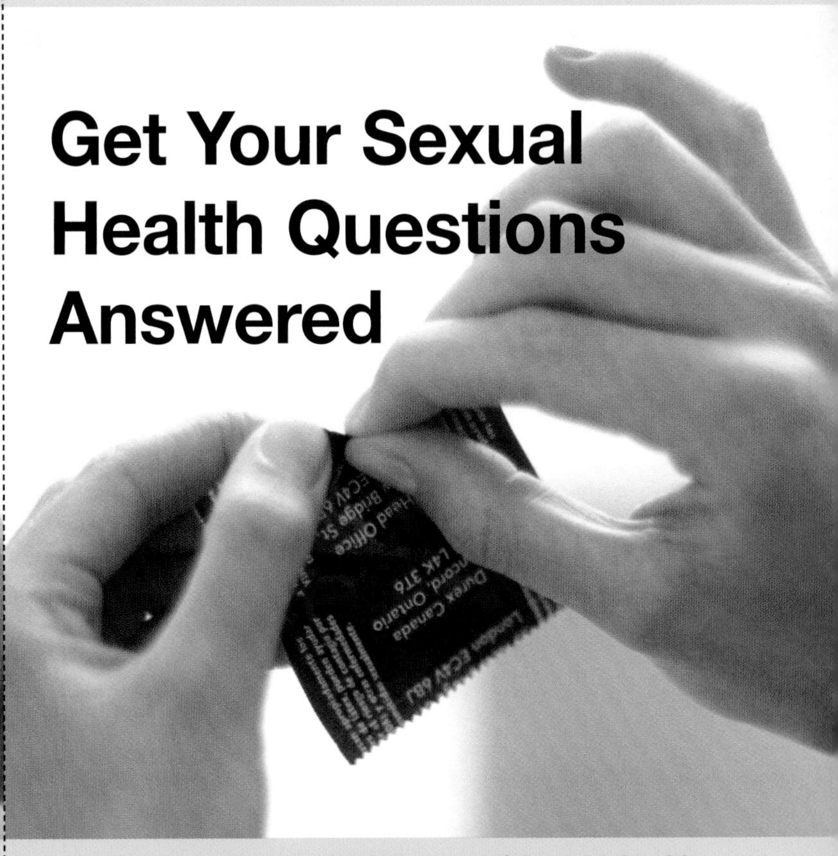

www.pearsonhighered.com/choosinghealth

Choose To...

Find Support for Lesbian, Gay, Bisexual, or Transgendered Students

Lesbian, gay, bisexual, or transgendered students may sometimes feel isolated on campus. If you are seeking support:

- Check out www.campuspride.org, a nationwide online resource for lesbian, gay, bisexual, or transgendered (LGBT) college students.

- Visit www.itgetsbetterproject.com to view video testimonials by members of the LGBT community as well as straight friends and supporters.

- Seek out LGBT resource centers on campus, where students of various orientations can find support.

- Ask your student health center if it has care providers and resources to address the sexual health needs of LGBT students.

Choose To...

Power Through PMS

If you are female and suffer from premenstrual syndrome, try the following strategies to reduce symptoms:

- Avoid smoking, alcohol, caffeine, and junk food.

- Get regular exercise.

- Get enough sleep—try for 8 hours per night.

- Consider taking a multivitamin designed for women containing adequate levels of B vitamins, vitamin E, and magnesium.

Choose To...

Get Your Sexual Health Questions Answered

The following are a few suggested resources for learning more about sexual health issues:

- Planned Parenthood
  www.plannedparenthood.org

- Go Ask Alice
  www.goaskalice.columbia.edu

- American Social Health Association
  www.ashastd.org

- National Sexuality Resource Center
  http://nsrc.sfsu.edu

Also, consult your campus health center for advice on matters of sexual health.

Choose To...

Talk About Sex Before Having It

If you're thinking about having sex with someone, talk to him or her about it beforehand. Yes, it's awkward, but it is important.

- Set up a time to talk.

- Ask about your prospective partner's sexual history. Be prepared to answer your prospective partner's questions about your own sexual history.

- Pay attention to your partner's responses—not just the words, but also the body language.

- Discuss what you will do to prevent pregnancy and sexually transmitted infections. For example, will you both get tested for infections beforehand? What kind of contraception will you use?

- Recap the decisions you make together, and follow through.

Know How to Wash Your Hands Effectively

Protect Yourself from Colds and Flu

Reduce Your Risk of STIs

Reduce Your Risk of Contracting MRSA

Choose To...
Protect Yourself from Colds and Flu

Follow these tips to reduce your chances of catching a cold or the flu:

- Wash your hands often, especially after riding public transit or using a public bathroom.
- Avoid touching your eyes, nose, and mouth.
- Avoid close contact with people who are sick.
- Don't share utensils or drinking glasses with other people.
- Regularly clean and disinfect surfaces such as keyboards, phones, and kitchen counters.
- Get an annual flu vaccine.
- Get enough sleep, exercise, and eat nutritiously.

Choose To...
Know How to Wash Your Hands Effectively

Washing your hands is one of the best ways to prevent infections, but many people don't wash their hands effectively.

- Wet your hands with running water.
- Use soap. Lather up to your wrists.
- Rub your hands thoroughly for at least 20 seconds. Clean every inch of your hands, including your fingertips, your palms, the back of your hands, and underneath your fingernails.
- Dry your hands on a clean towel, a disposable paper towel, or an air dryer.

Choose To...
Reduce Your Risk of Contracting MRSA

Methicillin-resistant *Staphylococcus aureus* (MRSA) infections are a serious public health threat. To reduce your risk:

- Wash your hands often.
- Keep open wounds covered with dry, sterile bandages.
- Do not share personal items such as razors or towels.
- When in a gym, use a clean towel to create a barrier between your skin and any shared equipment, such as a weight-training bench.
- If you have a skin infection that does not seem to improve after a day or two, see a doctor and request to be tested for MRSA.

For more information, visit
http://cdc.gov/Features/MRSAinSchools/#q4.

Choose To...
Reduce Your Risk of STIs

A few simple steps can dramatically reduce your risk of contracting an uncomfortable, embarrassing, and potentially dangerous STI:

- Consider abstinence.
- Be faithful and be picky—fewer sexual partners means less risk.
- Always use a condom (or insist that your partner use one).
- Get tested for STIs. Many STIs may not have clear symptoms, especially in women.
- Get vaccinated for HPV and hepatitis B.

Choosing Health Preventing Cardiovascular Disease, Diabetes, and Cancer

Have a Snack That's Easy on Your Blood Sugar

Choosing Health Preventing Cardiovascular Disease, Diabetes, and Cancer

Lower Your Risk of Heart Disease

Choosing Health Preventing Cardiovascular Disease, Diabetes, and Cancer

Help Someone in Cardiac Arrest

Choosing Health Preventing Cardiovascular Disease, Diabetes, and Cancer

Lower Your Risk of Cancer

Choose To...
Lower Your Risk of Heart Disease

Some ways to reduce your risk of cardiovascular disease:

- Eat a heart-healthy diet: reduce your fat and cholesterol intake, decrease your sodium intake, eat brightly colored fruits and vegetables, and boost consumption of omega-3 fatty acids (found in fish like salmon).
- Stay physically active.
- Don't smoke.
- Get enough sleep—8 hours per night.
- Brush and floss regularly (yes, the health of your heart and mouth are connected).
- Limit alcohol intake. Even when people are young, heavy drinking is linked to a greater risk of problems such as hypertension.

Choose To...
Have a Snack That's Easy on Your Blood Sugar

Whether you have diabetes, want to reduce your risk, or just want to eat more healthfully, reach for these snack options (recommended by the American Diabetes Association):

- 3 celery sticks + 1 tablespoon of peanut butter
- 1 hard-boiled egg
- 1/4 cup fresh blueberries
- 1 cup of light popcorn
- 1/4 whole, fresh avocado

Choose To...
Lower Your Risk of Cancer

Some ways to reduce your risk of cancer:

- Don't smoke or use tobacco products.
- Eat a nutritious diet rich in fruits and vegetables.
- Stay physically active.
- Limit alcohol intake.
- Wear sunscreen with an SPF of at least 30. Wear clothing to cover as much of your skin as possible when outdoors.
- Practice safe sex.
- If female, consider an HPV vaccine to lower the risk of cervical cancer.
- Check your home for radon, which can cause lung cancer. Visit www.epa.gov/radon/healthrisks.html for more information.

Choose To...
Help Someone in Cardiac Arrest

If you suspect someone's heart has stopped:

- Call 911 immediately. Every minute counts.
- Check for a pulse in the neck after you call 911.
- If you don't find a pulse, begin CPR. If you don't know how, ask the 911 dispatcher for instructions.
- If you are in a public place, look for an automated external defibrillator (AED). They are designed for anyone to use, and come with instructions.

Know How to Select a Doctor

Prevent Medical Errors

Be a Smart Patient

Know Your Genetic Rights

Choose To...
Prevent Medical Errors

Communicate actively, and you'll reduce your chances of a medical mistake. Be sure to:

- Let your doctor know about ALL the medicines, supplements, and other substances you are taking.

- Share information with all members of your medical team, especially if you have multiple care-givers.

- Understand the potential side effects of any medication you are taking.

- When picking up prescriptions, be sure you've been given the right drug.

Choose To...
Know How to Select a Doctor

Finding and choosing a doctor can require some legwork. Begin by asking friends and family for recommendations, or by asking your insurance company for a list of doctors in your area. Questions to ask the office staff:

- What insurance plans does this office accept?

- Is this doctor board-certified?

- How does the office handle lab work? Is there a lab in-house or nearby, or will you have to travel to a different location for a procedure such as a blood test?

- Is this a group practice? If so, will you mostly see your doctor, or all the doctors in the group? If so, how many of them are there and what are their specialties?

- Who will care for you if your doctor is unavailable?

- Is this medical practice affiliated with any particular hospitals or specialty centers?

Choose To...
Know Your Genetic Rights

In the U.S., the federal Genetic Information Nondiscrimination Act helps protect your genetic information. Under GINA:

- Your genetic information cannot be used to deny you health insurance or set the price you pay for it.

- Your genetic information can't be used to deny you a job or to fire you, or as a reason to withhold raises or promotions.

- Insurers can't require you or your family to take a genetic test.

Choose To...
Be a Smart Patient

Get the most out of a doctor's appointment. Follow these tips:

- Inform your doctor about any past or current medical issues, even if they are embarrassing.

- Ask questions! Don't be afraid to ask for clarification if you do not understand anything.

- Be proactive. If you have new symptoms, or a reaction to a new medication, let your doctor know immediately. If you took a lab test and are still awaiting results, let the office know.

- Take information home with you. Ask your doctor or the office staff if they have handouts related to your medical issue.

Avoid Distracted Driving

Select the Right Bike Helmet

Know Who to Call in an Emergency

Stay Safe on Campus

Choose To...

Select the Right Bike Helmet

When shopping for a helmet, a high price doesn't necessarily mean the best for you. Look for:

- **The right size.** You need a snug fit and a helmet you can't pull off.

- **Straight alignment.** Your helmet should sit straight on your head. If you have long hair, look for one with a ponytail port.

- **Solid straps and a good buckle.** Straps should fit snugly.

- **A CSPC sticker.** These are found inside helmets meeting U.S. safety standards.

Choose To...

Avoid Distracted Driving

Trying to text and drive? You are eight times more likely to crash. Aim for distraction-free driving by taking these steps:

- Once you are in the car, put your phone or PDA out of reach.

- If you must talk or text, pull over first.

- Set up your music (radio station, iPod, volume, etc.) before you hit the road.

- Don't try to eat, put on makeup, or juggle a hot cup of coffee behind the wheel.

Choose To...

Stay Safe on Campus

Key tips for campus safety:

- Don't prop open access doors to campus buildings or shared housing, and don't let strangers in.

- Keep your building or room locked, and don't loan out your keys.

- Drink in moderation, if at all.

- Don't travel alone after dark.

- Don't use a shared computer when making purchases online.

Choose To...

Know Who to Call in an Emergency

Emergency numbers to keep on hand (besides 911):

- National Poison Control Center: 1-800-222-1222

- National Domestic Violence Hotline: 1-800-799-SAFE (7233)

- Direct number to your local police (911 calls from mobiles may go to Highway Patrol dispatchers instead): _____

- Campus security: _____

Reduce Pollutants in Your Home

Make Cleaning Greener

Protect Your Hearing

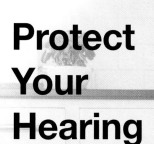

Ditch the Junk Mail

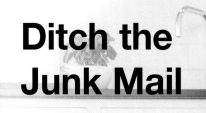

Choose To...
Make Cleaning Greener

Reach for these inexpensive, nontoxic choices the next time you clean:

- Baking soda cleans, deodorizes, and scours.
- Lemon juice has antibacterial properties.
- White vinegar cuts grease, cleans glass, removes mildew, and eliminates odors.
- Corn starch can help shampoo carpets and rugs.

Choose To...
Reduce Pollutants in Your Home

These strategies will help you protect your home from environmental pollutants:

- Test your home for radon. Visit www.epa.gov/radon/radontest.html.
- Install a carbon monoxide detector.
- Use only zero-VOC or low-VOC paint.
- Prevent mold by making sure bathrooms, kitchens, and basements have good air circulation and are cleaned often.
- When purchasing new furniture, mattresses, rugs, or carpeting, look for low-VOC options. Air these products out for a few days before using or installing them.
- Vacuum thoroughly and frequently.
- Don't allow smoking indoors.

Choose To...
Ditch the Junk Mail

Save trees and skip the barrage of advertisements in your snail-mail box:

- Go to www.dmachoice.org to stop direct mail advertising.
- Go to www.optoutprescreen.com to opt out of unsolicited credit card offers.
- Go to www.catalogchoice.org to stop receiving unwanted catalogs (a few companies don't work with Catalog Choice, so you'll need to contact those directly).

Choose To...
Protect Your Hearing

Give your ears a break:

- If you use earbuds, switch to over-the-ear styles and follow the 60/60 rule—don't go past 60% of the device's volume and don't listen for more than 60 minutes a day.
- At concerts, don't stand right next to the speakers.
- At bars and clubs with loud music, step outside periodically to give your ears a chance to recover.
- At loud workplaces, use noise-canceling headphones.

Protect Your Vision as You Age

Get Enough Calcium

Keep Your Brain Fit

Honor Loved Ones Creatively

Choose To...
Get Enough Calcium

Women may be at greater risk for osteoporosis than men, but we all need help maintaining strong bones as we age. Here are calcium recommendations based on age:

- Age 14–18 = 1,300 mg daily
- Age 19–50* = 1,000 mg daily
- Age 50+ = 1,200 mg daily

* If you are a woman who is pregnant or nursing, recommendations may be higher. Ask your doctor.

Choose To...
Protect Your Vision as You Age

To protect the health of your eyes:

- Have your vision checked by an optometrist at least once a year if you wear contacts or glasses.
- Have your vision checked every other year if you have 20/20 vision.

After age 40, ask your doctor about monitoring for:

- Presbyopia, or the loss of the eyes' ability to focus up close, especially in low light
- Glaucoma, caused by a buildup of pressure in the eye that can lead to blindness
- Cataracts, a clouding of the eye's lens that can dim vision
- Macular degeneration, retinal deterioration that can lead to blindness

Choose To...
Honor Loved Ones Creatively

When you've lost someone close to you, creative expressions of memories and feelings can help with grief. Try:

- Writing a letter to the person who died, saying everything you wish you could say now.
- Make a scrapbook.
- Paint pictures.
- Start an online memorial and ask other friends and family members of your loved one to post their own thoughts and photos.
- Plant flowers or trees.
- Get involved in activities that your loved one enjoyed or would have wanted to do.

Choose To...
Keep Your Brain Fit

Challenging your mind can prevent cognitive declines and slow memory loss. Give yourself a daily "brain workout" by:

- Completing a crossword puzzle
- Reading a book
- Playing a musical instrument
- Playing cards
- Writing in any form (e.g., email, letters, creative writing, journaling, blogging)
- Minimizing passive activities like watching television